PCAT®

2015–2016

STRATEGIES, PRACTICE, AND REVIEW

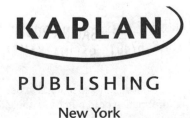

PUBLISHING

New York

Special thanks to the staff of Kaplan Test Prep who worked on this book.

Published by Kaplan Publishing, a division of Kaplan, Inc.
395 Hudson Street
New York, NY 10014

Printed in the United States of America

10 9 8 7 6 5 4 3 2 1

ISBN: 978-1-61865-888-3

Kaplan Publishing print books are available at special quantity discounts to use for sales promotions, employee premiums, or educational purposes. For more information or to purchase books, please call the Simon & Schuster special sales department at 866-506-1949.

TABLE OF CONTENTS

Note to International Students vii

How to Use This Book viii

SECTION I: PCAT STRATEGIES

Chapter 1: Introduction to the PCAT 3

Chapter 2: Studying Effectively 13

Chapter 3: Test Strategies 19

SECTION II: WRITING

Chapter 4: The PCAT Essay 29

Chapter 5: Usage and Style 35

Chapter 6: Practice Prompts 71

SECTION III: VERBAL ABILITY

Chapter 7: The Verbal Ability Section 89

Chapter 8: Analogies 95

Chapter 9: Sentence Completion 109

Chapter 10: Word Roots 123

Chapter 11: Vocabulary List 137

Chapter 12: Vocabulary Exercises 179

SECTION IV: BIOLOGY

Chapter 13: Cellular Biology 221

Chapter 14: Molecular Biology 239

Chapter 15: Genetics 253

Chapter 16: Evolution. 271

Chapter 17: Microorganisms 285

Chapter 18: Medical Microbiology. 293

Chapter 19: Integument and Immune Systems 299

Chapter 20: Nervous System 309

Chapter 21: Musculoskeletal System 325

Chapter 22: Circulatory and Respiratory Systems 337

Chapter 23: Digestive System 351

Chapter 24: Excretory System 359

Chapter 25: Endocrine System 367

Chapter 26: Reproductive System 379

SECTION V: GENERAL CHEMISTRY

Chapter 27: Atomic Structure 395

Chapter 28: The Periodic Table 411

Chapter 29: Chemical Bonding 425

Chapter 30: Stoichiometry 447

Chapter 31: Solutions 461

Chapter 32: Reaction Types 471

Chapter 33: Chemical Kinetics 479

Chapter 34: Equilibrium 495

Chapter 35: Phase Changes 505

Chapter 36: Gas Laws 517

Chapter 37: Acids and Bases 533

Chapter 38: Nuclear Chemistry 553

SECTION VI: ORGANIC CHEMISTRY

Chapter 39: Structural Formulas 567

Chapter 40: Isomers 583

Chapter 41: Bonding 605

Chapter 42: Alkanes 615

Chapter 43: Alkenes and Alkynes 629

Chapter 44: Aromatic Compounds 647

Chapter 45: Alcohols and Ethers 659

Chapter 46: Aldehydes and Ketones 675

Chapter 47: Carboxylic Acids 695

Chapter 48: Carboxylic Acid Derivatives 711

Chapter 49: Amines 737

Chapter 50: Spectroscopy 749

SECTION VII: BIOCHEMISTRY

Chapter 51: DNA and RNA.. 767

Chapter 52: Proteins.. 779

Chapter 53: Lipids 795

SECTION VIII: READING COMPREHENSION

Chapter 54: Reading Critically 805

Chapter 55: Question Types.. 813

Chapter 56: Practice Passages... 819

SECTION IX: QUANTITATIVE ABILITY

Chapter 57: Quantitative Strategies 837

Chapter 58: Basic Math 851

Chapter 59: Algebra 877

Chapter 60: Probability and Statistics................................. 897

Chapter 61: Precalculus... 917

Chapter 62: Calculus 927

INDEX 947

STUDY SHEETS

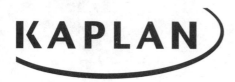

Available Online

kaptest.com/PCAT1516

Log in to Kaplan's PCAT online companion to access two full-length practice tests. You will be asked for a password derived from the text to access the online companion, so have your book available.

Late-Breaking Developments

kaplanpcat.com/testchange and **kaptest.com/publishing**

The material in this book is up-to-date at the time of publication. However, the test makers may release more information on test changes after this book is published. All test changes are posted at **kaplanpcat.com/testchange**. Be sure to read carefully the materials you receive when you register for the test. If there are any important late-breaking developments—or any changes or corrections to the Kaplan test preparation materials in this book—we will post that information online at **kaptest.com/publishing.**

Feedback and Comments

Email us: **booksupport@kaplan.com**

Ask us on Facebook: **facebook.com/KaplanPCAT**

Ask us on Twitter: **twitter.com/KaplanPCATPrep**

We would appreciate your comments and suggestions about this book. Please provide any feedback you have for the improvement of this book to **booksupport@kaplan.com**. Your feedback is extremely helpful as we continue to develop high-quality resources to meet your needs.

Note to International Students

If you are an international student hoping to attend a pharmacy school in the United States, Kaplan can help you explore your options. Here are some things to think about.

- If English is not your first language, most pharmacy schools will require you to take the TOEFL (Test of English as a Foreign Language) or provide some other evidence that you are proficient in English.
- Plan to take the PCAT. The majority of U.S. pharmacy schools require it.
- Begin the process of applying to pharmacy schools at least 12 months before the fall of the year you plan to start your studies. Most programs have only September start dates.
- You will need to obtain an I-20 Certificate of Eligibility from the school you plan to attend if you intend to apply for an F-1 Student Visa to study in the United States.
- If you've already completed a pharmacy degree outside the United States, get information from U.S. schools—some may have special programs for international graduates of pharmacy.

How to Use This Book

- Sign up for your PCAT Online Companion at **kaptest.com/PCAT1516,** which will give you access to your PCAT practice tests and their answers and explanations.

- Familiarize yourself with Kaplan's "Introduction to the PCAT" and "Studying Effectively" recommendations.

- Create a plan to study the Writing, Verbal Ability, Biology, General Chemistry, Organic Chemistry, Biochemistry, Reading Comprehension, and Quantitative Ability sections, using the end-of-chapter practice questions to assess your progress.

- When you are ready, take your first 4-hour, online PCAT Practice Test (available at **kaplanpcat.com** after you register for your PCAT Online Companion) to simulate the computer-based test-taking experience. Review your performance thoroughly. Use the recommendations from Kaplan's Smart Reports™ to help prioritize what you will need to do to improve your score.

- Take the second 4-hour, online PCAT Practice Test (also available at **kaplanpcat.com** after you register for your PCAT Online Companion). Compare your results on this test with your performance on the previous test. Continue to use Kaplan's Smart Reports™ to determine what you need to do to improve.

KAPLAN

Section I

PCAT STRATEGIES

CHAPTER ONE

Introduction to the PCAT

The Pharmacy College Admissions Test (PCAT) is a component of a complete application for admission to most pharmacy schools in the United States and Canada. The American Association of Colleges of Pharmacy (AACP) endorses the PCAT as the official preferred admissions test for entrance to pharmacy school. Scores earned by examinees are an important part of the pharmacy school admissions process because they provide a common factor for schools to use in comparing applications for admission. Your Kaplan program is designed to launch you along the path to your career in pharmacy by helping you achieve the best score possible on the PCAT.

The PCAT is likely different from any other test you encountered in your academic career. It is unlike the knowledge-based exams common in high schools and colleges that emphasize memorizing information; pharmacy schools can assess your academic prowess by looking at your transcript instead. The PCAT is not even like other standardized tests that focus on proving your general skills. Pharmacy schools use PCAT scores to assess whether you possess the foundation upon which to build a successful pharmacy career. Though you certainly need to know the content to do well, the focus is on thought processes. The PCAT emphasizes reasoning, critical thinking, reading comprehension, data analysis, and problem-solving skills.

The PCAT's power comes from its use as an indicator of your abilities: good scores can open up many opportunities for you. Your power comes from preparation and mindset. The key to PCAT success is knowing what you are up against. That's where this book helps. You'll learn the philosophy behind the test, review the sections one by one, attempt sample questions, master Kaplan's proven methods, and understand what the test makers really want. You'll get a handle on the process; find a confident, new perspective; and achieve your highest possible scores.

The PCAT should be viewed as an opportunity to show pharmacy schools who you are and what you can do, just like any other part of your application. Take control of your PCAT experience.

THE COMPUTER-BASED TEST

The PCAT is developed by Pearson Education, Inc. and is administered at Pearson VUE testing centers. The official PCAT website, where you can learn more about the PCAT and register to take the test, is at **http://pcatweb.info**. While there, download and read the *PCAT Candidate Information Booklet*, which contains detailed information about registration and the Test Day experience.

As of July 2011, the PCAT is administered exclusively on the computer and on test dates primarily in January, July, and September; in recent years, test dates with limited seating also have been added in October and November. To check in for your testing session, you will need your admission ticket (emailed to you as confirmation of your registration) and two forms of valid, nonexpired identification with signature, one of which must be government-issued and contain a photograph of you, such as a driver's license, passport, state ID, or military ID. The first and last names on your admission ticket must match your personal IDs exactly; however, IDs with only middle initial or with no middle name included will be accepted. At the testing center, a new photo, signature, and palm scan will be recorded as part of routine security procedures.

The test guidelines for the computer-based test are the same as for the original paper-and-pencil test: no strike-through or highlighting capabilities are provided, and calculators are not allowed at any time. Essays are typed with minimal editing functionality; copy, cut, and paste are available, but spell-check and grammar-check are not. The PCAT is not an adaptive test in which subsequent questions or sections are harder or easier depending on whether the examinee answers them correctly or not; instead, everyone taking the PCAT on the same day sees roughly the same test.

During the test, time is kept via a countdown timer in the corner of the screen. You will not be allowed to wear a watch and may not have access to a clock. One 15-minute rest break is scheduled for the middle of the test. You may take additional breaks with the permission of the proctor, but the test timer will continue running, and you will lose that time. Even if you are not at the computer, the test will continue to run itself, and successive sections will start automatically if time for the previous section has elapsed.

The testing center provides an erasable noteboard and marker to use for taking notes and writing out calculations. If you need to replace your noteboard or marker, you may ask the proctor for a new set any time during the test (although if this is during a section, your time will continue to elapse). You will not be allowed to bring your own writing utensils or paper.

CONTENT

The PCAT is, among other things, an endurance test. It consists of six sections and 232 multiple-choice questions. Add in the administrative details at both ends of the testing experience plus the break halfway through the test, and you can count on being in the test room for over four hours. It can be a grueling experience, to say the least. If you do not approach the PCAT with sufficient confidence and stamina, you may quickly lose your composure. That's why taking control of the test is so important.

The PCAT consists of six timed sections: Writing, Verbal Ability, Biology, Chemistry, Reading Comprehension, and Quantitative Ability. In this book, we'll take an in-depth look at each PCAT section with content review, sample questions, and specific, test-smart hints.

Writing

Time: 30 minutes

Format: problem-solving essay based on a given topic

What it tests: general composition skills and conventions of language; ability to communicate a solution to a problem

Verbal Ability

Time: 25 minutes (37.5 seconds per question)

Format: 40 multiple-choice questions

What it tests: general, nonscientific word knowledge using analogies (62.5%) and sentence completion (37.5%)

Biology

Time: 35 minutes (43.75 seconds per question)

Format: 48 multiple-choice questions

What it tests: knowledge of the concepts and principles of basic biology with an emphasis on general biology (50%), microbiology (20%), and human anatomy and physiology (A&P) (30%)

Specific content: cellular and molecular biology (17%), health (17%), microbiology (20%), diversity of life forms (17%), A&P structure (12%), and A&P systems (18%)

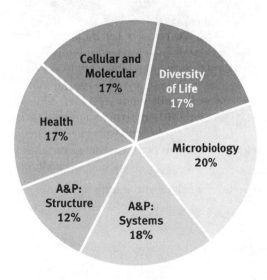

Figure 1.1

Chemistry

Time: 35 minutes (43.75 seconds per question)

Format: 48 multiple-choice questions

What it tests: knowledge of the concepts and principles of general inorganic chemistry (50%), organic chemistry (32%), and biochemistry (18%)

Specific content: atomic theory (8%), chemical bonding (8%), reactions (14%), kinetic theory (8%), solutions (8%), nuclear chemistry (4%), structure and properties of organic compounds (16%), reactions of organic compounds (16%), DNA & RNA (6%), proteins (6%), and lipids (6%)

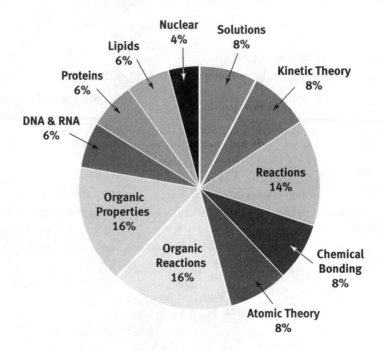

Figure 1.2

Reading Comprehension

Time: 50 minutes (8 minutes and 20 seconds per passage)

Format: 48 multiple-choice questions; 6 passages with 8 questions following each

What it tests: ability to comprehend, analyze, and interpret reading passages on scientific topics

KAPLAN

Quantitative Ability

Time: 45 minutes (56.25 seconds per question)

Format: 48 multiple-choice questions

What it tests: skills in arithmetic processes, including fractions, decimals, and percentages; ability to reason through and understand quantitative concepts and their relationships, including applications of basic math (14%), algebra (19%), probability and statistics (19%), precalculus (24%), and calculus (24%)

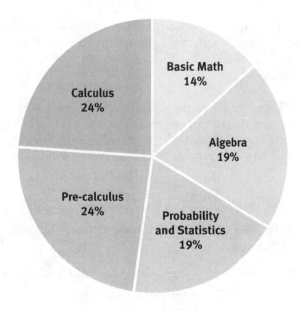

Figure 1.3

SCORING

Each PCAT section receives its own score. Each section except for Writing is scored on a scale ranging from 200 to 600 with 600 as the highest score and 400 as the median. The Writing section is scored numerically from 0 to 6 with 6 as the highest score and 4 as the approximate median. Your essay is evaluated by two essay graders who each assign a cumulative Writing score based on your appropriate use of grammar and style and your ability to create and support a solution to a problem. The Writing score you receive is an average of the scores given by the two graders. Note that if the scores given by the graders vary by more than one point, a third grader grades the essay in order to ensure that grading follows the set standardized rubric.

On the other sections of the test, the actual number of multiple-choice questions you answer correctly per section is your **raw score**. All multiple-choice questions are worth the same amount—one raw point—and there's no penalty for incorrect answers. That means you should always fill in an answer for every question whether you have time to fully invest in that question or not. Never let time run out on any section without filling in an answer for every question.

Note that most sections contain both operational (scored) and experimental (unscored) items. The experimental items are used to test questions for future administrations and have no bearing on your final results. Although some experimental items may look different than usual test questions, definitively determining which items are experimental is impossible on Test Day, so treat every item as if it will be scored while taking the actual test.

Your raw scores will not appear on your score report. Instead, they are converted to yield your **scaled scores**, the ones that fall somewhere in that 200–600 range. These scaled scores are reported to pharmacy schools as your PCAT scores.

In addition to scaled scores for individual sections, schools are also provided a **composite score**, which is a scaled score that factors in your performance on all the sections of the PCAT. Your composite score is not merely an average of the scores from all the sections but rather an evaluation of your performance on the entire test.

Your score report will tell you—and your potential pharmacy schools—not only your scaled scores but also the **percentile** ranking that corresponds with your scaled score in each section. A percentile ranking reflects how many test takers out of 100 scored at or below your level. For example, a percentile of 80 means that 80 percent of test takers did as well as or worse than you did and only 20 percent did better.

PCAT Scores and Equivalent Percentiles						
Percentile	Verbal Ability	Biology	Reading Comp.	Quant. Ability	Chemistry	Composite
≤49	≤394	≤392	≤394	≤392	≤393	≤394
50–64	395–409	393–409	395–409	393–409	394–409	395–409
65–79	410–412	410–412	410–412	410–412	410–412	410–412
80–94	413–443	413–444	413–441	413–443	413–442	413–443
≥95	≥443	≥445	≥442	≥444	≥443	≥444

Table 1.1

What's a Good Score?

What defines a good score can vary significantly based on personal situation. Much depends on the strength of the rest of your application (e.g., if your transcript is first-rate, then the pressure to do well on the PCAT isn't as intense) and on where you want to go to school (e.g., different schools have different score expectations).

For each PCAT administration, the average scaled scores are approximately 400 for each section; this equates to the 50th percentile. To be considered competitive, you'll likely want to score above the 50th percentile. Especially competitive schools may want scores above the 70th percentile range. It's important to check the scores for each individual school. One commonality is that most schools will consider scores that are evenly distributed across sections to be more favorable than a very high performance on one section offset by a very low performance on another section of the test. Performing consistently across the board is preferred.

KAPLAN

Because all of your section scores factor into your cumulative score, maximizing your performance on every question is important. Just a few questions one way or the other can make a big difference in your scaled score. Make an extra effort to score well on a test section if you did poorly in a corresponding class; the best revenge for getting a C in chemistry class is acing the Chemistry section of the PCAT!

WHAT THE PCAT REALLY TESTS

It's important to grasp not only the nuts and bolts of the PCAT (so you know what to do on Test Day) but also the underlying principles of the test (so you know why you're doing what you're doing). The straightforward facts tested by the PCAT are covered throughout this book, but now it's time to examine the heart and soul of the PCAT to see what it's really about.

The Myth

Most people preparing for the PCAT fall prey to the myth that the PCAT is a straightforward science test. They think something like this:

> *The PCAT covers the two years of science I had to take in school: biology, chemistry, and basic organic chemistry, plus math and freshman English. The important stuff is the science, though. After all, we're going to be pharmacists.*

Here's a little-known secret: the PCAT is not just a science test; it's also a critical thinking test. This means the test is designed to let you demonstrate your thought processes as well as your thought content. The implications are vast. Once you shift your test-taking paradigm to match the PCAT's, you'll find a new level of confidence and control over the test. You'll begin to work with the nature of the PCAT rather than against it. You'll be more efficient and insightful as you prepare for the test, and you'll be more relaxed on Test Day. In fact, you'll be able to see the PCAT for what it actually is rather than for what students fear it to be. We want your Test Day to feel familiar, not awkward!

The Zen of PCAT

Pharmacy schools do not need to rely on the PCAT to evaluate what content you already know; admission committees can measure your subject-area proficiency using your undergraduate coursework and grades. Schools are interested instead in the potential of your mind. In recent years, many pharmacy schools have shifted pedagogic focus away from an information-heavy curriculum to a concept-based curriculum. Currently, more emphasis is placed on problem solving, holistic thinking, and cross-disciplinary study. This trend affects you right now because it's reflected in the PCAT. Every good tool matches its task. In this case, the tool is the PCAT, which is used to measure you and other candidates, and the task is to quantify how likely it is you will succeed in pharmacy school. In fact, research shows the PCAT is correlated with success in pharmacy school, and, together with undergraduate GPA, is an excellent tool for pharmacy schools to determine which applicants are likely to be the top—and the bottom—pharmacy students.

Therefore, your intellectual potential—how skillfully you annex new territory into your mental boundaries, how quickly you build connections between ideas, and how confidently and creatively you solve problems—is far more important to admission committees than your ability to recite the pK_a for every acid known to humankind. Schools assume they can expand your knowledge base. They choose applicants carefully because expansive knowledge is not enough to succeed in pharmacy school or in the profession. There's something more, and it's this something more that the PCAT is trying to measure. Every section on the PCAT tests essentially the same higher-order thinking skills: analytical reasoning, abstract thinking, and problem solving. Most test takers get trapped into thinking they are being tested strictly about their knowledge of vocabulary, science, and math. Thus, they approach each section with a new outlook on what's expected. This constant mental shifting of gears can be exhausting and counterproductive. Instead of perceiving the PCAT as parsed into radically different sections, maintain your focus on the underlying nature of the test; each section presents a variation on the same theme. The PCAT is not just about what you know; it's also about how you think.

What About the Science?

With this perspective, you may be left asking questions: *What about the science? What about the content? Don't I need to know the basics?* The answer to each is a resounding *Yes!* You must be fluent in the different languages of the test. You cannot do well on the PCAT if you don't know the basics of biology, general chemistry, organic chemistry, biochemistry, and mathematics. The best approach to learning that content is to take one year each of biology, general chemistry, and organic chemistry and then review the content in this book thoroughly before taking the PCAT. Note that the biochemistry content you need for the PCAT is covered in introductory biology and chemistry courses and you should not need to take a separate biochemistry course (though taking one would not hurt you!). Knowing these basics is just the beginning of doing well on the PCAT, though. That's a shock to most test takers. They presume that once they relearn their undergraduate science they are ready to do battle against the PCAT. Wrong! Test takers with only this minimum of knowledge merely have directions to the battlefield and lack what they need to actually beat the test: an understanding of the test maker's battle plans. You won't merely be drilled on facts and formulas on the PCAT; you will need to demonstrate the ability to reason based on ideas and concepts. The science questions are painted with a broad brush to test your general understanding.

THE PCAT MINDSET

In addition to being a thinking test, the PCAT is a standardized test. As such, it has its own consistent patterns and idiosyncrasies, which can actually work in your favor. This is the key to why test preparation works: You have the opportunity to familiarize yourself with those consistent peculiarities and adopt the proper test-taking mindset.

The PCAT mindset is something to bring to every question, passage, and section you encounter. Being in the PCAT mindset means reshaping the test-taking experience so you are in control. Answer questions *when* you want to; feel free to skip tough but feasible passages and questions, coming back to them only after you've racked up points on easy ones. Answer questions *how* you want to; use Kaplan shortcuts and methods to get points quickly and confidently, even if those methods aren't exactly what the test makers had in mind when they wrote the test.

Some overriding principles of the PCAT mindset that will be covered in depth in the chapters to come are as follows:

- Read actively and critically.
- Translate prose into your own words.
- Save the toughest questions and passages for last.
- Know the test and its components inside and out.
- Do PCAT-style problems in each topic area after you've reviewed it.
- Allow your confidence to build on itself.

- Complete full-length practice tests to break down the mystique of the real experience.
- Know that you are going to make mistakes and learn from those mistakes to get the most out of your practice.
- Stick with the new methods you'll be learning. Some might take more practice than others, but when mastered, all will pay off on Test Day by saving you valuable time and earning you more points.
- Look at the PCAT as a challenge and the first step in your pharmacy career rather than as an arbitrary obstacle.

The PCAT mindset boils down to being proactive and taking control of the testing experience so you can get as many points possible as quickly and as easily as you can. Keep this in mind as you read and work through the material in this book and as you face the challenge on Test Day.

The Four Basic Principles of Good Test Mentality

Knowing the test content arms you with the tools you need to do well on the PCAT, but you must wield those tools with the right frame of mind and in the right spirit. Good test mentality involves taking a certain stance toward the entire test. Here's what's involved:

1. Test awareness

To do your best on the PCAT, always keep in mind that the test is like no other test you've taken before, both in terms of content and in terms of the scoring system. If you took a test in high school or college and got a number of the questions wrong, you generally wouldn't receive a perfect grade. However, on the PCAT, you can get a handful of questions wrong and still earn a fantastic—if not perfect—score. The test is geared so that only the very best test takers are able to finish every section, but even these people rarely get every question right.

What does this mean for you? Just as you shouldn't let one bad passage ruin an entire section, you shouldn't let what you consider to be a subpar performance on one section ruin your performance on the entire test. Often when you think you did not do well you are mistaken. If you allow a feeling of failure to rattle you, it can have a cumulative negative effect, setting in motion a downward spiral that does serious damage to your score. Losing a few points won't ruin your cumulative score, but losing your cool will. If you feel you did poorly on a section, don't sweat it: Chances are it was just a difficult section, and that factor will already be figured into the scoring curve. The point is to remain calm and collected. Do your best on each section, and, once a section is over, forget about it and move on.

2. Stamina

Improving your test-taking stamina can be just as beneficial as learning more content. Overall, the PCAT is a fairly grueling experience, and some test takers simply run out of mental endurance on the last section, which happens to be one of the toughest in terms of timing and mental capacity required: Quantitative Ability. To avoid running out of steam, prepare by taking full-length practice tests in the weeks before your exam so that, on Test Day, completing all seven sections will seem like a breeze. (Well, maybe not a breeze, but at least not a hurricane.) Taking online practice tests also ensures you are comfortable with the computer-based format and allows you to review the explanations and assess your performance. Although the scores you earn on your Kaplan practice tests will be quite realistic, the scores are far less important than the practice itself.

3. Confidence

Confidence feeds on itself; unfortunately, so does the opposite of confidence: self-doubt. Confidence in your ability leads to quick, sure answers and a sense of well-being that translates into more points. If you lack confidence, you may end up reading the sentences and answer choices two, three, or four times until you confuse yourself. This leads to timing difficulties, which only perpetuate the downward spiral, causing anxiety and a rush to finish each section.

However, if you subscribe to the right PCAT mindset, you'll gear all of your practice toward the major goal of taking control of the test. When you've achieved that goal, you'll be ready to face the PCAT with supreme confidence—armed with the principles, techniques, strategies, and approaches set forth in this book—and that's the one sure way to score your best on Test Day.

4. The right attitude

Those students who approach the PCAT as an obstacle, rail against the necessity of taking it, or make light of its importance rarely fare as well as those who see the PCAT as an opportunity to show off the reading and reasoning skills that pharmacy schools are looking for. Don't waste time making value judgments about the PCAT. It's not going away, so you have to deal with it. Those who look forward to doing battle with the PCAT—or, at least, who enjoy the opportunity to distinguish themselves from the rest of the applicants—tend to score better than do those who resent or dread it.

It may sound a little dubious, but attitude adjustment is a proven test-taking technique. Just as a successful athlete prepares mentally and uses positive visualization before a big game, so too should you. Here are a few steps you can take to make sure you develop the right PCAT attitude:

- Look at the PCAT as a challenge but don't obsess over it; you certainly don't want to psych yourself out of the game.
- Remember that, yes, the PCAT is important, but this one test will not single-handedly determine the outcome of your life (contrary to what some students think).
- Have fun with the test. Learning how to match your wits against the test makers' can be a very satisfying experience, and the reading and thinking skills you'll acquire will benefit you in pharmacy school as well as in your future pharmacy career.
- Remember that you're more prepared than most people. You're training with Kaplan. You will have the tools you need and know how to use them.
- Get in shape; you wouldn't run a marathon without working on your stamina well in advance of the race, and the same goes for taking the PCAT.

CHAPTER TWO

Studying Effectively

The first year of pharmacy school is a frenzied experience for most students. To meet the requirements of a rigorous work schedule, students either learn to prioritize and budget their time or else fall hopelessly behind. It's no surprise, then, that the PCAT, the test specifically designed to predict success in the first year of pharmacy school, is a high-speed, time-intensive test. The PCAT demands excellent time-management skills as well as grace under pressure, both during the test as well as while preparing for it. Having a solid plan of attack and sticking with it are key to giving you the confidence and structure you need to succeed.

CREATING A STUDY PLAN

The best time to create a study plan is at the beginning of your PCAT preparation. If you don't already use a calendar, you will want to start. You can purchase a planner from an office store, print out a free calendar from the internet, use a built-in calendar or app for one of your smart devices, or keep track using an interactive online calendar. Pick the option that is most practical for you and that you are most likely to see and use consistently.

Once you have a calendar, write in all your professional obligations: class sessions, work shifts, meetings, etc. Then add in personal obligations: appointments, lunch dates, family time, etc. As part of your personal obligations, schedule in specific time for family and friends, working out, or other hobbies. Making an appointment in your calendar for family dinner or going to see a movie may seem strange at first, but planning social activities in advance helps your loved ones cope with your busy schedule (soon to become even busier once you start pharmacy school!) and helps you balance your personal and professional obligations. When life gets busy, social appointments are often the first to be sacrificed, but this can lead to strained relationships and both physical and mental exhaustion. Having a happy balance allows you to be more focused and productive when it comes time to study, so stay well-rounded and don't neglect anything important to you.

Once you have established your calendar's framework, add in study blocks around your obligations, keeping your study schedule as consistent as possible across days and across weeks. Studying at the same time of day as your official test is ideal for promoting the best recall, but if that's not possible, then fit in study blocks whenever you can.

Next, plan in your full-length practice tests. Take one test earlier in your preparation, but save any remaining tests until you've reviewed all the content and are beginning to feel confident about the PCAT. Staggering your tests in this way allows you to form a baseline for comparison and to determine which areas to focus on right away, while also providing realistic feedback as to how you will perform on Test Day. For each test scheduled, set aside four hours to take the test and then another four hours the next day to thoroughly review the test (discussed more later in this chapter).

When planning your calendar, aim to finish your full-length practice tests and the majority of your studying by one week before Test Day, which will allow you to spend that final week completing a final, brief review of what you already know.

Study Blocks

To make studying as efficient as possible, block out short, frequent periods of study time throughout the week. From a learning perspective, studying one hour per day for six days per week is much more valuable than studying for six hours all at once one day per week. Spacing out your preparation allows your brain time to consolidate its new memories, and seeing the material repeatedly over a longer period of time makes recalling the information on Test Day easier and faster. Specifically, Kaplan recommends studying for no longer than three hours in one sitting. In fact, three hours is an ideal length of time to study: It's long enough to build up your stamina for the four-hour Test Day but not so long that you become overwhelmed with too much information.

Within those three-hour blocks, also plan to take 10-minute breaks every hour. Use these breaks to get up from your seat, do some quick stretches, get a snack and a drink, and clear your mind. Although 10 minutes of break for every 50 minutes of studying may sound like a lot, these breaks will allow you to deal with distractions and rest your brain so that, during the 50-minute study blocks, you can remain completely focused. Taking breaks more often than this, however, can be detrimental; research shows that becoming fully engaged in a mentally-taxing activity generally takes 10 minutes, so if you stop to check your email or social media, talk with your roommates, or grab yet another snack every ten minutes while studying, you will never be completely engaged and will not be using your time effectively.

If you would like to study for more than three hours in one day, space out your studying with a significant break in the middle. For example, you may study for three hours in the morning, take a two-hour break to have lunch with your friends, then study for another two hours in the afternoon.

If you are unable to study for a full three hours in one sitting, shorter amounts of time can work as well, but you'll get the most benefit from your studying if you immerse yourself in the material uninterrupted for at least one hour. For brief practice when you only have a few minutes, use the Study Sheets located at the back of this book. These sheets contain the most important information to memorize before Test Day, so take them with you wherever you go or put them somewhere you'll see them frequently. These can be a great way to fit in extra studying when you wouldn't be doing anything productive otherwise, such as when waiting for the bus to arrive or a class or meeting to start or even while brushing your teeth (you can hang them up on your bathroom mirror!). Even five or ten minutes per day quickly adds up to hours of additional studying over the course of a few weeks.

The total amount of time you spend studying each week will depend on your schedule and your test date, but it is recommended that you spend 200–250 hours before taking the official PCAT. One way you could break this down is to study for three hours per day, five days per week, for three months. But this is just one way. You might study six days per week (though avoid studying every day!) or might study for more than three hours per day. You might study over a longer period of time if you don't have as much time to study each week. Or you might find that you need more or fewer hours based on your personal performance and goal scores.

One way you could use this book is to complete at least one chapter per day. Note that the length of each chapter varies considerably, so only use this as a rough guideline, remembering each week to spend additional time practicing, memorizing vocabulary, and reviewing material previously covered. Furthermore, for best studying, don't just review all of the chapters in order; instead, start thinking about all of the sections of the test right away and reinforce long-term learning by staggering the material.

No matter what your plan is, ensure you complete enough practice to feel completely comfortable with the PCAT and its content. A good sign you're ready for Test Day is when you begin to earn your goal score consistently in practice.

Time Off

Taking some time off can be just as important as studying. Just as you should take breaks during study blocks, take breaks during the week as well. Kaplan recommends taking at least one full day off per week, ideally from all of your professional obligations but at minimum from studying for the PCAT. Taking this time allows you to recharge mentally, and any fun or relaxing activities you plan for those days give you something to look forward to during the rest of the week.

HOW TO STUDY

The PCAT covers a large amount of material, so studying for Test Day can initially seem daunting. To put studying more into your control, break the content down into specific goals for each day and each week instead of attempting to approach the test as a whole. A goal of "I want to increase my cumulative score by 100 points" is too big, abstract, and difficult to measure on the small scale. More reasonable goals are "I will read one chapter each day this week" or "I will be able to recite all the digestive enzymes by Friday." Goals like these are much less overwhelming and help break studying into manageable pieces. As you achieve these smaller goals, you may be surprised to see how quickly you begin achieving your bigger goals, too.

Once you've established your next short-term goals, you will want to achieve them as efficiently and effectively as possible, which means making the most of your study time. Always take notes when reading and practicing. Don't just passively read this book. Instead, read actively: Use the free margin spaces to jot down important ideas, draw diagrams, and make charts as you read. Active participation increases your retention and makes rereading your notes at a later date a great way to refresh your memory.

As you go through your Kaplan program, much of the information may be familiar to you. After all, you have probably seen most of the content before. However, be very careful: Familiarity with a subject does not necessarily translate to knowledge or mastery of that subject. Do not assume that if you recognize a concept you actually know it and can apply it quickly at an appropriate level. Frequently stop and ask yourself questions while you read (e.g., *What is the main point? How does this fit into the overall scheme of things? Could I thoroughly explain this to someone else?*). By making connections and focusing on the grander scheme, not only will you ensure you know the essential content, but you will also prepare yourself for the level of critical thinking required by the PCAT.

If you are limited by only having a minimal amount of time to prepare before Test Day, focus on your biggest areas of opportunity first. You likely won't have time to take detailed notes for every page of this book; instead, use your results from practice questions and tests to determine which areas are your biggest opportunities and seek those out. Skim over content matter for which you are already demonstrating proficiency, pausing to read more thoroughly when something looks unfamiliar or particularly difficult. If you are already feeling confident with the topic of a specific chapter, consider starting with the Review Problems at the end of the chapter. If you can get all of those questions correct within a reasonable amount of time, you may be able to quickly skim through that chapter, but if the questions prove to be more difficult, then you may need to spend time reading the chapter or certain subsections of that chapter more thoroughly, taking notes.

Leave time to review your practice questions and your notes from previous chapters, too. You lead a busy life in addition to preparing for the PCAT, and fitting in so much study time can often feel difficult. You may be tempted to push ahead and cover new material as quickly as possible, but failing to schedule ample time for review will actually throw away your greatest opportunity to improve your performance. The brain rarely remembers anything it sees or does only once. When you build a connection in the brain and then don't follow up on it, that knowledge may still be in your memory somewhere but not in the accessible way you need it to be on Test Day. When you carefully review notes you've taken or problems you've solved (and the explanations for them), the process of retrieving that information reopens and reinforces the connections you've built in your brain. This builds long-term retention and repeatable skill sets—exactly what you need to beat the PCAT!

While reviewing, take notes about the specific reasons why you missed questions you got wrong or you had to guess on, such as by using a spreadsheet like the one below in Table 2.1. Keep adding to the same Why I Missed It Sheet (WIMIS) as you complete more practice, and periodically review your WIMIS to identify any patterns you see, such as consistently missing questions in certain content areas or falling for the same test-maker traps.

Section	Q #	Topic or Type	Wrong Answer Chosen	Why I Missed It
Chemistry	42	Nuclear Chem.	Opposite	Didn't read "not" in question stem
Chemistry	47	K_{eq}	Miscalculation	Need to memorize Kaplan steps
Reading Comp.	2	Detail	Opposite	Didn't read "not" in answer choice; slow down!
Reading Comp.	4	Inference	Out of Scope	Forgot to make a prediction

Table 2.1

As you move through your PCAT program, adjust your study plan based on your available study time and the results of your practice questions. Your strengths and weaknesses are likely to change over the course of this program. Keep addressing the areas that are most important to your score, shifting your focus as those areas change.

Where to Study

One often-overlooked aspect of studying is the environment where the learning actually occurs. Although studying at home is many students' first choice, several problems can arise in this environment, chief of which are distractions. At home, many people have easy access to family, roommates, books, television, movies, food, the Internet, chores yet to be completed, and the list goes on. Studying can be a mentally draining process, so as time passes these distractions become ever more tempting as escape routes. As discussed earlier, the moment you lose focus due to one of these distractions you also lose the time it takes to return to the level of concentration you just had (not to mention any time clearly spent not studying!).

Although you may have considerable willpower, there's no reason to make staying focused harder than it must be. Instead of studying at home, head to a library, quiet coffee shop, or similar location whenever possible. This will eliminate many of the usual distractions and also promote efficient studying; instead of studying off and on at home over the course of an entire day, you can stay at the library for three hours of effective studying and enjoy the rest of the day off from the PCAT.

If you must study at home, consider ways to prevent distractions. Give copies of your schedule to family and friends and ask them not to interrupt your study blocks. Complete all the essential tasks you can before studying so they do not become distractions. If the Internet is a distraction for you, consider temporarily disabling your social media accounts or downloading an extension for your Internet browser that blocks certain websites while you are studying. Rather than fighting distractions with willpower alone, remove as many distractions as possible in advance to avoid the problem entirely.

An additional advantage of studying at libraries, however, is that their environments tend to be akin to those of the PCAT testing centers. Similar to a library, your testing center will be quiet but not completely silent. Not everyone at the test center will be taking the PCAT, and not everyone will start at exactly the same time. While you are in the middle of a multiple choice section, other test takers may be entering the testing room to start their tests, taking breaks, typing essays, or talking with their proctors. Practicing in this type of environment (as opposed to in complete silence or while listening to music at home) means you will be less distracted in the actual testing center on Test Day.

Finally, no matter where you study, make your practice as much like Test Day as possible. Just as required during the official test, don't have snacks or chew gum during your intense, 50-minute study blocks. Turn off your music, television, and phone. Practice on the computer to simulate the computer-based test environment. When completing practice questions, do your work on scratch paper or noteboard sheets rather than writing directly on any printed materials since you won't have that option on Test Day. Study at the same time of day as your official test, especially on the same day of the week, to get in the habit of thinking about the PCAT at those times. Because memory is tied to all of your senses, the more test-like you can make your studying environment, the easier it will be on Test Day to recall the information you're putting in so much work to learn.

In the end, you want to personalize your studying to be as effective as possible for you individually, follow a strict calendar that contains your study blocks and breaks, and make the most of those study blocks by focusing on your opportunity areas while simulating the testing environment. In this way, you'll learn more and at a faster rate than you could otherwise. Sticking with your efficient plan leads to effectively learning the material you need to ace the PCAT—this way, you can do well the first time and not need to study for the PCAT again. Being committed now will definitely pay off in the end.

KAPLAN)

CHAPTER THREE

Test Strategies

Even someone with perfect knowledge of all the science, math, and vocabulary on the PCAT is unlikely to achieve a perfect score without adequate test strategies. Understanding the PCAT question formats and having a clear plan for how to tackle each question while finishing every section on time can be just as important as content knowledge. In fact, using Kaplan's strategies allows you to use the test in your favor and determine correct answers even without knowledge of all the content. Specific strategies for each test section will be covered in the corresponding sections of this book, but this chapter will serve as an introduction to several overarching principles to apply throughout the PCAT.

KAPLAN QUESTION STRATEGY

Aside from the Writing Sample, the PCAT only has one question type: multiple choice. You won't find any fill-in-the-blank, matching, short response, or true/false problems on the PCAT. Instead, every question will provide you with the option to select one of four answer choices. Every time. This means two important things. First, you won't need to prepare your knowledge in such a way that you can recite vocabulary, facts, or statistics from rote memory. Instead, all you'll need to do is recognize and apply those ideas using the choices provided. This means your focus when studying and answering questions should be on recognizing relationships and patterns more than on memorizing lists. Second, the fact that every question is multiple choice means you can identify patterns among the questions and answer choices to help you choose the correct answer even when you're not completely confident regarding the content. Chapters 8, 9, 55, and 57 outline specific strategies for how to use question types and answer choices to your advantage with Analogies, Sentence Completion, Reading Comprehension, and Quantitative Ability questions, respectively.

All the specific strategies for each section start with one key process: Stop-Think-Predict-Match. Although you will make slight modifications to this strategy depending on which question type you are tackling, the core ideas remain the same: Carefully analyze each question and determine what the correct answer will look like *before* reading the corresponding answer choices. This will allow you to use the question format to your advantage. You will quickly bypass wrong answer choices without needing to analyze them fully or falling for the test makers' trap choices, and you also will be leaving yourself open to using alternative strategies such as the process of elimination when necessary. Each step of Stop-Think-Predict-Match is outlined in more detail below.

Stop

Your very first step when attempting any question is to Stop: Don't fully read the question or answers choices but instead **triage**, analyzing the question's subject matter, length, and difficulty to determine if you should tackle it immediately, later, or not at all. For most questions, you will also use this opportunity to characterize the answer choices (e.g., as vocabulary terms, sentences, equations, numbers with units, graphs, etc.).

As discussed later in this chapter, the Stop step allows you to make the most of the limited amount of time you have available. Determining each question's general characteristics before tackling it also allows you to get in the right mindset for that question. If you know you will need to calculate a specific value, you may list the variables you see on your noteboard as you read the question stem; if you know the answer will instead be a graph, you may sketch a quick plot of the variables instead of listing them.

Think

Once you've characterized the question stem and answer choices and decided to tackle a problem, the next step is to actually read the question stem—but still don't read the answer choices yet. While reading the question, don't just read passively; instead, paraphrase as you read so you can determine what the question is really asking. You won't be able to answer the question correctly if you misunderstand what the question is asking you to do, so don't minimize the importance of this step. This step ensures that you do not rush through the question, potentially leading to additional work that is not needed. Establish what the correct answer will look like as specifically as possible (e.g., velocity on the *x*-axis in meters per second) while being careful to note any negative words such as *not*, *except*, or *false*.

Predict

Once you have a clear idea of what the question is asking and have all the information you need to answer it, your next step is to formulate a framework of what the correct answer will look like. At this point, you still should not have read the answer choices, so you are essentially treating the problem as a fill-in-the-blank question. A great prediction will answer the question as thoroughly as possible; however, if you're not certain what to expect from wordy answer choices or don't have strong content knowledge for the subject being tested, a simpler prediction could be nearly as useful and is always better than no prediction at all.

Although the Stop-Think-Predict-Match strategy may sound like a radical change to the way you approach a multiple-choice test, chances are it's not entirely different from what you normally do. The major difference is likely the order: Most test takers who are not Kaplan students read the answer choices first and then determine what the correct answer will be. However, the advantages of predicting before reviewing the answer choices are many. First, making a prediction saves you time. Instead of analyzing all four answer choices, you can quickly skip the wrong choices that don't match your prediction without needing to disprove them specifically. Second, having a clear idea of what the correct answer will look like helps you avoid wrong answer choices that might otherwise be tempting. For example, although choice A of a hypothetical Reading Comprehension question might have sounded reasonable had you read it first, after making a prediction you instead realize it doesn't answer the question and in fact wasn't mentioned in the passage at all. In this way, you avoid the trap of "that sounds good" and hone in on the correct answer right away instead. Finally, you will feel much more confident with your answer if you predict it and then find it among the choices. As discussed in Chapter 1, confidence builds upon itself, so this aspect of the Predict step is great for Test Day.

Match

After preparing a prediction, your last step is to select the answer choice that truly meets the requirements of your prediction. When matching, your goal is not to judge each answer choice based on its own merits but rather to identify if a choice corresponds with the framework you predicted. To that end, answer choices will fall into one of three categories:

- *The choice matches your prediction:* In this case, read the entire choice thoroughly to ensure all components of the choice are correct, paraphrasing as needed. If the choice looks completely correct, select it and move on to the next question.

- *The choice is clearly the opposite of your prediction or otherwise incorrect:* If at any point you realize a choice is definitely incorrect, stop reading that choice and mark it as eliminated on your noteboard (see noteboard strategies later in this chapter). If one component of a choice is incorrect, the entire choice must be incorrect, so there's no need to read the entire option.

- *The choice does not match your prediction:* When an answer choice is not obviously wrong but also doesn't align with what you were anticipating, skip that choice. Don't spend time at this point attempting to definitively prove the choice is incorrect; one of the other answer choices is likely to match your prediction instead, meaning you won't ever need to determine why this option is incorrect.

  Note that just because a choice doesn't match your prediction doesn't mean you should eliminate it right away. In some cases, you may find that no answer choice matches your original prediction. When this happens, you will need to return to the Think and Predict steps, incorporating more information to modify your prediction by making it more general or more specific as needed. Using this modified prediction, you can then complete the Match step again on the choices you did not already eliminate.

As you first start using the Stop-Think-Predict-Match strategy, you may find yourself moving through questions more slowly, especially when you need to modify your predictions, but don't give up! With practice, you will begin to perform these steps automatically and find both your speed and accuracy increased. Because mastery of all the PCAT strategies does require practice, use them consistently throughout your practice tests and questions so you can use them effectively by Test Day.

TEST TIMING

For complete PCAT success, you must answer as many questions correctly as possible in the time allotted. Knowing the content and question strategies is important but not enough; you also must hone your time management skills so you have the opportunity to use those strategies on as many questions as possible. It's one thing to answer a Reading Comprehension question correctly; it's quite another to answer all 48 of them correctly in only 50 minutes. The same applies for the other sections; it's a completely different experience to move from handling an individual passage or problem at leisure to handling a full section under timed conditions. Time is a factor that affects every test taker, and the good news is that you can easily improve your scores by adhering to the following basic principles.

The Four Basic Principles of Test Timing

On some tests, if a question seems particularly difficult, you can spend significantly more time on it because you are given more points for correctly answering hard questions. This is not true on the PCAT. Every PCAT question, no matter how difficult, is worth a single point. There's no partial credit. Because there are so many questions to do in so little time, you can seriously hurt your score by spending five minutes earning one point for a hard question and then not having time to get several quick points from easier questions later in the section.

Given this combination—limited time and all questions equal in weight—you must manage the test sections to ensure you earn as many points possible as quickly and easily as you can.

1. Feel free to skip around

One of the most valuable strategies to help you finish sections in time is recognizing and dealing with the questions and passages that are easier and more familiar to you first. That means temporarily skipping those that promise to be more difficult and time-consuming. You can always come back to these at the end, and, if you run out of time, you're much better off having spent time on the questions that will definitely earn you points rather than those you might have gotten incorrect anyway. Because there's no guessing penalty, always fill in an answer to every question on the test whether you have time to fully attempt it or not.

This strategy is difficult for most test takers; we're conditioned to do things in order, but it just doesn't pay off on the PCAT. Don't let your ego sabotage your score by wasting time on questions you can't do. Sometimes it isn't easy to give up on a tough, time-consuming question, but often it's better simply to move on. The computer won't be impressed if you get the toughest question right. If you dig in your heels on a tough question, refusing to move on until you've cracked it, you're letting your ego get in the way of your test score. A test section is too short to waste on lost causes. There's no point of honor at stake here, but there are PCAT points at stake.

Give skipping around a try when you practice. Remember, if you do the test in the exact order given, you're letting the test makers control you. Be mindful of the clock, and don't get bogged down with the tough questions. On the computer-based test, you can skip around within a section but not among sections.

2. Seek out questions you can answer correctly

Being able to identify which questions will be most difficult for you personally is essential to making decisions about which ones to skip. Unlike items on some other standardized tests, questions and passages on the PCAT are not presented in order of difficulty. There's no rule that says you have to work through the questions within a section in any particular order; in fact, the test makers scatter the easy and difficult questions throughout the section, in effect rewarding those who actually get to the end. Don't lose sight of what you're being tested for along with your reading and thinking skills: efficiency and cleverness. If general chemistry questions are your area of expertise, head straight for them when you first begin the chemistry section and save the organic chemistry and biochemistry questions until the end of that section.

Ideally, you'll be able to determine if a question is easier or more difficult and time-consuming within the first five seconds. If you only realize a question is difficult after spending two minutes working on it, you've already lost time there and forfeited much of the advantage of skipping around.

When evaluating difficulty of a question, consider factors such as length of question stem and answer choices, type of question, type of answer choices provided (e.g., numbers, expressions, terms, or sentences), vocabulary used, content area being tested, etc. Also consider how long a question will take you; even if you know exactly how to perform a calculation, if it involves multiple steps and will take you several minutes, you may want to skip that question initially. If you do decide you can't do a question or realize you won't get to it, guess! Fill in an answer—any answer—for every question. There's no penalty if you're wrong, but you score a point if you're right. Note that no answer choice is any more commonly correct on the PCAT than any other, so avoid looking for big-picture patterns and instead make educated guesses based on logic and elimination.

3. Use the process of elimination judiciously

There are two ways to get all the answers right on the PCAT: You either know all the right answers, or you know all the wrong answers. Because there are three times as many wrong answers, you should be able to eliminate some, if not all, of them. Therefore, if you don't know the right answer, eliminate as many wrong answers as you can. By doing so, you either get to the correct response or increase your chances of guessing the correct response. You start out with a 25 percent chance of picking the right answer, and with each eliminated answer your odds go up. Eliminate one choice, and you have a $33\frac{1}{2}$ percent chance of picking the right answer; eliminate two choices, and you have a 50 percent chance; and so on. Remember to look for wrong-answer traps when eliminating. Some answers are designed to seduce you by distorting the correct answer and therefore can be quickly eliminated. For more information about common wrong answer pathologies, see Chapter 55, Question Types.

However, note that using the process of elimination can be slow. If you attempt to use the process of elimination on every question, you undoubtedly will run out of time before getting to all the questions. Evaluating four choices is much more time consuming than directly homing in on the correct answer and picking it without worrying about why all the wrong choices are incorrect. The process of elimination can be a powerful tool, but save it as a backup for when tackling the question directly with Stop-Think-Predict-Match has not yielded the correct answer.

4. Keep track of time

While working on a section, maintain a general sense of your timing without constantly looking at the clock. For most multiple choice sections, you must average approximately 35 seconds per question in order to finish in time (the exception is Quantitative Ability, during which you have closer to 55 seconds per question—but this still is not much time, considering all the math you will need to complete!). These are averages, though; you will be able to answer some basic questions in 15 seconds, whereas other questions, such as those that involve lengthy calculations, may take over 60 seconds. Especially because of such discrepancies, constantly looking at the countdown timer after every question can be unnecessarily stressful and potentially misleading; you may have just tackled a particularly difficult question for which taking more time was perfectly acceptable, so trying to stick too closely to the average for every question can be counterproductive. Nevertheless, to ensure you finish each section, you still shouldn't spend a wildly disproportionate amount of time on any one question or group of questions.

A good strategy, therefore, is to look at the clock every 5 or 10 minutes with a specific goal, such as "I should have finished 16 questions when the countdown timer shows 20 minutes left in the Chemistry section" (meaning 10 minutes has elapsed). Having specific guidelines in mind helps avoid spending time calculating how much time is left out of the total, which can use up valuable testing time.

When planning out your time, leave at least 30 seconds at the end of each section to review any questions you intended to come back to later and make quick educated guesses for questions you left blank (if any). The last thing you want to happen is for time to elapse for a particular section before you've gotten to half the questions. Therefore, it's essential that you pace yourself, keeping in mind the general guidelines for how long to spend on any individual question or passage. With practice, you will develop an innate sense of how long you have to complete each question so you know when you're exceeding the limit and should start to move faster.

Section-Specific Pacing

Let's now look at the section-specific timing requirements and some tips for meeting them. As described previously, keep in mind that the times per question or passage are only averages; some questions are bound to take less time, whereas others will take more. Try to stay balanced. Every question is of equal worth, so don't get hung up on any one. Think about it: If a question is so hard that it takes you a long time to answer it, chances are you may get it wrong anyway. In that case, you'd have nothing to show for your extra time but a lower score.

Reading Comprehension

Allow yourself approximately eight minutes per passage set, which includes reading a passage and answering the associated questions. On average, give yourself 3–4 minutes to read a passage and then 4–5 minutes to answer the eight corresponding questions. Some longer passages may take more time to read, but limit yourself to four minutes as a maximum so you have time to answer the questions, which are what actually contribute to your overall score.

Do the easiest passages first. This may mean avoiding topics that are extremely unfamiliar or passages that seem to include a lot of challenging vocabulary. For passage-based questions, choose an answer based only on the information given. Be careful not to overthink the question by inserting too much of your own logic. Passages might generate their own data. Your answer choices must be consistent with the information in the passage, even if that means an answer choice is inconsistent with the science of ideal, theoretical situations.

Verbal Ability, Biology, Chemistry, and Quantitative Ability

As previously mentioned, you have about 35 seconds per question for Verbal, Biology, and Chemistry questions and about 55 seconds for each Quantitative Ability question. Some questions will take more time and some less. Again, the rule is to do your best work first. Know also that you may not need a deep understanding of all the details of a question stem or topic to answer a question because a lot of information provided may be extraneous. Work to overcome your perfectionism and use your time wisely.

NOTEBOARD STRATEGIES

Other resources to maximize on Test Day are your erasable noteboard and marker. Finding a balance between using the noteboard when you need it but not so much that you waste your limited time is important. One efficient strategy is to make an elimination table, such as at the top of Figure 3.1. Rather than rewriting the letters A, B, C, and D for each question, write them only once and use a table to keep track of which choices you have eliminated. This has the added benefit of clearly retaining which choices you have eliminated for any given question, which is helpful for those questions you plan to return to later. As discussed previously, don't use elimination for every question since it can be time-consuming even with this shortcut.

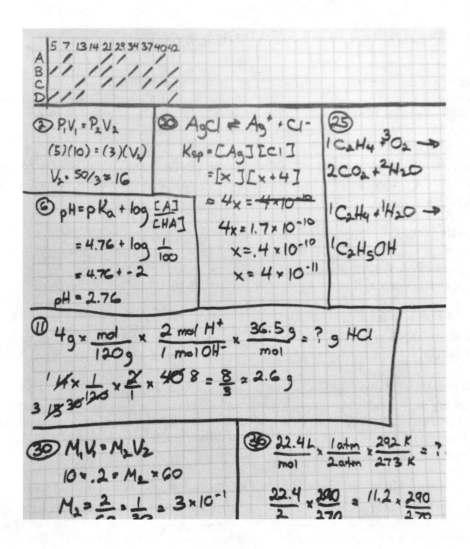

Figure 3.1

Write clearly on your noteboard. Conserve space by keeping all your work for a given problem in the same area. Number each question and box off its notes when you are finished so you can come back to it later if needed and so you do not confuse your work for one question with the work for another. If your noteboard fills up during a section, erase the bottom work, but keep your elimination table until you finish that section. When you do finish a section, completely erase your noteboard or ask your proctor for a new one (and a new marker if you sense yours is beginning to run out of ink).

KAPLAN'S TOP TEN PCAT STRATEGIES

1. **Relax!**

   Just by reading the first few chapters of this book you are already ahead of your competition. By the time Test Day arrives, you will have mastered the Kaplan strategies and PCAT content needed to conquer the exam. Have fun with the process; you're almost in pharmacy school already!

2. **Know what the PCAT tests.**

   Never forget the purpose of the PCAT: to test your powers of analytical reasoning. You need to know the content because each section has its own particular language, but the underlying PCAT intention is consistent throughout the test.

3. **Develop the PCAT mindset.**

   The PCAT is designed to let you show off everything you've learned so far. Don't let your spirit fall, or your attitude will slow you down. Don't let yourself worry about a question or section once you've finished it but instead change your mindset and tackle the next item as if you're just starting the day.

4. **Build your stamina.**

   Prepare your mind for Test Day by completing practice tests and studying for 3-hour blocks while remembering to take breaks every hour and one day off per week.

5. **Master the art of predicting.**

   Kaplan's Stop-Think-Predict-Match strategy allows you to break up each question into manageable steps. Carefully determine what a question is really asking, then anticipate answers before you read the answer choices. This helps protect you from persuasive, tricky, and time-consuming incorrect choices.

6. **Skip around within each section by seeking out questions you can answer correctly.**

   Attack each section confidently. You're in charge. Since every question is worth one point each, work your best areas first to maximize your opportunity for PCAT points. Don't be a passive victim of the test structure, and don't let any one question drag you down!

7. **Use process of elimination judiciously.**

   Most wrong answer choices are logical twists on the correct choice. Quickly move past any obvious traps to more easily match your prediction but only use the full process of elimination when you cannot find a match.

8. **Keep track of time.**

   Pace yourself to avoid spending too much time on any individual question. Don't let the clock add stress to Test Day; it's just another tool designed to help you.

9. **Make the most of your noteboard.**

   Keep track of all the notes you need on your noteboard by being neat and methodical. You aren't given many resources to use on Test Day, so take full advantage of those provided.

10. **Have the right attitude.**

    Your attitude toward the test really does affect your performance. You don't necessarily have to think nice thoughts about the PCAT, but work to develop confidence and a positive mental stance toward the test. You can do this!

Section II

WRITING

CHAPTER FOUR

The PCAT Essay

The Writing section of the test is your chance to demonstrate how adept you are at conveying a point clearly and concisely in essay form. Essays are assigned a score by two graders, each from 1–6, with 6 representing the highest score possible for a superior essay. Scores of 0 (invalid) are assigned to writing samples left blank, written in a language other than English, or completely off topic. The two grader's scores are then averaged (rounding to the nearest tenth) to assign a final score. Even if you do not consider yourself a strong writer, you can still master the basic skills the Writing section tests, especially if you follow Kaplan's Five-Step Method for success on the writing sample. If you are willing to work and practice, then you can score a 6.

The PCAT Writing section will require you to write a **problem-solving** essay in 30 minutes. A problem-solving topic will present a problem in the field of health, science, society, culture, or politics and ask you to write about a possible solution by performing four tasks:

1. Explain the prompt.
2. Suggest a solution and support it.
3. Offer and assess alternative solutions.
4. Wrap up with a strong conclusion.

These tasks should be accomplished in a unified essay that flows well, remains focused, and has minimal mistakes. Your essay will be assessed both for its ability to adhere to appropriate conventions of language (grammar, style, and usage) as well as its problem-solving capabilities (develop a logical argument with convincing support).

KAPLAN'S 5-STEP METHOD FOR THE WRITING SAMPLE

Kaplan's Five-Step Method, if followed correctly, will help you prepare an essay that meets, if not exceeds, expectations. Table 4.1, below, outlines the purpose of each step as well as the amount of time you should spend on each.

Step	Time
Step 1: Read and Annotate Purpose: Clarify what the given statement or problem means.	1 minute
Step 2: Prewrite Purpose: Sketch out a sensible solution, counterexample, and resolution.	6 minutes
Step 3: Clarify Main Idea and Plan Purpose: Make sure the main idea is stated concisely and that it is the centerpiece of your essay.	1 minute
Step 4: Write Purpose: Build a unified essay based on your prewritten tasks.	20 minutes
Step 5: Proofread Purpose: Detect errors, especially those that affect clarity.	2 minutes
Total Time:	30 minutes

Table 4.1

Below is an example of a problem-solving writing topic. Refer to this topic as you navigate through the Kaplan Five-Step Method.

> *Discuss a solution to the problem of increased levels of greenhouse gases, such as carbon dioxide, and the possibility of global climate change.*

Step 1: Read and Annotate

This first step may seem obvious but is essential. You should not simply read the topic and immediately begin writing. Instead, take a moment to digest the topic in full, considering each word as a possible source of ideas. Note any key words or phrases. Certain terms can be interpreted differently; consider how you interpret each word in the context of the given topic, remembering that you must support your interpretation with concrete examples. Look at the topic from all possible angles and jot down as any notes you need.

Step 2: Prewrite

After you have a clear idea of what the statement means and how you will begin to explain it, you are ready to brainstorm different solutions and prewrite each implied task. This will help you solidify your interpretation of the statement and is the key to using your time effectively and writing clearly. Note that the first solution you think of may not be the easiest to write about or support with examples; coming up with multiple solutions allows you to choose the easiest and gives you ideas for alternative solutions, too.

Task 1: Explanation

Explain the elements of the problem, making sure to define key concepts and words in the statement of the problem. For example, based on the above prompt, it would be important to discuss the meaning of the phrase *global climate change*, the sources of greenhouse gases, and the relationship between such gases and climate change. Also discuss *why* greenhouse gases and climate change are problems and what additional issues may arise if they are left unchecked.

Task 2: Solution

Explain the key elements of your solution. Also provide a brief example that demonstrates your solution, such as when a similar solution was used to solve a comparable problem in the past. For example, you could state that other sources of energy need to be more widely employed to reduce the sources of greenhouse gases and support this solution with the example of the effectiveness of recent, smaller-scale shifts of some power plants from coal to natural gas or biomass.

A strong writing sample also uses this task as an opportunity to explain and refute anticipated criticism by pointing out a potential weakness of an element of the solution but then providing a rebuttal. For the above solution, you might focus on the cost of implementing a new program but explain how this can be covered by carbon taxes on those entities that choose not to comply.

Task 3: Alternative Solution

In order to achieve the maximum score on your writing sample, you must also include one or more alternative solutions in addition to your main solution. These solutions should also be expanded upon with evidence and details but to a lesser extent than your main solution. For example, you might discuss changes individuals can make, such as driving less often, creating less waste, and purchasing energy-efficient devices.

Task 4: Conclusion

Finish your essay with a strong conclusion that shows why your main solution is the best of all those proposed. Use this opportunity to quickly summarize the overall issue and why it's a problem. Include a solid closing sentence to leave a strong impression with your graders as they are assigning your score.

Step 3: Clarify Main Idea and Plan

If you have budgeted your time wisely in the first two tasks, you should have at least one minute left to clarify your main idea and to discard ideas that do not belong or that detract from the cohesiveness of your essay plan. As you review your plan, ensure that your ideas work together and that the primary tasks are balanced. This is your chance to envision how all the major points will work together and to plan the overall flow of your argument.

Step 4: Write

After formulating a great plan, actually writing your essay is often the easiest step. Use the ideas from your prewrite as your outline. Stay with the prewrite and be careful not to veer off track. Introducing a new idea, no matter how good, is a surefire way to start digressing from the central focus of the paragraphs and run out of time, leaving behind an essay that is incomplete and not cohesive. While writing, avoid language that is too complex and that could detract from unity. Start with a basic, four-paragraph structure with one paragraph for each of the four implied tasks. Use simple, straightforward language and strong reasoning.

Step 5: Proofread

Your last few minutes should be devoted to correcting any errors that obscure your key points. The Kaplan strategy recommends at least two minutes, but this is a minimum; the more time you have to proofread, the better your essay will become. As you review your essay, look out for critical word omissions, run-on sentences, subject-verb agreement, and any other mistakes that make understanding your essay more difficult. Also correct any other spelling and grammar errors you notice, but ensure your initial focus is on the big picture; although these kinds of mistakes can affect your score, it's even more important that your argument makes sense. Type your corrections accurately and delete only what you mean to delete. Do not use this opportunity to rewrite entire paragraphs or make other major changes to structure since you may run out of time and end up with a confusing essay.

WRITING SAMPLE SCORING

Unlike some other scoring systems, PCAT essay scores don't start at a perfect score and have points taken off for errors. Instead, each level has to be earned. You cannot earn a 5 if you haven't earned a 4. Scores of 1–2 represent essays that fail to meet the basic instructions, a score of 3 describes an essay that is adequate in all categories and completes the assignment, and scores of 4–6 are assigned to essays that not only follow the tasks but have progressively stronger style, flow, and ideas. The following scoring rubric demonstrates how the PCAT graders judge your writing skills.

	6 Superior	5 Proficient	4 Effective	3 Satisfactory	2 Marginal	1 Inadequate
Conventions of Language	• Few, if any, errors made in sentence formation, usage, or mechanics. • No errors serious enough to interfere with meaning or flow.	• Some mistakes in sentence formation, usage, and mechanics present. • Errors do not interfere with essay's meaning or flow.	• Mistakes in sentence formation, usage, and mechanics interfere with flow but not meaning.	• Several mistakes in sentence formation, usage, and mechanics interfere with flow and meaning.	• Patterns of mistakes in sentence formation, usage, and mechanics detract from the essay. • Meaning of the response may be impaired.	• Frequent and serious mistakes in sentence formation, usage, and mechanics make the response difficult to understand.

	6	5	4	3	2	1
	Superior	*Proficient*	*Effective*	*Satisfactory*	*Marginal*	*Inadequate*
Problem Solving	• Main tenets of the problem are discussed in detail. • Solution clearly relates to the problem and is developed with convincing support. • Alternative solutions are included with clear discussions. • Argument is logical and effectively organized.	• Problem and evidence are discussed clearly. • Solution relates to the problem and is supported with relevant details. • Response lacks detailed, in-depth support. • Alternative solutions are discussed with some attempt at analysis. • Argument is logical and clear.	• Problem is discussed with reasonable clarity. • Solution discussed generally relates to the problem, and most of the support is appropriate. • Argument is loosely organized and may contain digressions in the structure that weaken its effectiveness.	• Presentation may be too general to be convincing. • Discussion of the problem and solution is adequate. • Solution is related to the prompt, and most of the support is relevant. • Argument may be logical, but loose organization results in digressions or redundancies.	• Response may not always be cohesive. • Writer may seem overly concerned with self-expression. • Problem is discussed. • Solution may be implicit. • Support is vague and interrupted with redundancies and digressions. • Organization is haphazard.	• Problem or solution does not clearly relate to the prompt. • Support is fragmentary, unconvincing, and irrelevant. • Chaotic organization makes following the logic difficult. • If no solution can be found, then the essay cannot exceed to a higher point.

Table 4.2

As described above, essays that score a 3 address each task and are clear and logical. They follow the directions. An essay that receives a 2 lacks at least one of these qualities. The difference is objective: tasks completed versus not completed. The criteria for higher scores become increasingly demanding, but there's no reason to be in the 1–2 range; simply following the directions prevents that from happening.

Practice Makes Perfect

The best way to learn is to practice writing an essay, such as those found in Chapter 6, then score your essay yourself based on the scoring rubric. Once you feel confident with your essays and can reliably finish on time, have someone else score your latest essay to ensure your ideas translate well to others. Give your work to others whose writing skills you respect: friends, instructors, or family members. Tell them about the nature of the assignment and the time limit. If your readers are not knowledgeable about the PCAT essay section, show them both the rubric above as well as the student essays and evaluations found in Chapter 6. In that way, your readers will become better critics of your work.

When you do find someone to comment on your work, do your best to take the criticism with a cool head. To get the most out of these practice essays, you must put aside your emotional attachment to your writing and achieve a certain degree of objectivity. Remember that your evaluators are not trying to tear you down when they point out certain areas where you need further practice. Through that practice, you will master the four tasks and the Kaplan 5-Step Method to ensure great success on Test Day.

CHAPTER FIVE

Usage and Style

The writing process is about producing a clearly developed and well-organized essay. Don't worry excessively about writing mechanics, but do train yourself out of poor habits and remember to proofread your essays for obvious errors. Your objective in taking the PCAT is admission to pharmacy school, and to achieve that objective you must give the pharmacy schools what they want. Many students mistakenly believe that their essays will be downgraded for such mechanical errors as misplaced commas, poor choice of words, misspellings, faulty grammar, and so on. Occasional problems of this type won't dramatically affect your PCAT essay score; the test readers understand that you are writing first-draft essays. They will not take points off for such errors, provided you don't have a demonstrable pattern of such errors. If your essays are littered with misspellings and incorrect usage, though, then a more serious communication problem is indicated.

Although the essay scorers do not expect eloquence in a thirty-minute assignment, they do expect effectiveness. To help you achieve this effectiveness in your essay, follow three broad objectives:

- Be **CONCISE**
- Be **FORCEFUL**
- Be **CORRECT**

An effective essay is concise: It wastes no words. An effective essay is forceful: It makes its point. And an effective essay is correct: It conforms to the generally accepted rules of grammar and form. The principles of concise and forceful writing are generally not as rigid as the principles of grammatically correct writing; conciseness and forcefulness are matters of art and personal style as well as common sense and tradition. However, on the PCAT Writing Sample, sticking closely to the principles of standard English writing will be the easiest way to produce a concise, forceful, and correct essay. Studies have shown that a writer's style improves dramatically when the writer knows what he or she is going to say. The message is that you should not generate too much anxiety over your writing style but instead make a solid plan and remain confident about it. Your goal here is not to create a publishable work but only to produce a solid, thirty-minute, first-draft essay about solutions to a problem.

The following pages break down the three broad objectives of conciseness, forcefulness, and correctness into twenty-three specific principles. However, the three objectives are interrelated;

for example, a forceful sentence is usually not verbose, and correct sentences tend to be more forceful than incorrect ones. Many of these rules will already be familiar to you, and you will have many chances to practice with the exercises and practice essays. Note that the best strategy is to study this section and work the exercises in short, manageable blocks interspersed with the study of other PCAT subjects. When studying, use your time wisely; don't do all the examples if you are confident you already understand the point. Instead, move on and spend extra time on those areas that give you trouble.

Most importantly, *keep it simple.* This applies to word choice, sentence structure, and overall argument. Obsession with how to spell a word correctly can throw off your flow of thought; instead, choose words with which you are comfortable and for which you clearly know the spellings and meanings. The more complicated your sentences, the more likely they will be plagued by errors. Recall that *simple* does not mean *simplistic.* A clear, straightforward approach can still be sophisticated.

BE CONCISE

Principle 1. Avoid Junk Phrases

Do not use several words when one word will achieve the same goal. Junk phrases are like junk food: They are empty "calories" and have no real value. Many people make the mistake of writing *at the present time* or *at this point in time* instead of the simpler *now* or writing *take into consideration* instead of simply *consider* in an attempt to make their prose seem more scholarly or formal. It does not work; their prose instead ends up seeming inflated and pretentious. Writing junk phrases is a waste of words, a waste of limited time, and a distraction from the point of the essay.

WORDY: I am of the opinion that the aforementioned managers should be advised that they will be evaluated with regard to the utilization of responsive organizational software for the purpose of devising a responsive network of customers.

CONCISE: We should inform the managers that we will evaluate their use of flexible computerized databases to develop a customer's network.

Exercise for Principle 1: Junk Phrases

Improve the following sentences by omitting or replacing junk phrases.

1. The agency is not prepared to undertake expansion at this point in time.
2. In view of the fact that John has prepared with much care for this presentation, it would be a good idea to award him with the project.
3. The airline has a problem with always having arrivals that come at least an hour late, despite the fact that the leaders of the airline promise that promptness is a goal that has a high priority for all the employees involved.
4. In spite of the fact that she only has a little bit of experience in photography right now, she will probably do well in the future because she has a great deal of motivation to succeed in her chosen profession.
5. The United States is not in a position to spend more money to alleviate the suffering of the people of other countries, considering the problems of its own citizens.

Principle 2. Avoid Redundancy

Redundancy means that the writer needlessly repeats an idea because he fails to realize the scope of a word or phrase that has already been used; for example, "a beginner lacking experience" (the word *beginner* already implies lack of experience). You can eliminate redundant words or phrases without changing the meaning of the sentence.

Here are some common redundancies:

REDUNDANT	CONCISE
refer back	refer
few in number	few
small-sized	small
grouped together	grouped
end result	result
serious crisis	crisis
new initiatives	initiatives

Redundancy often results from carelessness, but you can easily eliminate redundant elements in the proofreading stage by watching out for words that add nothing to the sense of the sentence.

Exercise for Principle 2: Redundancy

Repair the following sentences by marking out redundant elements.

1. All these problems have combined together to create a serious crisis.
2. A staff that large in size needs an effective supervisor who can get the job done.
3. He knows how to follow directions, and he knows how to do what he is told.
4. The writer's technical skill and ability do not mask his poor plot line.
5. That monument continues to remain a significant tourist attraction.

Principle 3. Avoid Needless Qualification

Since the goal of your essay is to convince your reader your solution would be effective, you will want to adopt a reasonable tone. There will likely be no single, clear-cut answer to the essay topic, so you should not overstate your case. Occasional use of such modifiers as *fairly, rather, somewhat, relatively* and of such expressions as *seems to be, a little,* and *a certain amount of* will let the reader know you are reasonable, but using such modifiers too often weakens your argument. Excessive qualification makes you sound hesitant; like junk phrases, they add bulk without adding substance.

WORDY: This rather serious breach of etiquette may possibly shake the very foundations of the corporate world.

CONCISE: This serious breach of etiquette may shake the foundations of the corporate world.

Just as bad is the overuse of the word *very*. Some writers use this intensifying adverb before almost every adjective in an attempt to be more forceful. If you need to add emphasis, look for a stronger adjective (or verb) instead.

WEAK:	Novak is a very good pianist.
STRONG:	Novak is a virtuoso pianist.
	or
	Novak plays beautifully.

And don't try to modify words that are already absolute.

WRONG	CORRECT
more unique	unique
the very worst	the worst
completely full	full

Exercise for Principle 3: Excessive Qualification

Although reasonable qualification benefits an essay, excessive qualification debilitates your argument. Though the qualification in some of the sentences below might be appropriate in certain contexts, use these sentences to practice achieving concision by eliminating qualification.

1. She is a fairly excellent teacher.
2. Ferrara seems to be sort of a slow worker.
3. There are very many reasons technology has not permeated all countries equally.
4. It is rather important to pay attention to all the details of a murder trial as well as to the larger picture.
5. You yourself are the very best person to decide what you should do for a living.

Principle 4. Avoid Unnecessary Sentences

This principle suggests several tenets:

- Do not write a sentence that gets you nowhere.
- Do not ask a question only to answer it (unless you have hit upon a brilliant exception!).
- Do not merely copy the essay's directions.
- Do not write a whole sentence only to announce that you're changing the subject.

If you have something to say, say it without preamble. If you need to smooth over a change of subject, do so with a transitional word or phrase rather than a meaningless sentence. If proofreading reveals unintentional, wasted sentences, delete them.

WORDY:	Which idea of the author's is more in line with what I believe? This is a very interesting question . . .

CONCISE:	The author's second theory more closely mirrors reality.

The author of the wordy example above is wasting words and limited time while getting nowhere. Get to the point quickly and stay there. Simplicity and clarity, not verbosity, win points.

BE FORCEFUL

Principle 5. Avoid Needless Self-Reference

Self-reference is another form of unnecessarily qualifying what you say, so do not make repeated references to yourself in your essay. Avoid such unnecessary phrases as *I believe*, *I feel*, and *in my opinion*. Self-reference is generally superfluous and therefore detracts from your essay's concision and forcefulness by constantly reminding your reader that you are expressing an opinion rather than fact. Practice expressing self-confidence in your writing. Your opinion is legitimate and deserves to be stated.

WEAK: I am of the opinion that air pollution is a more serious problem than the government has led us to believe.

STRONG: Air pollution is a more serious problem than the government has led us to believe.

Note that self-references are perfectly acceptable if you are providing a specific, personal story as supporting evidence. For example, in support of a similar solution you are proposing on the national level as part of your essay, you might correctly state, "When I instituted a mixed-stream recycling program in my apartment building, we saw a 40% reduction in trash sent to the landfill, and the money saved in garbage disposal fees caused the project to pay for itself."

Exercise for Principle 5: Needless Self-Reference

Repair the following sentences by marking out needless self-reference.

1. I feel we ought to pay teachers more than we pay senators.
2. The author, in my personal opinion, is stuck in the past.
3. I do not think this argument can be generalized to most business owners.
4. My own experience shows me that food is the best social lubricant.
5. I doubt more people would vote even if they had more information about candidates.

Principle 6. Avoid the Passive Voice

In the active voice, the subject performs the action (we should do it . . .). In the passive voice, the subject is the receiver of the action and is often only implied (it should be done . . .). Using the passive voice is another way writers avoid accountability, so avoid the passive voice and put verbs in the active voice whenever possible.

PASSIVE: The estimate of this year's tax revenues was prepared by the General Accounting Office.

ACTIVE: The General Accounting Office prepared the estimate of this year's tax revenues.

To change from the passive to the active voice, ask yourself who or what is performing the action. In the case above, the General Accounting Office (GAO) is performing the action. Therefore, the GAO should be the subject of the sentence. Weak sentences are usually the product of writing before thinking. Your prewriting, especially outlining ideas for sentences, should give you an idea of your sentence's purpose, so take a few seconds at that point to determine what each sentence is going to do before you actually write it.

Exercise for Principle 6: Undesirable Passives

Change the following sentences from passive to active voice.

1. The Spanish-American War was fought by brave but misguided men.
2. The bill was passed by Congress, but it was not signed by the President until the time for action had passed.
3. Advice is usually requested by those who need it least; it is not sought out by the truly lost and ignorant.
4. That building should be relocated to where it can be appreciated by the citizens.
5. Garbage collectors should be generously rewarded for their dirty, smelly labors.

Principle 7. Avoid Weak Openings

Do not begin a sentence with *There is*, *There are*, or *It is*. These are roundabout ways of getting to the main point of the sentence and usually indicate to your reader that you are trying to distance yourself from the position you are taking. Again, whatever the appearance, the problem usually results from writing before thinking about the sentence.

Exercise for Principle 7: Weak Openings

Rewrite the following sentences to avoid weak openings.

1. It would be unwise for businesses to ignore the illiteracy problem.
2. It can be seen that in many fields experience is more important than training.
3. There are several reasons why this plane is obsolete.
4. It would be of no use to fight a drug war without waging a battle against demand for illicit substances.
5. There are many strong points in the candidate's favor; intelligence, unfortunately, is not among them.

Principle 8. Avoid Vague Language

Choose specific, descriptive words. Vague language weakens your writing because it forces the reader to guess what you mean instead of allowing the reader to concentrate fully on the ideas you are presenting. The essay topic will supply you with an abundance of specifics; your argument will be more forceful if you use similar specifics to replace vague phrases with the particular facts at hand.

WEAK: Ms. Brown is highly educated.

STRONG: Ms. Brown has a master's degree in business administration.

WEAK: She is a great communicator.

STRONG: She speaks persuasively.

Notice that sometimes, to be more specific and concrete, you will have to use more words than you might with vague language. This principle is not in conflict with the general objective of concision. Being concise means eliminating *unnecessary* words; avoiding vagueness sometimes means adding *necessary* words.

Principle 9. Avoid Clichés

Clichés are commonly used expressions that may once have seemed powerful but now have lost much of their original meaning and effect because of overuse. When working under time pressure, you can easily let trite phrases slip into your writing. A reliance on vague or meaningless clichés will suggest you are a lazy thinker; keep them out of your essay.

WEAK: That painting cost an arm and a leg, but it's the real McCoy.

STRONG: The museum paid $10,000 for that painting, but it is a genuine work by Salvador Dali.

Putting a cliché in quotation marks in order to indicate your distance from the cliché does not strengthen the sentence; if anything, it merely calls attention to the weakness. If you do use a cliché, be aware that you are using one, and ask yourself whether the reader will understand what you mean and whether the cliché says exactly what you intend.

Exercise for Principle 9: Clichés

Make the following sentences more forceful by replacing clichés.

1. Beyond the shadow of a doubt, Jefferson was a great leader.
2. I have a sneaking suspicion that families spend less time together than they did fifteen years ago.
3. The pizza delivery man arrived in the sequestered jury's hour of need.
4. Trying to find the employee responsible for this embarrassing information leak is like trying to find a needle in a haystack.
5. Both strategies would be expensive and completely ineffective, so it's six of one and half a dozen of the other.

Principle 10. Avoid Jargon

Jargon describes the specialized vocabulary only used by a particular group, such as doctors, lawyers, or baseball coaches, that can be difficult for outsiders to understand. This can also include informal speech used in everyday conversation or typing, including acronyms such as *IMHO* (in my humble opinion) or emoticons such as :) (to represent smiling or happiness).

A similar category to avoid is the overly inflated and complex language that burdens many students' essays. You will not impress anyone with big words that do not fit the tone or context of your essay, especially if you misuse them. If you are not certain of a word's meaning or appropriateness, leave it out. An appropriate vocabulary, even if simple, will add impact to your argument.

Also remember that your essay scorers are human and may not have knowledge of every word in the English language. One proofreading technique is to ask yourself as you come across words you are unsure of, "Would a reader in a different field be able to understand exactly what I mean from the words I've chosen?" If you ever are not sure, change the word or phrase to a simpler and clearer version.

WEAK: Her patent foramen ovale was the root of her hypoxia.

STRONG: Her heart defect caused her to not have enough oxygen in her body.

Exercise for Principle 10: Jargon

Replace the jargon in the following sentences with more appropriate language.

1. Allow me to elucidate my position: This horse is the epitome, the very quintessence, of equine excellence.
2. In the case of the recent railway disaster, it is clear that governmental regulatory agencies obfuscated the materials for release to the public through both the electronic and print media.
3. Having been blindsided by innumerable unforeseen crises, this office has not been able to prepare for the aforementioned exigencies.
4. U need practice b4 u can match my l33t skills.
5. Pursuant to your being claimed as a dependent on the returns of another taxpayer or resident wage earner, you may not consider yourself exempt if your current nonwage income exceeds five hundred dollars or if your nonwage income combined with current wage income amounts to or exceeds five hundred dollars.

Principle 11. Vary Sentences in Length and Structure

Even when writing is clear and correct, sentences that are all similar in length and structure can be tedious to read. Your ideas will make more of an impact if you break up a series of complicated sentences by occasionally inserting a short and simple one. Usually you can do this by cutting one long, convoluted sentence into two shorter sentences. Take the following passage:

> The author suggests that a conflict exists between devoting limited resources to many people who would be affected positively or to a needy few for whom the effects would be less impressive. This conflict underlies many political arguments in the United States today about education, welfare, healthcare, and other issues that are costly and complex. We should direct resources where they will have the broadest impact if taxpayers are willing to devote only a limited portion of their income to the "general welfare" of the American people.

Each sentence, taken singly, is adequate stylistically and grammatically, but the passage lacks force because the same construction is repeated in each sentence. Each sentence is more than twenty-five words long and begins with the subject (*the author, this conflict, we*). This makes the content seem monotonous and suggests that the writer lacks imagination.

Compare the passage above with the following revised version:

> According to the author, a conflict exists between devoting limited resources to many people who would be affected positively or to a needy few for whom the effects would be less impressive. This conflict underlies many political arguments in the United States today. People fight about how to distribute resources for education, welfare, healthcare, and other issues that are costly and complex. However, taxpayers are willing to devote only a limited portion of their income to the

"general welfare" of the American people. As long as this is true, we should direct those resources where they will have the broadest impact.

The two passages contain the same information, often use the same phrasing, and are roughly the same length, yet the second passage is more interesting and persuasive because it is varied. Sentence length ranges from eleven to thirty-two words, and structure is varied by the use of dependent clauses.

BE CORRECT

Correctness is perhaps the most difficult objective for writers to achieve. The complex rules of standard English usage can leave you feeling unsure of your writing and more than a bit confused. Remember, though, that your readers will not expect perfection, so just think of the principles of correctness as providing you with general ideas to keep in mind rather than as rules you must completely memorize.

As you work through this section, you will come across a few technical words that describe particular functions that words have in a sentence. You will not be expected to know these terms, only to understand the essence of a word's function in the sentence so you can recognize an error when you see one. You do *not* need to memorize these terms; the use of grammatical terms here merely allows for simplification of what would otherwise be needlessly roundabout explanations.

PRINCIPLES OF CONSISTENCY

Many of the rules of English usage are designed to force the writer to stick with one structure or usage throughout a sentence or even an entire essay in order to give the reader as many clues as possible about meaning.

Principle 12. Do Not Shift Narrative Voice

Principle 5 advises you to avoid needless self-reference. Since you are asked to write an explanatory essay, however, an occasional self-reference may be appropriate. You may call yourself "I" if you keep the number of first-person pronouns to a minimum. Less egocentric ways of referring to the narrator include "we" and "one." If these more formal ways of writing seem stilted, stay with "I."

> *I* suggest . . .
>
> *We* can see . . .
>
> *One* must admit . . .

The method of self-reference you select is called the narrative voice of your essay. Any of the above narrative voices are acceptable. Nevertheless, whichever you choose, do not shift to a different narrative voice in your essay once you have begun. If you use *I* in the first sentence of a paragraph, for example, do not use *we* in a later sentence.

INCORRECT: I suggest that individuals best cherish principles of free speech when such principles are challenged. We can see how a free society can get too complacent when free speech is taken for granted.

To correct the above sentence, change one pronoun to agree with the other, such as:

CORRECT: "*We* suggest that individuals . . . " (to agree with "We can see how . . . ")

CORRECT: "*I* can see how . . . "(to agree with "I suggest that individuals . . . ")

Exercise for Principle 12: Shifting Narrative Voice

Rewrite these sentences to give them consistent points of view.

1. I am disgusted with the waste we tolerate in this country. One cannot simply stand by without adding to such waste. Living here makes you wasteful.

2. You must take care not to take these grammar rules too seriously since one can often become bogged down in details and forget why he is writing at all.

3. We all must take a stand against waste in this country; how else will one be able to look at oneself in the mirror?

4. You can readily see how politicians have a vested interest in pleasing powerful interest groups, though one should not generalize about this tendency.

Principle 13. Match Verb and Subject

Singular subjects and plural subjects take different forms of the verb in the present tense. Usually the difference lies in the presence or absence of a final –s (e.g., he becomes and they become), but sometimes the difference is more radical (e.g., he is, they are). If you are a native speaker of English, you can usually trust your ear to give you the correct verb form, but certain situations cause difficulty: when the subject and verb are separated by a number of words, when the subject is an indefinite pronoun, and when the subject consists of more than one noun.

- A verb must agree with its subject in number regardless of intervening phrases.

Do not let the words that come between the subject and the verb confuse you about the number (singular or plural) of the subject. Usually one word can be pinpointed as the grammatical subject of the sentence; the verb, no matter how far removed, must agree with that subject in number.

INCORRECT: The joys of climbing mountains, especially if one is a novice climber without the proper equipment, escapes me.

CORRECT: The *joys* of climbing mountains, especially if one is a novice climber without the proper equipment, *escape* me.

INCORRECT: A group of jockeys who have already finished the first race and who wish to have their pictures taken are blocking my view of the horses.

CORRECT: A *group* of jockeys who have already finished the first race and who wish to have their pictures taken *is* blocking my view of the horses. (The long prepositional phrase beginning with the preposition *of* qualifies the noun *group*. The subject of the sentence is the noun *group*, which takes the singular verb *is*.)

In both examples, the phrases and clauses between subject and verb do not affect the grammatical relationship between subject and verb. An intervening phrase that is plural does not change a singular subject into a plural one. In particular, look out for prepositional phrases intervening between subjects and verbs. These phrases often start with the following prepositions:

> in, out, up, down, over, under, between, off, on, behind, of, with, about,
> to, from, by, onto, before, after, through, despite, concerning, against

Also, watch out for collective nouns like *group*—such nouns are often plural in meaning but are nevertheless grammatically singular. Note that the word *number* takes a singular verb when preceded by *the* and a plural verb when preceded by *a*:

CORRECT: A *number* of fans *hope* for a mere glimpse of his handsome face; unfortunately, they are rarely satisfied with a mere glimpse.

CORRECT: The *number* of fans who catch a glimpse of his handsome face *seems* to grow exponentially each time the tabloids write a story of his seclusion.

- A subject that consists of two or more nouns connected by *and* takes the plural form of the verb.

CORRECT: *Karl,* who is expert in cooking Hunan spicy duck, and *George,* who is expert in eating Hunan spicy duck, *have* combined their expertise to start a new restaurant.

- When the subject consists of two or more nouns connected by *or* or *nor,* the verb agrees with the CLOSEST noun.

CORRECT: Either the senators or the president *is* misinformed.

CORRECT: Either the president or the senators *are* misinformed.

Some connecting phrases look as though they should make a group of words into a plural but actually do not. The only connecting word that can made a series of singular nouns into a plural subject is *and.* In particular, the following connecting words and phrases do NOT result in a plural subject:

> along with, besides, together with, as well as, in addition to

INCORRECT: The president, along with the secretary of state and the director of the CIA, are misinformed.

CORRECT: The president, along with the secretary of state and the director of the CIA, is misinformed.

A note on the subjunctive: After verbs such as *recommend, require, suggest, ask, demand,* and *insist* and after expressions of requirement, suggestion, and demand (for example, *I demand that*), use the subjunctive form of the verb—that is, the form of the verb used after such expressions as *I want to* _____."

CORRECT: I recommend that the chocolate cake *be* reinstated on your menu.

CORRECT: It is essential that the reader *understand* what you are trying to say.

Exercise for Principle 13: Subject-Verb Agreement

Repair the incorrect verbs.

1. The logical structure of his complicated and rather tortuous arguments are always the same.

2. The majority of the organization's members is over sixty years old.

3. Both the young child and her grandfather was depressed for months after discovering that the oldest ice cream parlor in the city had closed its doors forever.

4. Hartz brought the blueprints and model that was still on the table instead of the ones that Mackenzie had returned to the cabinet.

5. A case of bananas have been sent to the local distributor in compensation for the fruit that was damaged in transit.

Principle 14. Beware of Faulty Parallelism

A common style problem, faulty parallelism, results from not seeing the structure of the sentence you are constructing. Matching constructions must be expressed in parallel form. It is often rhetorically effective to use a particular construction several times in succession, in order to provide emphasis. The technique is called parallel construction, and it is effective only when used sparingly. If your sentences are varied, a parallel construction will stand out. If your sentences are already repetitive, a parallel structure will further obscure your meaning. As an example of how parallel construction should be used, look at the following sentence:

As a leader, Lincoln inspired a nation to throw off the chains of slavery; *as a philosopher,* he proclaimed the greatness of the little man; *as a human being,* he served as a timeless example of humility.

The repetition of the *italicized* construction provides a strong sense of rhythm and organization to the sentence and alerts the reader to yet another aspect of Lincoln's character.

Writers often use a parallel structure for dissimilar items.

INCORRECT: They are sturdy, attractive, and cost only a dollar each. (The phrase *they are* makes sense preceding the adjectives *sturdy* and *attractive,* but it cannot be used before *cost only a dollar each.*)

CORRECT: They are sturdy and attractive, and they cost only a dollar each.

Parallel constructions must be expressed in parallel grammatical form. In other words, each segment of the parallel must be in similar form to the other segments: they must be all nouns, all infinitives, all gerunds, all prepositional phrases, or all clauses.

INCORRECT: All business students should learn word processing, accounting, and how to program computers.

CORRECT: All business students should learn word processing, accounting, and computer programming.

This principle applies to any words that might begin each item in a series: prepositions (*in, on, by, with,* etc.), articles (*the, a, an*), helping verbs (*had, has, would,* etc.) and possessives (*his, her, our,* etc.). Either repeat the word before every element in a series or include it only in the first item. Anything else violates the rules of parallelism.

In effect, your treatment of the second element of the series determines the form of all subsequent elements:

INCORRECT: He invested his money in stocks, in real estate, and a home for retired performers.

CORRECT: He invested his money in stocks, in real estate, and in a home for retired performers.

CORRECT: He invested his money in stocks, real estate, and a home for retired performers.

When proofreading, check that each item in the series agrees with the word or phrase that begins the series. In the above example, *invested his money* is the common phrase that each item shares. You would read, "He invested his money in real estate, *invested his money in stocks, and invested his money in a home for retired performers.*"

A number of constructions call for you to always express ideas in parallel form. These constructions include:

X is as _____ as *Y*.

X is more _____ than *Y*.

X is less _____ than *Y*.

Both *X* and *Y* . . .

Either *X* or *Y* . . .

Neither *X* nor *Y* . . .

Not only *X* but also *Y* . . .

X and *Y* can stand for as little as one word or as much as a whole clause, but in any case the grammatical structure of *X* and *Y* must be identical.

INCORRECT: The view from this apartment is not nearly as spectacular as from that mountain lodge.

CORRECT: *The view from this apartment* is not nearly as spectacular as *the one from that mountain lodge.*

Exercise for Principle 14: Parallelism

Correct the faulty parallelism in the following sentences.

1. This organization will not tolerate the consumption, trafficking, or promoting the use of drugs.
2. The dancer taught her understudy how to move, how to dress, and how to work with choreographers and deal with professional competition.
3. The student's knowledge of chemistry is as extensive as what the professor knows.
4. They should not allow that man either to supervise the project or assist another supervisor, since he has proven himself to be thoroughly incompetent.
5. Either the balloon business will have to expand or declare bankruptcy.

Principle 15. Ensure Pronouns Refer Clearly and Properly to Their Antecedents

A pronoun is a word that replaces a noun in a sentence. Every time you write a pronoun—*he, him, his, she, her, it, its, they, their, that,* and *which*—be sure there can be absolutely no doubt about which particular noun the pronoun refers to (the antecedent). Careless use of pronouns can obscure your intended meaning.

WEAK: The teacher told the student he was lazy. (Does *he* refer to *teacher* or *student*?)

WEAK: Sara knows more about history than Irina because she learned it from her father. (Does *she* refer to *Sara* or *Irina*?)

You can usually rearrange a sentence to avoid ambiguous pronoun reference.

STRONG: The student was lazy, and the teacher told him so.

STRONG: The teacher considered himself lazy and told the student so.

STRONG: Since Sara learned history from her father, she knows more than Irina does.

STRONG: Because Irina learned history from her father, she knows less about it than Sara does.

If you are worried that a pronoun reference will be ambiguous, rewrite the sentence so that there is no doubt. Do not be afraid to repeat the antecedent (the noun that the pronoun refers to) if necessary:

WEAK: I would rather settle in Phoenix than in Albuquerque, although it lacks wonderful restaurants.

STRONG: I would rather settle in Phoenix than in Albuquerque, although Phoenix lacks wonderful restaurants.

A reader must be able to pinpoint the pronoun's antecedent. Even if you think the reader will know what you mean, do not use a pronoun without a clear and appropriate antecedent.

WEAK: When you are painting, be sure not to get it on the floor. (*It* could refer only to the noun *paint*; pronouns cannot refer to implied nouns.)

STRONG: When you are painting, be sure not to get any paint on the floor.

Avoid using *this, that, it,* or *which* to refer to a whole phrase, sentence, or idea. Even when these pronouns are placed very close to their intended antecedent, the references may still be unclear.

WEAK: United States consumers use larger amounts of nonrecyclable diapers every year. This will someday turn the Earth into a giant trashcan.

STRONG: United States consumers use larger amounts of nonrecyclable diapers every year. This ever-growing mass of waste products will someday turn the Earth into a giant trashcan. (A good rule of thumb is to try not to begin a sentence with *that* or *this* unless accompanying a noun.)

WEAK: The salesman spoke loudly, swayed back and forth, and tapped the table nervously, which made his customers extremely nervous.

STRONG: The salesman spoke loudly, swayed back and forth, and tapped the table nervously, mannerisms which made his customers extremely nervous.

Also, unless you are talking about the weather, avoid beginning a sentence with *it*. (See Principle 7: Avoid weak openings.)

WEAK: It is difficult to distinguish between the rights of criminals and those of victims.

STRONG: Distinguishing between the rights of criminals and those of victims is difficult.

Some nouns and pronouns are singular in one context and plural in another, depending on the number of the antecedent.

A few of the indefinite pronouns that can be either singular or plural are *some, all, most, any,* and *none*. When using one of these words as the subject, check to see whether the antecedent is singular or plural.

CORRECT: He was unable to finish his *work* last night. *Some remains* to be done today. *None* of it *is* easy. (Read: *Some* of his work *remains; none* of his work *is*)

CORRECT: His *superiors* have been following his progress. *Some are* more impressed than others. *None are* overwhelmed. (Read: *Some* of his superiors *are; none* of his superiors *are*)

Other indefinite pronouns are invariable in number:

SINGULAR:	anybody	everybody	somebody	either	one
	anyone	everyone	someone	neither	each
	anything	everything	something	no one	

(NOTE: Just remember that *-body*, *-one*, and *-thing* pronouns are singular.)

PLURAL:	both	few	many	several

A related problem has arisen recently because of concern over using gender-specific words to describe individuals or groups that are not necessarily of one gender. The writer will often mistakenly substitute the traditional generic singular pronoun *he* with the plural form *they*. But other methods exist to avoid using *he* as a generic pronoun.

INCORRECT: The author makes a strong statement about the individual: Each *person* must protect *their* individuality if *one* wants to remain individual.

CORRECT: The author makes a strong statement about individualism: *People* must protect *their* individuality if *they* want to remain individuals.

Beware of using the wrong form of the pronoun in a sentence.

When writing a sentence containing a relative clause (one that begins with the relative pronoun *who, whom, that,* or *which*), authors often become confused about which pronoun to use.

CORRECT: Those people, whom I have been calling all day, never returned my call.

CORRECT: Those people, who have been calling all day, are harassing me.

A useful technique for choosing the correct pronoun is to turn the clause into a question. In the first sentence, you would mentally ask, "I have been calling *who* or *whom*?" Answer your question, substituting a pronoun: "I have been calling *them*." In the second sentence, you would ask, "*Who* or *whom* has been calling all day?" Answer your question, substituting a pronoun: "*They* have been calling all day." If you use *me, her, him, them,* or *us* to answer the question, the appropriate relative pronoun is *whom*. If you use *I, she, he, they,* or *we* to answer the question, the appropriate relative pronoun is *who*.

That and *which* are often used interchangeably, but as a rule, *that* is a defining, or restrictive, pronoun, while *which* is a nondefining, or nonrestrictive, pronoun. Usually, this can be translated into a simple rule of thumb: If the relative clause is set off with commas (i.e., the clause is not crucial to the meaning of the sentence), use *which*. If the relative clause is not set off by commas (i.e., the clause *is* crucial to the meaning of the sentence), use *that*. (See also Principle 19: Use commas correctly when you punctuate.)

CORRECT: The movie, which was released two years behind schedule, was one of the few that were real box office hits this spring.

Exercise for Principle 15: Faulty Pronouns

Rewrite the following sentences to avoid ambiguous pronoun references or correct faulty pronoun references.

1. Clausen's dog won first place at the show because he was well bred.
2. The critic's review made the novel a commercial success. He is now a rich man.
3. The military advisor was more conventional than his commander, but he was a superior strategist.
4. Bertha telephoned her friends in California before going home for the night, which she had not done in weeks.
5. Although John hoped and prayed for the job, it did no good. He called him the next morning; they had hired someone else.

Principle 16. Use Clear Modification

In English, the position of the word within a sentence often establishes the word's relationship to other words in the sentence. This is especially true with modifying phrases. Modifiers, like pronouns, are generally connected to the nearest word that agrees with the modifier in person and number. If a modifier is placed too far from the word it modifies, the meaning may be lost or obscured. Notice in the following sentences that ambiguity results when the modifying phrases are misplaced in the sentence.

WEAK: Gary and Martha sat talking about the movie in the office.

WEAK: They wondered how much the house was really worth when they bought it.

Avoid ambiguity by placing modifiers as close as possible to the words they are intended to modify.

STRONG: Gary and Martha sat in the office talking about the movie.

STRONG: When they bought the house, they wondered how much it was really worth.

Modifiers can refer to words that either precede or follow them. Ambiguity can also result when a modifier is squeezed between two possible referents and the reader has no way of knowing which is the intended referent:

WEAK: The dentist instructed him regularly to brush his teeth.

WEAK: Tom said in the car he had a map of New Jersey.

Be sure that the modifier is closest to the intended referent and that there is no other possible referent on the other side of the modifier. If when proofreading your essay you find a misplaced modifier, just move it to its proper place in the sentence.

STRONG: The dentist instructed him to brush his teeth regularly.

STRONG: Tom said he had a map of New Jersey in the car.

All the ambiguous sentences above are examples of misplaced modifiers: modifiers whose placement makes the intended reference unclear. In addition to misplaced modifiers, watch for dangling modifiers: modifiers whose intended referents are not even present.

WEAK: Coming out of context, Peter was startled by Julia's perceptiveness.

The modifying phrase *coming out of context* is probably not intended to refer to *Peter,* but if not, then to whom or what? *Julia*? *Perceptiveness*? None of these makes sense as the referent of *coming out of context*. What came out of context was more likely a *statement* or *remark*. The sentence is incorrect because there is no word or phrase that can be pinpointed as the referent of the opening modifying phrase. Rearrangement and rewording solved the problem.

STRONG: Julia's remark, coming out of context, startled Peter with its perceptiveness.

Exercise for Principle 16: Faulty Modification

Clarify the following sentences by placing modifiers as close as possible to the intended referent.

1. Bentley advised him quickly to make up his mind.
2. I agree with the author's statements in principle.
3. Coming out of the woodwork, he was surprised to see termites.
4. The governor's conference met to discuss racial unrest in the auditorium.
5. Hernandez said in her office she had all the necessary documents.

OTHER THINGS TO WATCH

Principle 17. Avoid Colloquialisms

Conversational speech is filled with informal expressions that do not merit a place in the formal expository writing required for the PCAT Writing Sample. Slang terms and colloquialisms can be confusing to the reader since these expressions are not universally understood. Even worse, such informal writing may give readers the impression that you are poorly educated or arrogant.

WEAK: He is really into gardening.
STRONG: He enjoys gardening.

WEAK: She plays a wicked game of tennis.
STRONG: She excels in tennis.

WEAK: Myra has got to go to Memphis for a week.
STRONG: Myra must go to Memphis for a week.

WEAK: Joan has been doing science for eight years now.
STRONG: Joan has been a scientist for eight years now.

Many graders consider contractions to be too informal also. We recommend that you avoid contractions in your PCAT essay and spell out all words.

WEAK:	The blackened salmon's been one of the restaurant's most popular entrees.
STRONG:	The blackened salmon has been one of the restaurant's most popular entrees.

WEAK:	He hasn't missed a deadline in years.
STRONG:	He has not missed a deadline in years.

The English language has such a rich vocabulary that you should never have to resort to using a colloquialism to make a point. With a little thought you will find the right word. Using informal language is risky; play it safe by sticking to standard usage.

Exercise for Principle 17: Colloquialisms

Replace the informal elements of the following sentences with more appropriate terms.

1. Cynthia Larson sure knows her stuff.
2. The crowd was really into watching the fire-eating juggler, but then the dancing horse grabbed their attention.
3. As soon as the personnel department checks out his résumé, I am sure we will hear gales of laughter issuing from the office.
4. Having something funny to say seems awfully important in our culture.
5. The chef had a nice way with salmon: His sauce was simple but the effect was sublime.

Principle 18. Avoid Sentence Fragments and Run-On Sentences

The time pressure of the PCAT Writing Sample could cause you to lose track of what you are writing and cause you to end up with a sentence fragment or a run-on sentence. A sentence fragment has no independent clause; a run-on sentence has two or more independent clauses that are improperly connected. As you edit your practice essays, check your sentence constructions, noting any tendency toward fragments or run-on sentences.

Sentence fragments

Every sentence in formal expository writing must have an independent clause: a clause that contains a subject and a predicate and does *not* begin with a subordinate conjunction such as:

after	if	so that	whenever
although	in order that	than	where
as	provided that	though	whether
because	since	unless	while
before		until	

When you proofread your essays, make sure that every sentence has at least one independent clause.

INCORRECT:	Global warming. That is what the scientists and journalists are worried about this month.
CORRECT:	Global warming *is* the cause of concern for scientists and journalists this month.

INCORRECT:	Seattle is a wonderful place to live. Having mountains, ocean, and forests all within easy driving distance. If you can ignore the rain.
CORRECT:	Seattle is a wonderful place to live, with mountains, ocean, and forests all within easy driving distance, but it certainly does rain often.
INCORRECT:	Why do I think the author's position is preposterous? Because he makes generalizations that I know are rarely true.
CORRECT:	I think the author's position is preposterous because he makes generalizations that I know are rarely true.

Beginning single-clause sentences with coordinate conjunctions—*and, but, or, nor,* and *for*—is allowed according to the rule of grammar, but some readers may object on style grounds. To be safe, avoid or minimize this practice.

CORRECT:	Most people would agree that indigent patients should receive wonderful health-care. But every treatment has its price.

Run-on sentences

Time pressure may also cause you to write two or more sentences as one. When you proofread your essays, watch out for independent clauses that are not joined with any punctuation at all or are only joined with a comma.

RUN-ON:	Current insurance practices are unfair they discriminate against the people who need insurance most.
RUN-ON:	Current insurance practices are unfair, they discriminate against the people who need insurance most.

You can repair run-on sentences in any one of three ways. First, you could use a period to make separate sentences of the independent clauses.

CORRECT:	Current insurance practices are unfair. They discriminate against the people who need insurance most.

Second, you could use a semicolon. A semicolon is a weak period: It separates independent clauses but signals to the reader that the ideas in the clauses are related.

CORRECT:	Current insurance practices are unfair; they discriminate against the people who need insurance most.

The third method of repairing a run-on sentence is usually the most effective. Use a conjunction to turn an independent clause into a dependent one and to make explicit how the clauses are related.

CORRECT:	Current insurance practices are unfair, in that they discriminate against the people who need insurance most.

One common way to end up with a run-on sentence is to try to use transitional adverbs like *however, nevertheless, furthermore, likewise,* and *therefore* as conjunctions.

INCORRECT:	Current insurance practices are discriminatory, furthermore they make insurance too expensive for the poor.
CORRECT:	Current insurance practices are discriminatory. Furthermore, they make insurance too expensive for the poor.
INCORRECT:	Current insurance practices are discriminatory, however they make insurance too expensive for the poor.
CORRECT:	Current insurance practices are discriminatory; however, they make insurance too expensive for the poor.

Exercise for Principle 18: Sentence Fragments and Run-On Sentences

Repair the following by eliminating sentence fragments and run-on sentences.

1. The private academy has all the programs Angie will need. Except that the sports program has been phased out.

2. Leadership ability. This is the elusive quality that our current government employees have yet to capture.

3. Antonio just joined the athletic club staff this year but Barry has been with us since 1975, therefore we would expect Barry to be more skilled with the weight-lifting equipment. What a surprise to find Barry pinned beneath a barbell on the weight-lifting bench with Antonio struggling to lift the 300-pound weight from poor Barry's chest.

4. However much she tries to act like a Southern belle, she cannot hide her roots. The daughter of a Yankee fisherman, taciturn and always polite.

5. There is always time to invest in property ownership. After one has established oneself in the business world, however.

PRINCIPLES OF PUNCTUATION

Principle 19. Use Commas Correctly

When using the comma, follow these rules:

A. Use commas to separate items in a series. If more than two items are listed in a series, they should be separated by commas; the final comma, the one that precedes the word *and,* is optional.

CORRECT:	My recipe for buttermilk biscuits contains flour, baking soda, salt, shortening, and buttermilk.
CORRECT:	My recipe for chocolate cake contains flour, baking soda, sugar, eggs, milk, and chocolate.

B. Do not place commas before the first element of a series or after the last element.

INCORRECT:	My investment advisor recommended that I construct a portfolio of, stocks, bonds, commodities futures, and precious metals.

INCORRECT: The elephants, tigers, and dancing bears, were the highlights of the circus parade.

C. Use commas to separate two or more interchangeable adjectives before a noun; do not use a comma after the last adjective in the series.

CORRECT: I can't believe you sat through that long, dull, uninspired movie three times.

INCORRECT: The manatee is a round, blubbery, bewhiskered, creature whose continued presence in American waters is endangered by careless boaters.

D. Use commas to set off parenthetical clauses and phrases. (A parenthetical expression is one that is not necessary to the main idea of the sentence.)

CORRECT: Gordon, who is a writer by profession, bakes an excellent cheesecake.

The main idea is that Gordon bakes an excellent cheesecake. The intervening clause merely serves to identify Gordon; thus, it should be set off with commas.

CORRECT: The newspaper that has the most insipid editorials is the *Daily Times*.

CORRECT: The newspaper, which has the most insipid editorials of any I have read, won numerous awards last week.

In the first of these examples, the clause beginning with *that* defines which paper the author is discussing. In the second example, the main point is that the newspaper won numerous awards; the intervening clause beginning with *which* identifies the paper.

E. Use commas after introductory participial or prepositional phrases.

CORRECT: Having watered his petunias every day during the drought, Harold was very disappointed when his garden was destroyed by insects.

CORRECT: After the banquet, Harold and Martha went dancing.

F. Use commas to separate independent clauses (clauses that could stand alone as complete sentences) connected by a coordinate conjunction such as *and, or, but, not,* or *yet.*

CORRECT: Susan's old car has been belching blue smoke from the tailpipe for two weeks, but it has not broken down yet.

CORRECT: Zachariah's pet frog eats fifty flies a day, yet it has never gotten indigestion.

Make sure the comma separates two *independent* clauses, each containing its own subject and verb. It is incorrect to use a comma to separate the two parts of a compound verb.

INCORRECT: Barbara went to the grocery store, and bought two quarts of milk.

INCORRECT: Zachariah's pet frog eats fifty flies a day, and never gets indigestion.

Exercise for Principle 19: Commas

Correct the punctuation errors in the following sentences.

1. Peter wants me to bring music games candy and soda to his party.
2. I need, lumber, nails, a hammer and a saw to build the shelf.
3. It takes a friendly energetic person to be a successful salesman.
4. I was shocked to discover that a large, modern, glass-sheathed, office building had replaced my old school.
5. The country club, a cluster of ivy-covered whitewashed buildings was the site of the president's first speech.

Principle 20. Use Semicolons Correctly

A. Use a semicolon instead of a coordinate conjunction such as *and, or,* or *but* to link two closely related independent clauses.

CORRECT: Whooping cranes are an endangered species; there are only fifty whooping cranes in New Jersey today.

CORRECT: Whooping cranes are an endangered species, and they are unlikely to survive if we continue to pollute.

INCORRECT: Whooping cranes are an endangered species; and they are unlikely to survive if we continue to pollute.

B. Use a semicolon between independent clauses connected by words like *therefore, nevertheless,* and *moreover.*

CORRECT: The staff meeting has been postponed until next Thursday; therefore, I will be unable to get approval for my project until then.

CORRECT: Farm prices have been falling rapidly for two years; nevertheless, the traditional American farm is not in danger of disappearing.

Exercise for Principle 20: Semicolons

Correct the punctuation errors in the following sentences.

1. Morgan has five years' experience in karate; but Thompson has even more.
2. Very few students wanted to take the class in physics, only the professor's kindness kept it from being canceled.
3. You should always be prepared when you go on a camping trip, however you must avoid carrying unnecessary weight.

Principle 21. Use Colons Correctly

A. In formal writing the colon is used only as a means of signaling that what follows is a list, definition, explanation, or concise summary of what has gone before. The colon usually follows an independent clause, and it will frequently be accompanied by a reinforcing expression like *the following, as follows,* or *namely,* or by an explicit demonstrative like *this.*

CORRECT:	Your instructions are as follows: read the passage carefully, answer the questions on the last page, and turn over your answer sheet.
CORRECT:	This is what I found in the refrigerator: a moldy lime, half a bottle of stale soda, and a jar of peanut butter.
CORRECT:	The biggest problem with America today is apathy: the corrosive element that will destroy our democracy.

B. Do not separate a verb from its direct object with a colon.

INCORRECT:	I want: a slice of pizza and a small green salad.
CORRECT:	This is what I want: a slice of pizza and a small green salad. (The colon serves to announce that a list is forthcoming.)
CORRECT:	I don't want much for lunch: just a slice of pizza and a small green salad. (Here, what follows the colon defines what "don't want much" means.)

C. Context will occasionally make clear that a second independent clause is closely linked to its predecessor even without an explicit expression like those used above. Here, too, a colon is appropriate, although a period will always be correct as well.

CORRECT:	We were aghast: The "charming country inn" that had been advertised in such glowing terms proved to be a leaking cabin full of mosquitoes.
CORRECT:	We were aghast. The "charming country inn" that had been advertised in such glowing terms proved to be a leaking cabin full of mosquitoes.

Exercise for Principle 21: Colons

Correct the punctuation errors in the following sentences.

1. I am sick and tired of: your whining, your complaining, your nagging, your teasing, and most of all, your barbed comments.
2. The chef has created a masterpiece, the pasta is delicate yet firm, the mustard greens are fresh, and the medallions of veal are melting in my mouth.
3. In order to write a good essay, you must: get plenty of sleep, eat a good breakfast, and practice until you drop.

Principle 22. Use Hyphens and Dashes Correctly

A. Use a hyphen with the compound numbers twenty-one through ninety-nine and with fractions used as adjectives.

CORRECT: Sixty-five students constituted a majority.

CORRECT: A two-thirds vote was necessary to carry the measure.

B. Use a hyphen with the prefixes *ex, all,* and *self* and with the suffix *elect.*

CORRECT: The constitution protects against self-incrimination.

CORRECT: The president-elect was invited to chair the meeting.

C. Use a hyphen with a compound adjective when it comes BEFORE the word it modifies but not when it comes after the word it modifies.

CORRECT: The no-holds-barred argument continued into the night.

CORRECT: The argument continued with no holds barred.

D. Use a hyphen with any prefix used before a proper noun or adjective.

CORRECT: His pro-African sentiments were heartily applauded.

CORRECT: They believed that his activities were un-American.

E. Use a hyphen to separate component parts of a word in order to avoid confusion with other words or to avoid the use of a double vowel.

CORRECT: The sculptor was able to re-form the clay after the dog knocked over the bust.

CORRECT: They had to be re-introduced, since it had been so long since they last met.

F. Use a dash to indicate an abrupt change of thought. In general, however, formal writing is best when you think out what you want to say in advance and avoid abrupt changes of thought.

CORRECT: The inheritance must cover the entire cost of the proposal—Gail has no other money to invest.

CORRECT: To get a high score—and who doesn't want to get a high score—you need to devote yourself to prolonged and concentrated study.

Exercise for Principle 22: Hyphens and Dashes

Correct the punctuation errors in the following sentences.

1. The child was able to count from one to ninety nine.
2. The adults only movie was banned from commercial TV.
3. It was the first time she had seen a movie that was for adults-only.
4. John and his ex wife remained on friendly terms.
5. A two thirds majority would be needed to pass the budget reforms.

Principle 23. Use Apostrophes Correctly

A. Use the apostrophe with contracted forms of verbs to indicate that one or more letters have been eliminated in writing (just as sounds have been eliminated or shortened in speaking). However, as discussed in Principle 17, it's generally better to completely avoid using contractions on the PCAT since their use can be seen as too informal.

CONTRACTED:	you're	it's	you've	the boy's
	Harry's	we'd	wasn't	

FULL FORMS:	you are	it is	you have	the boy is
	Harry has	we would	was not	

One of the most common errors involving use of the apostrophe is using it in the contraction *you're* or *it's* to indicate the possessive form of *you* or *it*. When you write *you're*, ask yourself whether you mean *you are*. If not, the correct word is *your*. Similarly, are you sure you mean *it is*? If not, use the possessive form *its*.

INCORRECT:	You're chest of drawers is ugly.
INCORRECT:	The dog hurt it's paw.
CORRECT:	Your chest of drawers is ugly.
CORRECT:	The dog hurt its paw.

B. Use the apostrophe to indicate the possessive form of a noun.

NOT POSSESSIVE:	the boy	Harry	the children	the boys

POSSESSIVE:	the boy's	Harry's	the children's	the boys'

Note that the word *boy's* could have one of three meanings:

- The boy's an expert at chess. (The boy is . . .)
- The boy's left for the day. (The boy has . . .)
- The boy's face was covered with pie. (possessive: the face of the boy)

The word *boys'* can have only one meaning: a plural possessive (the . . . of the boys).

CORRECT:	I caught a glimpse of the fox's red tail as the hunters sped by. (The *'s* ending indicates that one fox is the owner of the tail.)
CORRECT:	Ms. Fox's office is on the first floor. (One person possesses the office.)

CORRECT: The Foxes' apartment has a wonderful view. (There are several people named Fox living in the same apartment. First form the plural, then add the apostrophe to indicate possession.)

C. The apostrophe is used to indicate possession only with nouns; in the case of pronouns there are separate possessives for each person and number.

my, mine	our, ours
your, yours	your, yours
him, his	their, theirs
her, hers	it, its

The exception is the neutral *one*, which forms its possessive by adding an apostrophe and an *s*.

Exercises for Principle 23: Apostrophes

Correct the punctuation errors in the following sentences.

1. The Presidents limousine had a flat tire.
2. You're tickets for the show will be at the box office.
3. The opportunity to change ones lifestyle does not come often.
4. The desks' surface was immaculate, but it's drawers were messy.
5. The cat on the bed is hers'.

ANSWERS TO EXERCISES

Answers to Exercise 1: Junk Phrases

1. The agency is not prepared to expand now.
2. Since John has prepared for this presentation so carefully, we should award him the project.
3. Flights are always at least an hour late on this airline, though its leaders promise that promptness is a high priority for all its employees.
4. Although she is inexperienced in photography, she will probably succeed because she is motivated.
5. The United States cannot spend more money to help other countries when its own citizens suffer.

Answers to Exercise 2: Redundancy

1. All these problems have combined to create a crisis.
2. A staff that large needs an effective supervisor.
3. He knows how to follow directions.
4. The writer's technical skill does not mask his poor plot line.
5. That monument remains a significant tourist attraction.

Answers to Exercise 3: Excessive Qualification

1. She is a good teacher.
2. Ferrara is a slow worker.
3. There are many reasons technology has not permeated all countries equally.
4. In a murder trial, it is important to pay attention to all the details as well as to the larger picture.
5. You are the best person to decide what you should do for a living.

Answers to Exercise 5: Needless Self-Reference

1. We ought to pay teachers more than we pay senators.
2. The author is stuck in the past.
3. This argument cannot be generalized to most business owners.
4. Food is perhaps the best social lubricant.
5. More people would not vote even if they had more information about candidates.

Answers to Exercise 6: Undesirable Passives

1. Brave but misguided men fought the Spanish-American War.
2. Congress passed the bill, but the President did not sign it until the time for action had passed.
3. Those who need advice least usually request it; the truly lost and ignorant do not seek it at all.
4. We should relocate that building to where citizens can appreciate it.
5. City government should generously reward garbage collectors for their dirty, smelly labors.

Answers to Exercise 7: Weak Openings

1. Businesses cannot ignore the illiteracy problem without suffering.
2. Experience is more important than training in many fields.
3. This plane is obsolete for several reasons.
4. The government cannot fight a drug war effectively without waging a battle against demand for illicit substances.
5. The candidate has many strong points; intelligence, unfortunately, is not among them.

Answers to Exercise 9: Clichés

1. Jefferson was certainly a great leader.
2. Families probably spend less time together than they did fifteen years ago.
3. The pizza delivery man arrived just when the sequestered jury most needed him.
4. Trying to find the employee responsible for this embarrassing information leak is a difficult task.
5. Both strategies would be expensive and completely ineffective: They have an equal chance of failing.

Answers to Exercise 10: Jargon

1. This is an exceptional horse.
2. Government regulatory agencies were not honest in their press releases about the recent railway accident.
3. Having spent our time responding to many unexpected problems this month, we have not been able to prepare for these longer-term needs.
4. With practice, you can match my level of expertise.
5. If someone claims you as a dependent on a tax return, you may still have to pay taxes on your income in excess of five hundred dollars.

Answers to Exercise 12: Shifting Narrative Voice

1. I am disgusted with the waste we tolerate in this country. People cannot simply stand by without adding to such waste: Living here makes all of us wasteful.
2. You must take care not to take these grammar rules too seriously, since you can often become bogged down in details and forget why you are writing at all. (Or use *one* consistently.)
3. We all must take a stand against waste in this country; how else will we be able to look at ourselves in the mirror? (When using *we*, use the plural form of verbs and pronouns.)
4. You can readily see how politicians have a vested interest in pleasing powerful interest groups, though you should not generalize about this tendency. (Or use *one* consistently.)

Answers to Exercise 13: Subject-Verb Agreement

1. The logical *structure* of his complicated and rather tortuous arguments *is* always the same.
2. The *majority* of the organization's members *are* over sixty years old.
3. *Both* the young child and her grandfather *were* depressed for months after discovering that the oldest ice cream parlor in the city had closed its doors forever.

4. Hartz brought the *blueprints* and *model* that *were* still on the table instead of the ones that Mackenzie had returned to the cabinet. (The restrictive phrase beginning with *that* defines the noun phrase *blueprints and model.*)

5. A *case* of bananas *has* been sent to the local distributor in compensation for the fruit that was damaged in transit.

Answers to Exercise 14: Parallelism

1. This organization will not tolerate the consumption, trafficking, or promotion of drugs.

2. The dancer taught her understudy how to move, dress, work with choreographers, and deal with professional competition.

3. *The student's knowledge* of chemistry is as extensive as *the professor's knowledge.*

4. They should not allow that man *either to supervise* the project or *to assist* another supervisor, since he has proven himself to be thoroughly incompetent.

5. The balloon business will have to either expand or declare bankruptcy.

Answers to Exercise 15: Faulty Pronouns

1. The structure of the sentence might leave us wondering whether Clausen or his dog was well bred. Instead, use the impersonal *it.*

   Sample Rewrite: Clausen's dog won first place at the show because it was well bred.

2. *He* is probably meant to refer to the author of the book reviewed by the critic, but the context makes *he* appear to refer to *the critic,* who could be an author as well as a critic.

   Sample Rewrite: The critic's review made the novel a commercial success, and the novelist is now a rich man.

3. We cannot tell from the context whether the military advisor or his superior was the superior strategist.

   Sample Rewrite: The military advisor was more conventional than his commander, but the advisor was a superior strategist.

4. *Which* is the problem here: We do not know whether Bertha had not spent the night at home in weeks or whether she had not telephoned her friends in weeks.
   Sample Rewrite: Because she had not telephoned her California friends in weeks, Bertha called them before she went home for the night.

5. Referring to some ambiguous *they* without identifying who *they* are beforehand is incorrect.
   Sample Rewrite: John wanted the job badly, but when he called the employer the next morning he found that the company had hired someone else.

Answers to Exercise 16: Faulty Modification

1. *Quickly* is sandwiched between two verbs, and it could refer to either one.
   Sample Rewrite: Bentley advised him to make up his mind quickly.

2. *In principle* probably modifies *agreed,* but its placement makes it appear to modify *statement.*
   Sample Rewrite: I agree in principle with the author's statements.

3. Termites are probably coming out of the woodwork, not the man, but an introductory modifying phrase always refers to the grammatical subject of the sentence.
   Sample Rewrite: He was surprised to see termites coming out of the woodwork.

4. Was the racial unrest in the auditorium, or was the conference merely held there?
   Sample Rewrite: The governor's conference met in the auditorium to discuss racial unrest.

5. Did she say it in her office? Were the documents in her office? Or both?
   Sample Rewrite: Hernandez said that she had all the necessary documents in her office.

Answers to Exercise 17: Colloquialisms

1. Cynthia Larson is surely an expert. (It may go without saying that *knows her stuff* is a slang expression, but the substitution of *sure* for *surely* may be more difficult to identify as an error. *Sure* is an adjective, *surely* is an adverb, and an adverb is needed in this case, since the word is meant to modify *knows*.)

2 The crowd was absorbed in watching the fire-eating juggler, but then the dancing horse caught their attention.

3. As soon as the personnel department tries to verify his résumé, I am sure we will hear gales of laughter issuing from the office.

4. Having something funny to say seems to be very important in our culture.

5. The chef is skillful with salmon: His sauce was simple but the effect was sublime.

Answers to Exercise 18: Sentence Fragments and Run-On Sentences

1. In this context, *except* is a conjunction, and as such makes the clause to which it is attached a dependent one.
   Sample Rewrite: The private academy has all the programs Angie will need, except that the sports program has been phased out.

2. *Leadership ability* is a sentence fragment, since it has no predicate.
   Sample Rewrite: Leadership ability: this is the elusive quality that our current government employees have yet to capture.

3. Here we have both a run-on sentence (two independent clauses linked by *therefore* and a comma) and a sentence fragment ("What a surprise to find . . ." contains no subject or predicate).
   Sample Rewrite: Antonio just joined the athletic club staff this year, but Barry has been with us since 1975; therefore, we would expect Barry to be more skilled with the weight-lifting equipment. It was quite a surprise to find Barry pinned beneath a barbell on the weight-lifting bench with Antonio struggling to lift the 300-pound weight from poor Barry's chest.

4. *The daughter of a Yankee fisherman* is a sentence fragment, since the group of words contains no verb.
   Sample Rewrite: However much she tries to act like a Southern belle, she cannot hide her roots. She will always be the daughter of a Yankee fisherman, taciturn and ever polite.

5. The conjunction *after* makes the second group of words a sentence fragment.
   Sample Rewrite: There is always time to invest in property ownership after one has established oneself in the business world, however.

Answers to Exercise 19: Commas

1. Peter wants me to bring music, games, candy, and soda to his party.

2. I need lumber, nails, a hammer, and a saw to build the shelf.

3. It takes a friendly, energetic person to be a successful salesman.

4. I was shocked to discover that a large, modern, glass-sheathed office building had replaced my old school.

5. The country club, a cluster of ivy-covered whitewashed buildings, was the site of the president's first speech.

Answers to Exercise 20: Semicolons

1. Morgan has five years' experience in karate, but Thompson has even more.

2. Very few students wanted to take the class in physics; only the professor's kindness kept it from being canceled.

3. You should always be prepared when you go on a camping trip; however, you must avoid carrying unnecessary weight.

Answers to Exercise 21: Colons

1. I am sick and tired of your whining, your complaining, your nagging, your teasing, and most of all, your barbed comments.

2. The chef has created a masterpiece: The pasta is delicate yet firm, the mustard greens are fresh, and the medallions of veal are melting in my mouth.

3. In order to write a good essay, you must do the following: get plenty of sleep, eat a good breakfast, and practice until you drop.

Answers to Exercise 22: Hyphens and Dashes

1. The child was able to count from one to ninety-nine.

2. The adults-only movie was banned from commercial TV.

3. It was the first time she had seen a movie that was for adults only.

4. John and his ex-wife remained on friendly terms.

5. A two-thirds majority would be needed to pass the budget reforms.

Answers to Exercise 23: Apostrophes

1. The President's limousine had a flat tire.

2. Your tickets for the show will be at the box office.

3. The opportunity to change one's lifestyle does not come often.

4. The desk's surface was immaculate, but its drawers were messy.

5. The cat on the bed is hers.

LIST OF COMMONLY MISUSED WORDS

This list includes common diction errors and common idiomatic errors.

A diction error results from use of a word whose meaning does not fit in a particular context. Often the word that is needed and the word that is misused sound or look alike (e.g., *affect/effect*).

Idioms are established and accepted expressions. Idiomatic errors usually involve use of the wrong preposition (*different than* versus *different from*).

accept/except	To *accept* is to willingly receive; to *except* is to omit or exclude.
	Example: Peter was *accepted* by the college because, if you *except* his failing grades in two courses, his academic record is excellent.
	Except is usually used as a preposition meaning "with the exception of."
	Example: I'll be home every day *except* Friday, when I have a dance class.
adapt/adopt	To *adapt* is to change something to make it suitable for a certain purpose; to *adopt* is to make something one's own.
	Example: *To Have and Have Not* was adapted for the screen by William Faulkner.
	Example: The Robinsons have *adopted* a baby.
affect/effect	To *affect* is to influence or change; to *effect* is to cause or to make (something) happen.
	Example: The size of the harvest was *affected* by the lack of rainfall. The medicine Allen took *effected* a rapid recovery.
	Effect is usually used as a noun meaning "influence."
	Example: The illegible signs on this road have a bad *effect* on safety.
allusion/delusion/ illusion	An *allusion* is an indirect reference, a *delusion* is something that is falsely believed, and an *illusion* is a false, misleading, or deceptive appearance.
	Example: Mr. Harmon fills his talk with *allusions* to literature and art to create the *illusion* that he is very learned. He has *delusions* that he is quite a scholar.
among/between	In most cases, you should use *between* for two items and *among* for more than two. There are exceptions, however; *among* tends to be used for less definite or exact relationships, and *between* is used for specific spatial relationships.
	Example: The competition *between* Anne and Fred has grown more intense. He is always at his best *among* strangers.
	Exception: Plant the trees *between* the road, the wall, and the fence.

amount/number	*Amount* should be used to refer to a singular or non-countable word; *number* should be used to refer to a countable quantity.
	Example: The *amount* of cloth on the bolt was enough for several suits. I was not sure of the *number* of yards of cloth on the bolt.
another/the other	*Another* refers to any other; *the other* is more specific, referring to one particular other.
	Example: Put *another* log on the fire (any one). Put *the other* log on the fire (the last one). The men were passing the pipe from one to the *other* (two men, back and forth). They passed the pipe from one to *another* (three or more).
as/like	*Like* is a preposition; it introduces a prepositional phrase. A phrase is a group of words that does not contain a subject and verb. *As,* when functioning as a conjunction, introduces a subordinate clause. A clause is a part of a sentence containing a subject and verb.
	Example: She sings *like* an angel. She sings *as* an angel sings.
as . . . as . . .	The idiom *as . . . as . . .* shows an equivalent relationship.
	Example: That suit is *as* expensive *as* (NOT *than*) this one.
assure/ensure/insure	To *ensure* is to make certain, safe, or secure; to *insure* is to provide for financial payment in case of loss; and to *assure* is to inform positively.
	Example: Mr. Green *assured* his mother-in-law that he had *insured* his life for $30,000 to *ensure* his wife would not suffer poverty if he died.
because	To say "the reason is *because* . . ." is considered ungrammatical in formal English. Use *that* instead.
	Example: The reason I'm late is *that* my car refused to start. OR: I'm late *because* my car refused to start.
beside/besides	*Beside* means "next to" something; *besides* means "in addition to."
	Example: She sat *beside* me at the basketball game. *Besides* the basketball teams, there were only three other people in the gym.
between . . . and . . .	The idiom *between . . . and . . .* shows a range of options.
	Example: Call *between* five *and* (NOT *to*) six o'clock. He chose *between* meat *and* (NOT *or*) fish.
criteria/data	These are *plural* nouns that are often mistakenly used as singular nouns.
	Example: One *criterion* (not *criteria*) for employment in this company is a willingness to work with surly people. The recently collected *data prove* (NOT *proves*) our original hypothesis was correct.
different from	*Different* is usually used with the preposition *from* and not with *than*.

Example: Frank's attitude is *different* from Charlie's.

The correct idiom is *differ* from and never *differ than*. *Differ* can also be used with *with*.

Example: On that issue, I *differ* with you.

each other/ one another	In formal writing, *each other* is used to refer to two things, and *one another* is used for three or more. **Example:** Len and Amy love *each other*. Those three theories contradict *one another*.
eminent/imminent/ immanent	*Eminent* means prominent or outstanding; *imminent* means likely to happen soon, impending; *immanent* means existing within, intrinsic. **Example:** The whole school was excited about the *imminent* arrival of the *eminent* scientist. Scrooge was characterized by *immanent* selfishness.
fewer/less	Use *fewer* before a countable noun and *less* before a singular noun that represents an uncountable quantity. **Example:** This amazing product contains *less* fat, *less* salt, and *fewer* calories.
if/whether	*If* is used in conditional clauses. **Example:** *If* I have the money, I will go. I do not know *whether* to go. (Nothing is conditional in the second sentence.)
imply/infer	To *imply* is to state or indicate indirectly; to *infer* is to deduce or conclude. Authors and speakers *imply*; readers and listeners *infer*. **Example:** Pete sarcastically *implied* he was angry. Joe *inferred* from Mary's dejected look that she had failed the exam.
ingenious/ingenuous	*Ingenious* means intelligent, clever, or resourceful; *ingenuous* means innocent, naive, or simple. **Example:** The thief entered the bank vault by means of an *ingenious* magnetic device. Alice is so *ingenuous* that she refuses to believe anyone would deliberately do harm.
irregardless	The correct word is *regardless,* regardless of the context.
its/it's	*It's* is a contraction of it is; *its* is a possessive pronoun meaning something belongs to it. **Example:** *It's* obvious that something is wrong with that dog; *it's* whining and chewing *its* paw.
maybe	Don't use *maybe* to modify an adjective or other adverb. **Example:** That is potentially (NOT *maybe*) a dangerous thing to do.

neither . . . nor	The correlative conjunction is *neither . . . nor* and not *neither . . . or*.
	Example: He is *neither* strong *nor* flexible.
	Avoid the redundancy caused by *neither . . . nor* following a negative.
	Example: Unnoticed by Debby or Sue (not *neither* Debby *nor* Sue), Naomi left.
not only . . .	If you use *not only,* it must be followed by *but;* the word *also* is optional.
but (also)	The words following *not only* must be parallel to the words following *but also*.
	Example: The book is *not only* fascinating *but also* instructive.
number	*The number* should be followed by a singular verb; *a number* should be followed by a plural.
	Example: *The number* of errors in his statement is astounding. *A number* of us are going camping.
regard as	*Regard as* is the correct idiom; *regard to be* is wrong.
	Example: I regard you *as* (NOT *to be*) a close friend.
when/where	Only use *when* or *where* when referring to time or location, respectively. Often, *that* is more appropriate.
	Example: A convention is a meeting of people with something in common (NOT *a convention is where a number of people*). A diagram is a sketch *that* illustrates the parts of something (NOT *is when a sketch illustrates*).
their/they're/there	*Their* is a possessive pronoun meaning something belonging to them, *they're* is a contraction of *they are*, and *there* means *that place* (among other things)
	Example: *They're* placing *their* bets over *there* at the race track, but there's no chance they will win *their* money back.

CHAPTER SIX

Practice Prompts

Practice is as vital for the writing sample as it is for other sections of the PCAT. There is simply no substitute for tackling a test question under test conditions.

In the first section of this chapter, you will have opportunities to practice writing essays of your own on five topics that closely resemble the kind you are likely to see on Test Day. Follow Test Day conditions: don't allow yourself any extra minutes to complete an essay, and don't look at an essay topic or its sample student response in advance of taking a practice test. Spend thirty minutes and only thirty minutes answering each essay question. Use a computer to write your essay and take notes on a separate piece of paper, just as you will on Test Day. Be sure to turn off spell check, grammar check, and any auto-correct options as you will not be able to use these on the PCAT. Being tough on yourself now will give you an edge on Test Day.

After your 30 minutes elapse, judge your essay's merits, thinking about your performance in terms of the four implied tasks and Kaplan's 5 Step Method for the Writing Sample as described in Chapter 4 in order to assign yourself a score. Also ask yourself questions about your writing process: Could your initial approach to the topic have been better? Did you skip or skimp on any of the prewriting? Did you fail to finish your essay or to leave time to proofread? If so, practice the prewriting more in order to improve your ability to finish in the recommended time. You can become comfortable with this efficient method only by practicing. If you are not clear about any part of this method, go back to Chapter 4 to refresh your memory.

Following the prompts, you will find sample student essays responding to the same five topics. These sample essays have been evaluated using the PCAT writing rubric discussed in the writing sample lessons and include detailed descriptions of why each earned its corresponding score. When you do look at a sample student response, first form your own opinion of the essay's merits. Pretend you are a professional PCAT grader and give the essay a grade based on the writing sample rubric in Chapter 4. After you have decided on a score, compare that with how our graders evaluated the essay. Doing this will help you develop your own critical skills, a crucial step to becoming a good writer. Once you've assigned a sample essay a score, compare it with your own writing to identify takeaway points you can use next time to improve your own essays.

PRACTICE PROMPTS

Prompt 1: Discuss a solution to the problem of high drop-out rates in American schools.

Prompt 2: Discuss a solution to the problem of insufficient funding of scientific research.

Prompt 3: Discuss a solution to the problem of childhood obesity in America.

Prompt 4: Discuss a solution to the problem of unequal treatment of women in the American workplace.

Prompt 5: Discuss a solution to the problem of low voter turnout in US federal elections.

SAMPLE STUDENT RESPONSES

Student's Essay in Response to Prompt 1: A

Education is the most important thing. Students who dropped out of school regret it day after day since they find no job in bad economy. And on the other hand they go and steal money and do drugs and that cost society a lot. The government should give people who drop high school a job to keep them from becomming criminals and join gangs. They can work in the coal mines or farming. Why have illegal immigrants do all work if american people cant find jobs and become criminals? All students who quit high school say its because school is boring. The best solutions is to make school more fun. Maybe add more free time or have less homework or even cut the school day in half. Its better to learn less than nothing. But if somebody still drops out they should still go to the mines.

Evaluation

Score = 1

The essay poorly addresses the topic at hand. The student shows low understanding of the prompt by discussing what to do with high school dropouts instead of how to lower the drop-out rate. One solution is presented (make school more fun), but the student soon digresses into an irrelevant topic ("They can work in the coal mines").

Poor grammar and sentence structure cloud the student's ideas. Many spelling mistakes are present. The student fails to use proper contractions and punctuation marks. The essay is not organized into paragraphs, and the student does not correctly use transitions (such as "on the other hand").

Student's Essay in Response to Prompt 1: B

There are too many children in American schools who drop out before they graduate. This leads to uneducated adults who can't get a good job and could get into trouble. The problem is that most kids are bored in school or they don't like it for some other reason so they just leave. I will write what one solution is, which is to make schools more interesting so kids want to go their.

Interesting things in school could be classes like movie making, computer blogging, rap music and hiphop dances. Dancing is also good exercize so that could be a gym class. Schools also need to teach the academic stuff too of course but they could do both. If kids liked what they saw in school maybe theyd stay there and graduate. However teachers could be nicer to the students too. Instead of sending to detention they could do something more interesting like writing a blog that says what they did wrong and how they won't do it again.

There could be other solutions like making sure that all kids know good English so they can understand what's going on, and making parents have to come to school to take to their teacher. When I was a kid my mom talked to the teacher and came home and told me I'd better do better, which I did. So I know this works.

Kids need to graduate school so they can get good jobs. Some solutions to kids dropping out is to make school more interesting so they'll stick in class and graduate. When I graduated I felt really good about myself and that makes me want to do better in life.

Evaluation

Score = 2

The writer has presented a primary and secondary solution to the problem, but both are shallow and general. The presentation is vague and not thoroughly convincing but does focus on the problem. The organization is logical for the most part, but the relevance of the conclusion is questionable. More considered ideas, presented in greater and more relevant depth, such as with better examples, would improve the essay.

The many mistakes in grammar and style also impede the writer's ideas in some places. The grammar and spelling have mistakes, transition words are sparse, and punctuation is inconsistent. The style lacks subtlety ("I will write what one solution is"). Word choice and sentence structure avoid glaring mistakes but are casual and littered with personal examples that are minimally relevant, giving the essay a tone of informal discussion between friends rather than formal exhibition of good thinking and communication skills.

Student's Essay in Response to Prompt 1: C

National Statistics show that high school drop-out rate is increasing at an alarming rate. It goes without saying that students who drop out lose any kind of advantage in a competitive economy. The most common reasons for dropping out is the lack of interest in school work and absent parents who fail to monitor their kids.

One way to slow dropout rates is to make school interesting. This can be accomplished by adding more fun activities to the curriculum, such as dance and theatre classes. Students who play school sports are also found to have lower dropout rates. However, fun classes are not the only way to keep students motivated. Schools teachers should build relationships with students and that can only be accomplished with small size classes. Any students that has a standing relationship with a teacher or a counselar will be less likely to drop out.

Another way to slow dropout rates is to involve the parents in their kids schoolwork. If students realize that their parents will be told every time they fail a test or skip class, they will pay more attention in class, complete their homework and earn better grades. It is the parents' duty to help their kids realize the importance of good education. And if they work or don't have time, they can ask an aunt or an uncle to follow up on school work.

The necessity that every high school student in the world graduates is undeniable. The effect on the global economy and on society are too great to neglect. It's not too late to start implementing the steps suggested above to avoid a bigger problem in the future.

Evaluation

Score = 3

The student provides a background on the topic by explaining the main causes of school dropouts, presents two relevant solutions, and ends with an adequate conclusion. However, the support provided is largely vague, and neither of the solutions is developed in great depth. For example, the student posits that "Any student that has a standing relationship with a teacher ... will be less likely to drop out," but this is not supported with examples or evidence.

The organization of the essay is adequate with some digressions (such as focusing on the world in paragraph 3 instead of just America, which was part of the prompt). Some grammar and spelling mistakes are present, but they do not distract the reader from the author's main ideas.

Student's Essay in Response to Prompt 1: D

The increase in high school dropout rates has reached significant levels. This problem can no longer be ignored as it affects our society in a myriad of ways. The likelihood of finding a job without a high school diploma is slim to none, and the resulting unemployment is one of the leading cause of surges in crime rates as struggling teenagers join gangs and resort to violence. Furthermore, those without a high school education are more likely to be below the poverty line and require more government assistance, draining resources of the already-weakened U.S. economy. We must find the roots of this problem to resolve it. The two main reasons students quit school are the failed school systems of most inner cities and the financial situation of students.

Rebuilding the school system is going not only to improve student education but also to keep many students from dropping out. Students who feel cared for in class will show more interest in learning and it's the job of the teachers to nurture this interest. Teachers should be evaluated based on how much student interest they can generate and not only on how much material they can explain. Smaller classrooms will also allow teacher to pay more attention to each student and to monitor their progress.

However, rebuilding the school system will not stop every student from dropping out. Some students drop out to find jobs and support their families. Poor families should be given aid and social workers should visit to asess the situation of the kids and take steps to keep them from dropping out.

In conclusion, the state of our high school students should be examined before its too late. Failing to take proper steps towards improving the conditions under which they live and learn will only exacerbate the problem and compound it.

Evaluation

Score = 4

This essay addresses all of the major tasks: introduction of the problem, solution with support, additional solution, and conclusion. The essay starts with a thorough explanation of the problem but then tapers off with each subsequent paragraph becoming shorter. This happens most often when a strong writer realizes he is running out of time and has to hurry to finish. The student should have limited the length of his first paragraph (especially since it begins to delve into personal opinion) in order to have enough time to develop the remainder of the essay. Although not all are well-developed, the ideas the student did have time for are logical and do address the prompt and tasks.

The organization of this essay is strong with good use of transition words. Minor mistakes in grammar and spelling are present (especially near the end), but these are few and do not impede the overall argument. The student uses some interesting vocabulary words ("myriad" and "exacerbate"). However, some redundancies are present (such as using both exacerbate and compound).

Student's Essay in Response to Prompt 1: E

The increase in high school dropout rates has reached significant levels. This problem can no longer be ignored as it effects our society in a myriad of ways. First, the likelihood of finding a job without a high school diploma is slim to none. Second, unemployment is one of the leading cause of surges in crime rates as struggling teenagers join gangs and resort to violence. We must find the roots of this problem to resolve it. The two main reasons students quit school are the failed school systems of most inner cities and the financial situation of students.

Rebuilding the school system is going to not only improve student education but also to keep many students from dropping out from there. Students who feel cared for in class will show more interest in learning, and it's the job of the teachers to nurture this interest. Teachers should be evaluated based on how much student interest they can generate and not only on how much material they can explain. Smaller classrooms will also allow teacher to pay more attention to each student and to monitor each student's progress.

However, rebuilding the school system will not stop every student from dropping out. Some students drop out to find jobs and support their families. Students in this very unfortunate situation should be cared for by the state of the government. Poor families should be given aid and social workers should visit them to assess the situation of the students and take steps to keep them from dropping out. Local businesses can also provide part time employment with fair pay to disadvantaged students. After all, businesses can only profit if dropout rates and hence crime rates fall.

In conclusion, the state of our high school students should be examined before its too late. Failing to take proper steps towards improving the conditions under which they live, and learn will only exacerbate the problem. Nevertheless, some districts have already started implementing the steps mentioned above, generating hope that improvement can continue and the upward trend of dropping out can be reversed.

Evaluation

Score = 5

Each of the four tasks is covered in this essay. Ideas flow logically within each paragraph and from one paragraph to the next. Both the main solution and additional solution are explained in detail and supported with logic, but the student did not provide any concrete examples as support.

The student makes good use of transition words throughout the essay and uses sufficiently correct grammar and spelling to get his ideas across (besides very minor mistakes, such as not including commas in compound sentences and using its instead of it's). Although the writer uses some interesting vocabulary words ("myriad" and "exacerbate"), he overuses the word "student" instead of including more variety ("teenager," "young adult," etc.). Additionally, some of the sentence construction is awkward or too wordy, such as the first sentence of the second paragraph.

Student's Essay in Response to Prompt 1: F

America is no longer the world leader in education. A recent study showed that only 69% of our high school students earn diplomas each year. The main culprits responsible for this national drop-out epidemic are poverty, disinterest in school work, and an educational infrastructure that fails in most inner cities. Because 90% of new jobs require a college degree, the impact of this problem is severe if not disastrous. The economy is losing billions of dollars over the lifetime of drop-out students, the United States is relinquishing its standing as a world leader in education, and crime rates in inner cities, where the problem is most prominent, are sky-high. These implications justify immediately finding remedies to what ails our educational system.

To begin with, an overhaul of our school system and infrastructure is needed. Admittedly, this is a daunting task that draws much debate at the federal and state level. However, easy steps can yield immense influence on the quality of education and care of our students and hence lower drop-out rates. One step is to improve teaching quality, which has been shown to bear great repercussion on students' school experiences and their interest in completing diplomas. Currently, more than half of public school teachers resign by their fifth year. Higher salaries and more comprehensive benefits for teachers will attract and retain better teachers. Other steps, such as using smaller class sizes, offering free tutoring, and exploring experiential learning, will also be advantageous for recruiting and retaining teachers.

Additionally, because the highest drop-rates are in poor school districts where most students leave school to seek employment, increasing federal and state aid to low-income families would help alleviate the financial burden on students and their families. Some schools have also found great success in employing students during the summer or helping students find after-hour jobs. City governments should build on this success by widening the reach of these programs and providing tax incentives to businesses who provide part time jobs to local teenagers who are still in school.

The United States has one of the highest drop-out rates among all industrialized nations. Rectifying the problem cannot be achieved overnight, but brave steps taken by legislators, school administrators, and parents have the potential to remedy this phenomenon and avoid its dire consequences.

Evaluation

Score = 6

This essay clearly completes all of the required tasks and does so in a polished, sophisticated manner. Not only does the student provide two clearly thought-out examples, she provides statistics and concrete examples (such as in reference to schools that help students find jobs) to support her argument. If you cannot come up with specific examples or numbers of your own immediately on Test Day, consider your own personal experience and local events. If all else fails, you can include your best guess at the actual values or events instead.

The grammar and spelling of this essay are free of mistakes, and the vocabulary is high-level and varied. Transition words are used to good effect, and sentences vary in length and format.

Student's Essay in Response to Prompt 2

Technological advancement has been the staple of our time. We have become accustomed to learning of innovations in the fields of medicine, pharmaceuticals, and engineering every day. However, the rate of innovation has slowed in the last decade. This is in part because the proliferation of industrial laboratories and the general decline in the global economy have worked together to curtail the flow of funds to individual institutions. Unfortunately, these setbacks threaten to exacerbate the very problems that caused them, which is on track to lead to a downward spiral and allow important research that saves and improves lives to come to a halt.

Fortunately, all hope is not lost. Governments continue to invest funds into research; we simply need to increase how much. Federal U.S. institutions like the NIH are already supplying academic researchers with grants, but the aid must increase in magnitude and reach to keep up with the increasing demand. To do so, governments should divert money from defense expenditure toward research funding. This will prove many benefits in the long run: Innovations in the field of medicine, for example, will make patient care cheaper and more efficient, both for civilians and the military. The savings in programs like Medicare in the U.S. will provide funds to more research, and the positive effects will continue to grow.

Additionally, legislators also must address patent law. Currently, many private pharmaceutical, biotechnology, and engineering companies fund their research and development from their own profits. Even though these companies are responsible for many of the advancements we enjoy today, this model does not allow for innovations and discoveries in many fields deemed unprofitable. For example, research on male pattern baldness commands more funds than research on some rare cancers since a cure for baldness has more profit potential. The government should balance this disparity by giving companies incentives to diversify their research portfolios or to donate money to academic research.

Certainly scientific research is not in a happy state, yet there is reason for hope. The government and private sector were able to fuel scientific discoveries in the past, and, with a few changes in legislation to allow for more funding and modified patents, they can continue to support even better works.

Evaluation

Score = 6

This essay excels in covering all the tasks, especially in providing support through the use of specific examples (including the NIH, Medicare, and male pattern baldness). The solutions are well thought-out and even build upon another with the themes of government intervention and having hope. The vocabulary is varied and used appropriately, and no spelling or grammar mistakes are present.

Student's Essay in Response to Prompt 3

One out of every three children in America is either overweight or obese, and this is rising at an alarming rate. This epidemic has become too dangerous to be neglected. The main factors responsible for the prevalence of child obesity are the diets and lifestyles of parents, the proliferation of fast food restaurants as cheap alternatives to healthy food, and the lack of physical activity caused by increased acceptance of sedentary tasks. If left untreated, the rampant surge of childhood obesity will terribly impact the cost of healthcare, the economy, and the general wellbeing of the population. Fortunately, we can still address the causes of obesity and halt its rapid growth.

The ability of schools to limit students' access to high calorie foods is a huge part of reducing obesity rates. Although great strides have been made in reducing the number of calories in school meals and banning soft drinks dispensers in most public schools, more steps need to be taken. The number of calories in tomato paste on a pizza slice may have the same number of calories as a serving of vegetables, but it is not nearly as filling, which prompts students to consume a greater quantity. Schools should limit the amount of processed foods that their students consume by instituting strict lunchroom rules. Cafeteria personnel should trained to ensure school lunches are made to fit the guidelines of the food pyramid, and overall portions should be controlled.

Furthermore, school districts should join parents and local community organizations to promote exercising in younger generation. Efforts have been made by the NBA and NFL urging children to participate in sports activity, but a more forceful approach is needed. Elementary school children should be forced to exercise one hour every day. They could join a team or individual sports, go to the gym, or take dance classes. Forming healthy habits at a young age will eventually improve the future health of these children.

Childhood obesity should be recognized as a great danger to the welfare of our society. Obesity is an important risk factor for diabetes, liver disease, vascular problems, and ailments. Parents and schools must tackle this issue head-on with aggressive measures, including changes

Evaluation

Score = 6

This essay exhibits an exceptional grasp of the issue and presents cogent, high-level solutions. The student used a more urgent tone than in some other essays but supported it with specific examples of programs that have already been instituted (removing soda machines from schools, developing programs sponsored by the NBA and NFL). Citing similar solutions that have already worked is a great way to show support for your solution and brings interest to your essay.

Student's Essay in Response to Prompt 4

In the United States, women being equal to men in the workplace is a relatively new idea. Indeed, prior to World War II, working women, other than those in traditionally female jobs (secretary, teacher, telephone operator and, yes, prostitute), were only grudgingly accepted. Even when feminism became more widespread in the 1960s, with women starting to become lawyers, doctors, politicians, and mechanics, their pay and promotions were limited by discrimination occurring because of prejudice from the men still in charge. This inequality continues to contribute to the unfair treatment of women, which is a problem that requires changes both in workplace policy and enforcement.

To begin with, the federal and state non-discriminatory laws must be better enforced. Businesses must develop, disseminate, and enforce policies that ensure women are treated the same as men in both pay and promotion. These policies must come from the highest company level and be communicated to all workers through written material, online notices, in-house training, and similar methods. These policies must also be backed up by real and appropriate measures, up to and including terminating the employment of those proven to be in violation of said policies.

We must also open non-threatening channels through which women can make complaints, investigations can be launched, and action can be taken. Working women, smart, tough and capable though they may be, need advocates in American industry. High-level employees, perhaps one man and one woman per institution, should be chosen to oversee policy compliance. These people would be alert to potential infractions of policy, such as a woman with excellent annual reviews who has not been promoted. With a firm policy in place and all employees needing to follow it, women would have a better opportunity to be treated the same as their male counterparts.

An equally important solution, though harder to enforce, is that of changing the way we think about women in the workplace. People need to stop thinking of women as temporary employees who may leave the job as soon as they become pregnant, are threats to men in the office, and are less competent just because they are women. This requires sensitivity education starting in the early grades, an end to jokes at women's expense, and a clear understanding of the fact that, intellectually and socially, women are completely the equal of men. Such rethinking will force a change in workplace ethics.

The issue of unequal treatment of women on the job is one which involves not only policy and laws but also human understanding. These injustices will be difficult to rectify, but we can take steps in the right direction by recognizing the problem, creating and enforcing non-discrimination policies, and knowing that all men—and women—are created equal.

Evaluation

Score = 6

This argument is powerful and sophisticated with excellent background, detail, and support given for each idea. All the ideas are expressed and organized effectively. The primary and secondary solutions are well developed, supported, and evaluated. The entire effect is one of an excellent essay that exemplifies superior thinking and communication skills.

The writer has a clear ability to use correct conventions of language including sentence structure, usage, and mechanics. There are no spelling, grammar, or punctuation errors. Word choice is clear and appropriate. Style flows well with some creative use of language, such as the parentheses in paragraph one and the reworking of the quote in the end sentence.

Student's Essay in Response to Prompt 5

The indisputable measure of the citizens' involvement in the democratic process is voter turnout. A high voter turnout is an indicator of a healthy democracy and even dictators manufacture high turnout data to bestow legitimacy to their regimes. Unfortunately, the US voter turnout is sinking below levels seen in most industrialized countries. This decline in voter turnout is the symptom to very dangerous threats to our democratic process. These threats include voters' belief that they can't change the outcome of an election, and the disenfranchisement of the poor, minority and naturalized citizens.

The recent national elections showed that voter turnout is lowest in "blue" or "red" states and highest in "battleground" states. This data suggest that voters in red and blue states have surrendered to the notion that their votes won't sway the results of elections. Democrats will not turn out heavily in red states, and neither will Republicans in blue states. The decentralization of the two major political parties will galvanize voters in all states. The current structures of the Democratic and Republican parties consist mainly of powerful national committee and elected officials and weak committees at the state levels. Shifting the power structure to give more funding and autonomy to local, state level committees will give help them disseminate their message and maybe win some local and federal seats. Red states with Democratic senators/governors and blue states with Republican senators/governors all have strong local leaderships and well as higher voter participation.

Voter ID laws are cited as reasons why some citizens fail to vote in national elections. The issue is highly debatable and while the constitutionality of such laws remain unclear there are still ways to overcome all hurdles they cause to minority groups as well as to the poor. The federal and state governments should provide funding for non profit organizations that help poor voters obtain all required paperwork and provide means of transportation to and from voting facilities.

The United States has a long history in attracting immigrants from all parts of the world. Millions of immigrants gained citizenship status in the last ten years. Even though all naturalized citizens are given a voting card application form and are encouraged to vote, statistics show that their turnout rate is considerably lower than natural born citizens especially for immigrants coming from third world countries where their democratic rights have been subjugated by totalitarian regimes. Involving these voters in the democratic process will improve overall voter turnout. National political parties should address this fraction of the American population, create a dialogue about their role in national and local politics and emphasize the freedom of expression that they now enjoy.

The recent decline in voter turnout is a real problem that threatens the standing of the United State as a model democracy. The burden to amend the recent voting turnouts falls not only on the government and political parties but also on each one of us.

Evaluation

Score = 6

As with any 6 essay, the writing here is clear and free of any major mistakes. Note that this student used two paragraphs to discuss the main solution. This task is one of the most important, so expanding on the main solution is one of the best uses for extra time on test day. Nevertheless, a shorter essay that covers similar points could receive a score of 6 as well.

Section III

VERBAL ABILITY

CHAPTER SEVEN

The Verbal Ability Section

The Verbal Ability section of the PCAT tests vocabulary, critical thinking, and strategy. You have 30 minutes to answer 40 questions in two formats: **Analogies** and **Sentence Completions**. Questions 1–25 are Analogies, and questions 25–40 are Sentence Completions, so you will always know in what order the questions will appear.

All 40 questions count toward your score (and each counts for the same number of points), so a big part of your success on the PCAT Verbal section is pacing and strategy to ensure you complete all of the questions in time. Spend an average of 45 seconds per Sentence Completion and 30 seconds per Analogy question. Following this guideline means not only ensuring you have enough time to get to all of the questions in the Verbal Ability section but also identifying questions that are too time-consuming or difficult for you. Spending three minutes on one question (and getting mad at yourself for it) is not worth the time or effort, especially when you could have skipped that question and correctly answered four other, more manageable questions instead. Success in Verbal Ability is not just a matter of knowing vocabulary and answering questions correctly; it's also about recognizing which questions aren't worth your time.

Both of the question types in the Verbal Ability section are vocabulary-intense, but these questions are just as susceptible to the Stop-Think-Predict-Match strategies as the math and science questions. The Verbal Ability questions are predictable. They follow specific patterns, and these patterns can be used to eliminate answer choices and guess strategically even when the vocabulary is extremely tough. You can answer questions correctly without knowing all the vocabulary.

This is not to say that you don't need to study vocabulary. In fact, building your vocabulary is a vital component of your mastery of the Verbal Ability section.

BUILDING YOUR VOCABULARY

The English language contains over 490,000 words, and it would be nearly impossible to learn them all. Thankfully, you don't have to for the PCAT. Only a very small percentage of words ever appear on the test. The Comprehensive Vocabulary List in Chapter 11, a compilation of 1,600 of the most difficult words you need to know, is a good place to start learning words for the test, and you can supplement it with your own reading.

Study at least twenty vocabulary words from the list for a few minutes each day. Read the words and their definitions until you feel you know them. Then, cover the definitions with a piece of paper and quiz yourself. Study something else for a while and then quiz yourself again. At the end of each week, test yourself on all the words you've studied so far. If you feel comfortable with all of them, reward yourself with a break from studying. If not, review them and test yourself again.

Besides memorizing specific words, it's also helpful to learn what *types* of words the test-makers prefer to use. Some are the classic, tough vocabulary terms; you know the type: long, semi-scholarly, abstract words that sound like they came from Latin or Greek (as many of them did). A knowledge of word roots often helps to cut these words down to more manageable—and understandable—sizes. For example, if you know that CIRCUM means "around" and LOC means "speak," you can make a pretty good guess at the meaning of *circumlocution* (excessive use of vague words to evade the subject; talking circles around something). One word root can help you come to grips with many related words. CIRCUM and LOC, for example, appear in *circumscribe*, *circumspect*, *eloquent*, and *colloquial*. Studying both the vocabulary words and the word roots in the next chapters will help you recognize and understand other, related words when they appear on the exam.

But there is another kind of difficult word on the exam. The test-makers also like to use familiar words with less familiar, secondary meanings. When *flag* appeared on a recent analogy question, the word didn't refer to a national banner. Instead, it was used as a verb meaning "to slacken or decline." Some of the words on our vocabulary list were included because of such unfamiliar secondary definitions, so read the definition(s) before you skip what seems like an easy word.

Finally, here's some good news. One of the most difficult aspects of vocabulary use isn't tested at all on the exam: You won't have to distinguish between words with very similar meanings or between words that differ only in nuance. For example, you won't have to master the subtle differences between *loquacious*, *verbose*, and *garrulous*. If you see any of those words, you will simply need to know that they have to do with being wordy or talkative. Again, the test format will provide context clues to make your job easier.

Best Practices for Studying Verbal Ability

- The key to building your vocabulary is to study small batches of words throughout the weeks ahead. Develop a game plan; a great vocabulary can't be built overnight. You can't cram all your study into a week and expect to remember much. You'll only remember the words you learn if you take the time to review them. Repetition and reinforcement are critical. Start studying now and don't let up until Test Day.
- While studying for the PCAT, your aim should be word recognition. You won't have to define words on a blank piece of paper, use them in an essay, or spout them in conversation. The most effective vocabulary study is tailored to your ability to build your word sense rather than your absolute knowledge. This often requires a variety of techniques as opposed to just straightforward memorization.
- Personalize your study methods. Try several techniques and pick the ones that work best for you. If you learn well by seeing, make flash cards of new words (or groups of words) and run through them whenever you have a few spare minutes. If you learn better by hearing, make a vocabulary recording on your computer that you can listen to later.
- Complete the vocabulary exercises in Chapter 12. As you encounter unfamiliar words, in that chapter or otherwise, look up their definitions and add them to your personal study list.

- Keep building your vocabulary whenever you read. Whether you're reading for school or for pleasure, jot down unfamiliar words and look them up when you get a chance. Keep a list and review it from time to time.

- Supplement your vocabulary study by learning the word roots in Chapter 10. Each day, familiarize yourself with a few roots from the list and the vocabulary examples that accompany them. Look up any unfamiliar words in the vocabulary list.

- Indulge in dictionary browsing. When looking up a new word, check to see whether other words on the same page are related. Don't limit yourself to definitions; take advantage of all the information in a word entry, including the etymology.

- Become an omnivorous reader, reading from as many different sources as you can. Make a habit of reading newspaper editorials, syndicated columns, and news magazines; all are good sources of words.

A Few Words to Get You Started

You're more likely to remember a word if you can remember something interesting about it (that's why, when you're learning a foreign language, you always remember the dirty words). Here are some words with interesting stories behind them that may help you remember them. Look them up in the vocabulary list or in a dictionary for even more background. If the stories don't help, don't worry about memorizing them, but you may find that a few of these words stick with you.

cavalier

Originally, a cavalier was a horseman, a knight, or an aristocrat. People like that could afford to be "proud" or "careless."

chimerical

A chimera is a mythical beast with the head of a lion, the body of a goat, and the tail of a snake. It also breathes fire. It's not surprising that chimerical means "unrealistic."

juggernaut

The original Juggernaut was an idol representing the Hindu god Krishna. It was drawn on a huge cart through the streets of Puri, India, in an annual festival, and sometimes people were crushed beneath its wheels accidentally. The word now means "overpowering" and "forceful."

maudlin

This word comes from the name of Mary Magdalene, the penitent prostitute in the New Testament. Some paintings of Mary weeping for her sins are very maudlin ("overly sentimental" and "tearful") indeed.

ostracism

This word sounds a little like oyster, and in fact there is a tenuous connection. In ancient Athens, ostracism was temporary banishment or "exclusion," and it was imposed upon a citizen by popular vote. In those days, the Athenians used potsherds, bits of broken pottery, as ballots for voting. Since potsherds often look somewhat like oyster shells, the Greek word for potsherd (*ostrikon*) derives from the Greek word for oyster (*ostreion*), which is also where the English word oyster comes from.

laconic, spartan

These words derive from Laconia and Sparta, which are two different names for the same place: a city-state in Ancient Greece. The Spartans, or Laconians, were famous for their "curt" manner of speech and "austere" way of life.

sybaritic

The citizens of Sybaris, an ancient Greek city, were just the opposite of the Spartans, or Laconians. The Sybarites were famous for being "devoted to luxury and pleasure."

choleric, melancholy, phlegmatic, sanguine

These words derive from the same source: ancient medical theory. Up until approximately the seventeenth century, it was believed that physical and mental health depended upon the proper balance of four humors or bodily fluids. Too much bile, or choler, caused "irritability"; black bile, or melan chole caused "sadness"; too much phlegm caused "apathy" or "sluggishness"; too much blood, or sanguis, caused excessive "cheerfulness." Although this theory was rejected centuries ago, the words remain.

serendipity

Serendip is an old name for Sri Lanka. An eighteenth-century English writer named Horace Walpole wrote an otherwise forgotten story about three princes of Serendip who had a knack for "making valuable discoveries by accident."

Now that you've seen how interesting some words' backstories can be, look up these words in a dictionary and note the derivation of each term as well as its meaning:

apocryphal

behemoth

cherubic

cynic

gargantuan

hackneyed

masochist

pariah

posh

quixotic

seraphic

stoic

utopia

Master Strategies to Supplement Vocabulary

Building your word sense is an essential skill in the Verbal Ability section. When you recognize the vocabulary in the question stem and the answer choices, your job is that much easier. Strong word sense allows you to move through the section quickly and efficiently. Chapters 10, 11, and 12 are a great resource for your vocabulary studies.

Equally important to your Verbal Ability success, however, are the strategies you will use to attack the two different question types in the section. Good strategy can help you determine the correct answer to a question when you don't know all the vocabulary. Plus, the better you understand what each type of question expects in a correct answer, what classic traps you are likely to see in the wrong answers, and what techniques are needed to distinguish correct from incorrect choices, the more confident you will be in the Verbal Ability section. Not only will you move faster through the section, you will also be able to quickly determine which questions are worth skipping, ultimately leading to more points on Test Day. Use the following chapters to master both strategies and vocabulary, and you are certain to find success on Test Day.

CHAPTER EIGHT

Analogies

Typical Analogy questions, such as the one below, provide two **stem** words with a specific, necessary relationship and a third **prompt** word; your task is to find the answer choice that has that same relationship with the prompt word. All four answer choices will be words that relate in some way to the prompt word, but only the correct answer will have the same specific, necessary relationship as the stem words. On the PCAT, question numbers 1–25 in the Verbal Ability section comprise the thirty Analogy questions. Aim to spend about 30 seconds on average per Analogy question.

> AIRPLANE : HANGAR :: BOAT:
>
> **(A)** Depot
> **(B)** Sail
> **(C)** Dock
> **(D)** Station

In this chapter, you will be introduced to the Kaplan strategy for this question type, learn what each step of the strategy means in greater detail, identify the six kinds of relationships, or bridges, the stem words have, and apply the strategy to practice questions.

KAPLAN QUESTION STRATEGY FOR ANALOGIES

Just like during the other sections of the PCAT, you will use Kaplan's Stop-Think-Predict-Match strategy to tackle Analogy questions. To maximize the effectiveness of this strategy, each step can be made more specific for Analogies:

Stop

Scan the stem and prompt words for familiarity.

Think

What is the bridge between the stem words?

Predict

Apply the bridge to the prompt word and predict an answer.

Match

Select the answer that matches your prediction, broadening or narrowing your bridge if necessary.

Each step is described in more detail below.

Stop: Scan the stem and prompt words for familiarity.

Analogies are a vocabulary-heavy question type. There is no context or keywords to help you; however, you can depend on the fact that the words will have a strong, necessary relationship, and by the end of this chapter you'll even know what kinds of relationships are possible. The ideal for any Analogy question is when you recognize both of the words in the stem—this makes it much easier to build a bridge. When you don't recognize one (or both) of the words in the stem, there are still strategies you can employ to narrow down the answer choices or guess strategically—more on that later in the chapter.

Think: What is the bridge between the stem words?

The two words in the stem must have a clear, necessary relationship. The "bridge" is a short sentence that explains how the two words relate. Are they opposites? Do they depend on each other in some specific way? Because the relationship between the stem words is a necessary one, you should be able to insert words like "always" or "by definition" into the sentence. There are six kinds of bridges that occur regularly on the PCAT: Synonyms, Antonyms, Association, Classification, Part/Whole, and Characteristic.

Predict: Apply the bridge to the prompt word and predict an answer.

Once you come up with a bridge describing the relationship between the stem words, plug the prompt word in place of the first stem word in your sentence. This will allow you to predict what kind of word has the same relationship to the prompt word. Don't get too caught up in predicting the perfect PCAT word; as long as you have a sense of the kind of word that fits the relationship correctly, you'll be able to evaluate the answer choices.

Match: Select the answer that matches your prediction, broadening or narrowing your bridge if necessary.

Again, the ideal is that you are familiar with the vocabulary in the answer choices, can quickly identify the answer choice that matches your prediction, and/or can eliminate the words that don't fit into the bridge. Sometimes small adjustments to the bridge are necessary; making the bridge more general or less general may be required to find the correct match in the answer choices.

Analogy Practice

Try out the Kaplan Question Strategy with the question from the beginning of the chapter:

AIRPLANE : HANGAR :: BOAT:

(A) Depot
(B) Sail
(C) Dock
(D) Station

Stop: Scan the stem and prompt words for familiarity.

Fortunately, the words here are straightforward—all referring to airplanes, boats, and places or things related to airplanes and boats. This is definitely the type of Analogy question that should be attacked right away!

Think: What is the bridge between the stem words?

What is the relationship between AIRPLANE and HANGAR? Remember, look for a specific, necessary relationship—if you can put the phrase "by definition" in the sentence, so much the better! A HANGAR, by definition, is a place to keep an AIRPLANE.

Predict: Apply the bridge to the prompt word and predict an answer.

Now let's take away airplanes and hangars, and put the prompt word, boats, in place of airplanes (make sure you always put the prompt word in the correct corresponding place in the sentence you've created.) A _____, by definition, is a place to keep a BOAT. Where do you keep boats? There are several words that may spring to mind; again, don't worry about making a specific prediction, as long as you know the correct answer choice is definitely a place to keep boats.

Match: Select the answer that matches your prediction, broadening or narrowing your bridge if necessary.

Looking at the answer choices, **(C)** is the clear match. A dock, by definition, is a place to keep boats. You *might* keep boats at a depot or a station, but those words have no *necessary* relationship with boats; that's what you need—a necessary relationship. Answer choice **(B)** can be eliminated for a different reason. A sail is, by definition, part of a boat, but that's an entirely different relationship than the relationship between airplanes and hangars.

THE SIX BRIDGE TYPES

The Analogy above with airplanes and hangars is an Association bridge. There are six kinds of bridges that occur frequently on the PCAT: Synonyms, Antonyms, Association, Classification, Part/Whole, and Characteristic. Familiarity with the different types of bridges will allow you to make predictions quickly and confidently on Test Day.

Synonyms

Synonym bridges are found for stem words with the same meaning or similar meanings with a slight change in degree. These stem words can fit into the sentences "A synonym for _____ is _____," or "A greater/lesser degree of _____ is _____." For example:

AUGUST : DIGNIFIED :: HAUGHTY :

(A) Timid
(B) Condescending
(C) Obnoxious
(D) Meek

AUGUST and DIGNIFIED mean basically the same thing, so you could fit them into the sentence "A synonym for AUGUST is DIGNIFIED." Plugging in the prompt word, then, gives "A synonym for HAUGHTY is _____." After making a prediction of something else that also means *arrogant*, you can see that answer choice (B), *condescending*, is the only answer that fits.

Antonyms

Antonym bridges are the opposite of a Synonym bridge. In an Antonym bridge, the two words in the stem will have meanings that contrast to fit the sentences "An antonym of _____ is _____," or "_____ is not _____." An example of an Antonym bridge is:

PLACID : AGITATED :: JOVIAL :

(A) Cheerful
(B) Unmanageable
(C) Surly
(D) Amiable

PLACID means to be calm, so it is the opposite of AGITATED. The bridge is "Something PLACID is not AGITATED." If you replace PLACID with JOVIAL, you get, "Something JOVIAL is not _____." JOVIAL means "happy" or "friendly," so the correct answer should be the opposite, which you see in choice (C), *surly*.

Association

Associations between stem words can appear in several ways. The words might have a cause-and-effect relationship, or one might be a by-product of the other. There might be a creator/creation relationship, or one might perform a function for the other. Though there are many kinds of Associations, keep in mind the relationship will always be a specific and necessary association between those two words, as in: "A HANGAR, by definition, is a place to keep AIRPLANES," "LUBRICATION, by definition, is used to reduce FRICTION," and "A NOVEL, by definition, is written by an AUTHOR." Take a look at this Association bridge:

OVEN : BAKER :: FABRIC :

(A) Artist
(B) Cloth
(C) Carpenter
(D) Tailor

How does OVEN relate to BAKER? "A BAKER uses an OVEN to bake." (Often Association bridges require a little more detail than other bridges and therefore frequently require adjustment during the Match step). Who has to use FABRIC to do what they do? Choice (D), *tailor*, does.

Classification

Classification bridges occur when one stem word is a type of the other stem word or both stem words can be categorized as different kinds of a bigger category. "A _____ is a type of _____," or "Both _____ and _____ are types of vehicles." Let's look at an example:

BOLOGNA: COLD CUT :: PARFAIT:

(A) Banana
(B) Dessert
(C) Pastrami
(D) Entree

What is the relationship between BOLOGNA and COLD CUT? BOLOGNA is a type of COLD CUT. Likewise, you can apply this relationship to the single word PARFAIT to find the answer: PARFAIT is a type of DESSERT.

Part/Whole

Part/whole relationships are just what they sound like: one of the stem words represents something that is part of the other stem word. "A _____ is part of a _____," or "_____ is made up of _____." It is important to note, however, that the parts and the whole must match up in the same order for both sets of words. A common wrong answer trap in Part/Whole bridges is when the stem words are given as PART : WHOLE and a wrong answer is given as WHOLE : PART. An example of this is:

ACTOR : CAST :: SHIP :

(A) Boat
(B) Fleet
(C) Mast
(D) Troupe

An ACTOR is part of a CAST. Applying this relationship to SHIP, you get "A SHIP is part of a _____." Only (B), *fleet*, fits. Always check which word is the part and which is the whole to ensure you apply the relationship correctly to the prompt word; choice (C), *mast*, represents a part of a ship, but this takes the relationship in the wrong direction.

Characteristic

A Characteristic bridge occurs when one stem word is a property of the other stem word. A Characteristic bridge can involve any attribute or quality that the other stem word has or lacks. "Something _____ is _____," or "A _____ lacks _____." Look at this Characteristic bridge:

MISER : ALTRUISM :: SKEPTIC :

(A) Loyalty
(B) Avarice
(C) Faith
(D) Doubt

A MISER lacks ALTRUISM. So what does a SKEPTIC lack? Predict *belief* to see that choice (C), *faith*, fits this relationship perfectly.

Identifying Bridges Practice

The ability to identify the classic bridges will allow you to move through the Analogy questions quickly, efficiently, and confidently. Identify the bridge types in the following exercise:

1. BAT : BASEBALL   Bridge type: _____

2. ILLICIT : LEGAL   Bridge type: _____

3. LITHE : GRACEFUL   Bridge type: _____

4. SCANDAL : LURID   Bridge type: _____

5. SCENE : PLAY   Bridge type: _____

6. HAIKU : POEM   Bridge type: _____

Answer key: 1. Association, 2. Antonym, 3. Synonym, 4. Characteristic, 5. Part/Whole, 6. Classification

KAPLAN'S TIPS FOR ANALOGIES

Determining a Good Bridge Helps Identify the Correct Answer

Here are some keys to building good bridges:
- Build a sentence that makes the relationship between the two words clear.
- Make sure the bridge expresses a direct and necessary relationship.
- Keep the sentence short and to the point.
- Avoid qualifying phrases such as *could, sometimes, may* or *may not*, etc.

A good bridge should help you predict the word that could plausibly complete the analogy. Build your bridge before looking at the answer choices; this will help you avoid answer traps or trick answers.

Practice building bridges for the following stem pairs:

PLATITUDE : TRITE

CINEMA : MOVIE

LUCIDITY : CLARITY

LETHARGY : LIVELINESS

FOAL : HORSE

Take a look at the following answers. Note that there are no qualifying words in these bridges and that they establish a definitive relationship. Your bridges may be slightly different but should express the same direct and clear relationship between the two words.

PLATITUDE is always TRITE. (Characteristic bridge)

CINEMA, by definition, is a place to show MOVIES. (Association bridge)

LUCIDITY is a synonym for CLARITY. (Synonym bridge)

LETHARGY is the antonym of LIVELINESS. (Antonym bridge)

FOAL is a young HORSE. (Classification bridge)

Once you have a precise bridge, such as the preceding ones, you can apply it to the second pairing in its question. Look at the single prompt word given in the question, say the bridge phrase to yourself, and then check each of the answer choices to see which one fits the relationship.

Anytime you feel the need to add words like *sometimes, maybe,* or *often,* you know that choice is wrong. The correct answer must have the same clear, necessary relationship to the prompt word, so don't try to make an answer choice fit if it does not. Any answer choice that uses those qualification words is a weak bridge.

When the vocabulary in the stem words is particularly difficult, you can at least eliminate any answer choices that make a weak bridge with the prompt word. Look at the following examples and determine whether they are strong bridges or weak bridges:

1. PRISONER : GUILTY

2. VIOLIN : INSTRUMENT

3. LOQUACIOUS : CHEERFUL

4. UNFORTUNATE : RESULT

5. EMANCIPATED : LIBERATED

6. PEN : MISSIVE

While 2 and 5 are strong bridges, 1, 3, 4, and 6 are weak bridges. A PRISONER is *often* GUILTY but not always, Likewise, someone LOQUACIOUS *can be* CHEERFUL but is not always by definition. A RESULT *can be* UNFORTUNATE, or it could be fortunate, and, while a PEN *can be* used to write a MISSIVE, so can a pencil. Identifying and eliminating answer choices that create weak bridges is one way to get around tough vocabulary.

Adjust the Bridge If Necessary

Sometimes, the bridge you come up with will not be specific enough to eliminate all the wrong answers. Other times, your bridge might be too specific, and none of the answers will seem correct. When either of these situations occur, adjusting the bridge will help.

When it seems as though more than one answer choice fits your bridge, you need to narrow your bridge (that is, add more detail back into the sentence). For example consider the question:

BAT : BALL :: STICK :

(A) Hockey
(B) Court
(C) Puck
(D) Net

If the bridge you came up with was something like "A BAT and a BALL are used to play games," this would leave several answer choices that could work with that bridge. So think more specifically: what do you do with a bat in a game? You use a BAT to hit the BALL. Now only answer choice (C), *puck*, fits the bridge.

On the other hand, if it seems like you are eliminating all of the answer choices because none of the answer choices fit your prediction, try generalizing your bridge more. A bridge of "You swing a BAT at ninety degrees to hit a BALL" would be too specific, so you need to remove the qualifier "at ninety degrees" to get to the general bridge you need.

On Test Day, you will come across questions for which you will need to adjust your bridge. If you write down your initial bridge in your scratchwork, it will make it that much easier to go back and adjust that bridge.

Work Backward When All Else Fails

What do you do if you can't build a bridge between the stem words? If you don't know some of the stem words? Or if you understand one half of the analogy but you don't know how to complete it? When the going gets tough, the tough work backward. Let's see how this is done.

The first thing to remember when you encounter a hard question is to skip it until you've answered all the questions that don't give you trouble. If you do have the time to go back to it, here are our tips for working backward:

1. If you can't build a bridge, pay attention to the parts of speech of the stem words.
2. Look for trap answer choices and eliminate them.
3. Try out the remaining answer choices and see if one of them makes sense.
4. If you're stuck, guess.

The first two strategies are the most important. These will help you narrow down the answer choices so you have a better chance of succeeding with the final two last-resort strategies of trying answers and guessing.

Pay Attention to Parts of Speech

If an analogy confuses you, take a look at the **parts of speech** in the question: that is, whether the words are **nouns**, **verbs**, **adjectives**, etc. With very few exceptions, parts of speech are always consistent between pairs within the same question. In other words, if the first word of one word pair is an adjective and the second word a noun, then the same is true for the other word pair. This means you can eliminate the answer choices that don't match the part of speech of the stem pair's second word. If you have time, you can also use the parts of speech to help you brainstorm new bridges.

Eliminate Trap Answer Choices

The right answer to an Analogy question will create the same strong bridge as between the stem pair. Wrong answer choices, on the other hand, come in two principal varieties: the first variety is exemplified by a weak bridge; the second by a strong but wrong bridge that does not share the same relationship as the stem pair. Revisit the example from earlier:

AIRPLANE : HANGAR :: BOAT

(A) Sail
(B) Station
(C) Dock
(D) Depot

Which answer choices can you eliminate? Without even referring to the stem pair, you can see that there is no strong bridge connection between BOAT and choices **(B)** and **(D)**, so these can be eliminated immediately. A strong bridge could be created between BOAT and SAIL, but this would be the wrong bridge. The right answer, choice **(C)**, is obvious if you know the relationship between the stem pair. If you don't know the stem pair relationship, then you have increased your chances of guessing correctly to 50% by simply eliminating the two most unlikely answers.

REVIEW PROBLEMS

Try the following Analogy questions using Kaplan's Question Strategy. Time yourself; on Test Day, you will have about 30 seconds to complete each question.

1. VIOLIN : INSTRUMENT :: MONARCH :
   - (A) Magnanimous
   - (B) Patriarch
   - (C) Butterfly
   - (D) Emperor

2. ALLEVIATE : ASSUAGE :: CONCEDE :
   - (A) Mitigate
   - (B) Relinquish
   - (C) Repudiate
   - (D) Argument

3. ELECTRON : ATOM :: SOURCE :
   - (A) Reference
   - (B) Origin
   - (C) Power
   - (D) Bibliography

4. EMANCIPATED : LIBERATED :: JUDICIOUS :
   - (A) Unfettered
   - (B) Imprudent
   - (C) Circumspect
   - (D) Trifling

5. CITIZENSHIP : PASSPORT :: PURCHASE :
   - (A) Receipt
   - (B) Product
   - (C) Ticket
   - (D) Visa

6. DRAWL : SPEAK :: LOPE :

   (A) Throw
   (B) Aim
   (C) Run
   (D) Slice

7. INVIDIOUS : OFFEND :: EVANESCENT :

   (A) Shock
   (B) Disappear
   (C) Grow
   (D) Rubbish

8. PANEGYRIC : CRITICAL :: POLEMIC :

   (A) Succinct
   (B) Impartial
   (C) Verbose
   (D) Direct

9. OPAQUE : TRANSPARENCY :: DEPRAVED :

   (A) Propriety
   (B) Wantonness
   (C) Effulgence
   (D) Hedonism

10. PERJURER : FABRICATION :: ORACLE :

   (A) Wisdom
   (B) Antiquity
   (C) Soothsayer
   (D) Prognostication

SOLUTIONS TO REVIEW PROBLEMS

1. C

Stop:	The vocabulary doesn't look too bad, a good one to do early.
Think:	A VIOLIN is a type of INSTRUMENT (Classification bridge).
Predict:	So, a MONARCH is a type of what? Ruler? Something else?
Match:	Get rid of choices (A) and (B) since they are weak bridges. Answer choice (D), *emperor*, seems relevant, but an emperor is a type of monarch, not the other way around—this is a strong but wrong bridge, so eliminate it. This leaves (C), *butterfly*, which fits the bridge perfectly: a MONARCH is a type of BUTTERFLY.

2. B

Stop:	Some tough vocabulary; this might be a good one to skip and come back to later.
Think:	ALLEVIATE is a synonym for ASSUAGE.
Predict:	What is a synonym of CONCEDE? Give in, accept, surrender, something like that.
Match:	Choices (A) and (D) are both weak bridges, so they can be eliminated. Answer choice (C) is an antonym to CONCEDE, which leaves (B), *relinquish*, as the correct match.

3. D

Stop:	Pretty straightforward vocabulary; do it now!
Think:	An ATOM is made up of ELECTRONS (Part/Whole bridge).
Predict:	What is made up of SOURCES? A list of some kind.
Match:	The only answer choice that is a list is (D), *bibliography*. Neither (B) nor (C) create strong bridges, and (A), *reference*, is a synonym for source.

4. C

Stop:	The vocabulary is moderately difficult; decide based on which words you recognize.
Think:	EMANCIPATED is a synonym for LIBERATED.
Predict:	What is a synonym of JUDICIOUS? Careful or sensible.
Match:	Choice (B) is an antonym, so eliminate that. Choices (A) and (D) make weak bridges, so (C) is the correct match.

5. A

Stop:	Straightforward vocabulary—go for it!
Think:	A PASSPORT is a proof of CITIZENSHIP.
Predict:	What is proof of PURCHASE? A receipt.
Match:	Choice (A) is an exact match.

6. C

Stop:	The vocabulary is not too bad in this one, though it would depend on what words you recognized.
Think:	To DRAWL is to SPEAK in a slow, drawn-out manner.
Predict:	To LOPE is to do what in a slow, drawn-out manner? Loping is a type of movement, like running.
Match:	Choice (C) is the perfect match.

7. B

Stop:	There's some tough vocabulary in this one—save it for later.
Think:	Something INVIDIOUS OFFENDS. Classic Characteristic bridge.
Predict:	So what is a characteristic action of something EVANESCENT? Something transitory that goes away quickly.
Match:	The only answer choice that matches is choice (B), *disappear*.

8. B

Stop:	Another one with difficult vocabulary.
Think:	A PANEGYRIC, a speech or written work that expresses praise, is the opposite of something CRITICAL.
Predict:	A POLEMIC, a work that expresses an argument, is the opposite of . . . something non-argumentative.
Match:	This prediction fits choice (B), *impartial*, exactly.

9. A

Stop:	Definitely some tough vocabulary in this one.
Think:	Something OPAQUE lacks TRANSPARENCY.
Predict:	So what does something DEPRAVED lack? Morality or good behavior.
Match:	Both choices (B) and (D) are the opposite of this prediction, and choice (C) doesn't make any bridge that makes sense. This leaves choice (A), *propriety*, which does match the prediction.

10. D

Stop:	The vocabulary here is somewhat difficult, maybe not the best one to do right away.
Think:	A PERJURER, someone who lies, speaks FABRICATIONS.
Predict:	What does an ORACLE speak? Prophecies.
Match:	This matches choice (D), *prognostication*. Choice (C), *soothsayer*, is tempting because an oracle is a soothsayer, but that's a different bridge.

CHAPTER NINE

Sentence Completion

A typical Sentence Completion question, such as the one below, provides a sentence with one or two missing words or phrases; your task is to find the answer that correctly fills the blanks. All four answer choices will be words that relate in some way to the sentence, but only the correct answer will fit the context and grammar of the sentence. On the PCAT, question numbers 26–40 in the Verbal Ability section comprise the eighteen Sentence Completion questions. You should aim to spend about 45 seconds on average per Sentence Completion question.

Although the initial cost of installing solar panels to produce electricity can be _____, the financial benefits are realized for years to come in the form of reduced electric bills.

(A) minimal
(B) exciting
(C) misleading
(D) exorbitant

In this chapter, you will be introduced to the Kaplan Strategy for this question type, both for one-blank and two-blank Sentence Completions, learn what each step means in greater detail, and apply them to practice questions.

KAPLAN QUESTION STRATEGY FOR ONE-BLANK SENTENCE COMPLETION

Stop

Is this a one-blank or a two-blank question?

Think

Read the sentence looking for clues.

What is the blank specifically referring to?

Predict

Predict a word to fit in the blank, using word charge to help formulate your prediction.

Match

Select the answer that matches your prediction.

Read the sentence with the selected answer plugged in to ensure it makes sense.

How the Kaplan Strategy Works

Now let's discuss how the Kaplan Strategy for Sentence Completions (one-blank) works.

Stop: Is this a one-blank or a two-blank question?

First, determine whether you are dealing with a one-blank or a two-blank sentence. Determining the number of blanks can help you decide whether to attack the question, skip it and come back later, or guess strategically if it looks difficult. This is especially important if you are starting to run out of time since two-blank sentences can be more time-consuming.

Think: Read the sentence looking for clues.

Every sentence completion question has clues contained in the sentence. **Structural keywords** help you understand how the parts of the sentence relate to each other. The three kinds of structural keywords are Contrast words, Continuation words, and Emphasis words.

Contrast words are just that: words that indicate part of the sentence is in contrast to another part of the sentence. When you see a Contrast keyword, the sentence might be going in a completely different direction, or one part of the sentence might be contradicting or qualifying another part of the sentence. Pay special attention to word charge, positive or negative, since Contrast keywords will influence the charge of that part of the sentence. Contrast keywords include words such as *but*, *despite*, *yet*, *however*, *unless*, *rather*, *although*, *while*, *on the other hand*, *unfortunately*, and *nonetheless*.

Continuation keywords indicate that the sentence is going to keep going in the direction that it already has been going. When you see a Continuation keyword, part of the sentence will often support or elaborate on another part of the sentence. The positive or negative tone of what follows is not changed by these clues. Continuation keywords include words such as *and*, *similarly*, *in addition*, *consequently*, *since*, *also*, *thus*, *because*, ; (semicolon), and *likewise*.

Emphasis keywords are also just what they sound like: They add emphasis to part of the sentence. When you see an Emphasis keyword, ask yourself what part of the sentence is more or less important. Pay special attention to degree; is something getting a little bit of emphasis or a lot? Emphasis keywords can vary a great deal from sentence to sentence, but they usually are vivid descriptors, such as *most important*, *unfortunate*, and *very likely*.

Think: What is the blank specifically referring to?

Knowing the different types of keywords and what they signify will help you determine the way the sentence is going and what kinds of words to predict for the blank(s). Before you predict, think about which words in the sentence the blank is referencing and what relationship the blank has to the rest of the sentence.

Predict: Predict a word to fit in the blank, using word charge to help formulate your prediction.

Once you locate the keywords and context relevant to the blank, predict the kind of word that should go in the blank. Don't feel you have to come up with a specific prediction or a PCAT-level word. Often, just the word charge of the blank is enough to answer the question. By predicting you save valuable time, avoiding the temptation to try out each answer choice in the sentence.

Match: Select the answer that matches your prediction.

Quickly go through the choices, identifying which choice most closely matches your prediction and eliminating choices that do not fit your prediction. If none of the choices match, use word charge to eliminate what you can and then plug in the remaining choices to see which sounds best.

Match: Read the sentence with the selected answer plugged in to ensure it makes sense.

Always read the sentence again, plugging in the answer choice you selected to ensure the sentence reads as both grammatically correct and logically consistent. This step is simply double-checking that you did your work correctly and that your answer choice is correct in context. If your answer makes sense when you read your choice back into the sentence, move on to the next question.

One-Blank Sentence Completion Practice

Try the Kaplan Question Strategy with the question from the beginning of the chapter:

Although the initial cost of installing solar panels to produce electricity can be _____, the financial benefits are realized for years to come in the form of reduced electric bills.

- **(A)** minimal
- **(B)** exciting
- **(C)** misleading
- **(D)** exorbitant

Stop: Is this a one-blank or a two-blank question?

This is a one-blank sentence, so it can be done fairly quickly. Additionally, it starts with a clear keyword—you should jump on this question! It's exactly the kind of Sentence Completion question you want to tackle right away during the test.

Think: Read the sentence looking for clues.

The keyword *Although* at the beginning of the sentence is a Contrast word, which tells you that the first part of the sentence (up until the comma) is going to oppose the second half of the sentence.

Think: What is the blank specifically referring to?

The blank is part of the first half of the sentence, which refers to the initial cost of solar panels, as opposed to the second half of the sentence, which refers to the long-term benefits of solar panels—reduced bills. This implies that the initial cost is high.

Predict: Predict a word to fit in the blank, using word charge to help formulate your prediction.

Since the blank is referring to the initial cost of the solar panels, and you know this is opposed to the long-term benefits, the blank should be at least somewhat negative. Notice you don't need to make a specific prediction here—you just need an idea of the kind of word that should go in the blank. Don't wrack your brains trying to come up with the perfect PSAT-vocabulary word. A prediction of charge (negative), or a simple word (high) will do nicely for most Sentence Completions.

Match: Select the answer that matches your prediction.

You can eliminate answer choices (A) and (B) right away, since they are the opposite of what you are looking for in the correct answer. This leaves choices (C) *misleading* and (D) *exorbitant*. While *misleading* is negative, it also adds meaning to the sentence that wasn't there before. There was no indication of falsehood or trickery in the original sentence. So answer choice (D) is the best match.

Match: Read the sentence with the selected answer plugged in to ensure it makes sense.

Reading answer choice (D) back into the sentence, you get: "Although the initial cost of installing solar panels to produce electricity can be *exorbitant*, the financial benefits are realized for years to come in the form of reduced electric bills." Choice (D) makes sense in context and is grammatically correct, so you can confirm this choice is correct and move on.

KAPLAN QUESTION STRATEGY FOR TWO-BLANK SENTENCE COMPLETION

Stop

Is this a one-blank or a two-blank question?

Think

Read the sentence looking for clues.

Which blank is easier to predict?

What is the blank specifically referring to?

Predict

Predict a word to fit in the blank, using word charge to help formulate your prediction.

Match

Eliminate the answer choices that don't match your prediction.

Repeat the Think and Predict steps for the remaining blank if necessary.

Read the sentence with the selected answers plugged in to ensure it makes sense.

In terms of approach, the main difference between the one-blank Sentence Completion and the two-blank Sentence Completion is that during the Think step, you have an additional task—identify which blank is easier to predict and focus on that blank first. Then you can make a prediction for that blank and eliminate anything that doesn't match. If needed, you can then go back and repeat the Think and

Predict steps with the remaining blank in order to eliminate the remaining wrong answers and find the correct match. Many PCAT students find two-blank Sentence Completions daunting because of their length, and they can be more time-consuming (something to consider during the Stop step when deciding whether to skip or not). However, with practice, the two-blank sentences can be managed in a reasonable amount of time. Think of it this way: Twice the number of blanks means twice as many opportunities to find something worth eliminating!

Two-Blank Sentence Completion Practice

Let's try the Kaplan Question Strategy on a two-blank Sentence Completion question:

Usually the biologist's presentations were extremely _____, but this week's lecture was strikingly muddled, even _____.

(A) eloquent . . . lucid

(B) cogent . . . incoherent

(C) wistful . . . curt

(D) convoluted . . . enigmatic

Stop: Is this a one-blank or a two-blank question?

This is a two-blank sentence, but it has several clear keywords, and the vocabulary is not too bad. You should be able to make good predictions for these blanks.

Think: Read the sentence looking for clues.

There are several excellent keywords in this sentence. Right away, the question starts with a *Usually* and then a Contrast keyword, *but*. So you know that the first half of the sentence is what usually happens, but the second half of the sentence contrasts with what usually happens. Since the first blank is in the first half of the sentence, and the second blank is in the second half of the sentence, the two blanks must be opposites.

Think: Which blank is easier to predict?

Muddled and *even* are vivid keywords leading straight to the second blank.

Think: What is the blank specifically referring to?

The answer for the second blank refers to something even stronger than *muddled*.

Predict: Predict a word to fit in the blank, using word charge to help formulate your prediction.

Something stronger than *muddled*, such as "very unclear."

Match: Eliminate the answer choices that don't match your prediction.

Eliminate choice (C), which has nothing to do with being unclear, and (A), which is the opposite of our prediction.

Repeat the Think and Predict steps for the remaining blank if necessary.

Now predict for the first blank: It should be the opposite of "unclear," such as "clear."

Match: Read the sentence with the selected answer plugged in to ensure it makes sense.

Choice (B) matches. Choice (D) *convoluted* is the opposite of what you're looking for in the first blank.

KAPLAN'S TIPS FOR SENTENCE COMPLETIONS

Look for Word Clues

Each sentence contains a few crucial clues that determine the answer. For a sentence to be used on the PCAT, the answer must already be in the sentence. Clues in the sentence limit the possible answers, and finding these clues will guide you to the correct answer.

For example, could the following sentence be on the PCAT?

The student thought the test was quite _____.

(A) long
(B) unpleasant
(C) predictable
(D) ridiculous

No. Because nothing in the sentence hints at which word to choose, it would be a terrible test question.

Now let's change the sentence to get a question that *could* be answered:

Since the student knew the form and content of the questions in advance, the test was quite _____ for her.

(A) long
(B) unpleasant
(C) predictable
(D) ridiculous

What are the important clues in this question? Well, the word *since* is a great structural clue. It indicates that the missing word follows logically from part of the sentence. Specifically, the missing word must follow from "knew the form and content . . . in advance." That means the test was predictable.

In the following examples, test your knowledge of Sentence Completion keywords by choosing the right answers from the choices in parentheses:

a. The winning argument was _____ *and* persuasive. (cogent, flawed)
b. The winning argument was _____ *but* persuasive. (cogent, flawed)
c. The populace _____ the introduction of the new taxes, *since* they had voted for them overwhelmingly. (applauded, despised)

    d.   *Despite* your impressive qualifications, I am _____ to offer you a position with our firm. (unable, willing)

    e.   Scientists have claimed that the dinosaurs became extinct in a single, dramatic event, *yet* new evidence suggests a _____ decline. (headlong, gradual)

    f.   The first wave of avant-gardists elicited _____ from the general population, *while* the second was completely ignored. (indifference, shock)

Answer Key: a. cogent, b. flawed, c. applauded, d. unable, e. gradual, f. shock

By concentrating on the keywords, it's easier to find your way through each question and arrive at the right answers.

Use Word Charge

Word charge is an excellent tool to help unlock tough Sentence Completions. You can use word charge to not only give you something to work with when you are unable to make an exact prediction but also to aid you in eliminating choices when you don't know exactly what a word means. Often you can eliminate many answer choices based on whether they are positive, negative, or neutral, even when you cannot remember the exact definition.

Word Charge Exercise

Predict the charge, positive (+) or negative (−), of the missing words in the following sentences:

    g.   The scientist's achievements and his seemingly _____ inventions made him world-famous.

    h.   While her initial reaction was _____, eventually she came to see the benefit of the new arrangement.

    i.   By the end of the century, sentimental literature faced complaints about the abundance of _____, and increasing lack of _____.

    j.   Since he wasn't very diligent in his studying, it's not surprising that his performance on the exam was _____.

    k.   The detective insisted on the _____ of the suspect, despite the initial evidence against him, completely convinced the _____ man was being falsely accused.

    l.   At least 80 percent of the population doesn't know enough about medical concepts to make _____ medical choices or to make _____ public policy decisions about healthcare.

Answer Key: g. positive, h. negative, i. negative, positive, j. negative, k. positive, positive, l. positive, positive

By noting word charge, you can save yourself time and get the answers even to questions with tough vocabulary!

Do Not Give Sentences Extra Meaning

You're not dealing with poetry here. These sentences aren't excerpted from the works of Toni Morrison or William Faulkner. The correct answer is the one most directly implied by the meanings of the words in the sentence. Read the sentence literally, not imaginatively. Pay attention to the meaning of the words, not associations or feelings that you have.

This is why it is also so important to read your answer choice back into the sentence. Words out of context can sound very tempting, but once you read them back in, you realize that answer choice adds to or changes the meaning of the sentence, which the correct answer will not do.

Determine the Relationship Between Blanks

Two-blank Sentence Completion questions can often be solved using the relationship between the two blanks. Even if you cannot predict either blank, understanding whether the blanks should be similar or opposite in charge and meaning can help you select the correct answer.

REVIEW PROBLEMS

1. The yearly financial statement of a large corporation may seem _____ at first, but the persistent reader soon finds its pages of facts and figures easy to decipher.

    (A) bewildering
    (B) surprising
    (C) inviting
    (D) misguided

2. The rise in the number of new housing starts in the final two quarters of last year suggests that the _____ economy should finally start to recover this year.

    (A) improbable
    (B) vigorous
    (C) sluggish
    (D) predictable

3. Organic farming is more labor intensive and thus initially more _____, but its long-term costs may be less than those of conventional farming.

    (A) uncommon
    (B) stylish
    (C) restrained
    (D) expensive

4. If the experiment is successful, it will represent a _____ leap forward in nanotechnology; not only _____ opportunities but also ushering in much new advancement.

    (A) miniscule . . . dispelling
    (B) prodigious . . . rejecting
    (C) necessary . . . creating
    (D) gargantuan . . . fostering

5. The governor's approval ratings had been _____ until a series of corruption scandals rocked his administration last year, causing the politician's career to _____.

    (A) lackluster . . . dwindle
    (B) robust . . . degenerate
    (C) exceptional . . . accelerate
    (D) prosaic . . . energize

6. After all the conclusive research that has been conducted in the last 30 years, it is _____ that there are many good reasons to _____ regular aerobic exercise.

    (A) dubious . . . implement

    (B) unequivocal . . . repudiate

    (C) apparent . . . engage in

    (D) jocular . . . acquiesce to

7. By the time she retires, she will have saved enough money to live _____, if not lavishly.

    (A) excessively

    (B) tolerably

    (C) reprehensibly

    (D) heedlessly

8. The newspaper reported that far too many homes were destroyed and severely _____ in the hurricane, indicating that the city was _____ the storm.

    (A) ameliorated . . . vulnerable to

    (B) subsidized . . . impervious to

    (C) tarnished . . . enamored of

    (D) marred . . . susceptible to

9. The more a product costs, whether it is a car or a handbag, the more likely it is to be _____ by consumers, who tend to associate price with quality.

    (A) esteemed

    (B) debased

    (C) canonized

    (D) rebuffed

10. The "green flash" is a _____ atmospheric refractive phenomenon whereby the top edge of a setting sun will momentarily turn green; rarely seen by the naked eye, it requires specific, _____ conditions to occur.

    (A) banal . . . superfluous

    (B) unique . . . prevalent

    (C) farcical . . . unusual

    (D) elusive . . . infrequent

SOLUTIONS TO REVIEW PROBLEMS

1. A

Stop: One blank, and the vocabulary is fairly straightforward—this is a good one to start with.

Think: You should recognize the keyword *but*, which indicates that the correct answer will mean the opposite of how the financial statement is described at the conclusion of the sentence, "easy to decipher."

Predict: In your own words, that opposite may be "difficult to understand."

Match: Choice (A), *bewildering*, is your answer. None of the other choices is an opposite of "easy to decipher" and can be eliminated.

2. C

Stop: Also a one-blank sentence. This is a pretty straightforward Sentence Completion.

Think: The keywords here are the phrase *suggests that* and the word *finally*. *Suggests that* indicates a cause-and-effect relationship between the parts of the sentence. This means that now that the housing numbers are up, the economy is finally recovering—and prior to this, the economy wasn't doing well.

Predict: You can fairly assert that the recovering economy was not moving before, so you're looking for something "slow" or "inactive."

Match: When you look for a synonym for "slow" in the answer choices, you should recognize *sluggish*, (C), as your answer.

3. D

Stop: Another one-blank sentence, with good keywords. Plus, the vocabulary is not too bad.

Think: The key word in this sentence is, again, *but*. That means the missing word will convey the opposite of the phrase after *but*, which is "long-term costs are less."

Predict: So your prediction should be something like "costly."

Match: *Expensive*, (D), is the opposite of lower costs. Actually, the word *costs* itself gives you a big clue, since *expensive* is the only answer that has anything to do with costs.

4. D

Stop: A two-blank sentence, but the vocabulary is not too bad, and there are several clear clues.

Think: Your road signs in this one are the semicolon in the middle of the sentence and the words *not only* just after. The semicolon tells you that the second half of the sentence elaborates on the first, so it is reiterating the idea that this experiment will lead to much new advancement.

Predict: So for the first blank, you are looking for something that indicates a huge advancement.

Match: So far, choices (B) and (D) fit this general idea, so move on to the second blank. *Not only* indicates that the blank will be similar to the word after *but also*, "ushering." Looking through the answers, only (D), *fostering*, fits.

5. B

Stop: Two blanks, but fairly tame vocabulary. This should be okay.

Think: The keywords here are *until* and *causing*, indicating a contrast and an effect. *Until* the corruption scandals, which are bad, the governor's rating's would have been the opposite—good. This *causes* something bad to happen to the governor's career.

Predict: The first blank should be something like "high" or "strong."

Match: Eliminate choices (A) and (D) since the first blank is an opposite. Now, predict that the second blank should be something bad—the governor's career is worse off than it was before the scandals. Eliminate (C) because *accelerate* is the opposite of what happened to the politician's career. Choice (B) must be correct.

6. C

Stop: Two blanks, some potentially difficult vocabulary, but the sentence itself is fairly straightforward—seems moderately difficult.

Think: The key word *After* indicates a cause-and-effect relationship. There are also several emphasis keywords—*conclusive* research and *good* reasons—the first blank should definitely be something positive.

Predict: The first blank should be something like "clear" or "obvious."

Match: Eliminate any choices whose first word isn't positive. This includes choices (A) and (D): *dubious*, which means doubtful, is the opposite of "clear," and *jocular* means laughable, which is too negative and doesn't match the prediction of "clear." The second blank is a verb—given that regular exercise is clearly a good idea, this verb should be positive as well. This eliminates (B), since *repudiate* means to deny or reject. The correct answer is (C).

7. B

Stop: A one-blank sentence, with somewhat difficult vocabulary in the answer choices.

Think: The keywords *if not* after the comma indicate the blank will be a less extreme version of *lavishly*. In other words, she'll have enough money, but not too much.

Predict: So, the blank should mean something like "good enough."

Match: Eliminate (C), *reprehensibly*, and (D), *heedlessly*, since they are both negative. Eliminate (A), *excessively*, because it's too strong—too close to "lavishly." Choice (B), *tolerably*, matches the prediction perfectly.

8. D

Stop: Two blanks with pretty clear keywords in the sentence. Do now.

Think: The emphasis keywords *far too many* and *severely* indicate something very bad happened to the homes in the hurricane. Predict for the first blank first.

Predict: The first blank should be something like "destroyed," "damaged," or something similar.

Match: Choices (A) and (B) can be eliminated right away since they are both positive. Looking at the second blank, the keywords *indicating that* imply that because *far too many* homes were damaged, the city was unprepared. "Unprepared" makes for a good prediction for the second blank, and eliminates (C), which is not related at all to the sentence. This makes (D) the correct answer.

9. A

Stop: One blank. Vocabulary is not the easiest but not terrible.

Think: The sentence is making a comparison between price and quality—the more a product costs, the more it is valued.

Predict: The blank should be something like "valued" or "prized."

Match: Choice (A) matches this prediction perfectly. Choices (B) and (D) are negative, so they can be quickly eliminated. Choice (C), *canonized*, is tempting, but it means to idolize or worship, which is too strong for this sentence.

10. D

Stop: Two blanks with some tough vocabulary. Definitely not one to do first.

Think: The semicolon indicates that the second half of the sentence will elaborate on the first half of the sentence, so the blanks should be similar in meaning.

Predict: The emphasis word *rarely* just after the semicolon reveals that the green flash is "rare" or "unusual," which is what should go in the first blank.

Match: Looking at the first blank, neither choices (A) nor (C) match the prediction of "rare"; eliminate. The second blank should be similar, so this eliminates (B), *prevalent*, which is the opposite of "rare." The correct answer is (D).

CHAPTER TEN

Word Roots

The Comprehensive Vocabulary List in Chapter 11 condenses the approximately 490,000 words of the English language into 1,600 words that will help you do well on the PCAT. But 1,600 words is still a lot to memorize. You can make this list more manageable by using word roots to help you learn related words. The root PATER, for example, gives you a convenient way to organize and memorize eight different words on the vocabulary list. Roots have a multiplier effect: Memorizing one root can help you understand a number of different words.

The root list in this chapter contains about 250 word roots, selected primarily for their usefulness as learning aids for examination-level words. The term root is used loosely here to include both prefixes and actual, etymological roots, often based on Greek or Latin words. While prefixes always introduce words (e.g., ANTE- in *antecedent* and NON- in *nonentity*), roots can be found at the beginning, middle, or end of words (e.g., ANIM in *animate* and *unanimous*).

Notice that some roots, especially certain short prefixes, change their forms slightly before certain letters. It's *exit*, but *egregious*; *inexorable*, but *impossible*. This is a common linguistic phenomenon: Certain sounds change or drop out before certain other sounds to make the words easier to pronounce.

This list does not include suffixes, which come at the end of words, because, in general, they don't say as much about words' meanings as roots do. For instance, the suffix -IOUS tells you that loquacious is an adjective, but it's more helpful to know that the root LOQU means "speak" if you're trying to figure out what loquacious means.

USING WORD ROOTS EFFECTIVELY

Word roots can help if you are confronted by an unfamiliar word on the PCAT. Suppose you see the word *circumnavigate* on the test, for example, but you don't know its meaning. If you recognize the root CIRCUM, you'll know that the word has something to do with a circle. If you also know the root NAV, meaning "sailing" (as in navy), you can guess that the word means "to sail around something," which is basically correct. Typically, it means to sail around the world.

A few words of warning are in order, though. Breaking a word down into its roots generally produces only an approximate definition, not a precise definition. Often, over the centuries, a word will have acquired a specific meaning that is not reflected in its etymology. For example, E means "out of," and GREG means "flock," but something *egregious* is "out of the flock" in a very specific, figurative way that you would not be able to figure out simply by breaking the word down into its roots; something egregious stands out by being conspicuously bad. Similarly, A means "not, without," and GNO means "know," but *agnostic* denotes a very specific kind of not knowing that pertains to religion. You therefore need to use a certain amount of caution when using word roots to figure out unfamiliar words, or the results can be misleading. A word may contain a combination of letters that looks like one of the roots on the root list but really means something different.

What does BELL mean in *belligerent*, *bellicose*, and *antebellum*? Does is mean the same thing in *belladonna*?

Think about what DEM means in *democracy*, *demographics*, and *demagogue*. Does it mean the same thing in *demolition*?

Sometimes two distinctly different roots look exactly the same, usually because they derive from different languages. There's no totally reliable way to tell them apart, though if you can partly understand a word through other word roots, context, or anything else, often common sense will do the rest.

In *antacid* and *antiperspirant*, does ANT mean "against" or "before"? How about in *antiquity* and *anticipate*?

In *homicide* does HOM mean "human being" or "same"? How about in *homogenize*, *homonym*, or *homosexual*?

What does PER mean in each of the following words: *perfidy*, *perimeter*, *permanent*, *perambulate*?

And finally, here's what is probably the most frequent example: in *inanimate*, *invisible*, and *inadvisable*, does IN mean "in" or "not"? How about in *invade*?

Use the word roots in this chapter to answer these questions, and continue coming up with your own questions as you study. This process will lead to deeper understanding of the meanings of words and therefore easier memorization, which will turn into more points on Test Day.

Root	Meaning	Examples
A, AN	not, without	amoral, atrophy, asymmetrical, anarchy, anesthetic, anonymity, anomaly, annul
AB, A	from, away, apart	abnegate, abortive, abrogate, abscond, absolve, abstemious, abstruse, avert, aversion, abnormal, abdicate, aberration, abhor, abject, abjure, ablution
AC, ACR	sharp, sour	acid, acerbic, exacerbate, acute, acuity, acumen, acrid, acrimony
AD, A	to, toward	adhere, adjacent, adjunct, admonish, adroit, adumbrate, advent, abeyance, abet, accede, accretion, acquiesce, affluent, aggrandize, aggregate, alleviate, alliteration, allude, allure, ascribe, aspersion, aspire, assail, assonance, attest
ALI, ALTR	another	alias, alienate, inalienable, altruism
AM, AMI	love	amorous, amicable, amiable, amity
AMBI, AMPHI	both	ambiguous, ambivalent, ambidextrous, amphibious
AMBL, AMBUL	walk	amble, ambulatory, perambulator, somnambulist
ANN, ENN	year	annual, annuity, superannuated, biennial, perennial
ANTE, ANT	before	antecedent, antediluvian, antebellum, antepenultimate, anterior, antiquity, antiquated, anticipate
ANTHROP	human	anthropology, anthropomorphic, misanthrope, philanthropy
ANTI, ANT	against, opposite	antidote, antipathy, antithesis, antacid, antagonist, antonym
AUD	hear	audio, audience, audition, auditory, audible
AUTO	self	autobiography, autocrat, autonomous
BELLI, BELL	war	belligerent, bellicose, antebellum, rebellion
BENE, BEN	good	benevolent, benefactor, beneficent, benign
BI	two	bicycle, bisect, bilateral, bilingual, biped
BIBLIO	book	Bible, bibliography, bibliophile

Root	Meaning	Examples
BIO	life	biography, biology, amphibious, symbiotic, macrobiotics
BURS	money, purse	reimburse, disburse, bursar
CAD, CAS, CID	happen, fall	accident, cadence, cascade, deciduous
CAP, CIP	head	captain, decapitate, capitulate, precipitous, precipitate, recapitulate
CAP, CAPT, CEPT, CIP	take, hold, seize	capable, capacious, captivate, deception, intercept, precept, inception, anticipate, emancipate, incipient, percipient
CARN	flesh	carnal, carnage, carnival, carnivorous, incarnate, incarnadine
CED, CESS	yield, go	cede, precede, accede, recede, antecedent, intercede, secede, cession, cease, cessation, incessant
CHROM	color	chrome, chromatic, monochrome
CHRON	time	chronology, chronic, anachronism
CIDE	murder	suicide, homicide, regicide, patricide
CIRCUM	around	circumference, circumlocution, circumnavigate, circumscribe, circumspect, circumvent
CLIN, CLIV	slope	incline, declivity, proclivity
CLUD, CLUS, CLAUS, CLOIS	shut, close	conclude, reclusive, claustrophobia, cloister, preclude, occlude
CO, COM, CON	with, together	coeducation, coagulate, coalesce, coerce, cogent, cognate, collateral, colloquial, colloquy, commensurate, commodious, compassion, compatriot, complacent, compliant, complicity, compunction, concerto, conciliatory, concord, concur, condone, conflagration, congeal, congenial, congenital, conglomerate, conjure, conjugal, conscientious, consecrate, consensus, consonant, constrained, contentious, contrite, contusion, convalescence, convene, convivial, convoke, convoluted, congress
COGN, GNO	know	recognize, cognition, cognizance, incognito, diagnosis, agnostic, prognosis, ignorant

Root	Meaning	Examples
CONTRA	against	controversy, incontrovertible, contravene, contradict
CORP	body	corpse, corporeal, corpulence
COSMO, COSM	world	cosmopolitan, cosmos, microcosm, macrocosm
CRAC, CRAT	rule, power	democracy, bureaucracy, theocracy, autocrat, aristocrat, technocrat
CRED	trust, believe	incredible, credulous, credence
CRESC, CRET	grow	crescent, crescendo, accretion
CULP	blame, fault	culprit, culpable, inculpate, exculpate
CURR, CURS	run	current, concur, cursory, precursor, incursion
DE	down, out, apart	depart, debase, debilitate, declivity, decry, deface, defamatory, defunct, delegate, demarcation, demean, demur, deplete, deplore, depravity, deprecate, deride, derivative, desist, detest
DEC	ten, tenth	decade, decimal, decathlon, decimate
DEMO, DEM	people	democrat, demographics, demagogue, epidemic, pandemic, endemic
DI, DIURN	day	diary, diurnal, quotidian
DIA	across	diagonal, diatribe, diaphanous
DIC, DICT	speak	diction, interdict, predict, abdicate, indict, verdict, dictum
DIS, DIF, DI	not, apart, away	disaffected, disband, disbar, disburse, discern, discordant, discredit, discursive, disheveled, disparage, disparate, dispassionate, dispirit, dissemble, disseminate, dissension, dissipate, dissonant, dissuade, distend, differentiate, diffidence, diffuse, digress, divert
DOC, DOCT	teach	doctrine, docile, doctrinaire
DOL	pain	condolence, doleful, dolorous, indolent
DUC, DUCT	lead	seduce, induce, conduct, viaduct, induct
EGO	self	ego, egoist, egocentric

Root	Meaning	Examples
EN, EM	in, into	enter, entice, encumber, endemic, ensconce, enthrall, entreat, embellish, embezzle, embroil, empathy
ERR	wander	erratic, aberration, errant
EU	well, good	eulogy, euphemism, euphony, euphoria, eurhythmic, euthanasia
EX, E	out, out of	exit, exacerbate, excerpt, excommunicate, exculpate, execrable, exhume, exonerate, exorbitant, exorcise, expatriate, expedient, expiate, expunge, expurgate, extenuate, extort, extremity, extricate, extrinsic, exult, evoke, evict, evince, elicit, egress, egregious
FAC, FIC, FECT, FY, FEA	make, do	factory, facility, benefactor, malefactor, fiction, fictive, beneficent, affect, confection, refectory, magnify, unify, rectify, vilify, feasible
FERV	boil	fervent, fervid, effervescent
FID	faith, trust	confident, diffidence, perfidious, fidelity
FLU, FLUX	flow	fluent, flux, affluent, confluence, effluvia, superfluous
FORE	before	forecast, foreboding, forestall
FRAG, FRAC	break	fragment, fracture, diffract, fractious, refract
FUS	pour	profuse, infusion, effusive, diffuse
GEN	birth, class, kin	generation, congenital, homogeneous, heterogeneous, ingenious, engender, progenitor, progeny
GRAD, GRESS	step	graduate, gradual, retrograde, centigrade, degrade, gradation, gradient, progress, congress, digress, transgress, ingress, egress
GRAPH, GRAM	writing	biography, bibliography, epigraph, grammar, epigram
GRAT	pleasing	grateful, gratitude, gratis, ingrate, congratulate, gratuitous, gratuity
GRAV, GRIEV	heavy	grave, gravity, aggravate, grieve, aggrieve, grievous
GREG	crowd, flock	segregate, gregarious, egregious, congregate, aggregate

Root	Meaning	Examples
HABIT, HIBIT	have, hold	habit, inhibit, cohabit, habitat
HAP	by chance	happen, haphazard, hapless, mishap
HELIO, HELI	sun	heliocentric, helium, heliotrope, aphelion, perihelion
HETERO	other	heterosexual, heterogeneous, heterodox
HOL	whole	holocaust, catholic, holistic
HOMO	same	homosexual, homogenize, homogeneous, homonym
HOMO	man	*Homo sapiens,* homicide, bonhomie
HYDR	water	hydrant, hydrate, dehydration
HYPER	too much, excess	hyperactive, hyperbole, hyperventilate
HYPO	too little, under	hypodermic, hypothermia, hypochondria, hypothesis, hypothetical
IN, IG, IL, IM, IR	not	incorrigible, indefatigable, indelible, indubitable, inept, inert, inexorable, insatiable, insentient, insolvent, insomnia, interminable, intractable, incessant, inextricable, infallible, infamy, innumerable, inoperable, insipid, intemperate, intrepid, inviolable, ignorant, ignominious, ignoble, illicit, illimitable, immaculate, immutable, impasse, impeccable, impecunious, impertinent, implacable, impotent, impregnable, improvident, impassioned, impervious, irregular
IN, IL, IM, IR	in, on, into	invade, inaugurate, incandescent, incarcerate, incense, indenture, induct, ingratiate, introvert, incarnate, inception, incisive, infer, infusion, ingress, innate, inquest, inscribe, insinuate, inter
INTER	between, among	intercede, intercept, interdiction, interject, interlocutor, interloper, intermediary, intermittent, interpolate, interpose, interregnum, interrogate, intersect, intervene
INTRA, INTR	within	intrastate, intravenous, intramural, intrinsic

Root	Meaning	Examples
IT, ITER	between, among	transit, itinerant, reiterate, transitory
JECT, JET	throw	eject, interject, abject, trajectory, jettison
JOUR	day	journal, adjourn, sojourn
JUD	judge	judge, judicious, prejudice, adjudicate
JUNCT, JUG	join	junction, adjunct, injunction, conjugal, subjugate
JUR	swear, law	jury, abjure, adjure, conjure, perjure, jurisprudence
LAT	side	lateral, collateral, unilateral, bilateral, quadrilateral
LAV, LAU, LU	wash	lavatory, laundry, ablution, antediluvian
LEG, LEC, LEX	read, speak	legible, lecture, lexicon
LEV	light	elevate, levitate, levity, alleviate
LIBER	free	liberty, liberal, libertarian, libertine
LIG, LECT	choose, gather	eligible, elect, select
LIG, LI, LY	bind	ligament, oblige, religion, liable, liaison, lien, ally
LING, LANG	tongue	lingo, language, linguistics, bilingual
LITER	letter	literate, alliteration, literal
LITH	stone	monolith, lithograph, megalith
LOQU, LOC, LOG	speech, thought	eloquent, loquacious, colloquial, colloquy, soliloquy, circumlocution, interlocutor, monologue, dialogue, eulogy, philology, neologism
LUC, LUM	light	lucid, illuminate, elucidate, pellucid, translucent
LUD, LUS	play	ludicrous, allude, delusion, allusion, illusory
MACRO	great	macrocosm, macrobiotics
MAG, MAJ, MAS, MAX	great	magnify, majesty, master, maximum, magnanimous, magnate, magnitude
MAL	bad	malady, maladroit, malevolent, malodorous
MAN	hand	manual, manuscript, emancipate, manifest
MAR	sea	submarine, marine, maritime

Root	Meaning	Examples
MATER, MATR	mother	maternal, matron, matrilineal
MEDI	middle	intermediary, medieval, mediate
MEGA	great	megaphone, megalomania, megaton, megalith
MEMOR, MEMEN	remember	memory, memento, memorabilia, memoir
METER, METR, MENS	measure	meter, thermometer, perimeter, metronome, commensurate
MICRO	small	microscope, microorganism, microcosm, microbe
MIS	wrong, bad, hate	misunderstand, misanthrope, misapprehension, misconstrue, misnomer, mishap
MIT, MISS	send	transmit, emit, missive
MOLL	soft	mollify, emollient, mollusk
MON, MONIT	warn	admonish, monitor, premonition
MONO	one	monologue, monotonous, monogamy, monolith, monochrome
MOR	custom, manner	moral, mores, morose
MOR, MORT	dead	morbid, moribund, mortal, amortize
MORPH	shape	amorphous, anthropomorphic, metamorphosis, morphology
MOV, MOT, MOB, MOM	move	remove, motion, mobile, momentum, momentous
MUT	change	mutate, mutability, immutable, commute
NAT, NASC	born	native, nativity, natal, neonate, innate, cognate, nascent, renascent, renaissance
NAU, NAV	ship, sailor	nautical, nauseous, navy, circumnavigate
NEG	not, deny	negative, abnegate, renege
NEO	new	neoclassical, neophyte, neologism, neonate
NIHIL	none, nothing	annihilation, nihilism
NOM, NYM	name	nominate, nomenclature, nominal, cognomen, misnomer, ignominious, antonym, homonym, pseudonym, synonym, anonymity

Root	Meaning	Examples
NOX, NIC, NEC, NOC	harm	obnoxious, noxious, pernicious, internecine, innocuous
NOV	new	novelty, innovation, novitiate
NUMER	number	numeral, numerous, innumerable, enumerate
OB	against	obstruct, obdurate, obfuscate, obnoxious, obsequious, obstinate, obstreperous, obtrusive
OMNI	all	omnipresent, omnipotent, omniscient, omnivorous
ONER	burden	onerous, onus, exonerate
OPER	work	operate, cooperate, inoperable
PAC	peace	pacify, pacifist, pacific
PALP	feel	palpable, palpitation
PAN	all	panorama, panacea, panegyric, pandemic, panoply
PATER, PATR	father	paternal, paternity, patriot, compatriot, expatriate, patrimony, patricide, patrician
PATH, PASS	feel, suffer	sympathy, antipathy, empathy, apathy, pathos, impassioned
PEC	money	pecuniary, impecunious, peculation
PED, POD	foot	pedestrian, pediment, expedient, biped, quadruped, tripod
PEL, PULS	drive	compel, compelling, expel, propel, compulsion
PEN	almost	peninsula, penultimate, penumbra
PEND, PENS	hang	pendant, pendulous, compendium, suspense, propensity
PER	through, by, for, throughout	perambulator, percipient, perfunctory, permeable, perspicacious, pertinacious, perturbation, perusal, perennial, peregrinate
PER	against, destruction	perfidious, pernicious, perjure
PERI	around	perimeter, periphery, perihelion, peripatetic
PET	seek, go toward	petition, impetus, impetuous, petulant, centripetal
PHIL	love	philosopher, philanderer, philanthropy, bibliophile, philology
PHOB	fear	phobia, claustrophobia, xenophobia

Root	Meaning	Examples
PHON	sound	phonograph, megaphone, euphony, phonetics, phonics
PLAC	calm, please	placate, implacable, placid, complacent
PON, POS	put, place	postpone, proponent, exponent, preposition, posit, interpose, juxtaposition, depose
PORT	carry	portable, deportment, rapport
POT	drink	potion, potable
POT	power	potential, potent, impotent, potentate, omnipotence
PRE	before	precede, precipitate, preclude, precocious, precursor, predilection, predisposition, preponderance, prepossessing, presage, prescient, prejudice, predict, premonition, preposition
PRIM, PRI	first	prime, primary, primal, primeval, primordial, pristine
PRO	ahead, forth	proceed, proclivity, procrastinator, profane, profuse, progenitor, progeny, prognosis, prologue, promontory, propel, proponent, propose, proscribe, protestation, provoke
PROTO	first	prototype, protagonist, protocol
PROX, PROP	near	approximate, propinquity, proximity
PSEUDO	false	pseudoscientific, pseudonym
PYR	fire	pyre, pyrotechnics, pyromania
QUAD, QUAR, QUAT	four	quadrilateral, quadrant, quadruped, quarter, quarantine, quaternary
QUES, QUER, QUIS, QUIR	question	quest, inquest, query, querulous, inquisitive, inquiry
QUIE	quiet	disquiet, acquiesce, quiescent, requiem
QUINT, QUIN	five	quintuplets, quintessence
RADI, RAMI	branch	radius, radiate, radiant, eradicate, ramification
RECT, REG	straight, rule	rectangle, rectitude, rectify, regular
REG	king, rule	regal, regent, interregnum
RETRO	backward	retrospective, retroactive, retrograde

Root	Meaning	Examples
RID, RIS	laugh	ridiculous, deride, derision
ROG	ask	interrogate, derogatory, abrogate, arrogate, arrogant
RUD	rough, crude	rude, erudite, rudimentary
RUPT	break	disrupt, interrupt, rupture, erupt
SACR, SANCT	holy	sacred, sacrilege, consecrate, sanctify, sanction, sacrosanct
SCRIB, SCRIPT, SCRIV	write	scribe, ascribe, circumscribe, inscribe, proscribe, script, manuscript, scrivener
SE	apart, away	separate, segregate, secede, sedition
SEC, SECT, SEG	cut	sector, dissect, bisect, intersect, segment, secant
SED, SID	sit	sedate, sedentary, supersede, reside, residence, assiduous, insidious
SEM	seed, sow	seminar, seminal, disseminate
SEN	old	senior, senile, senescent
SENT, SENS	feel, think	sentiment, nonsense, assent, sentient, consensus, sensual
SEQU, SECU	follow	sequence, sequel, subsequent, obsequious, obsequy, non sequitur, consecutive
SIGN	mark, sign	signal, designation, assignation
SIM, SEM	similar, same	similar, semblance, dissemble, verisimilitude
SIN	curve	sine curve, sinuous, insinuate
SOL	sun	solar, parasol, solarium, solstice
SOL	alone	solo, solitude, soliloquy, solipsism
SOMN	sleep	insomnia, somnolent, somnambulist
SON	sound	sonic, consonance, dissonance, assonance, sonorous, resonate
SOPH	wisdom	philosopher, sophistry, sophisticated, sophomoric
SPEC, SPIC	see, look	spectator, circumspect, retrospective, perspective, perspicacious
SPER	hope	prosper, prosperous, despair, desperate
SPERS, SPAR	scatter	disperse, sparse, aspersion, disparate

Root	Meaning	Examples
SPIR	breathe	respire, inspire, spiritual, aspire, transpire
STRICT, STRING	bind	strict, stricture, constrict, stringent, astringent
STRUCT, STRU	build	structure, construe, obstruct
SUB	under	subconscious, subjugate, subliminal, subpoena, subsequent, subterranean, subvert
SUMM	highest	summit, summary, consummate
SUPER, SUR	above	supervise, supercilious, supersede, superannuated, superfluous, insurmountable, surfeit
SURGE, SURRECT	rise	surge, resurgent, insurgent, insurrection
SYN, SYM	together	synthesis, sympathy, synonym, syncopation, synopsis, symposium, symbiosis
TACIT, TIC	silent	tacit, taciturn, reticent
TACT, TAG, TANG	touch	tact, tactile, contagious, tangent, tangential, tangible
TEN, TIN, TAIN	hold, twist	detention, tenable, tenacious, pertinacious, retinue, retain
TEND, TENS, TENT	stretch	intend, distend, tension, tensile, ostensible, contentious
TERM	end	terminal, terminus, terminate, interminable
TERR	earth, land	terrain, terrestrial, extraterrestrial, subterranean
TEST	witness	testify, attest, testimonial, testament, detest, protestation
THE	god	atheist, theology, apotheosis, theocracy
THERM	heat	thermometer, thermal, thermonuclear, hypothermia
TIM	fear, frightened	timid, intimidate, timorous
TOP	place	topic, topography, utopia
TORT	twist	distort, extort, tortuous
TORP	stiff, numb	torpedo, torpid, torpor
TOX	poison	toxic, toxin, intoxication
TRACT	draw	tractor, intractable, protract

Root	Meaning	Examples
TRANS	across, over, beyond	transport, transgress, transient, transitory, through, translucent, transmutation, transpire, intransigent
TREM, TREP	shake	tremble, tremor, tremulous, trepidation, intrepid
TURB	shake	disturb, turbulent, perturbation
UMBR	shadow	umbrella, umbrage, adumbrate, penumbra
UNI, UN	one	unify, unilateral, unanimous
URB	city	urban, suburban, urbane
VAC	empty	vacant, evacuate, vacuous
VAL, VAIL	value, strength	valid, valor, ambivalent, convalescence, avail, prevail, countervail
VEN, VENT	come	convene, contravene, intervene, venue, convention, circumvent, advent, adventitious
VER	true	verify, verity, verisimilitude, veracious, aver, verdict
VERB	word	verbal, verbose, verbiage, verbatim
VERT, VERS	turn	avert, convert, pervert, revert, incontrovertible, divert, subvert, versatile, aversion
VICT, VINC	conquer	victory, conviction, evict, evince, invincible
VID, VIS	see	evident, vision, visage, supervise
VIL	base, mean	vile, vilify, revile
VIV, VIT	life	vivid, vital, convivial, vivacious
VOC, VOK, VOW	call, voice	vocal, equivocate, vociferous, convoke, evoke, invoke, avow
VOL	wish	voluntary, malevolent, benevolent, volition
VOLV, VOLUT	turn, roll	revolve, evolve, convoluted
VOR	eat	devour, carnivorous, omnivorous, voracious

CHAPTER ELEVEN

Vocabulary List

This list is based on the hardest vocabulary words that were likely to appear on actual exams in the past five years. Use this as a condensed mini-dictionary to look up new words you encounter during this course. Each word is followed by a short, simple definition. We've dispensed with longer definitions, pronunciation guides, and other dictionary-type information because your primary concern right now is word recognition. However, you should occasionally supplement your vocabulary study with judicious use of your regular dictionary.

ABANDON (n.)	total lack of inhibition	ABORTIVE	interrupted while incomplete
ABASE	to humble, disgrace	ABRIDGE	to condense, shorten
ABATEMENT	decrease, reduction		
ABDICATE	to give up a position, right, or power	ABROGATE	to abolish or invalidate by authority
ABERRATION	something different from the usual or normal	ABSCOND	to depart secretly
		ABSOLVE	to forgive, free from blame
ABET	to aid, act as accomplice	ABSTEMIOUS	moderate in appetite
ABEYANCE	temporary suppression or suspension	ABSTRACT (adj.)	theoretical; complex, difficult
ABHOR	to loathe, detest	ABSTRUSE	difficult to comprehend
ABJECT	miserable, pitiful	ACCEDE	to express approval; agree to
ABJURE	to reject, abandon formally	ACCESSIBLE	attainable, available; approachable
ABLUTION	act of cleansing		
ABNEGATE	to deny, renounce	ACCESSORY	attachment, ornament; accomplice, partner
ABOLITIONIST	one who opposes the practice of slavery		

ACCOLADE	praise, distinction	AERODYNAMIC	relating to objects moving through the air
ACCOST	to approach and speak to someone		
ACCRETION	growth in size or increase in amount	AESTHETIC	pertaining to beauty or art
ACCRUE	to accumulate, grow by additions	AFFABLE	friendly, easy to approach
ACERBIC	bitter, sharp in taste or temper	AFFECTED (adj.)	pretentious, phony
ACME	highest point; summit	AFFINITY	fondness, liking; similarity
ACQUIESCE	to agree, comply quietly	AFFLUENT	rich, abundant
ACQUITTAL	release from blame	AFFRONT (n.)	personal offense, insult
ACRID	harsh, bitter	AGENDA	plan, schedule
ACRIMONY	bitterness, animosity	AGGRANDIZE	to make larger or greater in power
ACUITY	sharpness	AGGREGATE (n.)	collective mass or sum; total
ACUMEN	sharpness of insight	AGGRIEVE	to afflict, distress
ACUTE	sharp, pointed	AGILE	well-coordinated, nimble
ADAGE	old saying or proverb		
ADAMANT	uncompromising, unyielding	AGITATION	commotion, excitement; uneasiness
ADAPT	to accommodate, adjust	AGNOSTIC	one doubting that people can know God
ADHERE	to cling or follow without deviation	AGRARIAN	relating to farming or rural matters
ADJACENT	next to	ALACRITY	cheerful willingness, eagerness; speed
ADJUNCT	something added, attached, or joined		
ADMONISH	to caution or reprimand	ALCHEMY	medieval chemical philosophy based on changing metal into gold
ADROIT	skillful, accomplished, highly competent	ALGORITHM	mechanical problem-solving procedure
ADULATION	high praise	ALIAS	assumed name
ADULTERATE	to corrupt or make impure	ALIENATED	distanced, estranged
ADUMBRATE	to sketch, outline in a shadowy way	ALIGNED	precisely adjusted; committed to one side or party
ADVANTAGEOUS	favorable, useful	ALLAY	to lessen, ease, or soothe
ADVERSARIAL	antagonistic, competitive		
ADVERSE	unfavorable, unlucky, harmful	ALLEGORY	symbolic representation
		ALLEVIATE	to relieve, improve partially
AERIAL	having to do with the air	ALLITERATION	repetition of the beginning sounds of words
AERIE	nook or nest built high in the air		

ALLOCATION	allowance, portion, share	AMPLIFY	to increase, intensify
ALLURE (v.)	to entice by charm; attract	AMULET	ornament worn as a charm against evil spirits
ALLUSION	indirect reference	ANACHRONISM	something chronologically inappropriate
ALLUSIVENESS	quality of making many indirect references	ANACHRONISTIC	outdated
ALOOF	detached, indifferent	ANALOGOUS	comparable, parallel
ALTERCATION	noisy dispute	ANARCHY	absence of government or law; chaos
ALTRUISM	unselfish concern for others' welfare	ANATHEMA	ban, curse; something shunned or disliked
AMALGAM	mixture, combination, alloy	ANCILLARY	accessory, subordinate, helping
AMBIDEXTROUS	able to use both hands equally well	ANECDOTE	short, usually funny account of an event
AMBIGUOUS	uncertain; subject to multiple interpretations	ANGULAR	characterized by sharp angles; lean and gaunt
AMBIVALENCE	attitude of uncertainty; conflicting emotions	ANIMATION	enthusiasm, excitement
AMELIORATE	to make better, improve	ANIMOSITY	hatred, hostility
AMENABLE	agreeable, cooperative	ANNUL	to cancel, nullify, declare void, or make legally invalid
AMEND	to improve or correct flaws in	ANODYNE	something that calms or soothes pain
AMENITY	pleasantness; something increasing comfort	ANOINT	to apply oil to, especially as a sacred rite
AMIABLE	friendly, pleasant, likable	ANOMALY	irregularity or deviation from the norm
AMICABLE	friendly, agreeable	ANONYMITY	condition of having no name or an unknown name
AMITY	friendship		
AMORAL	unprincipled, unethical	ANTAGONIST	foe, opponent, adversary
AMOROUS	strongly attracted to love; showing love	ANTEBELLUM	existing before a war, prewar
AMORPHOUS	having no definite form	ANTECEDENT (adj.)	coming before in place or time
AMORTIZE	to diminish by installment payments	ANTEDILUVIAN	prehistoric, ancient beyond measure
AMPHIBIAN (n.)	creature equally at home on land or in water	ANTEPENULTIMATE	third from last
		ANTERIOR	preceding, previous, before, prior (to)
AMPHITHEATER	arena theater with tiers rising around a central open space	ANTHOLOGY	collection of literary works
AMPLE	abundant, plentiful	ANTHROPOMORPHIC	attributing human qualities to non-humans

ANTIPATHY	dislike, hostility; extreme opposition or aversion	ARDOR	great emotion or passion
ANTIQUATED	outdated, obsolete	ARDUOUS	extremely difficult, laborious
ANTIQUITY	ancient times; the quality of being old or ancient	ARID	extremely dry or deathly boring
ANTITHESIS	exact opposite or direct contrast	ARRAIGN	to call to court to answer a charge
APATHETIC	indifferent, unconcerned	ARROGATE	to demand, claim arrogantly
APATHY	lack of feeling or emotion	ARSENAL	ammunition storehouse
APHASIA	inability to speak or use words	ARTICULATE (adj.)	well-spoken, expressing oneself clearly
APHELION	point in a planet's orbit that is farthest from the sun	ARTIFACT	historical relic, item made by human craft
		ARTISAN	craftsperson; expert
APHORISM	old saying or short pithy statement	ASCEND	to rise or climb
APOCRYPHAL	not genuine; fictional	ASCENDANCY	state of rising, ascending; power or control
APOSTATE (n.)	one who renounces a religious faith	ASCERTAIN	to determine, discover, make certain of
APOSTROPHE	speech to the reader or someone not present	ASCETIC (adj.)	self-denying, abstinent, austere
APOTHEOSIS	glorification; glorified ideal	ASCRIBE	to attribute to, assign
		ASHEN	resembling ashes; deathly pale
APPEASE	to satisfy, placate, calm, pacify	ASKEW	crooked, tilted
APPROBATION	praise; official approval	ASPERSION	false rumor, damaging report, slander
APPROPRIATE (v.)	to take possession of		
AQUATIC	belonging or living in water	ASPIRE	to have great hopes; to aim at a goal
ARABLE	suitable for cultivation	ASSAIL	to attack, assault
ARBITRARY	depending solely on individual will; inconsistent	ASSENT (v.)	to express agreement
		ASSERT	to affirm, attest
ARBITRATOR	mediator, negotiator	ASSIDUOUS	diligent, persistent, hard-working
ARBOREAL	relating to trees; living in trees	ASSIGNATION	appointment for lovers' meeting; assignment
ARBORETUM	place where trees are displayed and studied	ASSIMILATION	act of blending in, becoming similar
ARCANE	secret, obscure, known only to a few	ASSONANCE	resemblance in sound, especially in vowel sounds; partial rhyme
ARCHAIC	antiquated, from an earlier time; outdated		
ARCHIPELAGO	large group of islands	ASSUAGE	to make less severe, ease, relieve
ARDENT	passionate, enthusiastic, fervent	ASTRINGENT	harsh, severe, stern

ASTUTE	having good judgment		AWRY	crooked, askew, amiss
ASUNDER (adv.)	into different parts		AXIOM	premise, postulate, self-evident truth
ASYMMETRICAL	not corresponding in size, shape, position, etc.		BALEFUL	harmful, with evil intentions
ATONE	to make amends for a wrong		BALK (v.)	to refuse, shirk; prevent
ATROCIOUS	monstrous, shockingly bad, wicked		BALLAD	folk song, narrative poem
ATROPHY (v.)	to waste away, wither from disuse		BALM	soothing, healing influence
ATTAIN	to accomplish, gain		BAN (v.)	to forbid, outlaw
ATTENUATE	to make thin or slender; weaken		BANAL	trite and overly common
ATTEST	to testify, stand as proof of, bear witness		BANE	something causing ruin, death, or destruction
AUDACIOUS	bold, daring, fearless			
AUDIBLE	capable of being heard		BANTER	playful conversation
AUDIT (n.)	formal examination of financial records		BASTION	fortification, stronghold
AUDITORY	having to do with hearing		BAY (v.)	to bark, especially in a deep, prolonged way
AUGMENT	to expand, extend		BECALM	to make calm or still; keep motionless by lack of wind
AUGURY (adj.)	prophecy, prediction of events			
AUGUST	dignified, awe-inspiring, venerable		BECLOUD	to confuse; darken with clouds
AUSPICIOUS	having favorable prospects, promising		BEGUILE	to deceive, mislead; charm
AUSTERE	stern, strict, unadorned		BEHEMOTH	huge creature
AUTHORITARIAN	extremely strict, bossy		BELABOR	to insist repeatedly or harp on
AUTOCRAT	dictator		BELATED	late
AUTONOMOUS	separate, independent		BELEAGUER	to harass, plague
AUXILIARY	supplementary, reserve		BELFRY	bell tower, room in which a bell is hung
AVARICE	greed			
AVENGE	to retaliate, take revenge for an injury or crime		BELIE	to misrepresent; expose as false
			BELITTLE	to represent as unimportant, make light of
AVER	to declare to be true, affirm		BELLICOSE	warlike, aggressive
AVERSION	intense dislike		BELLIGERENT	hostile, tending to fight
AVERT	to turn (something) away; prevent		BELLOW	to roar, shout
AVIARY	large enclosure housing birds		BEMUSE	to confuse, stupefy; plunge deep into thought
AVOW	to state openly or declare		BENCHMARK	standard of measure

BENEFACTOR	someone giving aid or money	BONANZA	extremely large amount; something profitable
BENEFICENT	kindly, charitable; doing good deeds; producing good effects	BONHOMIE	good-natured geniality; atmosphere of good cheer
BENIGHTED	unenlightened	BOON	blessing, something to be thankful for
BENIGN	kindly, gentle or harmless	BOOR	crude person, one lacking manners or taste
BEQUEATH	to give or leave through a will; to hand down	BOTANIST	scientist who studies plants
BERATE	to scold harshly	BOUNTIFUL	plentiful
BESEECH	to beg, plead, implore	BOURGEOIS	middle-class
BESTIAL	beastly, animal-like	BOVINE	cow-like; relating to cows
BESTOW	to give as a gift		
BETOKEN	to indicate, signify, give evidence of	BRAZEN	bold, shameless, impudent; of or like brass
BEVY	group	BREACH	act of breaking, violation
BIAS	prejudice, slant		
BIBLIOGRAPHY	list of books	BRIGAND	bandit, outlaw
BIBLIOPHILE	book lover	BROACH	to mention or suggest for the first time
BILATERAL	two-sided		
BILK	to cheat, defraud	BRUSQUE	rough and abrupt in manner
BILLET	board and lodging for troops	BUFFET (v.)	to strike, hit
BIPED	two-footed animal	BUFFOON	clown or fool
BISECT	to cut into two (usually equal) parts	BULWARK	defense wall; anything serving as defense
BLANCH	to pale; take the color out of	BURGEON	to sprout or flourish
BLANDISH	to coax with flattery	BURLY	brawny, husky
BLASPHEMOUS	cursing, profane, irreverent	BURNISH	to polish, make smooth and bright
BLATANT	glaring, obvious, showy	BURSAR	treasurer
BLIGHT (v.)	to afflict, destroy	BUSTLE	commotion, energetic activity
BLITHE	joyful, cheerful, or without appropriate thought	BUTT	person or thing that is object of ridicule
BLUDGEON	to hit as with a short heavy club	BUTTRESS (v.)	to reinforce or support
BOISTEROUS	rowdy, loud, unrestrained	BYWAY	back road
		CACOPHONOUS	jarring, unpleasantly noisy
BOMBASTIC	using high-sounding but meaningless language	CADENCE	rhythmic flow of poetry; marching beat
		CAJOLE	to flatter, coax, persuade

CALAMITOUS	disastrous, catastrophic	CAUSALITY	cause-and-effect relationship
CALLOUS	thick-skinned, insensitive	CAUSTIC	biting, sarcastic; able to burn
CALLOW	immature, lacking sophistication	CAVALIER (adj.)	carefree, happy; with lordly disdain
CALUMNY	false and malicious accusation, misrepresentation, slander	CAVORT	to frolic, frisk
CANDOR	honesty of expression	CEDE	to surrender possession of something
CANNY	smart; founded on common sense	CELEBRITY	fame, widespread acclaim
CANONIZE	to declare a person a saint; raise to highest honors	CENSORIOUS	severely critical
		CENTRIPETAL	directed or moving toward the center
CANVASS	to examine thoroughly; conduct a poll	CERTITUDE	assurance, certainty
CAPACIOUS	large, roomy; extensive	CESSATION	temporary or complete halt
CAPITULATE	to submit completely, surrender	CESSION	act of surrendering something
CAPRICIOUS	impulsive, whimsical, without much thought	CHAGRIN	shame, embarrassment, humiliation
CARDIOLOGIST	physician specializing in diseases of the heart	CHALICE	goblet, cup
		CHAMPION (v.)	to defend or support
CARICATURE	exaggerated portrait, cartoon	CHAOTIC	extremely disorderly
CARNAL	of the flesh	CHARLATAN	quack, fake
CARNIVOROUS	meat-eating	CHARY	watchful, cautious, extremely shy
CARP (v.)	to find fault, complain constantly	CHASTISE	to punish, discipline, scold
CARTOGRAPHY	science or art of making maps	CHERUBIC	sweet, innocent, resembling a cherub angel
CAST (n.)	copy, replica		
CAST (v.)	to fling, to throw	CHICANERY	trickery, fraud, deception
CASTIGATE	to punish, chastise, criticize severely	CHIDE	to scold, express disapproval
CATALYST	something causing change without being changed	CHIMERICAL	fanciful, imaginary, visionary, impossible
CATEGORICAL	absolute, without exception	CHOLERIC	easily angered, short-tempered
CATHARSIS	purification, cleansing	CHOICE (adj.)	specially selected, preferred
CATHOLIC	universal; broad and comprehensive	CHORTLE	to chuckle
CAUCUS	smaller group within an organization; a meeting of such a group	CHROMATIC	relating to color
		CHRONICLER	one who keeps records of historical events
CAULK	to make watertight	CIRCUITOUS	roundabout

CIRCUMFERENCE	boundary or distance around a circle or sphere	COGNOMEN	family name; any name, especially a nickname
CIRCUMLOCUTION	roundabout, lengthy way of saying something	COHABIT	to live together
		COHERENT	intelligible, lucid, understandable
CIRCUMNAVIGATE	to sail completely around	COLLATERAL	accompanying
CIRCUMSCRIBE	to encircle; set limits on, confine	COLLOQUIAL	characteristic of informal speech
CIRCUMSPECT	cautious, wary	COLLOQUY	dialogue or conversation, conference
CIRCUMVENT	to go around; avoid	
CISTERN	tank for rainwater	COLLUSION	collaboration, complicity, conspiracy
CITADEL	fortress or stronghold	COMELINESS	physical grace and beauty
CIVIL	polite; relating to citizens	COMMEND	to compliment, praise
CIVILITY	courtesy, politeness	COMMENSURATE	proportional
CLAIRVOYANT (adj.)	having extrasensory perception, psychic	COMMISSION	fee payable to an agent; authorization
CLAMOR (v.)	to make a noisy outcry	COMMODIOUS	roomy, spacious
CLAMOR (n.)	noisy outcry	COMMONPLACE	ordinary, found every day
CLANDESTINE	secretive, concealed for a darker purpose	COMMUNICABLE	transmittable
CLARITY	clearness; clear understanding	COMMUTE	to change a penalty to a less severe one
CLAUSTROPHOBIA	fear of small, confined places	COMPATRIOT	fellow countryman
CLEAVE	to split or separate OR to stick, cling, adhere	COMPELLING (adj.)	having a powerful and irresistible effect
CLEMENCY	merciful leniency	COMPENSATE	to repay or reimburse
CLOISTER (v.)	to confine, seclude	COMPLACENT	self-satisfied, smug, affable
COAGULATE	to clot or change from a liquid to a solid	COMPLEMENT	to complete, perfect
COALESCE	to grow together or cause to unite as one	COMPLIANT	submissive and yielding
CODDLE	to baby, treat indulgently	COMPLICITY	knowing partnership in wrongdoing
COERCE	to compel by force or intimidation	COMPOUND (adj.)	complex; composed of several parts
COFFER	strongbox, large chest for money	COMPOUND (v.)	to combine, add to
		COMPRESS (v.)	to reduce, squeeze
COGENT	logically forceful, compelling, convincing	COMPULSIVE	obsessive, fanatic
COGNATE	related, similar, akin	COMPUNCTION	feeling of uneasiness caused by guilt or regret
COGNITION	mental process by which knowledge is acquired	CONCAVE	curving inward
		CONCEDE	to yield, admit

CONCEPTUALIZE	to envision, imagine	CONSOLIDATE	to combine, incorporate
CONCERTO	musical composition for orchestra and soloist(s)	CONSONANT (adj.)	consistent with, in agreement with
CONCILIATORY	overcoming distrust or hostility	CONSTITUENT	component, part; citizen, voter
CONCORD	agreement	CONSTRAINED	forced, compelled; confined, restrained
CONCUR	to agree		
CONDONE	to pardon or forgive; overlook, justify, or excuse a fault	CONSTRAINT	something that forces or compels; something which restrains or confines
CONDUIT	tube, pipe, or similar passage	CONSTRUE	to explain or interpret
CONFECTION	something sweet to eat	CONSUMMATE (adj.)	accomplished, complete, perfect
CONFISCATE	to appropriate, seize	CONSUMMATE (v.)	to complete, fulfill
CONFLAGRATION	big, destructive fire	CONTEND	to battle, clash; compete
CONFLUENCE	meeting place; meeting of two streams		
CONFOUND	to baffle, perplex	CONTENTIOUS	quarrelsome, disagreeable, belligerent
CONGEAL	to become thick or solid, as a liquid freezing	CONTINENCE	self-control, self-restraint
CONGENIAL	similar in tastes and habits	CONTRAVENE	to contradict, deny, act contrary to
CONGENITAL	existing since birth	CONTRITE	deeply sorrowful and repentant for a wrong
CONGLOMERATE	collected group of varied things	CONTUSION	bruise
CONGRESS	formal meeting or assembly	CONUNDRUM	riddle, puzzle, or problem with no solution
CONGRUITY	correspondence, harmony, agreement	CONVALESCENCE	gradual recovery after an illness
CONJECTURE	speculation, prediction	CONVENE	to meet, come together, assemble
CONJUGAL	pertaining to marriage	CONVENTIONAL	typical, customary, commonplace
CONJURE	to evoke a spirit, cast a spell	CONVEX	curved outward
CONNIVE	to conspire, scheme	CONVIVIAL	sociable; fond of eating, drinking, and people
CONSANGUINEOUS	of the same origin; related by blood		
CONSCIENTIOUS	governed by conscience; careful and thorough	CONVOKE	to call together, summon
		CONVOLUTED	twisted, complicated, involved
CONSECRATE	to declare sacred; dedicate to a goal	COPIOUS	abundant, plentiful
CONSENSUS	unanimity, agreement of opinion or attitude	COQUETTE	woman who flirts
CONSIGN	to commit, entrust	CORPOREAL	having to do with the body; tangible, material
CONSOLATION	something providing comfort or solace for a loss or hardship	CORPULENCE	obesity, fatness, bulkiness

CORRELATION	association, mutual relation of two or more things	CULPABLE	guilty, responsible for wrong
CORROBORATE	to confirm, verify	CULPRIT	guilty person
CORRUGATE	to mold in a shape with parallel grooves and ridges	CUMULATIVE	resulting from gradual increase
		CUPIDITY	greed
COSMETIC (adj.)	relating to beauty; affecting the surface of something	CURATOR	caretaker and overseer of an exhibition, esp. in a museum
COSMOGRAPHY	science that deals with the nature of the universe	CURMUDGEON	cranky person
		CURSORY	hastily done, superficial
COSMOPOLITAN	sophisticated, free from local prejudices	CURT	abrupt, blunt
		CURTAIL	to shorten
COSSET	to pamper, treat with great care	CUTLERY	cutting instruments; tableware
COTERIE	small group of persons with a similar purpose	CYGNET	young swan
COUNTENANCE (n.)	facial expression; look of approval or support	CYNIC	person who distrusts the motives of others
COUNTENANCE (v.)	to favor, support	DAUNT	to discourage, intimidate
COUNTERMAND	to annul, cancel, make a contrary order	DEARTH	lack, scarcity, insufficiency
COUNTERVAIL	to counteract, to exert force against	DEBASE	to degrade or lower in quality or stature
COVEN	group of witches	DEBAUCH	to corrupt, seduce from virtue or duty; indulge
COVERT	hidden; secret		
COVET	to desire strongly something possessed by another	DEBILITATE	to weaken, enfeeble
		DEBUNK	to discredit, disprove
CRASS	crude, unrefined	DEBUTANTE	young woman making debut in high society
CRAVEN	cowardly		
CREDENCE	acceptance of something as true or real	DECAPITATE	to behead
		DECATHLON	athletic contest with ten events
CREDIBLE	plausible, believable		
CREDULOUS	gullible, trusting	DECIDUOUS	losing leaves in the fall; short-lived, temporary
CREED	statement of belief or principle		
CRESCENDO	gradual increase in volume of sound	DECLIVITY	downward slope
		DECOROUS	proper, tasteful, socially correct
CRITERION	standard for judging, rule for testing	DECORUM	proper behavior, etiquette
CRYPTIC	puzzling		
CUISINE	characteristic style of cooking	DECRY	to belittle, openly condemn
CULMINATION	climax, final stage	DEFACE	to mar the appearance of, vandalize

DEFAMATORY	slanderous, injurious to the reputation	DENOUNCE	to accuse, blame
DEFENDANT	person required to answer a legal action or suit	DENUDE	to make bare, uncover, undress
DEFERENTIAL	respectful and polite in a submissive way	DENUNCIATION	public condemnation
		DEPICT	to describe, represent
DEFILE	to dirty, spoil; to disgrace, dishonor	DEPLETE	to use up, exhaust
DEFINITIVE	clear-cut, explicit or decisive	DEPLORE	to express or feel disapproval of; regret strongly
DEFLATION	decrease, depreciation	DEPLOY	to spread out strategically over an area
DEFORM	to disfigure, distort	DEPOSE	to remove from a high position, as from a throne
DEFT	skillful, dexterous		
DEFUNCT	no longer existing, dead, extinct	DEPRAVITY	sinfulness, moral corruption
DELECTABLE	appetizing, delicious	DEPRECATE	to belittle, disparage
DELEGATE (v.)	to give powers to another	DEPRECIATE	to lose value gradually
DELETERIOUS	harmful, destructive, detrimental	DERIDE	to mock, ridicule, make fun of
DELINEATION	depiction, representation	DERIVATIVE	copied or adapted; not original
DELTA	tidal deposit at the mouth of a river	DERIVE	to originate; take from a certain source
DELUGE (n.)	flood	DEROGATE	to belittle, disparage
DELUGE (v.)	to submerge, overwhelm	DESECRATE	to abuse something sacred
DEMAGOGUE	leader, rabble-rouser, usually using appeals to emotion or prejudice	DESICCATE	to dry completely, dehydrate
		DESIST	to stop doing something
DEMARCATION	borderline; act of defining or marking a boundary or distinction	DESPONDENT	feeling discouraged and dejected
		DESPOT	tyrannical ruler
DEMEAN	to degrade, humiliate, humble	DESTITUTE	very poor, poverty-stricken
DEMOGRAPHICS	data relating to study of human population	DESULTORY	at random, rambling, unmethodical
DEMOTE	to reduce to a lower grade or rank	DETER	to discourage; prevent from happening
DEMOTION	lowering in rank or grade	DETERMINATE	having defined limits; conclusive
DEMUR	to express doubts or objections	DETRIMENTAL	causing harm or injury
		DEVIATE	to stray, wander
DEMYSTIFY	to remove mystery from, clarify	DEVIATION	departure, exception, anomaly
DENIGRATE	to slur or blacken someone's reputation	DEVOID	totally lacking
		DEVOUT	deeply religious

DEXTEROUS	skilled physically or mentally	DISCREDITED	disbelieved, discounted; disgraced, dishonored
DIABOLICAL	fiendish; wicked	DISCREPANCY	difference between
DIALECT	regional style of speaking	DISCRETIONARY	subject to one's own judgment
DIAPHANOUS	allowing light to show through; delicate	DISCURSIVE	wandering from topic to topic
DIATRIBE	bitter verbal attack	DISDAIN	to regard with scorn and contempt
DICHOTOMY	division into two parts	DISDAINFUL	contemptuous, scornful
DICTUM	authoritative statement; popular saying	DISENGAGED	disconnected, disassociated
DIDACTIC	excessively instructive	DISGORGE	to vomit, discharge violently
DIFFERENTIATE	to distinguish between two items	DISHEVELED	untidy, disarranged, unkempt
DIFFIDENCE	shyness, lack of confidence	DISINCLINED	averse, unwilling, lacking desire
DIFFRACT	to cause to separate into parts, esp. light	DISPARAGE	to belittle, speak disrespectfully about
DIFFUSE	widely spread out	DISPARATE	dissimilar, different in kind
DIGRESS	to turn aside; to stray from the main point	DISPARITY	contrast, dissimilarity
DILAPIDATED	in disrepair, run down, neglected	DISPASSIONATE	free from emotion; impartial, unbiased
DILATE	to enlarge, swell, extend	DISPEL	to drive out or scatter
DILATORY	slow, tending to delay	DISPENSE	to distribute, administer
DILUVIAL	relating to a flood	DISPENSE WITH	to suspend the operation of, do without
DIMINUTIVE	small	DISPERSE	to break up, scatter
DIPLOMACY	discretion, tact	DISPIRIT	to dishearten, make dejected
DIRGE	funeral hymn	DISREPUTE	disgrace, dishonor
DISAFFECTED	discontented and disloyal	DISSEMBLE	to pretend, disguise one's motives
DISARRAY	clutter, disorder	DISSEMINATE	to spread far and wide
DISBAND	to break up	DISSENSION	difference of opinion
DISBAR	to expel from legal profession	DISSIPATE	to scatter; to pursue pleasure to excess
DISBURSE	to pay out	DISSOCIATE	to separate; remove from an association
DISCERN	to perceive something obscure	DISSONANT	harsh and unpleasant sounding
DISCLAIM	to deny, disavow	DISSUADE	to persuade someone to alter original intentions
DISCLOSE	to confess, divulge		
DISCONCERTING	bewildering, perplexing, slightly disturbing		
DISCORDANT	harsh-sounding, badly out of tune		
DISCREDIT	to dishonor or disgrace		

DISTEND	to swell, inflate, bloat	DURABILITY	strength, sturdiness
DISTRAUGHT	very worried and distressed	DURATION	period of time that something lasts
DISTRUST (n.)	disbelief and suspicion	DURESS	threat of force or intimidation; imprisonment
DITHER (v.)	to move or act confusedly or without clear purpose		
DIURNAL	daily	DYSPEPTIC	suffering from indigestion; gloomy and irritable
DIVINE (v.)	to foretell or know by inspiration	EBB (v.)	to fade away, recede
DIVISIVE	creating disunity or conflict	EBULLIENT	exhilarated, full of enthusiasm and high spirits
DOCILE	tame, willing to be taught	ECLECTIC	selecting from various sources
DOCTRINAIRE	rigidly devoted to theories	ECSTATIC	joyful
DOGGED (adj.)	persistent, stubborn	EDDY	air or wind current
DOGMATIC	rigidly fixed in opinion, opinionated	EDICT	law, command, official public order
DOLEFUL	sad, mournful	EDIFICE	building
DOLT	idiot, dimwit, foolish person	EDIFY	to instruct morally and spiritually
DOMINEER	to rule over something in a tyrannical way	EDITORIALIZE	to express an opinion on an issue
DONOR	benefactor, contributor	EFFACE	to erase or make illegible
DORMANT	at rest, inactive, in suspended animation	EFFERVESCENT	bubbly, lively
DOTARD	senile old person	EFFICACIOUS	effective, efficient
DOTING	excessively fond, loving to excess	EFFIGY	stuffed doll; likeness of a person
DOUR	sullen and gloomy; stern and severe	EFFLUVIA	outpouring of gases or vapors
DOWRY	money or property given by a bride to her husband	EFFRONTERY	impudent boldness; audacity
		EFFULGENT	brilliantly shining
DRAFT (v.)	to plan, outline; to recruit, conscript	EFFUSIVE	expressing emotion without restraint
DRIVEL	stupid talk; slobber	EGOCENTRIC	acting as if things are centered around oneself
DROLL	amusing in a wry, subtle way		
DROSS	waste produced during metal smelting; garbage	EGREGIOUS	conspicuously bad
		EGRESS	exit
		ELATION	exhilaration, joy
DULCET	pleasant sounding, soothing to the ear	ELEGY	mournful poem, usually about the dead
DUPE (v.)	to deceive, trick	ELICIT	to draw out, provoke
DUPE (n.)	fool, pawn	ELOQUENCE	fluent and effective speech
DUPLICITY	deception, dishonesty, double-dealing		

ELUCIDATE	to explain, clarify
EMACIATED	skinny, scrawny, gaunt, esp. from hunger
EMANCIPATE	to set free, liberate
EMBELLISH	to ornament, make attractive with decoration or details; add details to a statement
EMBEZZLE	to steal money in violation of a trust
EMBROIL	to involve in; cause to fall into disorder
EMEND	to correct a text
EMINENT	celebrated, distinguished; outstanding, towering
EMOLLIENT	having soothing qualities, especially for skin
EMOTIVE	appealing to or expressing emotion
EMPATHY	identification with another's feelings
EMULATE	to copy, imitate
ENCIPHER	to translate a message into code
ENCORE	additional performance, often demanded by audience
ENCUMBER	to hinder, burden, restrict motion
ENDEMIC	belonging to a particular area, inherent
ENDURANCE	ability to withstand hardships
ENERVATE	to weaken, sap strength from
ENGENDER	to produce, cause, bring about
ENIGMATIC	puzzling, inexplicable
ENJOIN	to urge, order, command; forbid or prohibit, as by judicial order
ENMITY	hostility, antagonism, ill-will
ENNUI	boredom, lack of interest and energy
ENORMITY	state of being gigantic or terrible

ENSCONCE	to settle comfortably into a place
ENSHROUD	to cover, enclose with a dark cover
ENTAIL	to involve as a necessary result, necessitate
ENTHRALL	to captivate, enchant, enslave
ENTITY	something with its own existence or form
ENTOMOLOGIST	scientist who studies insects
ENTREAT	to plead, beg
ENUMERATE	to count, list, itemize
ENUNCIATE	to pronounce clearly
EPHEMERAL	momentary, transient, fleeting
EPICURE	person with refined taste in food and wine
EPIGRAM	short, witty saying or poem
EPIGRAPH	quotation at the beginning of a literary work
EPILOGUE	concluding section of a literary work
EPITOME	representative of an entire group; summary
EPOCHAL	very significant or influential; defining an epoch or time-period
EQUANIMITY	calmness, composure
EQUESTRIAN (n.)	one who rides on horseback
EQUINE	relating to horses
EQUIVOCAL	ambiguous, open to two interpretations
EQUIVOCATE	to use vague or ambiguous language intentionally
ERADICATE	to erase or wipe out
ERRANT	straying, mistaken, roving
ERUDITE	learned, scholarly
ESCHEW	to abstain from, avoid
ESOTERIC	understood only by a learned few
ESPOUSE	to support or advocate; to marry

ESTRANGE	to alienate, keep at a distance	EXHUME	to remove from a grave; uncover a secret
ETHEREAL	not earthly, spiritual, delicate	EXIGENT	urgent; excessively demanding
ETHOS	beliefs or character of a group	EXONERATE	to clear of blame
ETYMOLOGY	origin and history of a word; study of words	EXORBITANT	extravagant, greater than reasonable
EULOGY	high praise, often in a public speech	EXORCISE	to expel evil spirits
EUPHEMISM	use of an inoffensive word or phrase in place of a more distasteful one	EXOTIC	foreign; romantic, excitingly strange
EUPHONY	pleasant, harmonious sound	EXPANSIVE	sweeping, comprehensive; tending to expand
EUPHORIA	feeling of well-being or happiness	EXPATRIATE (n.)	one who lives outside one's native land
EURYTHMICS	art of harmonious bodily movement	EXPATRIATE (v.)	to drive someone from his/her native land
EUTHANASIA	mercy-killing; intentional, easy, and painless death	EXPEDIENT (adj.)	convenient, efficient, practical
EVADE	to avoid, dodge	EXPIATE	to atone for, make amends for
EVANESCENT	momentary, transitory, short-lived	EXPIRE	to come to an end; die; breathe out
EVICT	to put out or force out	EXPLICABLE	capable of being explained
EVINCE	to show clearly, display, signify	EXPLICIT	clearly defined, specific; forthright in expression
EVOKE	to inspire memories; to produce a reaction	EXPLODE	to debunk, disprove; blow up, burst
EXACERBATE	to aggravate, intensify the bad qualities of	EXPONENT	one who champions or advocates
EXASPERATION	irritation	EXPOUND	to elaborate; to expand or increase
EXCERPT (n.)	selection from a book or play	EXPUNGE	to erase, eliminate completely
EXCOMMUNICATE	to bar from membership in the church	EXPURGATE	to censor
EXCRUCIATING	agonizing, intensely painful	EXTEMPORANEOUS	unrehearsed, on the spur of the moment
EXCULPATE	to clear of blame or fault	EXTENUATE	to lessen the seriousness, strength, or effect of
EXECRABLE	utterly detestable	EXTINCTION	end of a living thing or species
EXHILARATION	state of being energetic or filled with happiness	EXTOL	to praise
EXHORT	to urge or incite by strong appeals	EXTORT	to obtain something by threats

EXTRANEOUS	irrelevant, unrelated, unnecessary	FEIGN	to pretend, give a false impression; to invent falsely
EXTREMITY	outermost or farthest point	FEISTY	excitable, easily drawn into quarrels
EXTRICATE	to free from, disentangle, free	FELICITOUS	suitable, appropriate; well-spoken
EXTRINSIC	not inherent or essential, coming from without	FELL (v.)	to chop, cut down
EXUBERANT	lively, happy, and full of good spirits	FERVID	passionate, intense zealous
		FETID	foul-smelling, putrid
EXUDE	to give off, ooze	FETTER	to bind, chain, confine
EXULT	to rejoice	FIASCO	disaster, utter failure
FABRICATE	to make or devise; construct	FICTIVE	fictional, imaginary
FABRICATED	constructed, invented; faked, falsified	FIDELITY	loyalty
		FILCH	to steal
FACADE	face, front; mask, superficial appearance	FILIBUSTER	use of obstructive tactics in a legislative assembly to prevent adoption of a measure
FACILE	very easy		
FACILITATE	to aid, assist		
FACILITY	aptitude, ease in doing something	FINICKY	fussy, difficult to please
		FISSION	process of splitting into two parts
FALLACIOUS	wrong, unsound, illogical	FITFUL	intermittent, irregular
FALLOW	uncultivated, unused	FLACCID	limp, flabby, weak
FANATICISM	extreme devotion to a cause	FLAGRANT	outrageous, shameless
FARCICAL	absurd, ludicrous	FLAMBOYANT	flashy, garish; exciting, dazzling
FASTIDIOUS	careful with details	FLAMMABLE	combustible, being easily burned
FATHOM (v.)	to measure the depth of, gauge	FLAUNT	to show off
FATUOUS	stupid; foolishly self-satisfied	FLEDGLING	young bird just learning to fly; beginner, novice
FAULT	break in a rock formation; mistake or error		
FAWN (v.)	to flatter excessively, seek the favor of	FLORA	plants
		FLORID	gaudy, extremely ornate; ruddy, flushed
FAZE	to bother, upset, or disconcert	FLOUNDER	to falter, waver; to muddle, struggle
FEASIBLE	possible, capable of being done	FLOUT	to treat contemptuously, scorn
FECKLESS	ineffective, careless, irresponsible	FLUCTUATE	to alternate, waver
		FODDER	raw material; feed for animals
FECUND	fertile, fruitful, productive	FOIBLE	minor weakness or character flaw
FEDERATION	union of organizations; union of several states, each of which retains local power	FOIL (v.)	to defeat, frustrate
		FOLIATE	to grow, sprout leaves

FOMENT	to arouse or incite	FRAUGHT	full of, accompanied by
FORBEARANCE	patience, restraint, leniency	FRENETIC	wildly frantic, frenzied, hectic
FORD (v.)	to cross a body of water at a shallow place	FRENZIED	feverishly fast, hectic, and confused
FOREBODING	dark sense of evil to come	FRIVOLOUS	petty, trivial; flippant, silly
FORECLOSE	to rule out; to seize debtor's property for lack of payments	FROND	leaf
		FRUGAL	thrifty; cheap
FORENSIC	relating to legal proceedings; relating to debates	FULSOME	excessive, overdone, sickeningly abundant
FORENSICS	study of argumentation and debate	FUNEREAL	mournful, appropriate to a funeral
FORESTALL	to prevent, delay; anticipate	FURTIVE	secret, stealthy
FORETHOUGHT	anticipation, foresight	FUSION	process of merging things into one
FORGO	to go without, refrain from	GALL (n.)	bitterness; careless nerve
FORLORN	dreary, deserted; unhappy; hopeless, despairing	GALL (v.)	to exasperate and irritate
FORMULATE	to conceive, devise; to draft, plan; to express, state	GAMBOL	to dance or skip around playfully
		GAME (adj.)	courageous
FORSAKE	to abandon, withdraw from	GARGANTUAN	giant, tremendous
		GARNER	to gather and store
FORSWEAR	to repudiate, renounce, disclaim, reject	GARRULOUS	very talkative
FORTE (n.)	strong point, something a person does well	GAUNT	thin and bony
		GAVEL	mallet used for commanding attention
FORTUITOUS	happening by luck, fortunate	GENRE	type, class, category
FOSTER (v.)	to nourish, cultivate, promote	GERMINATE	to begin to grow (used of a seed or idea)
FOUNDATION	groundwork, support; institution established by donation to aid a certain cause	GESTATION	growth process from conception to birth
		GIBE (v.)	to make heckling, taunting remarks
FOUNDER (v.)	to fall helplessly; sink	GIRTH	distance around something
FRACAS	noisy dispute	GLIB	fluent in an insincere manner; off-hand, casual
FRACTIOUS	unruly, rebellious	
FRAGMENTATION	division, separation into parts, disorganization	GLOBAL	involving the entire world; relating to a whole
FRANK	honest and straightforward	GLOWER	to glare, stare angrily and intensely
FRAUD	deception, hoax	GLUTTONY	eating and drinking to excess
FRAUDULENT	deceitful, dishonest, unethical	GNARL	to make knotted, deform

GNOSTIC	having to do with knowledge		HARROWING	extremely distressing, terrifying
GOAD	to prod or urge		HASTEN	to hurry, to speed up
GRADATION	process occurring by regular degrees or stages; variation in color		HAUGHTY	arrogant and condescending
GRANDILOQUENCE	pompous talk, fancy but meaningless language		HEADSTRONG	reckless; insisting on one's own way
			HEATHEN	pagan; uncivilized and irreligious
GRANDIOSE	magnificent and imposing; exaggerated and pretentious		HECTIC	hasty, hurried, confused
GRANULAR	having a grainy texture		HEDONISM	pursuit of pleasure as a goal
GRASP (v.)	to perceive and understand; to hold securely		HEGEMONY	leadership, domination, usually by a country
GRATIS	free, costing nothing		HEIGHTEN	to raise
GRATUITOUS	free, voluntary; unnecessary and unjustified		HEINOUS	shocking, wicked, terrible
GRATUITY	something given voluntarily, tip		HEMICYCLE	semicircular form or structure
GREGARIOUS	outgoing, sociable		HEMORRHAGE (n.)	heavy bleeding
GRIEVOUS	causing grief or sorrow; serious and distressing		HEMORRHAGE (v.)	to bleed heavily; to lose something vital at a rapid rate
GRIMACE	facial expression showing pain or disgust		HERETICAL	opposed to an established religious orthodoxy
GRIMY	dirty, filthy		HERMETIC	tightly sealed
GROSS (adj.)	obscene; blatant, flagrant		HETERODOX	unorthodox, not widely accepted
GROSS (n.)	total before deductions		HETEROGENEOUS	composed of unlike parts, different, diverse
GROVEL	to humble oneself in a demeaning way		HEW	to cut with an ax
GUILE	trickery, deception		HIATUS	break, interruption, vacation
GULLIBLE	easily deceived			
GUSTATORY	relating to sense of taste		HIDEBOUND	excessively rigid; dry and stiff
HABITAT	dwelling place		HINDSIGHT	perception of events after they happen
HACKNEYED	worn out by over-use		HINTERLAND	wilderness
HALLOW	to make holy; treat as sacred		HOARY	very old; whitish or gray from age
HAMLET	small village		HOLISTIC	emphasizing importance of the whole and interdependence of its parts
HAPLESS	unfortunate, having bad luck			
HARBINGER	precursor, sign of something to come		HOLOCAUST	widespread destruction, usually by fire
HARDY	robust, vigorous			

HOMAGE	public honor and respect	IMMACULATE	spotless; free from error
HOMOGENEOUS	composed of identical parts	IMMATERIAL	extraneous, inconsequential, nonessential; not consisting of matter
HOMONYM	word identical in pronunciation but different in meaning	IMMENSE	enormous, huge
HONE	to sharpen	IMMERSE	to bathe, dip; to engross, preoccupy
HONOR (v.)	to praise, glorify, pay tribute to	IMMOBILE	not moveable; still
HUMANE	merciful, kindly	IMMUNE	exempt; protected from harm or disease; unresponsive to
HUSBAND (v.)	to farm; manage carefully and thriftily	IMMUNOLOGICAL	relating to immune system
HUTCH	pen or coop for animals; shack, shanty	IMMUTABLE	unchangeable, invariable
HYDRATE	to add water to	IMPAIR	to damage, injure
HYGIENIC	clean, sanitary	IMPASSE	blocked path, dilemma with no solution
HYMN	religious song, usually of praise or thanks	IMPASSIONED	with passion
HYPERBOLE	purposeful exaggeration for effect	IMPASSIVE	showing no emotion
HYPERVENTILATE	to breath abnormally fast	IMPEACH	to charge with misdeeds in public office; accuse
HYPOCHONDRIA	unfounded belief that one is often ill	IMPECCABLE	flawless, without fault
HYPOCRITE	person claiming beliefs or virtues he or she doesn't really possess	IMPECUNIOUS	poor, having no money
HYPOTHERMIA	abnormally low body temperature	IMPEDIMENT	barrier, obstacle; speech disorder
HYPOTHESIS	assumption subject to proof	IMPERATIVE	essential; mandatory
HYPOTHETICAL	theoretical, speculative	IMPERIOUS	arrogantly self-assured, domineering, overbearing
ICONOCLAST	one who attacks traditional beliefs	IMPERTINENT	rude
IDEALISM	pursuit of noble goals	IMPERTURBABLE	not capable of being disturbed
IDIOSYNCRASY	peculiarity of temperament, eccentricity	IMPERVIOUS	impossible to penetrate; incapable of being affected
IGNOBLE	dishonorable, not noble in character	IMPETUOUS	quick to act without thinking
IGNOMINIOUS	disgraceful and dishonorable	IMPIOUS	not devout in religion
ILK	type or kind	IMPLACABLE	inflexible, incapable of being pleased
ILLICIT	illegal, improper	IMPLANT	to set securely or deeply; to instill
ILLIMITABLE	limitless	IMPLAUSIBLE	improbable, inconceivable
ILLUSORY	unreal, deceptive	IMPLICATE	to involve in a crime, incriminate
ILLUSTRIOUS	famous, renowned		
IMBUE	to infuse; dye, wet, moisten		

IMPLICIT	implied, not directly expressed
IMPORTUNE	to ask repeatedly, beg
IMPOSE	to inflict, force upon
IMPOSING	dignified, grand
IMPOTENT	powerless, ineffective, lacking strength
IMPOUND	to seize and confine
IMPOVERISH	to make poor or bankrupt
IMPRECATION	curse
IMPREGNABLE	totally safe from attack, able to resist defeat
IMPRESSIONABLE	easily influenced or affected
IMPROMPTU	spontaneous, without rehearsal
IMPROVIDENT	without planning or foresight, negligent
IMPUDENT	arrogant and rude
IMPUGN	to call into question, attack verbally
IMPULSE	sudden tendency, inclination
IMPULSIVE	spontaneous, unpredictable
INADVERTENTLY	unintentionally
INANE	foolish, silly, lacking significance
INAUGURATE	to begin or start officially; to induct into office
INCANDESCENT	shining brightly
INCARCERATE	to put in jail; to confine
INCARCERATION	imprisonment
INCARNADINE	blood-red in color
INCARNATE	having bodily form
INCENDIARY	combustible, flammable, burning easily
INCENSE (v.)	to infuriate, enrage
INCEPTION	beginning
INCESSANT	continuous, never ceasing
INCHOATE	just begun; disorganized

INCIPIENT	beginning to exist or appear; in an initial stage
INCISIVE	perceptive, penetrating
INCLINATION	tendency toward
INCLUSIVE	comprehensive, all-encompassing
INCOGNITO	in disguise, concealing one's identity
INCONCEIVABLE	impossible, unthinkable
INCONSEQUENTIAL	unimportant, trivial
INCONTROVERTIBLE	unquestionable, beyond dispute
INCORRIGIBLE	incapable of being corrected
INCREDULOUS	skeptical, doubtful
INCULCATE	to teach, impress in the mind
INCULPATE	to blame, charge with a crime
INCUMBENT (adj.)	holding a specified office, often political; required, obligatory
INCURSION	sudden invasion
INDEFATIGABLE	never tired
INDEFENSIBLE	inexcusable, unforgivable
INDELIBLE	permanent, not erasable
INDICATIVE	showing or pointing out, suggestive of
INDICT	to accuse formally, charge with a crime
INDIGENOUS	native, occurring naturally in an area
INDIGENT	very poor
INDIGNANT	angry, incensed, offended
INDOLENT	habitually lazy, idle
INDOMITABLE	fearless, unconquerable
INDUBITABLE	unquestionable
INDUCE	to persuade; bring about
INDUCT	to place ceremoniously in office
INDULGE	to give in to a craving or desire

INDUSTRY	business or trade; diligence, energy	INJECT	to force into; to introduce into conversation
INEBRIATED	drunk, intoxicated	INJUNCTION	command, order
INEPT	clumsy, awkward	INKLING	hint; vague idea
INERT	unable to move, tending to inactivity	INNATE	natural, inborn
INESTIMABLE	too great to be estimated	INNATENESS	state of being natural or inborn
INEVITABLE	certain, unavoidable	INNOCUOUS	harmless; inoffensive
INEXORABLE	inflexible, unyielding	INNOVATE	to invent, modernize, revolutionize
INEXTRICABLE	incapable of being disentangled	INNUENDO	indirect and subtle criticism, insinuation
INFALLIBLE	incapable of making a mistake	INNUMERABLE	too many to be counted
INFAMY	reputation for bad deeds	INOFFENSIVE	harmless, innocent
INFANTILE	childish, immature	INOPERABLE	not operable; incurable by surgery
INFATUATED	strongly or foolishly attached to, inspired with foolish passion, overly in love	INQUEST	investigation; court or legal proceeding
INFER	to conclude, deduce	INSATIABLE	never satisfied
INFILTRATE	to pass secretly into enemy territory	INSCRUTABLE	impossible to understand fully
INFINITESIMAL	extremely tiny	INSENTIENT	unfeeling, unconscious
INFIRMITY	disease, ailment	INSIDIOUS	sly, treacherous, devious
INFRINGE	to encroach, trespass; to transgress, violate	INSINUATE	to suggest, say indirectly, imply
INFURIATE	to anger, provoke, outrage	INSIPID	bland, lacking flavor; lacking excitement
INFURIATING	provoking anger or outrage	INSOLENT	insulting and arrogant
INGENIOUS	original, clever, inventive	INSOLUBLE	not able to be solved or explained
INGENUOUS	straightforward, open; naive and unsophisticated	INSOLVENT	bankrupt, unable to pay one's debts
INGRATE	ungrateful person	INSTIGATE	to incite, urge, agitate
INGRATIATE	to bring oneself purposely into another's good graces	INSUBSTANTIAL	modest, insignificant
INGRESS	entrance	INSULAR	isolated, detached
INHIBIT	to hold back, prevent, restrain	INSUPERABLE	insurmountable, unconquerable
INIMICAL	hostile, unfriendly	INSURGENT (adj.)	rebellious, insubordinate
INIQUITY	sin, evil act	INSURRECTION	rebellion
INITIATE	to begin, introduce; to enlist, induct	INTEGRAL	central, indispensable
		INTEGRITY	decency, honest; wholeness
		INTEMPERATE	not moderate
		INTER	to bury

INTERDICT	to forbid, prohibit	INVIDIOUS	likely to provoke ill-will, offensive
INTERJECT	to interpose, insert	INVINCIBLE	invulnerable, unbeatable
INTERLOCUTOR	someone taking part in a dialogue	INVIOLABLE	safe from violation or assault
INTERLOPER	trespasser; meddler in others' affairs	INVOKE	to call upon, request help
INTERMINABLE	endless	IOTA	very tiny amount
INTERMITTENT	starting and stopping	IRASCIBLE	easily angered
INTERNECINE	deadly to both sides	IRIDESCENT	showing many colors
INTERPOLATE	to insert; change by adding new words or material	IRRESOLVABLE	unable to be resolved; not analyzable
INTERPOSE	to insert; to intervene	IRREVERENT	disrespectful
INTERREGNUM	interval between reigns	IRREVOCABLE	conclusive, irreversible
INTERROGATE	to question formally	ITINERANT	wandering from place to place, unsettled
INTERSECT	to divide by passing through or across	ITINERARY	route of a traveler's journey
INTERSPERSE	to distribute among, mix with	JADED	tired by excess or over-use; slightly cynical
INTIMATION	clue, suggestion	JANGLING	clashing, jarring; harshly unpleasant (in sound)
INTRACTABLE	not easily managed		
INTRAMURAL	within an institution like a school	JARGON	nonsensical talk; specialized language
INTRANSIGENT	uncompromising, re-fusing to be reconciled	JAUNDICE	yellowish discolor-ation of skin
INTREPID	fearless	JAUNDICED	affected by jaundice; prejudiced or embit-tered
INTRINSIC	inherent, internal		
INTROSPECTIVE	contemplating one's own thoughts and feelings	JETTISON	to cast off, throw cargo overboard
INTROVERT	someone given to self-analysis	JINGOISM	belligerent support of one's country
INTRUSION	trespass, invasion of another's privacy	JOCULAR	jovial, playful, humorous
INTUITIVE	instinctive, untaught	JUBILEE	special anniversary
INUNDATE	to cover with water; overwhelm	JUDICIOUS	sensible, showing good judgment
INURE	to harden; accustom; become used to	JUGGERNAUT	huge force destroying everything in its path
INVALIDATE	to negate or nullify	JUNCTURE	point where two things are joined
INVECTIVE	verbal abuse		
INVESTITURE	ceremony conferring authority	JURISPRUDENCE	philosophy of law
		JUXTAPOSITION	side-by-side placement
INVETERATE	confirmed, long-standing, deeply rooted	KEEN	having a sharp edge; intellectually sharp, perceptive

KERNEL	innermost, essential part; seed grain, often in a shell
KEYNOTE	note or tone on which a musical key is founded; main idea of a speech, program, etc.
KINDLE	to set fire to or ignite; excite or inspire
KINETIC	relating to motion; characterized by movement
KNELL	sound of a funeral bell; omen of death or failure
KUDOS	fame, glory, honor
LABYRINTH	maze
LACERATION	cut or wound
LACHRYMOSE	tearful
LACKADAISICAL	idle, lazy; apathetic, indifferent
LACONIC	using few words
LAGGARD	dawdler, loafer, lazy person
LAMENT (v.)	to deplore, grieve
LAMPOON (v.)	to attack with satire, mock harshly
LANGUID	lacking energy, indifferent, slow
LAP (v.)	to drink using the tongue; to wash against
LAPIDARY	relating to precious stones
LARCENY	theft of property
LARDER	place where food is stored
LARGESS	generosity; gift
LARYNX	organ containing vocal cords
LASSITUDE	lethargy, sluggishness
LATENT	present but hidden; potential
LAUDABLE	deserving of praise
LAXITY	carelessness
LEERY	suspicious
LEGERDEMAIN	trickery
LEGIBLE	readable

LEGISLATE	to decree, mandate, make laws
LENIENT	easygoing, permissive
LETHARGY	indifferent inactivity
LEVITATE	to rise in the air or cause to rise
LEVITY	humor, frivolity, gaiety
LEXICON	dictionary, list of words
LIBERAL (adj.)	tolerant, broad-minded; generous, lavish
LIBERATION	freedom, emancipation
LIBERTARIAN	one who believes in unrestricted freedom
LIBERTINE	one without moral restraint
LICENTIOUS	immoral; unrestrained by society
LIEN	right to possess and sell the property of a debtor
LIMPID	clear, transparent
LINEAGE	ancestry
LINGUISTICS	study of language
LINIMENT	medicinal liquid used externally to ease pain
LIONIZE	to treat as a celebrity
LISSOME	easily flexed, limber, agile
LISTLESS	lacking energy and enthusiasm
LITERATE	able to read and write; well-read and educated
LITHE	moving and bending with ease; graceful
LITIGATION	lawsuit
LIVID	discolored from a bruise; reddened with anger
LOATHE	to abhor, despise, hate
LOCOMOTION	movement from place to place
LOGO	corporate symbol
LOITER	to stand around idly
LOQUACIOUS	talkative

LOW (v.)	to make a sound like a cow, moo	MALFUNCTION (v.)	to fail to work
LUCID	clear and easily understood	MALFUNCTION (n.)	breakdown, failure
		MALICE	animosity, spite, hatred
LUDICROUS	laughable, ridiculous	MALINGER	to evade responsibility by pretending to be ill
LUGUBRIOUS	sorrowful, mournful		
LUMBER (v.)	to move slowly and awkwardly	MALNUTRITION	under-nourishment
		MALODOROUS	foul-smelling
LUMINARY	bright object; celebrity; source of inspiration	MANDATORY	necessary, required
		MANIFEST (adj.)	obvious
LUMINOUS	bright, brilliant, glowing	MANIFOLD	diverse, varied, comprised of many parts
LUNAR	relating to the moon		
LURID	harshly shocking, sensational; glowing	MANNERED	artificial or stilted in character
		MANUAL (adj.)	hand-operated; physical
LURK	to prowl, sneak	MAR	to damage, deface; spoil
LUSCIOUS	very good-tasting		
LUXURIANCE	elegance, lavishness	MARGINAL	barely sufficient
LYRICAL	suitable for poetry and song; expressing feeling	MARITIME	relating to the sea or sailing
		MARTIAL	war-like, pertaining to the military
MACHINATION	plot or scheme		
MACROBIOTICS	art of prolonging life by special diet of organic non-meat substances	MARTINET	strict disciplinarian, one who rigidly follows rules
		MARTYR	person dying for his/her beliefs
MACROCOSM	system regarded as an entity with subsystems		
		MASOCHIST	one who enjoys pain or humiliation
MAELSTROM	whirlpool; turmoil; agitated state of mind	MASQUERADE	disguise; action that conceals the truth
MAGNANIMOUS	generous, noble in spirit		
		MATERIALISM	preoccupation with material things
MAGNATE	powerful or influential person	MATRICULATE	to enroll as a member of a college or university
MAGNITUDE	extent, greatness of size		
		MATRILINEAL	tracing ancestry through mother's line rather than father's
MALADROIT	clumsy, tactless		
MALADY	illness		
MALAPROPISM	humorous misuse of a word	MAUDLIN	overly sentimental
		MAWKISH	sickeningly sentimental
MALCONTENT	discontented person, one who holds a grudge	MEDDLER	person interfering in others' affairs
		MEDIEVAL	relating to the Middle Ages
MALEDICTION	curse		
MALEFACTOR	evil-doer; culprit		
MALEVOLENT	ill-willed; causing evil or harm to others	MEGALITH	huge stone used in prehistoric structures

MEGALOMANIA	mental state with delusions of wealth and power	MISANTHROPE	person who hates human beings
MELANCHOLY	sadness, depression	MISAPPREHEND	to misunderstand, fail to know
MELODY	pleasing musical sounds; tune	MISCONSTRUE	to misunderstand, fail to discover
MENAGERIE	various animals kept together for exhibition	MISERLINESS	extreme stinginess
MENDACIOUS	dishonest	MISGIVING	apprehension, doubt, sense of foreboding
MENDICANT	beggar	MISHAP	accident; misfortune
MENTOR	experienced teacher and wise adviser	MISNOMER	an incorrect name or designation
MERCENARY (n.)	soldier for hire in foreign countries	MISSIVE	note or letter
MERCENARY (adj.)	motivated only by greed	MITIGATE	to soften, or make milder
MERCURIAL	quick, shrewd, and unpredictable	MNEMONIC	relating to memory; designed to assist memory
MERETRICIOUS	gaudy, falsely attractive	MOBILITY	ease of movement
MERIDIAN	circle passing through the two poles of the earth	MOCK (v.)	to deride, ridicule
		MODERATE (adj.)	reasonable, not extreme
MERITORIOUS	deserving reward or praise	MODERATE (v.)	to make less excessive, restrain; regulate
METAMORPHOSIS	change, transformation	MOLLIFY	to calm or make less severe
METAPHOR	figure of speech comparing two different things	MOLLUSK	sea animal with soft body
METICULOUS	extremely careful, fastidious, painstaking	MOLT (v.)	to shed hair, skin, or an outer layer periodically
METRONOME	time-keeping device used in music	MONASTIC	extremely plain or secluded, as in a monastery
METTLE	courageousness; endurance		
MICROBE	microorganism	MONOCHROMATIC	having one color
MICROCOSM	tiny system used as analogy for larger system	MONOGAMY	custom of marriage to one person at a time
		MONOLITH	large block of stone
MIGRATORY	wandering from place to place with the seasons	MONOLOGUE	dramatic speech performed by one actor
		MONTAGE	composite picture
MILITATE	to operate against, work against	MOOT	debatable; previously decided
MINIMAL	smallest in amount, least possible	MORBID	gruesome; relating to disease; abnormally gloomy
MINUSCULE	very small	MORES	customs or manners
MIRTH	frivolity, gaiety, laughter	MORIBUND	dying, decaying

MOROSE	gloomy, sullen, or surly	NOCTURNAL	pertaining to night; active at night
MORSEL	small bit of food	NOISOME	stinking, putrid
MOTE	small particle, speck	NOMADIC	moving from place to place
MOTLEY	many-colored; composed of diverse parts	NOMENCLATURE	terms used in a particular science or discipline
MOTTLE	to mark with spots		
MULTIFACETED	having many parts, many-sided	NOMINAL	existing in name only; negligible
MULTIFARIOUS	diverse	NON SEQUITUR	conclusion not following from apparent evidence
MUNDANE	worldly; commonplace		
MUNIFICENT	generous	NONDESCRIPT	lacking interesting or distinctive qualities; dull
MUNITIONS	ammunition		
MUTABILITY	changeability		
MYOPIC	near-sighted	NOTORIETY	fame; unfavorable fame
MYRIAD	immense number, multitude	NOVICE	apprentice, beginner
NADIR	lowest point	NOVITIATE	beginner or novice
NARRATIVE	account, story	NOXIOUS	harmful, unwholesome
NASCENT	starting to develop, coming into existence	NUANCE	shade of meaning
NATAL	relating to birth	NULLIFY	to make legally invalid; to counteract the effect of
NEBULOUS	vague, cloudy		
NECROMANCY	black magic	NUMISMATICS	coin collecting
NEFARIOUS	vicious, evil	NUPTIAL	relating to marriage
NEGLIGENT	careless, inattentive	NUTRITIVE	relating to nutrition or health
NEGLIGIBLE	not worth considering		
NEOLOGISM	new word or expression	OBDURATE	stubborn
		OBFUSCATE	to confuse, obscure
NEONATE	newborn child	OBLIQUE	indirect, evasive; misleading, devious
NEOPHYTE	novice, beginner		
NETHER	located under or below	OBLITERATE	demolish completely, wipe out
NETTLE (v.)	to irritate		
NEUTRALITY	disinterest, impartiality	OBLIVIOUS	unaware, inattentive
		OBSCURE (adj.)	dim, unclear; not well-known
NEUTRALIZE	to balance, offset		
NICETY	elegant or delicate feature; minute distinction	OBSCURITY	place or thing that's hard to perceive
		OBSEQUIOUS	overly submissive, brown-nosing
NICHE	recess in a wall; best position for something	OBSEQUY	funeral ceremony
NIHILISM	belief that existence and all traditional values are meaningless	OBSESSIVE	preoccupying, all-consuming
		OBSOLETE	no longer in use

OBSTINATE	stubborn	ORNITHOLOGIST	scientist who studies birds
OBSTREPEROUS	troublesome, boisterous, unruly	OSCILLATE	to move back and forth
OBTRUSIVE	pushy, too conspicuous	OSSIFY	to turn to bone; to become rigid
OBTUSE	insensitive, stupid, dull	OSTENSIBLE	apparent
OBVIATE	to make unnecessary; to anticipate and prevent	OSTENTATIOUS	showy
OCCLUDE	to shut, block	OSTRACISM	exclusion, temporary banishment
ODIOUS	hateful, contemptible	OUSTER	expulsion, ejection
OFFICIOUS	too helpful, meddlesome	OVERSTATE	to embellish, exaggerate
OFFSHOOT	branch	OVERTURE	musical introduction; proposal, offer
OMINOUS	menacing, threatening, indicating misfortune	OVERWROUGHT	agitated, overdone
OMNIPOTENT	having unlimited power	PACIFIC	calm, peaceful
OMNISCIENT	having infinite knowledge	PACIFIST	one opposed to war
OMNIVOROUS	eating everything; absorbing everything	PACIFY	to restore calm, bring peace
ONEROUS	burdensome	PALATIAL	like a palace, magnificent
ONTOLOGY	theory about the nature of existence	PALAVER	idle talk
OPALESCENT	iridescent, displaying colors	PALEONTOLOGY	study of past geological eras through fossil remains
OPAQUE	impervious to light; difficult to understand	PALETTE	board for mixing paints; range of colors
OPERATIVE	functioning, working	PALISADE	fence made up of stakes
OPINE	to express an opinion	PALL (n.)	covering that darkens or obscures; coffin
OPPORTUNE	appropriate, fitting	PALL (v.)	to lose strength or interest
OPPORTUNIST	one who takes advantage of circumstances	PALLIATE	to make less serious, ease
OPPROBRIOUS	disgraceful, contemptuous	PALLID	lacking color or liveliness
OPULENCE	wealth	PALPABLE	obvious, real, tangible
ORACLE	person who foresees the future and gives advice	PALPITATION	trembling, shaking, irregular beating
ORATION	lecture, formal speech	PALTRY	pitifully small or worthless
ORATOR	lecturer, speaker	PANACEA	cure-all
ORB	spherical body; eye	PANACHE	flamboyance, verve
ORCHESTRATE	to arrange music for performance; to coordinate, organize	PANDEMIC	spread over a whole area or country
ORDAIN	to make someone a priest or minister; to order		

PANEGYRIC	elaborate praise; formal hymn of praise	PATRICIDE	murder of one's father
PANOPLY	impressive array	PATRIMONY	inheritance or heritage derived from one's father
PANORAMA	broad view; comprehensive picture	PATRONIZE	to condescend to, disparage; to buy from
PARADIGM	ideal example, model		
PARADOX	contradiction, incongruity; dilemma, puzzle	PAUCITY	scarcity, lack
		PAUPER	very poor person
PARADOXICAL	self-contradictory but true	PAVILION	tent or light building used for shelter or exhibitions
PARAGON	model of excellence or perfection	PECCADILLO	minor sin or offense
PARAMOUNT	supreme, dominant, primary	PECULATION	theft of money or goods
PARAPHRASE	to reword, usually in simpler terms	PEDAGOGUE	teacher
		PEDANT	uninspired, boring academic
PARASITE	person or animal that lives at another's expense	PEDESTRIAN (adj.)	commonplace
PARCH	to dry or shrivel	PEDIATRICIAN	doctor specializing in children and their ailments
PARE	to trim		
PARIAH	outcast	PEDIMENT	triangular gable on a roof or facade
PARITY	equality	PEER (n.)	contemporary, equal, match
PARLEY	discussion, usually between enemies	PEERLESS	unequaled
PAROCHIAL	of limited scope or outlook, provincial	PEJORATIVE	having bad connotations; disparaging
PARODY	humorous imitation	PELLUCID	transparent; translucent; easily understood
PAROLE	conditional release of a prisoner	PENANCE	voluntary suffering to repent for a wrong
PARRY	to ward off or deflect	PENCHANT	inclination
PARSIMONY	stinginess	PENDING (prep.)	during, while awaiting
PARTISAN (n.)	strong supporter	PENITENT	expressing sorrow for sins or offenses, repentant
PARTISAN (adj.)	biased in favor of		
PASTICHE	piece of literature or music imitating other works	PENSIVE	thoughtful
		PENULTIMATE	next to last
PATENT (adj.)	obvious, unconcealed	PENUMBRA	partial shadow
PATENT (n.)	official document giving exclusive right to sell an invention	PENURY	extreme poverty
		PERAMBULATOR	baby carriage
PATERNITY	fatherhood; descent from father's ancestors	PERCIPIENT	discerning, able to perceive
PATHOGENIC	causing disease	PERDITION	complete and utter loss; damnation
PATHOS	pity, compassion		
PATRICIAN	aristocrat	PEREGRINATE	to wander from place to place

PERENNIAL	present throughout the years; persistent
PERFIDIOUS	faithless, disloyal, untrustworthy
PERFUNCTORY	done in a routine way; indifferent
PERIHELION	point in orbit nearest to the sun
PERIPATETIC	moving from place to place
PERJURE	to tell a lie under oath
PERMEABLE	penetrable
PERNICIOUS	very harmful
PERPETUAL	endless, lasting
PERSONIFICATION	act of attributing human qualities to objects or abstract qualities
PERSPICACIOUS	shrewd, astute, keen-witted
PERT	lively and bold
PERTINACIOUS	persistent, stubborn
PERTINENT	applicable, appropriate
PERTURBATION	disturbance
PERUSAL	close examination
PERVERT (v.)	to cause to change in immoral way; to misuse
PESTILENCE	epidemic, plague
PETULANCE	rudeness, peevishness
PHALANX	massed group of soldiers, people, or things
PHILANDERER	pursuer of casual love affairs
PHILANTHROPY	love of humanity; generosity to worthy causes
PHILISTINE	narrow-minded person, someone lacking appreciation for art or culture
PHILOLOGY	study of words
PHLEGMATIC	calm in temperament; sluggish
PHOBIA	anxiety, horror
PHOENIX	mythical, immortal bird which lives for 500 years, burns itself to death, and rises from its ashes

PHONETICS	study of speech sounds
PHONIC	relating to sound
PIETY	devoutness
PILFER	to steal
PILLAGE	to loot, especially during a war
PINNACLE	peak, highest point of development
PIOUS	dedicated, devout, extremely religious
PIQUE	fleeting feeling of hurt pride
PITHY	profound, substantial; concise, succinct, to the point
PITTANCE	meager amount or wage
PLACATE	to soothe or pacify
PLACID	calm
PLAGIARIST	one who steals words or ideas
PLAINTIFF	injured person in a lawsuit
PLAIT	to braid
PLATITUDE	stale, overused expression
PLEBEIAN	crude, vulgar, low-class
PLENITUDE	abundance, plenty
PLETHORA	excess, overabundance
PLIANT	pliable, yielding
PLUCK	to pull strings on musical instrument
PLUCKY	courageous, spunky
PLUMMET	to fall, plunge
PLURALISTIC	including a variety of groups
PLY (v.)	to use diligently; to engage; to join together
PNEUMATIC	relating to air; worked by compressed air
POACH	to steal game or fish; cook in boiling liquid
PODIUM	platform or lectern for orchestra conductors or speakers
POIGNANT	emotionally moving
POLAR	relating to a geographic pole; exhibiting contrast

POLARIZE	to tend towards opposite extremes	PREDATOR	one that preys on others, destroyer, plunderer
POLEMIC	controversy, argument; verbal attack	PREDICAMENT	difficult situation
POLITIC	shrewd and practical, diplomatic	PREDICATE (v.)	to found or base on
POLYGLOT	speaker of many languages	PREDICTIVE	relating to prediction, indicative of the future
PONDEROUS	weighty, heavy, large	PREDILECTION	preference, liking
PONTIFICATE	to speak in a pretentious manner	PREDISPOSITION	tendency, inclination
PORE (v.)	to study closely or meditatively	PREEMINENT	celebrated, distinguished
POROUS	full of holes, permeable to liquids	PREFACE	introduction to a book; introductory remarks to a speech
PORTENT	omen	PREMEDITATE	to consider, plan beforehand
PORTLY	stout, dignified	PREMONITION	forewarning; presentiment
POSIT	to put in position; to suggest an idea	PREPONDERANCE	majority in number; dominance
POSTERIOR	bottom, rear	PREPOSSESSING	attractive, engaging, appealing
POSTERITY	future generations; all of a person's descendants	PREPOSTEROUS	absurd, illogical
POTABLE	drinkable	PRESAGE	to foretell, indicate in advance
POTENTATE	monarch or ruler with great power	PRESCIENT	having foresight
PRAGMATIC	practical; moved by facts rather than abstract ideals	PRESCRIBE	to set down a rule; to recommend a treatment
PRATTLE	meaningless, foolish talk	PRESENTIMENT	premonition, sense of foreboding
PRECARIOUS	uncertain	PRESTIDIGITATION	sleight of hand
PRECEPT	principle; law	PRESUMPTUOUS	rude, improperly bold
PRECIPICE	edge, steep overhang	PRETEXT	excuse, pretended reason
PRECIPITATE (adj.)	sudden and unexpected	PREVALENT	widespread
PRECIPITATE (v.)	to throw down from a height; to cause to happen	PREVARICATE	to lie, evade the truth
		PRIMEVAL	ancient, primitive
PRECIPITOUS	hasty, quickly, with too little caution	PRIMORDIAL	original, existing from the beginning
PRÉCIS	short summary of facts	PRISTINE	untouched, uncorrupted
PRECISION	state of being precise	PRIVATION	lack of usual necessities or comforts
PRECLUDE	to rule out		
PRECOCIOUS	unusually advanced at an early age	PROBITY	honesty, high-mindedness
PRECURSOR	forerunner, predecessor	PROCLIVITY	tendency, inclination

PROCRASTINATOR	one who continually and unjustifiably postpones
PROCURE	to obtain
PRODIGAL	wasteful, extravagant, lavish
PRODIGIOUS	vast, enormous, extraordinary
PROFANE	impure; contrary to religion; sacrilegious
PROFICIENT	expert, skilled in a certain subject
PROFLIGATE	corrupt, degenerate
PROFUSE	lavish, extravagant
PROGENITOR	originator, forefather, ancestor in a direct line
PROGENY	offspring, children
PROGNOSIS	prediction of disease outcome; any prediction
PROGRESSIVE	favoring progress or change; moving forward, going step-by-step
PROLIFERATION	propagation, reproduction; enlargement, expansion
PROLIFIC	productive, fertile
PROLOGUE	introductory section of a literary work or play
PROMONTORY	piece of land or rock higher than its surroundings
PROMULGATE	to make known publicly
PROPENSITY	inclination, tendency
PROPINQUITY	nearness
PROPITIATE	to win over, appease
PROPITIOUS	favorable, advantageous
PROPONENT	advocate, defender, supporter
PROSAIC	relating to prose; dull, commonplace
PROSCRIBE	to condemn; to forbid, outlaw
PROSE	ordinary language used in everyday speech

PROSECUTOR	person who initiates a legal action or suit
PROSELYTIZE	to convert to a particular belief or religion
PROSTRATE	lying face downward, lying flat on ground
PROTAGONIST	main character in a play or story, hero
PROTEAN	readily assuming different forms or characters
PROTESTATION	declaration
PROTOCOL	ceremony and manners observed by diplomats
PROTRACT	to prolong, draw out, extend
PROTRUSION	something that sticks out
PROVINCIAL	rustic, unsophisticated, limited in scope
PROVOCATION	cause, incitement to act or respond
PROWESS	bravery, skill
PROXIMITY	nearness
PROXY	power to act as substitute for another
PRUDE	one who is excessively proper or modest
PRUDENT	careful, cautious
PRURIENT	lustful, exhibiting lewd desires
PRY	to intrude into; force open
PSEUDONYM	pen name; fictitious or borrowed name
PSYCHIC (adj.)	perceptive of non-material, spiritual forces
PUERILE	childish, immature, silly
PUDGY	chubby, overweight
PUGILISM	boxing
PUGNACIOUS	quarrelsome, eager and ready to fight
PULCHRITUDE	beauty
PULVERIZE	to pound, crush, or grind into powder; destroy

PUMMEL	to pound, beat	QUOTIDIAN	occurring daily; commonplace
PUNCTILIOUS	careful in observing rules of behavior or ceremony	RACONTEUR	witty, skillful storyteller
PUNGENT	strong or sharp in smell or taste	RADICAL (adj.)	fundamental; drastic
		RAIL (v.)	to scold with bitter or abusive language
PUNITIVE	having to do with punishment	RALLY (v.)	to assemble; recover, recuperate
PURGATION	process of cleansing, purification	RAMBLE (v.)	to roam, wander; to babble, digress
PURGE (v.)	to cleanse or free from impurities	RAMIFICATION	implication, out-growth, or conse-quence
PURITANICAL	adhering to a rigid moral code		
PURPORT	to profess, suppose, claim	RAMSHACKLE	likely to collapse
		RANCID	spoiled, rotten
QUACK (n.)	faker; one who falsely claims to have medical skill	RANCOR	bitter hatred
		RANT	to harangue, rave, forcefully scold
QUADRILATERAL	four-sided polygon		
QUADRUPED	animal having four feet	RAPPORT	relationship of trust and respect
QUAGMIRE	marsh; difficult situation	RAPT	deeply absorbed
		RAREFY	to make thinner, purer, or more refined
QUALIFY	to provide with needed skills; modify, limit	RASH (adj.)	careless, hasty, reckless
QUANDARY	dilemma, difficulty	RATIFY	to approve formally, confirm
QUARANTINE	isolation period, originally 40 days, to prevent spread of disease	RATIOCINATION	methodical, logical reasoning
		RATION (n.)	portion, share
QUATERNARY	consisting of or relat-ing to four units or members	RATION (v.)	to supply; to restrict consumption of
		RATIONAL	logical, reasonable
QUELL	to crush or subdue	RAUCOUS	harsh-sounding; boisterous
QUERULOUS	inclined to complain, irritable		
QUERY (n.)	question	RAVAGE	to destroy, devastate
QUIBBLE	to argue about insig-nificant and irrelevant details	RAVENOUS	extremely hungry
		RAVINE	deep, narrow gorge
		RAZE	to tear down, demolish
QUICKEN	to hasten, arouse, excite	REACTIONARY (adj.)	marked by extreme conservatism, esp. in politics
QUIESCENCE	inactivity, stillness		
QUINTESSENCE	most typical example; concentrated essence	REBUFF (n.)	blunt rejection
		REBUKE (v.)	to reprimand, scold
QUIVER (v.)	to shake slightly, tremble, vibrate	REBUT	to refute by evidence or argument
QUIXOTIC	overly idealistic, impractical	RECALCITRANT	resisting authority or control

RECANT	to retract a statement, opinion, etc.	RELISH (v.)	to enjoy greatly
RECAPITULATE	to review with a brief summary	REMEDIABLE	capable of being corrected
RECEPTIVE	open to others' ideas; congenial	REMEDY (v.)	to cure, correct
RECLUSIVE	shut off from the world	REMINISCENCE	remembrance of past events
RECONDITE	relating to obscure learning; known to only a few	REMISSION	lessening, relaxation
		REMIT	to send (usually money) as payment
RECOUNT (v.)	to describe facts or events	REMOTE	distant, isolated
RECRUIT (v.)	to draft, enlist; to seek to enroll	REMUNERATION	pay or reward for work, trouble, etc.
RECTIFY	to correct	RENASCENT	reborn, coming into being again
RECTITUDE	moral uprightness	RENEGADE	traitor, person abandoning a cause
RECURRENCE	repetition		
REDRESS (n.)	relief from wrong or injury	RENEGE	to go back on one's word
REDUNDANCY	unnecessary repetition	RENOUNCE	to give up or reject a right, title, person, etc.
REFECTORY	room where meals are served	RENOWN	fame, widespread acclaim
REFLECTION	image, likeness; opinion, thought, impression	REPAST	meal or mealtime
		REPEAL	to revoke or formally withdraw (often a law)
REFORM (v.)	to change, correct	REPEL	to rebuff, repulse; disgust, offend
REFRACT	to deflect sound or light		
REFUGE	escape, shelter	REPENT	to regret a past action
REFURBISH	to renovate	REPENTANT	apologetic, guilty, remorseful
REFUTE	to contradict, discredit	REPLETE	abundantly supplied
REGIMEN	government rule; systematic plan	REPLICATE	to duplicate, repeat
		REPOSE	relaxation, leisure
REGRESS	to move backward; revert to an earlier form or state	REPRESS	to restrain or hold in
		REPRESSION	act of restraining or holding in
REHABILITATE	to restore to good health or condition; reestablish a person's good reputation	REPREHENSIBLE	blameworthy, disreputable
		REPRISE	repetition, esp. of a piece of music
REITERATE	to say again, repeat	REPROACH (v.)	to find fault with; blame
REJOINDER	response		
REJUVENATE	to make young again; renew	REPROBATE	morally unprincipled person
RELEGATE	to assign to a class, especially an inferior one	REPROVE	to criticize or correct
RELINQUISH	to renounce or surrender something	REPUDIATE	to reject as having no authority

REPULSE	repel, fend off; sicken, disgust	RETROSPECTIVE	looking back to the past
REQUIEM	hymns or religious service for the dead	REVELRY	boisterous festivity
REQUITE	to return or repay	REVERE	to worship, regard with awe
RESCIND	to repeal, cancel	REVERT	to backslide, regress
RESIDUE	remainder, leftover, remnant	REVILE	to criticize with harsh language, verbally abuse
RESILIENT	able to recover quickly after illness or bad luck; able to bounce back to shape	REVITALIZE	to renew; give new energy to
		REVOKE	to annul, cancel, call back
RESOLUTE	determined; with a clear purpose	REVULSION	strong feeling of repugnance or dislike
RESOLVE (n.)	determination, firmness of purpose	RHAPSODY	emotional literary or musical work
RESOLVE (v.)	to conclude, determine	RHETORIC	persuasive use of language
RESONATE	to echo		
RESPIRE	to breathe	RHYTHM	regular pattern or variation of sounds and stresses
RESPITE	interval of relief		
RESPLENDENT	splendid, brilliant	RIBALD	humorous in a vulgar way
RESTITUTION	act of compensating for loss or damage	RIDDLE (v.)	to make many holes in; permeate
RESTIVE	impatient, uneasy, restless	RIFE	widespread, prevalent; abundant
RESTORATIVE	having the power to renew or revitalize	RISQUÉ	bordering on being inappropriate or indecent
RESTRAINED	controlled, repressed, restricted	ROBUST	strong and healthy; hardy
RESUSCITATE	to revive, bring back to life	ROCOCO	very highly ornamented
RETAIN	to hold, keep possession of	ROOT (v.)	to dig with a snout (like a pig)
RETARD (v.)	to slow, hold back		
RETICENT	not speaking freely; reserved	ROSTRUM	stage for public speaking
RETINUE	group of attendants with an important person	ROTUND	round in shape; fat
		RUE	to regret
RETIRING	shy, modest, reserved	RUMINATE	to contemplate, reflect upon
RETORT	cutting response	RUSTIC	rural
RETRACT	to draw in or take back	SACCHARINE	excessively sweet or sentimental
RETRENCH	to regroup, reorganize		
RETRIEVE	to bring, fetch; reclaim	SACROSANCT	extremely sacred; beyond criticism
RETROACTIVE	applying to an earlier time	SAGACIOUS	shrewd, wise
RETROGRADE	having a backward motion or direction	SALIENT	prominent or conspicuous

SALLOW	sickly yellow in color
SALUBRIOUS	healthful
SALUTATION	greeting
SANCTION	permission, support; law; penalty
SANCTUARY	haven, retreat
SANGUINE	ruddy; cheerfully optimistic
SARDONIC	cynical, scornfully mocking
SATIATE	to satisfy
SAUNTER	to amble; walk in a leisurely manner
SAVANT	learned person
SAVORY	agreeable in taste or smell
SCABBARD	sheath for sword or dagger
SCALE (v.)	to climb to the top of
SCATHING	harshly critical; painfully hot
SCENARIO	plot outline; possible situation
SCINTILLA	very small amount
SCINTILLATE	to sparkle, flash
SCOFF	to deride, ridicule
SCORE (n.)	notation for a musical composition
SCORE (v.)	to make a notch or scratch
SCRIVENER	professional copyist
SCRUPULOUS	restrained; careful and precise
SCRUTINY	careful observation
SCURRILOUS	vulgar, low, indecent
SECANT	straight line intersecting a curve at two points
SECEDE	to withdraw formally from an organization
SECLUDED	isolated and remote
SECTARIAN	narrow-minded; relating to a group or sect
SECULAR	not specifically pertaining to religion
SEDENTARY	inactive, stationary; sluggish

SEDITION	behavior promoting rebellion
SEISMOLOGY	science of earthquakes
SEMINAL	relating to the beginning or seeds of something
SENESCENT	aging, growing old
SENSUAL	satisfying or gratifying the senses; suggesting sexuality
SENTENTIOUS	having a moralizing tone
SENTIENT	aware, conscious, able to perceive
SEQUEL	anything that follows
SEQUESTER	to remove or set apart; put into seclusion
SERAPHIC	angelic, pure, sublime
SERENDIPITY	habit of making fortunate discoveries by chance
SERENITY	calm, peacefulness
SERPENTINE	serpent-like; twisting, winding
SERRATED	saw-toothed, notched
SERVILE	submissive, obedient
SHARD	piece of broken glass or pottery
SHEEPISH	timid, meek or bashful
SHIRK	to avoid a task due to laziness or fear
SIGNIFY	denote, indicate; symbolize
SIMIAN	ape-like; relating to apes
SIMPER	to smirk, smile foolishly
SINECURE	well-paying job or office that requires little or no work
SINGE	to burn slightly, scorch
SINUOUS	winding; intricate, complex
SKEPTICAL	doubtful, questioning
SKULK	to move in a stealthy or cautious manner; sneak
SLIGHT	to treat as unimportant; insult

SLIPSHOD	careless, hasty
SLOTH	sluggishness, laziness
SLOUGH	to discard or shed
SLOVENLY	untidy, messy
SLUGGARD	lazy, inactive person
SMELT (v.)	to melt metal in order to refine it
SNIPPET	tiny part, tidbit
SOBRIETY	seriousness
SOBRIQUET	nickname
SODDEN	thoroughly soaked; saturated
SOJOURN	visit, stay
SOLACE	comfort in distress; consolation
SOLARIUM	room or glassed-in area exposed to the sun
SOLECISM	grammatical mistake
SOLICITOUS	concerned, attentive; eager
SOLIDARITY	unity based on common aims or interests
SOLILOQUY	literary or dramatic speech by one character, not addressed to others
SOLIPSISM	belief that the self is the only reality
SOLSTICE	shortest or longest day of the year
SOLUBLE	capable of being solved or dissolved
SOMBER	dark and gloomy; melancholy, dismal
SOMNAMBULIST	sleepwalker
SOMNOLENT	drowsy, sleepy; inducing sleep
SONIC	relating to sound
SONOROUS	producing a full, rich sound
SOPHIST	person good at arguing deviously
SOPHISTRY	deceptive reasoning or argumentation
SOPHOMORIC	immature and overconfident

SOPORIFIC	sleepy or tending to cause sleep
SORDID	filthy; contemptible and corrupt
SOVEREIGN	having supreme power
SPARTAN	austere, severe, grave; simple, bare
SPAWN	to generate, produce
SPECULATION	contemplation; act of taking business risks for financial gain
SPECULATIVE	involving assumption; uncertain; theoretical
SPONTANEOUS	on the spur of the moment, impulsive
SPORADIC	infrequent, irregular
SPORTIVE	frolicsome, playful
SPRIGHTLY	lively, animated, energetic
SPUR (v.)	to prod
SPURIOUS	lacking authenticity; counterfeit, false
SPURN	to reject or refuse contemptuously; scorn
SQUALID	filthy; morally repulsive
SQUANDER	to waste
STACCATO	marked by abrupt, clear-cut sounds
STAGNANT	immobile, stale
STAID	self-restrained to the point of dullness
STALK (v.)	to hunt, pursue
STAND (n.)	group of trees
STARK	bare, empty, vacant
STASIS	motionless state; standstill
STIFLE	to smother or suffocate; suppress
STIGMA	mark of disgrace or inferiority
STILTED	stiff, unnatural
STINT (n.)	period of time spent doing something
STINT (v.)	to be sparing or frugal
STIPEND	allowance; fixed amount of money paid regularly

STOCKADE	enclosed area forming defensive wall
STOIC	indifferent to or unaffected by emotions
STOLID	having or showing little emotion
STRATAGEM	trick designed to deceive an enemy
STRATIFY	to arrange into layers
STRICTURE	something that restrains; negative criticism
STRIDENT	loud, harsh, unpleasantly noisy
STRINGENT	imposing severe, rigorous standards
STULTIFY	to impair or reduce to uselessness
STUNTED	having arrested growth or development
STUPEFY	to dull the senses of; stun, astonish
STYLIZE	to fashion, formalize
STYMIE	to block or thwart
SUAVE	smoothly gracious or polite; blandly ingratiating
SUBDUED	suppressed, stifled
SUBJECTION	dependence, obedience, submission
SUBJUGATE	to conquer, subdue; enslave
SUBLIME	awe-inspiring; of high spiritual or moral value
SUBLIMINAL	subconscious; imperceptible
SUBMISSIVE	tending to be meek and submit
SUBPOENA	notice ordering someone to appear in court
SUBSEQUENT	following in time or order
SUBTERFUGE	trick or tactic used to avoid something
SUBTERRANEAN	hidden, secret; underground
SUBTLE	hard to detect or describe; perceptive

SUBVERT	to undermine or corrupt
SUCCINCT	terse, brief, concise
SUCCULENT	juicy; full of vitality or freshness
SUFFERABLE	bearable
SUFFRAGIST	one who advocates extended voting rights
SULLEN	brooding, gloomy
SULLY	to soil, stain, tarnish; taint
SUMPTUOUS	lavish, splendid
SUPERANNUATED	too old, obsolete, outdated
SUPERCILIOUS	arrogant, haughty, overbearing, condescending
SUPERFICIAL	hasty; shallow and phony
SUPERFLUOUS	extra, more than necessary
SUPERSEDE	to take the place of; replace
SUPERVISE	to direct or oversee the work of others
SUPPLANT	to replace, substitute
SUPPLE	flexible, pliant
SUPPLICANT	one who asks humbly and earnestly
SURFEIT	excessive amount
SURLY	rude and bad-tempered
SURMISE	to make an educated guess
SURMOUNT	to conquer, overcome
SURPASS	to do better than, be superior to
SURPLUS	excess
SURREPTITIOUS	characterized by secrecy
SURVEY (v.)	to examine in a comprehensive way
SUSCEPTIBLE	vulnerable, unprotected
SUSPEND	to defer, interrupt; dangle, hang
SUSTAIN	support, uphold; endure, undergo

SWARTHY	having a dark complexion	TEMPERANCE	restraint, self-control, moderation
SYBARITE	person devoted to pleasure and luxury	TEMPERED	moderated, restrained
SYCOPHANT	self-serving flatterer, yes-man	TEMPESTUOUS	stormy, raging, furious
		TENABLE	defensible, reasonable
SYLLABUS	outline of a course	TENACIOUS	stubborn, holding firm
SYMBIOSIS	cooperation, mutual helpfulness	TENET	belief, doctrine
		TENSILE	capable of withstanding physical stress
SYMPOSIUM	meeting with short presentations on related topics	TENUOUS	weak, insubstantial
SYNCOPATION	temporary irregularity in musical rhythm	TEPID	lukewarm; showing little enthusiasm
		TERMINAL (adj.)	concluding, final; fatal
SYNOPSIS	plot summary	TERMINAL (n.)	depot, station
SYNTHESIS	blend, combination	TERRESTRIAL	earthly; down-to-earth, commonplace
SYNTHETIC	artificial, imitation		
TABLEAU	vivid description, striking incident or scene	TERSE	concise, brief, free of extra words
TACIT	silently understood or implied	TESTAMENT	statement of belief; will
TACITURN	uncommunicative, not inclined to speak much	TESTIMONIAL	statement testifying to a truth; something given in tribute to a person's achievement
TACTILE	relating to the sense of touch	TETHER (v.)	to bind, tie
TAINT	to spoil or infect; to stain honor	THEOCRACY	government by priests representing a god
TAINTED	stained, tarnished; corrupted, poisoned	THEOLOGY	study of God and religion
TALON	claw of an animal, esp. a bird of prey	THEORETICAL	abstract
		THERAPEUTIC	medicinal
TANG	sharp flavor or odor	THESAURUS	book of synonyms and antonyms
TANGENTIAL	digressing, diverting		
TANGIBLE	able to be sensed; perceptible, measurable	THESIS	theory or hypothesis; dissertation or long written composition
TANTAMOUNT	equivalent in value or significance; amounting to	THWART	to block or prevent from happening; frustrate
TARNISHED	corroded, discolored; discredited, disgraced	TIDINGS	news
TAWDRY	gaudy, cheap, showy	TIMOROUS	timid, shy, full of apprehension
TAXONOMY	science of classification	TINGE	to color slightly
TECHNOCRAT	strong believer in technology; technical expert	TIRADE	long violent speech; verbal assault
		TITAN	person of colossal stature or achievement

TOADY	flatterer, hanger-on, yes-man	TRIFLING	of slight worth, trivial, insignificant
TOLERANCE	capacity to respect different values; capacity to endure or resist something	TRITE	shallow, superficial
		TROUNCE	to beat severely, defeat
		TROUPE	group of actors
TOME	book, usually large and academic	TRUNCATE	to cut off, shorten by cutting
TONAL	relating to pitch or sound	TRYING	difficult to deal with
TOPOGRAPHY	art of making maps or charts	TRYST	agreement between lovers to meet; rendezvous
TORPID	lethargic; unable to move; dormant	TUMULT	state of confusion; agitation
TORRID	burning hot; passionate	TUNDRA	treeless plain found in arctic or subarctic regions
TORSION	act of twisting and turning	TURBULENCE	commotion, disorder
TORTUOUS	having many twists and turns; highly complex	TURGID	swollen, bloated
		TURPITUDE	inherent vileness, foulness, depravity
TOTTERING	barely standing	TYRO	beginner, novice
TOXIN	poison	UBIQUITOUS	being everywhere simultaneously
TRACTABLE	obedient, yielding		
TRANSCEND	to rise above, go beyond	UMBRAGE	offense, resentment
TRANSCENDENT	rising above, going beyond	UNADULTERATED	absolutely pure
		UNANIMITY	state of total agreement or unity
TRANSCRIPTION	copy, reproduction; record	UNAPPEALING	unattractive, unpleasant
TRANSGRESS	to trespass, violate a law	UNAVAILING	hopeless, useless
TRANSIENT (adj.)	temporary, short-lived, fleeting	UNCONSCIONABLE	unscrupulous; shockingly unfair or unjust
TRANSITORY	short-lived, existing only briefly	UNCTUOUS	greasy, oily; smug and falsely earnest
TRANSLUCENT	partially transparent	UNDERMINE	to sabotage, thwart
TRANSMUTE	to change in appearance or shape	UNDOCUMENTED	not certified, unsubstantiated
TRANSPIRE	to happen, occur; become known	UNDULATING	moving in waves
		UNEQUIVOCAL	absolute, certain
TRAVESTY	parody, exaggerated imitation, caricature	UNFROCK	to strip of priestly duties
TREMULOUS	trembling, quivering; fearful, timid	UNHERALDED	unannounced, unexpected, not publicized
TRENCHANT	acute, sharp, incisive; forceful, effective	UNIDIMENSIONAL	having one size or dimension, flat
TREPIDATION	fear and anxiety	UNIFORM (adj.)	consistent and unchanging; identical

UNIMPEACHABLE	beyond question	VENT (v.)	to express, say out loud
UNINITIATED	not familiar with an area of study	VERACIOUS	truthful, accurate
UNKEMPT	uncombed, messy in appearance	VERACITY	accuracy, truth
		VERBATIM	word for word
UNOBTRUSIVE	modest, unassuming	VERBOSE	wordy
UNSCRUPULOUS	dishonest	VERDANT	green with vegetation; inexperienced
UNSOLICITED	unrequested		
UNWARRANTED	groundless, unjustified	VERDURE	fresh, rich vegetation
UNWITTING	unconscious; unintentional	VERIFIED	proven true
		VERISIMILITUDE	quality of appearing true or real
UNYIELDING	firm, resolute		
UPBRAID	to scold sharply	VERITY	truthfulness; belief viewed as true and enduring
UPROARIOUS	loud and forceful		
URBANE	courteous, refined, suave	VERMIN	small creatures offensive to humans
USURP	to seize by force	VERNACULAR	everyday language used by ordinary people; specialized language of a profession
USURY	practice of lending money at exorbitant rates		
UTILITARIAN	efficient, functional, useful	VERNAL	related to spring
UTOPIA	perfect place	VERSATILE	adaptable, all-purpose
VACILLATE	to waver, show indecision	VESTIGE	trace, remnant
		VETO (v.)	to reject formally
VACUOUS	empty, void; lacking intelligence, purposeless	VEX	to irritate, annoy; confuse, puzzle
VAGRANT	poor person with no home	VIABLE	workable, able to succeed or grow
VALIDATE	to authorize, certify, confirm	VIADUCT	series of elevated arches used to cross a valley
VANQUISH	to conquer, defeat	VICARIOUS	substitute, surrogate; enjoyed through imagined participation in another's experience
VAPID	tasteless, dull		
VARIABLE	changeable, inconstant		
VARIEGATED	varied; marked with different colors	VICISSITUDE	change or variation; ups and downs
VAUNTED	boasted about, bragged about	VIE	to compete, contend
VEHEMENTLY	strongly, urgently	VIGILANT	attentive, watchful
VENDETTA	prolonged feud marked by bitter hostility	VIGNETTE	decorative design; short literary composition
VENERABLE	respected because of age	VILIFY	to slander, defame
		VIM	energy, enthusiasm
VENERATION	adoration, honor, respect	VINDICATE	to clear of blame; support a claim

VINDICATION	clearance from blame or suspicion	WALLOW	to indulge oneself excessively, luxuriate
VINDICTIVE	spiteful, vengeful, unforgiving	WAN	sickly pale
VIRILE	manly, having qualities of an adult male	WANTON	undisciplined, unrestrained, reckless
VIRTUOSO	someone with masterly skill; expert musician	WARRANTY	guarantee of a product's soundness
VIRULENT	extremely poisonous; malignant; hateful	WARY	careful, cautious
VISCOUS	thick, syrupy and sticky	WAYWARD	erratic, unrestrained, reckless
VITRIOLIC	burning, caustic; sharp, bitter	WEATHER (v.)	to endure, undergo
VITUPERATE	to abuse verbally	WHET	to sharpen, stimulate
VIVACIOUS	lively, spirited	WHIMSY	playful or fanciful idea
VIVID	bright and intense in color; strongly perceived	WILY	clever, deceptive
VOCIFEROUS	loud, vocal and noisy	WINDFALL	sudden, unexpected good fortune
VOID (adj.)	not legally enforceable; empty	WINSOME	charming, happily engaging
VOID (n.)	emptiness, vacuum	WITHDRAWN	unsociable, aloof; shy, timid
VOID (v.)	to cancel, invalidate	WIZENED	withered, shriveled, wrinkled
VOLITION	free choice, free will; act of choosing	WRIT	written document, usually in law
VOLLEY (n.)	flight of missiles, round of gunshots	WRY	amusing, ironic
VOLUBLE	speaking much and easily, talkative; glib	XENOPHOBIA	fear or hatred of foreigners or strangers
VOLUMINOUS	large; of great quantity; writing or speaking at great length	YOKE (v.)	to join together
		ZEALOT	someone passionately devoted to a cause
VORACIOUS	having a great appetite	ZENITH	highest point, summit
VULNERABLE	defenseless, unprotected; innocent, naive	ZEPHYR	gentle breeze
WAIVE	to refrain from enforcing a rule; to give up a legal right	ZOOLOGIST	scientist who studies animals

CHAPTER TWELVE

Vocabulary Exercises

One of the best ways to practice vocabulary is to learn definitions. Either through flashcards or studying the word list in Chapter 11, learning definitions is always a great way to build your vocabulary. Once you have a good start, use the following exercises to test your knowledge and improve your Verbal Ability skills.

VOCABULARY EXERCISE 1: DEFINITIONS

Directions: Match the words in the left-hand column with the definitions on the right.

1. **ABJECT**	_____	=	loud, vocal
2. **AUGUST**	_____	=	excessively sweet
3. **CONSONANT**	_____	=	faithless, disloyal
4. **INSULAR**	_____	=	swollen, bloated
5. **NOISOME**	_____	=	learned, scholarly
6. **PERFIDIOUS**	_____	=	in agreement with
7. **ERUDITE**	_____	=	dignified, awe-inspiring
8. **SACCHARINE**	_____	=	miserable, pitiful
9. **TURGID**	_____	=	isolated, detached
10. **VOCIFEROUS**	_____	=	foul-smelling, putrid

VOCABULARY EXERCISE 2: DEFINITIONS

Directions: Match each word on the left with its antonym on the right. Use each word only once.

1. **ESPOUSE** _____ erect

2. **EXONERATE** _____ abridge

3. **AMELIORATE** _____ palpable

4. **SUBJUGATE** _____ adore

5. **OBFUSCATE** _____ aver

6. **INCITE** _____ monochrome

7. **SULLY** _____ clarify

8. **ABHOR** _____ drench

9. **RAZE** _____ abjure

10. **DENY** _____ emancipate

11. **PROTRACT** _____ purify

12. **PARCH** _____ acme

13. **NADIR** _____ quell

14. **ETHEREAL** _____ inculpate

15. **OPALESCENT** _____ exacerbate

VOCABULARY EXERCISE 3: VOCABULARY IN CONTEXT

Directions: Fill in each blank with a word from the column on the right. One and only one of the words makes sense in each blank.

1. During the ceremony, the president of the university delivered a(n) _____ honoring the retiring professor.

2. Protesters argued that the government's aggressive foreign policy was not motivated by true patriotism, but by _____.

3. Despite his enormous girth, he was known by the _____ "Slim."

4. Art world _____ Louise Nevelson has influenced a generation of her fellow sculptors.

5. The expression "to wait an eternity" is an example of a(n) _____.

6. After the alarm clock rang, she grabbed a towel and performed her daily _____(s) in about five minutes.

7. Forgetting to introduce me to your friends was a mere _____ for which I gladly forgive you.

8. The crowd at the shopping mall was a(n) _____ of neighborhood residents and visitors from out of town.

9. The courageous adventurer was able to face the most dangerous situations with _____.

10. Much to the consternation of female executives, the exclusive club remained a(n) _____ of male privilege.

11. The governor granted the sick prisoners _____ and allowed them to be released so they could receive medical treatments not available in jail.

12. Though I express myself quite eloquently in private conversation, public speaking is not my _____.

13. The book was a critically acclaimed best-seller, but I found it to be utter _____.

14. Writer Richard Wright was an American-born _____ who lived in Paris for many years.

15. She steamed open the envelope and read the _____ addressed to her sister.

ABLUTION

AMALGAM

BASTION

CLEMENCY

DRIVEL

EQUANIMITY

EXPATRIATE

FORTE

HYPERBOLE

JINGOISM

LUMINARY

MISSIVE

PANEGYRIC

PECCADILLO

SOBRIQUET

VOCABULARY EXERCISE 4: WORD CHARGE

Directions: Draw an arrow toward the left from words on this list that relate to GOOD or VIRTUE. Draw an arrow toward the right from words that relate to BAD or EVIL.

GOOD   BAD

←————————— HONESTY

ALTRUISM

AVARICE

BENEFICENT

CUPIDITY

DEBAUCH

DEPRAVITY

DIABOLICAL

GLUTTONY

HEINOUS

INIQUITY

MALEFACTOR

MALEVOLENT

MENDACIOUS

PERDITION

PRISTINE

PROBITY

PROFANE

PROFLIGATE

PRURIENT

RECTITUDE

REPROBATE

SACROSANCT

SCRUPULOUS

SLOTH

SYBARITE

TURPITUDE

WANTON

VOCABULARY EXERCISE 5: WORD CHARGE

Directions: Draw an arrow toward the left from words on this list that suggest COORDINATION or SKILL. Draw an arrow toward the right from words that suggest AWKWARDNESS or CLUMSINESS.

COORDINATED   CLUMSY

ADROIT

AMBIDEXTROUS

DEFT

DEXTEROUS

LUMBER

MALADROIT

PONDEROUS

PROFICIENT

PROWESS

VIRTUOSO

VOCABULARY EXERCISE 6: WORD CHARGE

Directions: Draw an arrow toward the left from words on this list that are associated with SICKNESS or DISEASE. Draw an arrow toward the right from words associated with HEALTH or RECOVERY FROM ILLNESS.

SICKNESS   HEALTH

ATROPHY

CONVALESCENCE

HYPOCHONDRIA

HYPOTHERMIA

MALADY

PATHOGENIC

ROBUST

SALUBRIOUS

THERAPEUTIC

VIRULENT

WAN

VOCABULARY EXERCISE 7: DEFINITIONS

Directions: Match the words in the left-hand column with the definitions on the right.

1. **ALLAY**   _____ = to infuse; dye, moisten

2. **APPROPRIATE**   _____ = to evade responsibility by pretending to be ill

3. **BILK**

    _____ = to make unnecessary

4. **IMBUE**

    _____ = to lessen, ease, soothe

5. **INURE**

    _____ = to abuse verbally

6. **MALINGER**

    _____ = to take possession of

7. **OBVIATE**

    _____ = to happen; become known

8. **RUE**

    _____ = to harden; accustom; become used to

9. **TRANSPIRE**

10. **VITUPERATE**   _____ = to regret

    _____ = to cheat, defraud

VOCABULARY EXERCISE 8: DEFINITIONS

Directions: Match each word on the left with its antonym on the right. Use each word only once.

1. **SOPHOMORIC**	_____	morose
2. **SONOROUS**	_____	parsimony
3. **DOUR**	_____	feisty
4. **EBULLIENT**	_____	suave
5. **IMPLACABLE**	_____	adroit
6. **GARGANTUAN**	_____	sagacious
7. **INEPT**	_____	pliant
8. **GARRULOUS**	_____	adulterated
9. **LARGESS**	_____	somber
10. **BOORISH**	_____	taciturn
11. **INANE**	_____	minuscule
12. **PRISTINE**	_____	depravity
13. **PROBITY**	_____	rhapsodic
14. **JOCULAR**	_____	venerable
15. **PHLEGMATIC**	_____	raucous

VOCABULARY EXERCISE 9: VOCABULARY IN CONTEXT

Directions: Fill in each blank with a word from the column on the right. One and only one of the words makes sense in each blank.

1. Saying "polo bears" instead of "polar bears" is an example of a(n) _____.

2. I had a _____ that you would call me, so I'm not at all surprised to pick up the phone and hear your voice.

3. Orson Welles' radio enactment of H.G. Wells' novel *War of the Worlds* had such an air of _____ that many listeners thought Martians were actually landing on earth.

4. When you learn to sail, you also learn nautical _____: words like "port," "starboard," and "alee."

5. Plants require carbon dioxide to flourish and give off oxygen, while the opposite is true for mammals; thus, the two life forms live in a state of _____.

6. The hiker exercised a great deal of _____ in tiptoeing past the sleeping grizzly bears.

7. The conviction of the obviously innocent man on charges of murder was truly a _____ of justice.

8. The wealthy aristocrat, like most of his _____, lived comfortably and had no idea what life was like for those who were less fortunate than he.

9. For comatose patients with terminal illnesses, _____ may be better than unnecessary prolongation of life.

10. The judge ordered that construction of the new dam be held in _____ until its impact on the environment could be more thoroughly considered.

11. The _____ asked everyone who walked by for spare change.

12. After the corn kernels are removed from an ear of corn, the husk and cob are discarded as _____.

ABEYANCE

CIRCUMSPECTION

DROSS

EUTHANASIA

ILK

MALAPROPISM

MENDICANT

NOMENCLATURE

PRESENTIMENT

SYMBIOSIS

TRAVESTY

VERISIMILITUDE

VOCABULARY EXERCISE 10: WORD CHARGE

Directions: Draw an arrow toward the left from words on this list that are associated with INTELLIGENCE, WISDOM, or LEARNING. Draw an arrow toward the right from words associated with FOOLISHNESS, IGNORANCE, or STUPIDITY.

SMART   STUPID

ACUMEN

CANNY

ERUDITE

FATUOUS

INANE

JUDICIOUS

MENTOR

PERSPICACIOUS

PRATTLE

RECONDITE

SAGACIOUS

SAVANT

VOCABULARY EXERCISE 11: WORD CHARGE

Directions: Draw an arrow toward the left from words on this list that are associated with OLD AGE or EXPERIENCE. Draw an arrow toward the right from words associated with YOUTH, BIRTH, or INEXPERIENCE.

OLD   YOUNG

ANTEDILUVIAN

ANTIQUATED

ARCHAIC

CALLOW

DOTARD

FLEDGLING

NASCENT

NATAL

NEONATE

NOVITIATE

PRECOCIOUS

PRIMEVAL

PRIMORDIAL

RENASCENT

SENESCENT

SUPERANNUATED

TYRO

VENERABLE

WIZENED

VOCABULARY EXERCISE 12: DEFINITIONS

Directions: Match the words in the left-hand column with the definitions on the right.

1. **ABSTRUSE** _____ = gaudy; falsely attractive

2. **CRAVEN** _____ = extremely sacred; beyond criticism

3. **DESULTORY** _____ = quick, shrewd, unpredictable

4. **HACKNEYED** _____ = difficult to comprehend

5. **LACHRYMOSE** _____ = childish, immature

6. **MERCURIAL** _____ = obsolete, outdated

7. **MERETRICIOUS** _____ = worn out by over-use

8. **PUERILE** _____ = cowardly

9. **SACROSANCT** _____ = at random, rambling

10. **SUPERANNUATED** _____ = tearful

VOCABULARY EXERCISE 13: DEFINITIONS

Directions: Match each word on the left with its antonym on the right. Use each word only once.

1. **AMORPHOUS**	_____	aristocratic
2. **AVER**	_____	honest
3. **BELIE**	_____	shapely
4. **DILATORY**	_____	blame
5. **EXCULPATE**	_____	deny
6. **FLACCID**	_____	cowardice
7. **LAUDATORY**	_____	clear
8. **MENDACIOUS**	_____	explicit
9. **NEBULOUS**	_____	permanent
10. **PLEBEIAN**	_____	reveal
11. **TACIT**	_____	praise
12. **TRANSITORY**	_____	disparaging
13. **VILIFY**	_____	punctual
14. **METTLE**	_____	necessitate
15. **OBVIATE**	_____	firm

VOCABULARY EXERCISE 14: VOCABULARY IN CONTEXT

Directions: Fill in each blank with a word from the column on the right. One and only one of the words makes sense in each blank.

1. The behind-the-scenes _____(s) of powerful corporate heads ensured that legislation curbing industrial development would never be passed.

2. The kneeling _____ humbly asked God to forgive his sins.

3. The scholar's life work was a lengthy _____ that was difficult to carry, much less read.

4. Since I'd spent almost my entire paycheck on Christmas presents, receiving a holiday bonus was a real _____.

5. The dictator's _____ continued to report strong public support for government policies despite daily pro-democracy demonstrations in the capital.

6. The princess was known for her _____; painters begged to paint her portrait and scores of suitors proposed marriage.

7. He had the _____ to demand an apology from the woman he'd just insulted.

8. A stalactite begins as a small _____ of dissolved mineral deposits on the ceiling of a cave.

9. Not one to rely on _____, the newspaper editor insisted that the senator's rumored infidelities be more thoroughly investigated before a story was written.

10. The _____ of employment in rural areas forces many job seekers to leave their home towns in search of jobs.

11. Compared to her coworkers who had been on the job for years, the recently hired college graduate was an inexperienced _____.

12. The Swedish botanist Linnaeus invented the system of _____ used to classify all life forms into separate, distinct species.

ACCRETION

BOON

DEARTH

EFFRONTERY

INNUENDO

MACHINATION

NEOPHYTE

PULCHRITUDE

SUPPLICANT

TAXONOMY

TOADY

TOME

VOCABULARY EXERCISE 15: WORD CHARGE

Directions: Draw an arrow toward the left from words on this list that are associated with GROWTH or LIVING THINGS. Draw an arrow toward the right from words associated with LIMITING or PREVENTING GROWTH.

GROWING   LIMITING

ARID

BURGEON

CURTAIL

DESICCATE

FALLOW

FECUND

FOLIATE

GERMINATE

GESTATION

MORIBUND

PARCH

PROLIFIC

STIFLE

STULTIFY

STUNTED

TRUNCATE

VERDANT

VOCABULARY EXERCISE 16: WORD CHARGE

Directions: Draw an arrow toward the left from words on this list that are associated with ENERGY or MOVEMENT. Draw an arrow toward the right from words associated with LACK OF ENERGY or STILLNESS.

ENERGETIC   LAZY

APATHY
EFFERVESCENT
ENERVATE
ENNUI
GAMBOL
INDOLENT
INERT
LANGUID
LASSITUDE
LISTLESS
PEREGRINATE
PERIPATETIC
QUIESCENCE
RESTIVE
SPRIGHTLY
STAGNANT
STASIS
TORPID
VIM
VIVACIOUS

VOCABULARY EXERCISE 17: DEFINITIONS

Directions: Match the words in the left-hand column with the definitions on the right.

1. **ACME** _____ = origin and history of a word

2. **BONHOMIE** _____ = trace amount

3. **COMPLICITY** _____ = strict disciplinarian

4. **DIFFIDENCE** _____ = one who attacks traditional beliefs

5. **ETYMOLOGY** _____ = partial shadow

6. **HIATUS** _____ = knowing partnership in wrongdoing

7. **ICONOCLAST** _____ = highest point, summit

8. **MARTINET** _____ = shyness, lack of confidence

9. **PENUMBRA** _____ = break, interruption

10. **SCINTILLA** _____ = good-natured geniality

VOCABULARY EXERCISE 18: DEFINITIONS

When most people think of "hard" words, they think of long words, like antepenultimate or verisimilitude. However, not all hard words are long. Here are some words, each four letters or less, that many people find difficult.

Directions: Match each word on the left with its definition on the right.

1. **BALM**	_____	abundant
2. **BANE**	_____	to annoy, irritate
3. **BOON**	_____	to become boring or tiresome
4. **BOOR**	_____	blessing, gift
5. **CARP**	_____	to complain
6. **CEDE**	_____	crude person
7. **DEFT**	_____	to cut, chop, hack
8. **DOUR**	_____	pale
9. **EBB**	_____	to peel or trim
10. **EDDY**	_____	to recede, fade away
11. **HEW**	_____	to regret
12. **MOLT**	_____	to sharpen, hone
13. **PALL**	_____	to shed periodically
14. **PARE**	_____	skillful, dexterous
15. **RAZE**	_____	small whirlpool
16. **RIFE**	_____	causing harm
17. **RUE**	_____	healing or comforting
18. **VEX**	_____	sullen and gloomy
19. **WAN**	_____	to surrender possession
20. **WHET**	_____	to tear down, demolish

VOCABULARY EXERCISE 19: VOCABULARY IN CONTEXT

Directions: Fill in each blank with a word from the column on the right. One and only one of the words makes sense in each blank.

1. In Flannery O'Connor's humorous short story "A Good Man Is Hard to Find," the main character constantly recites _____ phrases like "it takes one to know one" and "another day, another dollar."

2. The outlaw had a _____ disregard for the legal system; there was no law he would not break.

3. The _____ humor in some of Shakespeare's plays sometimes escapes first-time readers who don't recognize the Elizabethan slang and obscenities he uses.

4. The Mayor's _____ nature is evident from his refusal to negotiate with community leaders who oppose his plans for the new business district.

5. Given his _____ manner, I'm not surprised that the televangelist is thought to be insincere and only concerned with money.

6. Plants flourished in the rich and _____ soil.

7. The television series was filled with _____ violence that served no purpose except to shock viewers with its brutality.

8. Those who attended the _____ funeral service had hardly a dry handkerchief among them.

9. It is not uncommon for passengers on crowded city buses to become _____ and fight over an empty seat.

10. The water was so _____ you could see every stone in the river bed.

11. The reclusive scholar specialized in an area of knowledge so _____ it was of little interest to anyone but a handful of specialists.

12. The sorcerer's _____ glance made me so afraid I shivered uncontrollably.

BALEFUL

FECUND

FRACTIOUS

GRATUITOUS

HACKNEYED

LACHRYMOSE

LIMPID

OBDURATE

RECONDITE

RIBALD

UNCTUOUS

WANTON

VOCABULARY EXERCISE 20: WORD CHARGE

Directions: Draw an arrow toward the left from words on this list that are associated with LOVE, FRIENDLINESS, or GOOD. Draw an arrow toward the right from words associated with HATE, HOSTILITY, or ANTAGONISM.

LOVE   HATE

AFFABLE

ALTERCATION

ALTRUISM

AMITY

AMOROUS

AVERSION

BALEFUL

BENIGN

CALUMNY

CIVILITY

CODDLE

COSSET

ENMITY

ESPOUSE

ESTRANGE

GLOWER

IMPRECATION

PHILANTHROPY

PUGNACIOUS

RANCOR

SOLICITOUS

WANTON

XENOPHOBIA

VOCABULARY EXERCISE 21: WORD CHARGE

Directions: Draw an arrow toward the left from words on this list that are associated with WAR, FIGHTING, or DISORDER. Draw an arrow toward the right from words associated with PEACE or AGREEMENT.

WAR   PEACE

ACRIMONY
ANTAGONIST
ANTIPATHY
ASSAIL
AVERSION
BELLICOSE
BILLET
CONCORD
CONSENSUS
EMBROIL
FRACAS
FRACTIOUS
INCURSION
INFILTRATE
INSURRECTION
MARTIAL
PACIFIST
PACIFY
PILLAGE
RAPPORT
RAVAGE

VOCABULARY EXERCISE 22: DEFINITIONS

Directions: Match the words in the left-hand column with the definitions on the right.

1. **ALTRUISTIC** _____ = harsh or loud

2. **CALLOW** _____ = unselfish

3. **CHARY** _____ = joking or jesting

4. **DOLEFUL** _____ = very hot, passionate

5. **JOCULAR** _____ = sorrowful, mournful

6. **PANORAMIC** _____ = lethargic; unable to move

7. **RAUCOUS** _____ = wordy

8. **TORRID** _____ = immature, lacking in sophistication

9. **TORPID** _____ = watchful, cautious, extremely shy

10. **VERBOSE** _____ = having a wide view

VOCABULARY EXERCISE 23: DEFINITIONS

Directions: Match the words in the left-hand column with the definitions on the right.

1. **LARCENY** _____ = merciful leniency

2. **PLAINTIFF** _____ = knowing partnership in wrongdoing

3. **RESTITUTION** _____ = feeling of uneasiness caused by guilt

4. **EXONERATE** _____ = guilty of wrongdoing

5. **INJUNCTION** _____ = guilty person

6. **CULPABLE** _____ = to acquit, clear from blame

7. **ARRAIGN** _____ = illegal

8. **ILLICIT** _____ = to charge formally with a crime

9. **CULPRIT** _____ = command, court order

10. **CLEMENCY** _____ = criminal theft

11. **COMPLICITY** _____ = lawsuit

12. **TRANSGRESS** _____ = to lie under oath

13. **PERJURE** _____ = to trespass, violate a law

14. **LITIGATION** _____ = injured person in a lawsuit

15. **COMPUNCTION** _____ = compensation for loss in a crime

VOCABULARY EXERCISE 24: WORD CHARGE

Directions: Draw an arrow toward the left from words on this list that are associated with HAPPINESS or HUMOR. Draw an arrow toward the right from words associated with SADNESS or GLOOM.

HAPPY   SAD

DESPONDENT

DIRGE

DOLEFUL

DOUR

DROLL

EBULLIENT

FUNEREAL

JOCULAR

KNELL

LACHRYMOSE

LEVITY

LUGUBRIOUS

MORBID

MOROSE

REVELRY

RIBALD

SOMBER

VOCABULARY EXERCISE 25: WORD CHARGE

Directions: Draw an arrow toward the left from words on this list that are associated with SIMPLICITY. Draw an arrow toward the right from words that are associated with COMPLEXITY or ORNAMENTATION.

SIMPLE   COMPLEX

AUSTERE

MONASTIC

ROCOCO

SERPENTINE

SINUOUS

SPARTAN

TORTUOUS

VOCABULARY EXERCISE 26: WORD CHARGE

Directions: Draw an arrow toward the left from words on this list that suggest IMPROVEMENT or being BETTER. Draw an arrow toward the right from words that suggest WORSENING.

BETTER   WORSE

ALLAY

ALLEVIATE

AMELIORATE

APPEASE

ASSUAGE

CONVALESCE

DEBASE

EXACERBATE

MOLLIFY

PACIFY

PALLIATE

PERVERT

SUBVERT

VOCABULARY EXERCISE 27: WORD CHARGE

Directions: Draw an arrow toward the left from words on this list that suggest being LARGE, BIG, or NUMEROUS. Draw an arrow toward the right from words that suggest being SMALL, TINY, or FEW.

BIG   SMALL

BEHEMOTH
BEVY
BOUNTIFUL
COPIOUS
DIMINUTIVE
GARGANTUAN
ILLIMITABLE
INESTIMABLE
INFINITESIMAL
INNUMERABLE
IOTA
JUGGERNAUT
MINUSCULE
MYRIAD
PITTANCE
PLETHORA
PRODIGIOUS
SCINTILLA
TITAN
TRIFLING
VOLUMINOUS

VOCABULARY EXERCISE 28: WORD CHARGE

Directions: Draw an arrow toward the left from words on this list that suggest being RICH or GENEROUS. Draw an arrow toward the right from words that suggest being POOR, CHEAP, or STINGY.

RICH   POOR

AFFLUENT

BENEFACTOR

DESTITUTE

IMPECUNIOUS

INDIGENT

INSOLVENT

LARGESS

MAGNANIMOUS

MENDICANT

MUNIFICENT

OPULENT

PALATIAL

PARSIMONIOUS

PAUCITY

PAUPER

PENURY

SUMPTUOUS

VOCABULARY EXERCISE 29: WORD CHARGE

Directions: Draw an arrow toward the left from words on this list that suggest PRAISE or SUPPORT. Draw an arrow toward the right from words that suggest BLAME, CRITICISM, or a PUT DOWN.

PRAISE   BLAME

ACCOLADE

ADMONISH

APPROBATION

BERATE

CASTIGATE

CENSORIOUS

CHASTISE

CHIDE

CONDONE

DECRY

DEMEAN

DEPLORE

DEPRECATE

DERIDE

DEROGATE

DIATRIBE

INCULPATE

KUDOS

LAUDABLE

RATIFY

REPROVE

UPBRAID

VILIFY

ANSWER KEY

Vocabulary Exercise 1

1. abject = miserable, pitiful
2. august = dignified, awe-inspiring
3. consonant = in agreement with
4. insular = isolated, detached
5. noisome = foul-smelling, putrid
6. perfidious = faithless, disloyal
7. erudite = learned, scholarly
8. saccharine = excessively sweet
9. turgid = swollen, bloated
10. vociferous = loud, vocal

Vocabulary Exercise 2

1. espouse — abjure
2. exonerate — inculpate
3. ameliorate — exacerbate
4. subjugate — emancipate
5. obfuscate — clarify
6. incite — quell
7. sully — purify
8. abhor — adore
9. raze — erect
10. deny — aver
11. protract — abridge
12. parch — drench
13. nadir — acme
14. ethereal — palpable
15. opalescent — monochrome

Vocabulary Exercise 3

1. panegyric
2. jingoism
3. sobriquet
4. luminary
5. hyperbole
6. ablution
7. peccadillo
8. amalgam
9. equanimity
10. bastion
11. clemency
12. forte
13. drivel
14. expatriate
15. missive

Vocabulary Exercise 4

GOOD	BAD
honesty	avarice
altruism	cupidity
beneficent	debauch
pristine	depravity
probity	diabolical
rectitude	gluttony
sacrosanct	heinous
scrupulous	iniquity
	malefactor
	malevolent
	mendacious
	perdition
	profane
	profligate
	prurient
	reprobate
	sloth
	sybarite
	turpitude
	wanton

Vocabulary Exercise 5

COORDINATED

adroit

ambidextrous

deft

dexterous

proficient

prowess

virtuoso

CLUMSY

lumber

maladroit

ponderous

Vocabulary Exercise 6

HEALTHY

convalescence

robust

salubrious

therapeutic

SICK

atrophy

hypochondria

hypothermia

malady

pathogenic

virulent

wan

Vocabulary Exercise 7

1. allay = to lessen, ease, soothe
2. appropriate = to take possession of
3. bilk = to cheat, defraud
4. imbue = to infuse; dye, moisten
5. inure = to harden; accustom
6. malinger = to evade responsibility by faking illness
7. obviate = to make unnecessary
8. rue = to regret
9. transpire = to happen
10. vituperate = to abuse verbally

Vocabulary Exercise 8

1. sophomoric — venerable
2. sonorous — raucous
3. dour — rhapsodic
4. ebullient — somber
5. implacable — pliant
6. gargantuan — minuscule
7. inept — adroit
8. garrulous — taciturn
9. largess — parsimony
10. boorish — suave
11. inane — sagacious
12. pristine — adulterated
13. probity — depravity
14. jocular — morose
15. phlegmatic — feisty

Vocabulary Exercise 9

1. malapropism
2. presentiment
3. verisimilitude
4. nomenclature
5. symbiosis
6. circumspection
7. travesty
8. ilk
9. euthanasia
10. abeyance
11. mendicant
12. dross

Vocabulary Exercise 10

SMART	STUPID
acumen	fatuous
canny	inane
erudite	prattle
judicious	
mentor	
perspicacious	
recondite	
sagacious	
savant	

Vocabulary Exercise 11

OLD	YOUNG
antediluvian	callow
antiquated	fledgling
archaic	nascent
dotard	natal
primeval	neonate
primordial	novitiate
senescent	precocious
superannuated	renascent
venerable	tyro
wizened	

Vocabulary Exercise 12

1. abstruse = difficult to comprehend
2. craven = cowardly
3. desultory = at random, rambling, unmethodical
4. hackneyed = worn out by over-use
5. lachrymose = tearful
6. mercurial = quick, shrewd, unpredictable
7. meretricious = gaudy; falsely attractive
8. puerile = childish, immature
9. sacrosanct = extremely sacred
10. superannuated = obsolete, outdated

Vocabulary Exercise 13

1. amorphous — shapely
2. aver — deny
3. belie — reveal
4. dilatory — punctual
5. exculpate — blame
6. flaccid — firm
7. laudatory — disparaging
8. mendacious — honest
9. nebulous — clear
10. plebeian — aristocratic
11. tacit — explicit
12. transitory — permanent
13. vilify — praise
14. mettle — cowardice
15. obviate — necessitate

Vocabulary Exercise 14

1. machinations
2. supplicant
3. tome
4. boon
5. toady
6. pulchritude
7. effrontery
8. accretion
9. innuendo
10. dearth
11. neophyte
12. taxonomy

Vocabulary Exercise 15

GROWING	LIMITING
burgeon	arid
fecund	curtail
foliate	desiccate
germinate	fallow
gestation	moribund
prolific	parch
verdant	stifle
	stultify
	stunted
	truncate

Vocabulary Exercise 16

ENERGETIC

effervescent

gambol

peregrinate

peripatetic

restive

sprightly

vim

vivacious

LAZY

apathy

enervate

ennui

indolent

inert

languid

lassitude

listless

quiescence

stagnant

stasis

torpid

Vocabulary Exercise 17

1. acme = highest point, summit
2. bonhomie = good-natured geniality
3. complicity = knowing partnership in wrongdoing
4. diffidence = shyness, lack of confidence
5. etymology = origin and history of a word
6. hiatus = break, interruption
7. iconoclast = one who attacks traditional beliefs
8. martinet = strict disciplinarian
9. penumbra = partial shadow
10. scintilla = trace amount

Vocabulary Exercise 18

1. balm = something soothing, healing, or comforting
2. bane = something causing death or harm
3. boon = blessing, gift
4. boor = crude person
5. carp = to complain
6. cede = to surrender possession of something
7. deft = skillful, dexterous
8. dour = sullen and gloomy
9. ebb = to recede, fade away
10. eddy = small whirlpool
11. hew = to cut, chop, hack
12. molt = to shed skin, hair, or feathers periodically
13. pall = to become boring or tiresome
14. pare = to peel or trim
15. raze = to tear down, demolish
16. rife = abundant
17. rue = to regret
18. vex = to annoy, irritate
19. wan = pale
20. whet = to sharpen, hone

Vocabulary Exercise 19

1. hackneyed
2. wanton
3. ribald
4. obdurate
5. unctuous
6. fecund
7. gratuitous
8. lachrymose
9. fractious
10. limpid
11. recondite
12. baleful

Vocabulary Exercise 20

LOVE	HATE
affable	altercation
altruism	aversion
amity	baleful
amorous	calumny
benign	enmity
civility	estrange
coddle	glower
cosset	imprecation
espouse	pugnacious
philanthropy	rancor
solicitous	wanton
	xenophobia

Vocabulary Exercise 21

WAR	PEACE
acrimony	concord
antagonist	consensus
antipathy	pacifist
assail	pacify
aversion	rapport
bellicose	
billet	
embroil	
fracas	
fractious	
incursion	
infiltrate	
insurrection	
martial	
pillage	
ravage	

Vocabulary Exercise 22

1. altruistic = unselfish
2. callow = immature, lacking in sophistication
3. chary = watchful, cautious, extremely shy
4. doleful = sorrowful, mournful
5. jocular = joking or jesting
6. panoramic = having a wide view
7. raucous = harsh or loud
8. torrid = very hot; passionate
9. torpid = lethargic, unable to move
10. verbose = wordy

Vocabulary Exercise 23

1. larceny = criminal theft
2. plaintiff = injured person in a lawsuit
3. restitution = compensation for a crime
4. exonerate = to acquit, clear from blame
5. injunction = command
6. culpable = guilty of wrongdoing
7. arraign = to charge formally with a crime
8. illicit = illegal
9. culprit = guilty person
10. clemency = merciful leniency
11. complicity = knowing partnership in wrongdoing
12. transgress = to trespass, violate a law
13. perjure = to lie under oath
14. litigation = lawsuit
15. compunction = feeling of uneasiness caused by guilt

Vocabulary Exercise 24

HAPPY	SAD
droll	despondent
ebullient	dirge
jocular	doleful
levity	dour
revelry	funereal
ribald	knell
	lachrymose
	lugubrious
	morbid
	morose
	somber

Vocabulary Exercise 25

SIMPLE	COMPLEX
austere	rococo
monastic	serpentine
spartan	sinuous
	tortuous

Vocabulary Exercise 26

BETTER	WORSE
allay	debase
alleviate	exacerbate
ameliorate	pervert
appease	subvert
assuage	
convalesce	
mollify	
pacify	
palliate	

Vocabulary Exercise 27

BIG	SMALL
behemoth	diminutive
bevy	infinitesimal
bountiful	iota
copious	minuscule
gargantuan	pittance
illimitable	scintilla
inestimable	trifling
innumerable	
juggernaut	
myriad	
plethora	
prodigious	
titan	
voluminous	

Vocabulary Exercise 28

RICH

affluent

benefactor

largess

magnanimous

munificent

opulent

palatial

sumptuous

POOR

destitute

impecunious

indigent

insolvent

mendicant

parsimonious

paucity

pauper

penury

Vocabulary Exercise 29

PRAISE

accolade

approbation

condone

kudos

laudable

ratify

BLAME

admonish

berate

castigate

censorious

chastise

chide

decry

demean

deplore

deprecate

deride

derogate

diatribe

inculpate

reprove

upbraid

vilify

Section IV

BIOLOGY

CHAPTER THIRTEEN

Cellular Biology

The cell is the fundamental unit of all living things. Every function in biology involves a process that occurs within cells or at the interface between cells. Therefore, to understand biology, you need to appreciate the structure and function of different parts of the cell.

CELL THEORY AND STRUCTURE

Cell Theory

The cell was not discovered or studied in detail until the development of the microscope in the 17th century. Since then, much more has been learned, and a unifying theory known as the Cell Theory has been proposed.

The Cell Theory may be summarized as follows:
- All living things are composed of cells.
- The cell is the basic functional unit of life.
- The chemical reactions of life take place inside the cell.
- Cells arise only from pre-existing cells.
- Cells carry genetic information in the form of **DNA**. This genetic material is passed from parent cell to daughter cell.

Cell Structure

The components of the cell are specialized in their structure and function. These organelles include the nucleus, ribosomes, endoplasmic reticulum, Golgi apparatus, vesicles, vacuoles, lysosomes, mitochondria, chloroplasts, and centrioles.

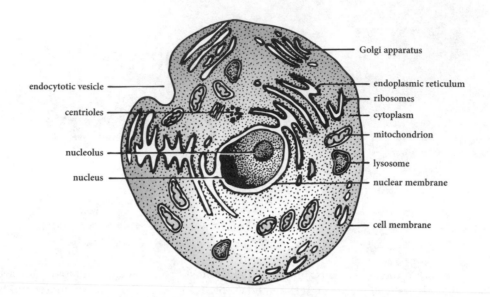

Figure 13.1

There are millions of species of "living things" that can be divided into six kingdoms: **Bacteria, Archaea, Protista, Fungi, Plantae,** and **Animalia.** Within these six kingdoms are two major types of cells: **prokaryotic** and **eukaryotic.** The word prokaryote means "before nucleus," and prokaryotic cells lack a membrane-bound nucleus. Note that scientists formerly divided life into only five kingdoms but recently separated the kingdom of Monera (Prokaryota) into Bacteria and Archaea due to differing evolutionary origins.

Cell membrane

The cell membrane (plasma membrane) encloses the cell and exhibits selective permeability; it regulates the passage of materials into and out of the cell. According to the generally accepted **fluid mosaic model**, the cell membrane consists of a phospholipid bilayer with proteins embedded throughout. The lipids and many of the proteins can move freely within the membrane.

The phospholipid bilayer has a specific structure that forms spontaneously. Phospholipid molecules are arranged such that the long, nonpolar, hydrophobic, "fatty" chains of carbon and hydrogen face each other, with the phosphorus-containing, polar, hydrophilic heads facing outward. The hydrophilic heads face the watery regions inside and outside the cell, while the hydrophobic tails face each other in a water-free region.

As a result of its lipid bilayer structure, a plasma membrane is readily permeable to both small, nonpolar hydrophobic molecules, such as oxygen, and small polar molecules, such as water. Small charged particles are usually able to cross the membrane through protein channels. However, charged ions and larger charged molecules cross the membrane with the assistance of **carrier proteins.**

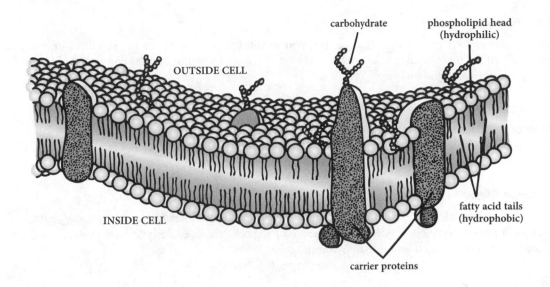

Figure 13.2

Nucleus

The nucleus controls the activities of the cell, including cell division. It is surrounded by a nuclear membrane. The nucleus contains DNA, which is complexed with structural proteins called **histones** to form **chromosomes**. DNA winds around histones to make it more compact, and these histones are also involved in regulation of gene transcription. The **nucleolus** is a dense structure in the nucleus where **ribosomal RNA** (rRNA) synthesis occurs (ribosomal RNA is necessary for protein synthesis at the ribosome).

Ribosome

Ribosomes are the sites of protein production and are synthesized by the nucleolus. Free ribosomes are found in the cytoplasm, whereas bound ribosomes line the outer membrane of the endoplasmic reticulum.

Endoplasmic reticulum

The endoplasmic reticulum (ER) is a network of membrane-enclosed spaces involved in the transport of materials throughout the cell, particularly those materials destined to be secreted by the cell. There are two kinds of endoplasmic reticuli, rough ER and smooth ER. **Smooth ER** does not contain ribosomes and so is not involved with protein synthesis but instead is involved with metabolism and the production of lipids. **Rough ER** contains ribosomes (which gives it a "rough" appearance under microscopy) and plays an important role in the production of proteins.

Golgi apparatus

The Golgi apparatus receives vesicles and their contents from the smooth ER and then modifies them (such as through glycosylation), repackages them into vesicles, and distributes them to the cell surface by exocytosis.

Mitochondria

Mitochondria are the sites of aerobic respiration within the cell and hence the suppliers of energy, especially in the form of adenosine triphosphate (ATP). Each mitochondrion is composed of an outer and inner phospholipid bilayer.

Cytoplasm

Most of the cell's metabolic activity occurs in the cytoplasm, which includes the **cytosol** (the cellular fluid contained within the cell membrane) and all the organelles of the cell. Transport within the cytoplasm occurs by **cyclosis** (streaming movement within the cell).

Vacuoles/Vesicles

Vacuoles and vesicles are membrane-bound sacs involved in the transport and storage of materials that are ingested, secreted, processed, or digested by the cell. Vacuoles are larger than vesicles and are more likely to be found in plant than in animal cells.

Centrioles

Centrioles are involved in spindle organization during cell division and are not bound by a membrane. Animal cells usually have a pair of centrioles oriented at right angles to each other that lie in a region called the centrosome. Plant cells do not contain centrioles.

Lysosomes

Lysosomes are membrane-bound vesicles that contain **hydrolytic enzymes** involved in intracellular digestion. Lysosomes break down material ingested by the cell. An injured or dying tissue may "commit suicide" by rupturing the lysosome membrane and releasing its hydrolytic enzymes; this process is called **autolysis**.

Cytoskeleton

The cytoskeleton supports the cell, maintains its shape, and aids in cell motility. It is composed of microtubules, microfilaments, and intermediate filaments.

Microtubules are hollow rods made up of polymerized **tubulin** that radiate throughout the cell and provide it with support. Microtubules provide a framework for organelle movement within the cell. Centrioles, which direct the separation of chromosomes during cell division, are composed of microtubules. **Cilia** and **flagella** are specialized arrangements of microtubules that extend from certain cells and are involved in cell motility and cytoplasmic movement.

Microfilaments are solid rods of **actin,** which are important in cell movement as well as support. Muscle contraction, for example, is based on the interaction of actin with myosin. Microfilaments move materials across the plasma membrane, for instance, in the contraction phase of cell division and in amoeboid movement.

CELLULAR TRANSPORT

Substances can move into and out of cells in various ways. Some methods occur passively, without energy, whereas others are active and require energy expenditure (via hydrolysis of ATP).

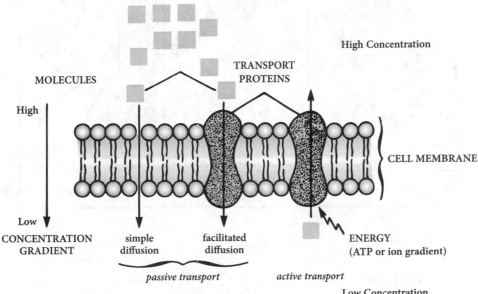

Figure 13.3

Simple Diffusion

Simple diffusion is the net movement of dissolved particles down their concentration gradients—from a region of higher concentration to a region of lower concentration. This is a passive process that requires no external source of energy.

Osmosis

Osmosis is the simple diffusion of water from a region of lower solute concentration to a region of higher solute concentration. When the cytoplasm of a cell has a lower solute concentration than the extracellular medium, the medium is said to be **hypertonic** to the cell, and water will flow out of the cell. This process, also called **plasmolysis**, will cause the cell to shrivel.

If the extracellular environment is less concentrated than the cytoplasm of the cell, the extracellular medium is said to be **hypotonic**, and water will flow into the cell, causing it to swell and **lyse** (burst). For example, red blood cells will burst if placed in distilled water. Freshwater protozoa have contractile vacuoles to pump out excess water and prevent bursting.

If the extracellular environment has the same concentration of solutes as the cell cytoplasm, the cell is said to be **isotonic** to the environment, and water will move back and forth in equal amounts across the cell membrane.

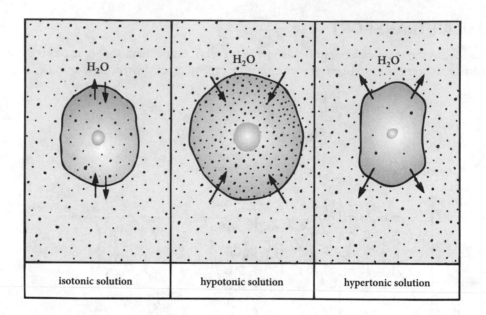

Figure 13.4

Facilitated Diffusion

Facilitated diffusion (passive transport) is the net movement of dissolved particles down their concentration gradient through special channels or carrier proteins in the cell membrane. This process, like simple diffusion, does not require energy.

Active Transport

Active transport is the net movement of dissolved particles against their concentration gradients with the help of transport proteins. Unlike diffusion, active transport requires energy. These carrier molecules or transport proteins aid in the regulation of the cell's internal content of ions and large molecules. The passage of specific ions and molecules is facilitated by these carrier molecules, which include the following:

- **Energy-independent carriers**: facilitate the movement of compounds along a concentration gradient
- **Symporters**: move two or more ions or molecules in the same direction across the membrane
- **Antiporters**: exchange one or more ions (or molecules) for another ion or molecule across the membrane
- **Pumps**: energy-dependent carriers (require ATP); e.g., sodium-potassium pump

Endocytosis

Endocytosis is a process in which the cell membrane invaginates, forming a vesicle that contains extracellular medium (see Figure 13.5). This allows the cell to bring large volumes of extracellular material inside the cell. **Pinocytosis** is the ingestion of fluids or small particles, and **phagocytosis** is the engulfing of large particles. Particles may bind to receptors on the cell membrane before being engulfed.

Exocytosis

In exocytosis, a vesicle within the cell fuses with the cell membrane and releases a large volume of contents to the outside. Fusion of the vesicle with the cell membrane can play an important role in cell growth and intercellular signaling (see Figure 13.5). For example, neurotransmitters, which act as signals to neighboring cells, are often released from neurons in this manner. Note that in both endocytosis and exocytosis, material never actually passes through the cell membrane.

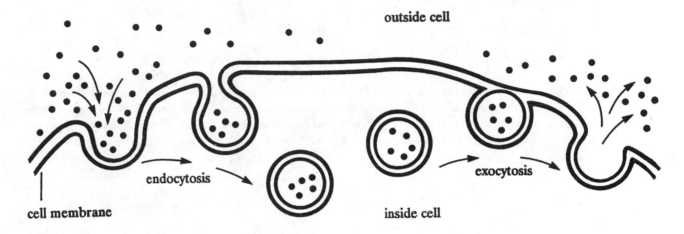

Figure 13.5

Intracellular Circulation

Materials move about within a cell in a number of ways. Some examples include the following:

- **Brownian movement**: Kinetic energy spreads small suspended particles throughout the cytoplasm of the cell.
- **Cyclosis or streaming**: The circular motion of cytoplasm around the cell transports molecules.
- **Endoplasmic reticulum**: The ER forms a network of channels throughout the cytoplasm and provides a direct continuous passageway from the plasma membrane to the nuclear membrane.

Extracellular Circulation

A number of systems deal with the movement of materials on a larger scale through the body of an organism. Examples include:

- **Diffusion**: If cells are in direct or close contact with the external environment, diffusion can serve as a sufficient means of transport for food and oxygen from the environment to the cells. In larger, more complex animals, diffusion is important for the transport of materials between cells and the interstitial fluid that bathes the cells.
- **Circulatory system**: Complex animals, whose cells are too far from the external environment to transport materials by diffusion, require a circulatory system. It generally includes vessels to transport fluid and a pump to drive the circulation. See Chapter 22 for more information.

CELL DIVISION

Cell division is the process by which a cell doubles its organelles and cytoplasm, replicates its DNA, and then divides in two. For **unicellular organisms**, cell division is a means of reproduction, whereas for **multicellular organisms**, it is a method of growth, development, and replacement of worn-out cells. Cell division can follow two different courses, mitosis or meiosis, but each is preceded by interphase. Together, these pieces constitute the **cell cycle,** the entire series of events leading to cellular replication.

Interphase

Interphase is a period of growth and chromosome replication. A cell normally spends at least 90 percent of its life in interphase. During this period, the cell performs its normal cellular functions, and each chromosome is replicated so that during division a complete copy of the genome can be distributed to both daughter cells. After replication, the chromosomes consist of two identical **sister chromatids** held together at a central region called the **centromere**. During interphase, the individual chromosomes are not visible; the DNA is instead uncoiled and called **chromatin**.

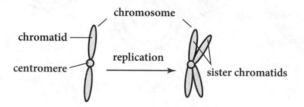

Figure 13.6

Interphase consists of the following three parts:

1. **G1**: This phase initiates interphase. It is described as the active growth phase and can vary in length. The cell increases in size and synthesizes proteins. The length of the G1 phase determines the length of the entire cell cycle.
2. **S**: This is the period of DNA synthesis.
3. **G2**: The cell prepares to divide in G2. It grows and synthesizes proteins.

The last phase of the cell cycle is the M phase. During M phase mitosis or meiosis occurs, generally resulting in either two identical or four non-identical daughter cells.

Mitosis

Mitosis is the division and distribution of the cell's DNA to its two daughter cells such that each cell receives a complete copy of the original genome. This type of cell division takes place in somatic cells (as opposed to gametes). Nuclear division (**karyokinesis**) is followed by cell division (**cytokinesis**).

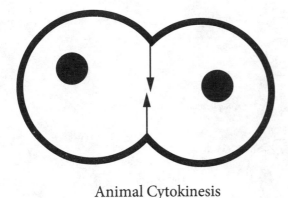

Animal Cytokinesis

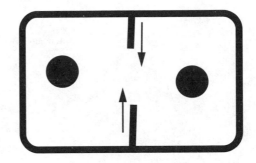

Plant Formation of Cell Plate

Figure 13.7

Prophase

During prophase, the chromosomes condense, and the centriole pairs (in animals) separate and move toward the opposite poles of the cell. The spindle apparatus forms between them, and the nuclear membrane dissolves, allowing the spindle fibers to interact with the chromosomes.

Metaphase

The centriole pairs are now at opposite poles of the cell. The fibers of the spindle apparatus attach to each chromatid at its corresponding **kinetochore**, a protein location on the centromere. The spindle fibers align the chromosomes at the center of the cell (equator), forming the **metaphase plate**.

Anaphase

The centromeres split so that each chromatid has its own distinct centromere, thus allowing sister chromatids to separate. The sister chromatids are pulled toward the opposite poles of the cell by the shortening of the spindle fibers. Spindle fibers are composed of microtubules.

Telophase

The spindle apparatus disappears. A nuclear membrane forms around each set of newly formed chromosomes. Thus, each nucleus contains the same number of chromosomes (the **diploid** number, $2N$) as the original or parent nucleus. The chromosomes uncoil, resuming their interphase form.

Cytokinesis

Near the end of telophase the cytoplasm divides into two daughter cells, each with a complete nucleus and its own set of organelles. In animal cells, a **cleavage furrow** forms, and the cell membrane indents along the equator of the cell, eventually pinching through the cell and separating the two nuclei. In plant cells a cell plate forms between the two nuclei, effectively splitting the plant cell in half and allowing the cell to divide.

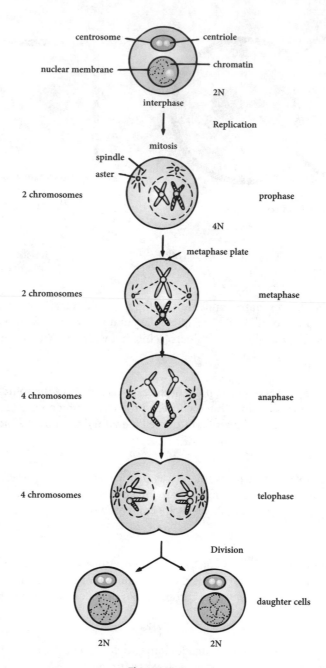

Figure 13.8

Meiosis

Sexual reproduction differs from asexual reproduction in that there are two parents involved. Sexual reproduction occurs via the fusion of two gametes—specialized sex cells produced by each parent. **Meiosis** is the process by which these sex cells are produced. Meiosis is similar to mitosis in that a cell duplicates its chromosomes before undergoing the process. However, whereas mitosis preserves the diploid number of the cell, meiosis produces **haploid (1N)** cells, halving the number of chromosomes. Meiosis involves two divisions of **primary sex cells**, resulting in four haploid cells called **gametes**.

Interphase

As in mitosis, the parent cell's chromosomes are replicated during interphase, resulting in the 2N number of sister chromatids.

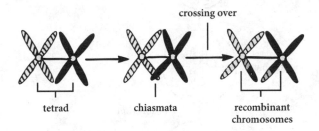

Figure 13.9

First meiotic division

The first division produces two intermediate daughter cells with N chromosomes and sister chromatids.

Prophase I: The chromatin condenses into chromosomes, the spindle apparatus forms, and the nucleoli and nuclear membrane disappear. Homologous chromosomes (chromosomes that code for the same traits, one inherited from each parent) come together and intertwine in a process called **synapsis**. Since at this stage each chromosome consists of two sister chromatids, each synaptic pair of homologous chromosomes contains four chromatids and is therefore often called a **tetrad**. Sometimes chromatids of homologous chromosomes break at corresponding points and exchange equivalent pieces of DNA; this process is called **crossing over**. The points of contact between these homologous chromosomes where crossing over can occur are called chiasmata. Note that crossing over occurs between homologous chromosomes and not between sister chromatids of the same chromosomes (the latter are identical, so **crossing over** would not produce any genetic variation). The chromatids involved are left with an altered but complete set of genes. Recombination among chromosomes results in increased genetic diversity within a species. Note that the two pairs of sister chromatids are no longer identical after recombination has occurred.

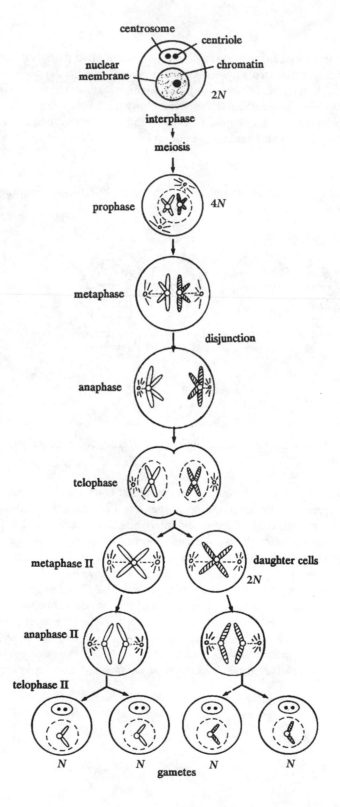

Figure 13.10

Metaphase I: Homologous pairs (tetrads) align at the equatorial plane, and each pair attaches to a separate spindle fiber at the kinetochore.

Anaphase I: The homologous pairs separate and are pulled to opposite poles of the cell. This process is called **disjunction**, and it accounts for a fundamental Mendelian law. During disjunction, each chromosome of paternal origin separates (or disjoins) from its homologue of maternal origin, and either chromosome can end up in either daughter cell. Thus, the distribution of homologous chromosomes to the two intermediate daughter cells is random with respect to parental origin. Each daughter cell will have a unique pool of genes from a random mixture of maternal and paternal origin.

Nondisjunction occurs when cells do not separate appropriately during meiosis. This results in the daughter cells having an incorrect number of chromosomes and is discussed in greater detail in Chapter 15.

Telophase I: A nuclear membrane forms around each new nucleus. At this point, each chromosome still consists of sister chromatids joined at the centromere.

Second meiotic division

This second division is very similar to mitosis, except that meiosis II is not preceded by chromosomal replication. The chromosomes align at the equator, separate and move to opposite poles, and are surrounded by a re-formed nuclear membrane. The new cells have the haploid number of chromosomes. Note that, in women, only one of these daughter cells becomes a functional gamete; the other two or three cells are destroyed by the body.

REVIEW PROBLEMS

1. All of the following are components of the Cell Theory EXCEPT the idea that

   (A) all living things are composed of cells.

   (B) all living things contain mitochondria.

   (C) cooperation among cells allows for complex functioning in living things.

   (D) all cells arise from pre-existing cells.

2. A eukaryotic cell contains organelles specialized for various activities. Name the organelles involved and the role they play in the following activities.

   (A) Ingestion

   (B) Digestion

   (C) Transport of proteins

3. Which of the following activities occurs in the Golgi apparatus?

   (A) Synthesis of proteins

   (B) Breakdown of lipids and carbohydrates

   (C) Catalysis of various oxidative reactions

   (D) Modification and packaging of proteins

4. Draw the fluid mosaic model of the cell membrane. How does this model account for the passage of materials across the membrane?

5. Prokaryotes and eukaryotes differ in a number of ways. Compare them in terms of the following characteristics.

   (A) Organization of genetic material

   (B) Site of cellular respiration

   (C) Presence of membrane-bound organelles

6. A researcher treats a solution containing animal cells with ouabain, a substance that interferes with the Na^+/K^+ pump embedded in the cell membrane and causes the cell to lyse. Which of the following statements best explains ouabain's mechanism of action?

   (A) Treatment with ouabain results in high levels of extracellular Ca_2^+.

   (B) Treatment with ouabain results in high levels of extracellular K^+ and Na^+.

   (C) Treatment with ouabain increases intracellular concentrations of Na^+.

   (D) Treatment with ouabain decreases intracellular concentrations of Na^+.

7. Prokaryotic cells and eukaryotic animal cells both have

   (A) DNA.

   (B) ribosomes.

   (C) a cell wall.

   (D) A and B.

8. What is the significance of the lysosomal membrane?

9. What roles do microtubules and microfilaments play in cell division?

10. If the haploid number of an organism is 13, what is its diploid number?

11. Fill in the blanks with the name of the appropriate stage of mitosis.
    (A) During _____, the chromosomes separate and move to opposite poles of the cell.
    (B) The nuclear membrane begins to dissolve during _____.
    (C) The centromeres of the replicated chromosomes have completely split by _____.
    (D) During _____, nucleoli disappear.
    (E) Chromosomes condense, shorten, and coil during _____.
    (F) Centromeres line up at the equatorial plate during _____.
    (G) During _____, a cleavage furrow is formed.

12. How do metaphase and anaphase of mitosis differ from metaphase I and anaphase I of meiosis?

SOLUTIONS TO REVIEW PROBLEMS

1. **B** Discussed in cell theory section of this chapter.

2. **A** Cellular ingestion is a function of the cell membrane and vesicles. The cell membrane invaginates around a food particle and pinches off, enclosing the material in a vesicle that can travel freely in the cytoplasm. This is known as endocytosis.

   B The organelles involved in digestion are lysosomes, vesicles, and mitochondria. A lysosome is a membrane-bound sac containing hydrolytic enzymes. It fuses with a vesicle, allowing its enzymes to chemically degrade the ingested material. The products of lysosomal digestion are released into the cytoplasm where they can be used by the cell. Glucose is metabolized in mitochondria via aerobic respiration.

   C The endoplasmic reticulum forms a long, interconnecting series of passageways through which proteins are transported. Smooth ER secretes proteins into cytoplasmic vesicles that are transported to the Golgi apparatus. Microtubules are involved in the transport of proteins in some specialized cells such as neurons.

3. **D** Discussed in cell biology section of this chapter.

4. According to the fluid mosaic model in Figure 13.2, the individual molecules of the lipid bilayer are in constant motion within the plane of the membrane. This fluidity allows ions and small molecules to diffuse directly across the cell membrane. However, large molecules cannot cross the membrane without the aid of special carrier protein molecules, which are embedded within the phospholipid bilayer. Some substances cannot cross the membrane at all. This selective permeability allows the cell membrane to tightly control the passage of materials into and out of the cell.

5. **A** In prokaryotes, the genetic material is composed of a single circular molecule of DNA localized in a region of the cell called the nucleoid. Eukaryotes have highly coiled linear strands of DNA organized into chromosomes within a membrane-bound nucleus.

   B In prokaryotes, cellular respiration occurs directly at the cell membrane, whereas in eukaryotes, cellular respiration occurs across the mitochondrial membrane and within the mitochondrion itself.

   C Prokaryotes do not contain any membrane-bound organelles, whereas eukaryotes contain a number of membrane-bound organelles, such as the nucleus, lysosomes, vesicles, ER, and mitochondria.

6. **C** This question requires an understanding of osmosis and the action of the Na^+/K^+ pump, also known as Na^+/K^+ adenosine triphosphatase (ATPase). When a cell is placed in a hypertonic solution (a solution having a higher solute concentration than the cell), fluid will diffuse out of the cell into the solution, resulting in cell shrinkage. When a cell is placed in a hypotonic solution (a solution having a lower solute concentration than the cell), fluid will diffuse from the solution into the cell, causing the cell to expand and possibly lyse. Na^+/K^+ ATPase moves three sodium ions out for every two potassium ions it lets into the cell. Therefore, inhibition of Na^+/K^+ ATPase by ouabain will cause a net increase in the Na^+ concentration inside the cell, and water will diffuse down its concentration gradient and into the cell, causing the cell to swell and then lyse.

7. **D** Discussed in cell biology section of this chapter.

8. The lysosomal membrane serves an important function. It protects the cell from the hydrolytic actions of the enzymes it contains. If the membrane were to burst, these enzymes would digest cellular components and ultimately kill the cell.

9. Microtubules and microfilaments play important roles in cell division. Microtubules form the mitotic spindle, which is responsible for separating sister chromatids. During prophase, a radial array of microtubules forms around the centrioles. The microtubules "push" the centrioles to opposite poles of the cell, forming the bipolar spindle apparatus. When the chromosomes align at the metaphase plate, these spindle fibers attach to the centromeres. During anaphase, the fibers shorten and pull on the centromeres, separating the sister chromatids and moving them toward opposite poles of the cell.

    After anaphase, microfilaments (actin filaments) and myosin filaments under the cell membrane contract, leading to the indentation of the membrane at the metaphase plate and the subsequent division of the parent cell into two daughter cells.

10. Haploid gametes are produced by meiosis, a process in which the chromosome number of the parent cell is reduced by one half. Thus, if the haploid number *(N)* of a particular organism is 13, then the diploid number *(2N)* must be 26.

11. **A** anaphase
    B prophase
    C anaphase
    D prophase
    E prophase
    F metaphase
    G telophase

12. In metaphase of mitosis, replicated chromosomes line up in single file; during anaphase, sister chromatids separate and move to opposite poles of the cell. In metaphase I of meiosis, homologous pairs of replicated chromosomes line up; during anaphase I, the homologous chromosomes separate, but sister chromatids remain attached to each other.

CHAPTER FOURTEEN

Molecular Biology

Humans use energy obtained from the digestion of food to maintain their internal environment and regulate the basic activities of life. The following terms are used to describe the acquisition, the conversion, and some of the uses of energy by a living organism:

- **Metabolism**: The sum of all chemical reactions that occur in the body. Metabolism can be divided into **catabolic reactions**, which break down large chemicals and release energy, and **anabolic reactions**, which build up large chemicals and require energy.

- **Ingestion**: The acquisition and consumption of food and other raw materials.

- **Digestion**: The process of converting food into a usable soluble form so it can pass through membranes in the digestive tract and enter the body.

- **Absorption**: The passage of nutrient molecules through the lining of the digestive tract into the body proper. Absorbed molecules pass through cells lining the digestive tract by diffusion or active transport.

- **Transport**: The circulation of essential compounds required to nourish the tissues and the removal of waste products from the tissues.

- **Assimilation**: The building up of new tissues from digested food materials.

- **Respiration**: The consumption of oxygen by the body. Cells use oxygen to convert glucose into ATP, a ready source of energy for cellular activities.

- **Excretion**: The removal of waste products (such as carbon dioxide, water, and urea) produced during metabolic processes like respiration and assimilation.

- **Synthesis**: The creation of complex molecules from simple ones (anabolism).

- **Regulation**: The control of physiological activities. The body's metabolism functions to maintain its internal environment in a changing external environment. The steady state of the internal environment is known as **homeostasis** and includes regulation by hormones and the nervous system. **Irritability** is the ability to respond to a stimulus and is part of regulation.

- **Growth**: An increase in size caused by cell division and synthesis of new materials.

- **Reproduction**: The generation of additional individuals of a species.

RESPIRATION

Respiration involves the conversion of the chemical energy in molecular bonds into the usable energy needed to drive the processes of living cells. All living cells need energy for growth, maintenance of homeostasis, defense mechanisms, repair, and reproduction. The cells of the human body and those of other organisms obtain this energy from aerobic respiration (in the presence of oxygen). Respiration refers to the use of **oxygen** by an organism. This process includes the intake of oxygen from the environment, the transport of oxygen in the blood, and the ultimate oxidation of fuel molecules in the cell. **External respiration** refers to the entrance of air into the lungs and the gas exchange between the alveoli and the blood (see Chapter 22). **Internal respiration** includes the exchange of gas between the blood and the cells and the intracellular processes of respiration.

Carbohydrates and fats are the favored **fuel** molecules in living cells. As hydrogen is removed, bond energy is made available. The C-H bond is energy rich; in fact, compared with other bonds, it is capable of releasing the largest amount of energy per mole. In contrast, carbon dioxide contains little usable energy. It is the stable, energy-exhausted end product of respiration.

During respiration, high-energy hydrogen atoms are removed from organic molecules. This is called **dehydrogenation** and is an oxidation reaction. The subsequent acceptance of hydrogen by a hydrogen acceptor (oxygen in the final step) is the reduction component of the redox reaction. Energy released by this reduction is used to form a high-energy phosphate bond in ATP. Although the initial oxidation step requires energy input, the net result of the redox reaction is energy production. If all of this energy was released in a single step, little could be harnessed. Instead, the reductions occur in a series of steps called the **electron transport chain.**

GLUCOSE CATABOLISM

The degradative oxidation of glucose occurs in two stages: **glycolysis** and **cellular respiration.**

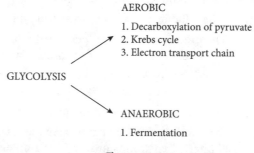

AEROBIC

1. Decarboxylation of pyruvate
2. Krebs cycle
3. Electron transport chain

GLYCOLYSIS

ANAEROBIC

1. Fermentation

Figure 14.1

Glycolysis

The first stage of glucose catabolism is glycolysis. Glycolysis is a series of reactions that leads to the oxidative breakdown of glucose into two molecules of **pyruvate** (the ionized form of pyruvic acid), the production of ATP, and the reduction of NAD^+ into NADH. All of these reactions occur in the **cytoplasm** and are mediated by specific enzymes.

The process of glycolysis is defined as the sequence of reactions that converts glucose into pyruvate with the concomitant production of ATP. Glycolysis begins when glucose reacts with hexokinase to form glucose 6-phosphate. When this compound interacts with the enzyme phosphoglucose isomerase, the compound fructose 6-phosphate is formed. Fructose 6-phosphate interacts with the enzyme phosphofructokinase to form the compound fructose 1,6-biphosphate. When interacted with aldolase, glyceraldehyde 3-phosphate is formed. After a number of enzymatic reactions, the compound phosphoenolpyruvate is formed. When acted upon by pyruvate kinase, pyruvate is formed, and the glycolytic pathway is completed.

Glycolytic pathway

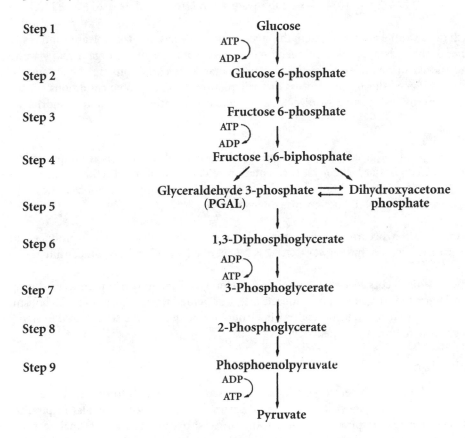

*Note: Steps 5–9 occur twice per molecule of glucose

Figure 14.2

Note that at step 4, fructose 1,6-biphosphate is split into two three-carbon molecules: **dihydroxyacetone phosphate** and **glyceraldehyde 3-phosphate (PGAL).** Dihydroxyacetone phosphate is isomerized into PGAL so that it can be used in subsequent reactions. Thus, two molecules of PGAL are formed per molecule of glucose, and all of the subsequent steps occur twice for each glucose molecule.

From one molecule of glucose (a six-carbon molecule), two molecules of pyruvate (a three-carbon molecule) are obtained. During this sequence of reactions, two ATP are used (in steps 1 and 3) and four ATP are generated (two in step 6 and two in step 9). Thus, there is a net production of two ATP per glucose molecule. This type of phosphorylation is called **substrate level phosphorylation** because ATP synthesis is directly coupled with the degradation of glucose without the participation of an intermediate molecule such as NAD^+. One NADH is produced per PGAL for a total of two NADH per glucose.

The net reaction for glycolysis is:

$$\text{Glucose} + 2\,\text{ADP} + 2\,P_i + 2\,NAD^+ \longrightarrow 2\,\text{Pyruvate} + 2\,\text{ATP} + 2\,\text{NADH} + 2\,H^+ + 2\,H_2O$$

At this stage much of the initial energy stored in the glucose molecule has not been released and is still present in the chemical bonds of pyruvate. Depending on the capabilities of the organism, pyruvate degradation can proceed in one of two directions. Under **anaerobic** conditions (in the absence of oxygen), pyruvate is reduced during the process of fermentation. Under aerobic conditions (in the presence of oxygen), pyruvate is further oxidized during cellular respiration in the mitochondria.

Fermentation

NAD^+ must be regenerated for glycolysis to continue in the absence of O_2. This is accomplished by reducing pyruvate into ethanol or lactic acid. Fermentation refers to all of the reactions involved in this process (i.e., glycolysis and the additional steps leading to the formation of ethanol or lactic acid). Fermentation produces only two ATP per glucose molecule.

Alcohol fermentation often occurs only in yeast and some bacteria. The pyruvate produced in glycolysis is converted to ethanol. In this way, NAD^+ is regenerated and glycolysis can continue.

Lactic acid fermentation occurs in certain fungi and bacteria and in human muscle cells during strenuous activity. When the oxygen supply to muscle cells lags behind the rate of glucose catabolism, the pyruvate generated is reduced to lactic acid. As in alcohol fermentation, the NAD^+ used in step 5 of glycolysis is regenerated when pyruvate is reduced.

Cellular Respiration

Cellular respiration is the most efficient catabolic pathway used by organisms to harvest the energy stored in glucose. Whereas glycolysis yields only **2 ATP** per molecule of glucose, cellular respiration can yield **36–38 ATP**. Cellular respiration is an **aerobic** process; **oxygen** acts as the final acceptor of electrons that are passed from carrier to carrier during the final stage of glucose oxidation. The metabolic reactions of cell respiration occur in the eukaryotic mitochondrion and are catalyzed by reaction-specific enzymes.

Cellular respiration can be divided into three stages: pyruvate decarboxylation, the citric acid cycle, and the electron transport chain.

Pyruvate decarboxylation

The pyruvate formed during glycolysis is transported from the cytoplasm into the mitochondrial matrix where it is decarboxylated (i.e., it loses a CO_2), and the acetyl group that remains is transferred to coenzyme A to form acetyl-CoA. In the process, NAD^+ is reduced to NADH.

Citric acid cycle

The citric acid cycle is also known as the **Krebs cycle**. The cycle begins when the two-carbon acetyl group from acetyl-CoA combines with oxaloacetate, a four-carbon molecule, to form the six-carbon citrate. Through a series of reactions, two CO_2 are released, and oxaloacetate is regenerated for use in another turn of the cycle.

For each turn of the citric acid cycle one ATP is produced by substrate-level phosphorylation via a GTP intermediate. In addition, electrons are transferred to NAD^+ and FAD, generating NADH and $FADH_2$, respectively. These coenzymes then transport the electrons to the electron transport chain, where more ATP is produced via oxidative phosphorylation (see below). Studying the cycle, we can do some bookkeeping; keep in mind that for each molecule of glucose, two pyruvate are decarboxylated and channeled into the citric acid cycle. Therefore, two of each type of molecular product at this stage of the cycle are created for each glucose molecule.

$$2 \times 3 \text{ NADH} \quad \rightarrow \quad 6 \text{ NADH}$$
$$2 \times 1 \text{ FADH}_2 \quad \rightarrow \quad 2 \text{ FADH}_2$$
$$2 \times 1 \text{ GTP (ATP)} \quad \rightarrow \quad 2 \text{ ATP}$$

The net reaction of the citric acid cycle per glucose molecule is:

$$2 \text{ acetyl-CoA} + 6 \text{ NAD}^+ + 2 \text{ FAD} + 2 \text{ GDP} + 2 \text{ P}_i + 4 \text{ H}_2\text{O} \longrightarrow$$
$$4 \text{ CO}_2 + 6 \text{ NADH} + 2 \text{ FADH}_2 + 2 \text{ GTP} + 4 \text{ H}^+ + 2\text{CoA}$$

Electron transport chain

The electron transport chain (ETC) is a complex carrier mechanism located on the inside of the **inner mitochondrial membrane.** During oxidative phosphorylation, ATP is produced when high-energy potential electrons are transferred from NADH and $FADH_2$ to oxygen by a series of carrier molecules located in the inner mitochondrial membrane. As the electrons are transferred from carrier to carrier, free energy is released, which is then used to form ATP. Most molecules of the ETC are **cytochromes**, electron carriers that resemble hemoglobin in the structure of their active site. The functional unit contains a central iron atom that is capable of undergoing a reversible redox reaction (i.e., it can be alternatively reduced and oxidized). Sequential redox reactions continue to occur as the electrons are transferred from one carrier to the next; each carrier is reduced as it accepts an electron and is then oxidized when it passes it on to the next carrier. The last carrier of the ETC passes its electron to the final electron acceptor, O_2. In addition to the electrons, O_2 picks up a pair of hydrogen ions from the surrounding medium, forming water.

$$2 \text{ H}^+ + 2 \text{ e}^- + \frac{1}{2} \text{ O}_2 \longrightarrow \text{H}_2\text{O}$$

Total Energy Production

To calculate the net amount of ATP produced per molecule of glucose, we need to tally the number of ATP produced by substrate-level phosphorylation and the number of ATP produced by oxidative phosphorylation.

Substrate-level phosphorylation

Degradation of one glucose molecule yields a net of two ATP from glycolysis and one ATP for each turn of the citric acid cycle. Thus, a total of four ATP are produced by substrate-level phosphorylation.

Oxidative phosphorylation

Oxidative phosphorylation is the process that produces more than 90 percent of the ATP used by the cells in our body. The major steps involved in this process occur within the ETC or respiratory chain of the mitochondria. The steps at the end of the electron transport chain where ATP is generated are as follows: Along the ETC, the respiratory enzymes continually pump hydrogen ions from the matrix of the mitochondria to the intermembrane space, which creates a large concentration gradient. At the end of the ETC, hydrogen ions pass through channels in the respiratory enzymes along the concentration gradient. As the hydrogen ions pass through these enzymes, the energy created is used to convert ADP to ATP. Now, specifically looking at the process of oxidative phosphorylation, two pyruvate decarboxylations yield one NADH each for a total of two NADH. Each turn of the citric acid cycle yields three NADH and one $FADH_2$, for a total of six NADH and two $FADH_2$ per glucose molecule. Each $FADH_2$ generates two ATP, as previously discussed. Each NADH generates three ATP except for the two NADH that were reduced during glycolysis. These NADH cannot cross the inner mitochondrial membrane and must transfer their electrons to an intermediate carrier molecule, which delivers the electrons to the second carrier protein complex, Q. Therefore, because one ATP is used in this transfer, these NADH generate only two ATP per glucose. So the two NADH of glycolysis yield four ATP, the other eight NADH yield 24 ATP, and the two $FADH_2$ produce four ATP, for a total of 32 ATP by oxidative phosphorylation.

The total amount of ATP produced during eukaryotic glucose catabolism is therefore four via substrate-level phosphorylation plus 32 via oxidative phosphorylation, for a total of 36 ATP. (For prokaryotes, the yield is 38 ATP because the two NADH of glycolysis don't have any mitochondrial membranes to cross and therefore don't lose energy.)

Eukaryotic ATP Production per Glucose Molecule

Glycolysis

2 ATP invested (steps 1 and 3)	− 2 ATP
4 ATP generated (steps 6 and 9)	+ 4 ATP (substrate)
2 NADH × 2 ATP/NADH (step 5)	+ 4 ATP (oxidative)

Pyruvate decarboxylation

2 NADH × 3 ATP/NADH	+ 6 ATP (oxidative)

Citric acid cycle

6 NADH × 3 ATP/NADH	+ 18 ATP (oxidative)
2 $FADH_2$ × 2 ATP/$FADH_2$	+ 4 ATP (oxidative)
2 GTP × 1 ATP/GTP	+ 2 ATP (substrate)
Total	+ 36 ATP

ALTERNATE ENERGY SOURCES

When glucose supplies run low, the body uses other energy sources. These sources are used by the body in the following preferential order: other carbohydrates, fats, and proteins. These substances are first converted to either glucose or glucose intermediates, which can then be degraded in the glycolytic pathway and the citric acid cycle.

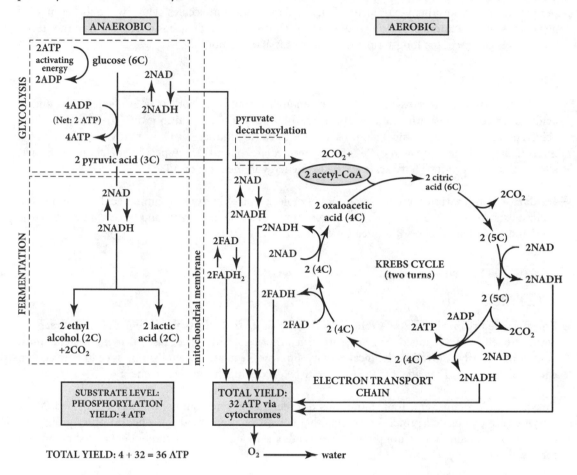

Figure 14.3

Carbohydrates

Disaccharides are hydrolyzed into monosaccharides, most of which can be converted into glucose or glycolytic intermediates. Glycogen stored in the liver can be converted, when needed, into a glycolytic intermediate.

Fats

Fat molecules are stored in adipose tissue in the form of triglycerides. When needed, they are hydrolyzed by **lipases** to **fatty acids** and **glycerol** and are carried by the blood to other tissues for oxidation. Glycerol can be converted into PGAL, a glycolytic intermediate. A fatty acid must first be "activated" in the cytoplasm; this process requires two ATP. Once activated, the fatty acid is transported into the mitochondrion and taken through a series of beta-oxidation cycles that convert it into two-carbon fragments, which are then converted into acetyl-CoA. Acetyl-CoA then enters the citric acid cycle. With each round of β-oxidation of a saturated fatty acid, one NADH and one $FADH_2$ are generated.

Of all the high-energy compounds used in cellular respiration, fats yield the greatest number of ATP per gram. This makes them extremely efficient energy storage molecules. Thus, while the amount of glycogen stored in humans is enough to meet the short-term energy needs of about a day, the stored fat reserves can meet the long-term energy needs for about a month.

Proteins

The body degrades proteins only when not enough carbohydrate or fat is available. Most amino acids undergo a **transamination reaction** in which they lose an amino group to form an α-keto acid. The carbon atoms of most amino acids are converted into acetyl-CoA, pyruvate, or one of the intermediates of the citric acid cycle. These intermediates enter their respective metabolic pathways, allowing cells to produce fatty acids, glucose, or energy in the form of ATP.

Oxidative deamination removes an ammonia molecule directly from the amino acid. **Ammonia** is a toxic substance in vertebrates. Fish can excrete ammonia, whereas insects and birds convert it to uric acid, and mammals convert it to urea for excretion.

ENZYMES

Enzymes are organic catalysts. A catalyst is any substance that affects the rate of a chemical reaction without itself being changed. Enzymes are crucial to living things because all living systems must have continuously controlled chemical activity. Enzymes regulate metabolism by speeding up certain chemical reactions. They affect the reaction rate by decreasing the activation energy.

Enzymes are proteins, and thus, thousands of different enzymes can conceivably be formed. Many enzymes are conjugated proteins (proteins that consist of amino acids attached to other groups via covalent bonds) and have a nonprotein **coenzyme**. In these cases, both components must be present for the enzyme to function.

Enzymes are very selective; they may catalyze only one reaction or one specific class of closely related reactions. The molecule upon which an enzyme acts is called the **substrate**. There is an area on each enzyme to which the substrate binds called the **active site**. The following characteristics are true for all enzymes:

- Enzymes do NOT alter the equilibrium constant.
- Enzymes are NOT consumed in the reaction. This means that they will appear in both the reactants and the products.
- Enzymes are pH and temperature sensitive, with optimal activity at specific pH ranges and temperatures.

Most enzyme-catalyzed reactions are reversible. The product synthesized by an enzyme can be decomposed by the same enzyme. An enzyme that synthesizes maltose from glucose can also hydrolyze maltose back to glucose. The two models that follow describe the binding of the enzyme to the substrate.

Lock and Key Theory

This theory holds that the spatial structure of an enzyme's active site is exactly complementary to the spatial structure of its substrate. The two fit together like a lock and key. In other words, receptors are large proteins that contain a recognition site (lock) that is directly linked to transduction systems. When a drug or endogenous substance (key) binds to the receptor, a sequence of events is started. Although this theory has been largely discounted, it is still frequently used as a teaching tool when explaining drug interactions with receptors and enzymes.

Induced Fit Theory

This more widely accepted theory describes the active site as having flexibility of shape. When the appropriate substrate comes in contact with the active site, the conformation of the active site changes to fit the substrate.

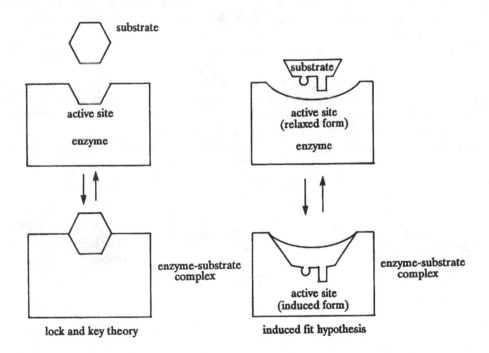

Figure 14.4

Enzyme Specificity

Enzyme action and the reaction rate depend on several environmental factors including temperature, pH, and the concentration of enzyme and substrate.

In general, as the temperature increases, the rate of enzyme action increases until an optimum temperature is reached (usually around 40°C). Beyond optimal temperature, heat alters the shape of the active site of the enzyme molecule and deactivates it, leading to a rapid drop in rate.

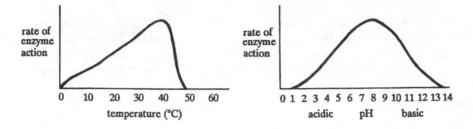

Figure 14.5

For each enzyme there is an optimal pH; above and below that, enzymatic activity declines. Maximal activity of many human enzymes occurs around pH 7.2, which is the pH of most body fluids. Exceptions include **pepsin**, which works best in the highly acidic conditions of the stomach (pH = 2), and pancreatic enzymes, which work optimally in the alkaline conditions of the small intestine (pH = 8.5). In most cases the optimal pH matches the conditions under which the enzyme operates.

The concentrations of substrate and enzyme greatly affect the reaction rate. When the concentrations of both enzyme and substrate are low, many of the active sites on the enzyme are unoccupied, and the reaction rate is low. Increasing the substrate concentration will increase the reaction rate until all of the active sites are occupied. After this point, further increase in substrate concentration will not increase the reaction rate, and the reaction is said to have reached the maximum velocity, V_{max}.

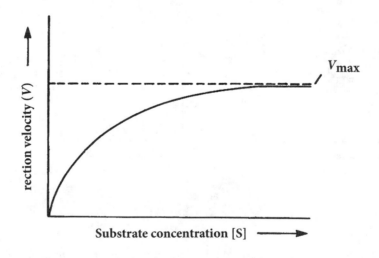

Figure 14.6

Competitive Inhibition

The active site of an enzyme is specific for a particular substrate or class of substrates. However, it is possible for molecules that are similar to the substrate to bind to the active site of the enzyme. If a similar molecule is present in a concentration comparable to the concentration of the substrate, it will compete with the substrate for binding sites on the enzyme and interfere with enzyme activity. This is known as competitive inhibition because the enzyme is inhibited by the inactive substrate, or competitor. If sufficient quantities of the substrate are introduced, however, the substrate can outcompete the competitor and will still be able to reach the V_{max}; however, this will require much higher concentrations of substrate than would be necessary without the competitor.

Noncompetitive Inhibition

A noncompetitive inhibitor is a substance that forms strong covalent bonds with an enzyme, making it unable to bind with its substrate, and consequently a noncompetitive inhibitor cannot be displaced by the addition of excess substrate. Therefore, noncompetitive inhibition is irreversible. Because this inhibition is noncompetitive, addition of excess substrate will not influence the rate of the reaction, and the reaction will never reach V_{max}. A noncompetitive inhibitor may be bound at, near, or far from the active site. When the inhibition takes place at a site other then the active site, this is called **allosteric inhibition**. (**Allosteric** means "other site" or "other structure.") The interaction of an inhibitor at an allosteric site changes the structure of the enzyme so that the active site is also changed.

Examples of enzyme activity

Every reaction in the body is regulated by enzymes. Some of the basic reaction types are listed below.

Hydrolysis reactions function to digest large molecules into smaller components. **Lactase** hydrolyzes lactose to the monosaccharides glucose and galactose. **Proteases** degrade proteins to amino acids, and **lipases** break down lipids to fatty acids and glycerol.

In multicellular organisms, digestion can begin outside of the cells in the gut. Other hydrolytic reactions occur within cells.

Synthesis reactions (including dehydrations) can be catalyzed by the same enzymes as hydrolysis reactions, but the directions of the reactions are reversed.

These reactions occur in different parts of the cell. For example, protein synthesis occurs in the ribosomes and involves dehydration reactions between amino acids.

Synthesis is required for growth, repair, regulation, protection, and production of food reserves such as fat and glycogen by the cell. The survival of an organism depends on its ability to ingest substances that it needs but cannot synthesize. Once ingested, these substances are converted into useful products.

Certain vitamin cofactors and essential amino acids cannot be synthesized by humans. If they are not available in the diet, deficiency diseases will occur.

Many enzymes require the incorporation of a nonprotein molecule to become active. These molecules, called **cofactors**, can be metal cations such as Zn^{2+} or Fe^{2+} or small organic groups called coenzymes. Most coenzymes cannot be synthesized by the body and are obtained from the diet as vitamin derivatives. Cofactors that bind to the enzyme by strong covalent bonds are called **prosthetic groups**.

REVIEW PROBLEMS

1. What is the net reaction for glycolysis? For the citric acid cycle?

2. In glucose catabolism

   (A) oxygen must be the final electron acceptor.
   (B) oxygen is necessary for any ATP synthesis.
   (C) inorganic phosphate is produced.
   (D) ATP is generated.

3. Fatty acids enter the degradative pathway in the form of

   (A) glycerol.
   (B) glucose.
   (C) acetyl-CoA.
   (D) brown adipose tissue.

4. How do ATP, NADH, and $FADH_2$ store energy?

5. How is NAD^+ regenerated and why is this important?

6. Describe the production of ATP via oxidative phosphorylation.

7. Which of the following is LEAST likely to occur during oxygen debt?

   (A) Buildup of lactic acid
   (B) Buildup of pyruvate
   (C) Decrease in pH
   (D) Fatigue

8. Describe the kinetic effects of increasing substrate concentration while enzyme concentration remains constant.

9. What determines enzyme specificity?

SOLUTIONS TO REVIEW PROBLEMS

1. The net reaction for glycolysis is:

    Glucose + 2ATP + 4ADP + 2P$_i$ + 2NAD$^+$ →

    2 Pyruvate + 2ADP + 4ATP + 2NADH + 2H$^+$ + 2H$_2$O

    The net reaction for the citric acid cycle is:

    2 Acetyl-CoA + 6NAD$^+$ + 2FAD + 2GDP + 2P$_i$ + 4H$_2$O →

    4CO$_2$ + 6NADH + 2FADH$_2$ + 2GTP + 4H$^+$ + 2CoA

2. **D** Although oxygen is necessary as the final electron receptor for aerobic catabolism (respiration), anaerobic catabolism (fermentation) can occur in the absence of oxygen to still consume ADP and inorganic phosphate as reactants to create ATP.

3. **C** Discussed in alternate energy sources section of this chapter.

4. Energy is stored in ATP as high-energy bonds created by the covalent bonding of three phosphates to adenosine. The hydrolysis of ATP to ADP releases inorganic phosphate (P$_i$) and 7 kcal of energy. Hydrolysis of ADP to AMP releases an additional 7 kcal. Alternatively, ATP hydrolysis to AMP + PP$_i$ releases 7 kcal.

    NADH and FADH$_2$ are reducing agents that carry chemical energy in the form of high-potential electrons, which can be transferred as hydride ions. In cellular respiration, these hydride ions are transferred to the electron transport chain, where energy release is coupled with ATP synthesis during a series of redox reactions.

5. Step 5 of glycolysis involves the reduction of NAD$^+$ to NADH. Because NAD$^+$ is necessary for glycolysis to continue, it must be regenerated in one of two ways. In the presence of oxygen, oxidative phosphorylation and the ETC can be used to oxidize NADH to NAD$^+$. Alternatively, alcohol or lactic acid fermentation can be used to regenerate NAD$^+$ under anaerobic conditions.

6. In the electron transport chain, the release of hydrogen ions is coupled with the transfer of electrons. H$^+$ ions accumulate in the mitochondrial matrix and are shuttled across the inner mitochondrial membrane, creating a proton gradient. To cross the inner membrane, the hydrogen ions must pass through ATP synthetases, which catalyze the phosphorylation of ADP into ATP.

7. **B** Discussed in fermentation section of this chapter.

8. When substrate concentration is low, the reaction proceeds slowly. Initial increases in substrate concentration greatly increase the reaction rate because of the binding of substrate to available active sites. Eventually, a point is reached at which all of the active sites are occupied, and the addition of more substrate will not hasten the reaction appreciably. Eventually, at very high levels of substrate, the reaction rate approaches a maximum, V_{max}.

9. Enzyme specificity is determined by the unique three-dimensional spatial structure of the active site. According to the induced fit hypothesis, an enzyme's active site is capable of undergoing a conformational change when the appropriate substrate comes into contact with it, such that the substrate is held in place to form an enzyme-substrate complex.

CHAPTER FIFTEEN

Genetics

Genetics is the study of how traits are inherited from one generation to the next. The basic unit of heredity is the **gene**. Genes are composed of DNA and are located on **chromosomes**. When a gene exists in more than one form, the alternative forms are called **alleles**. The genetic makeup of an individual is the individual's **genotype**; the physical manifestation of the genetic makeup is the individual's **phenotype**. Some phenotypes correspond to a single genotype, whereas other phenotypes correspond to several different genotypes. Knowledge of genetics will help clarify the concepts of evolution by the process of natural selection.

MENDELIAN GENETICS

In the 1860s Gregor Mendel developed the basic principles of genetics through his experiments with the garden pea. Mendel studied the inheritance of individual pea traits by performing **genetic crosses**. He took true-breeding individuals (which, if self-crossed, produce progeny only with the parental phenotype) with different traits, mated them, and statistically analyzed the inheritance of the traits in the progeny.

Mendel's First Law: Law of Segregation

Mendel postulated four principles of inheritance:

1. Genes exist in alternative forms (now referred to as alleles). A gene controls a specific trait in an organism.

2. An organism has two alleles for each inherited trait, one inherited from each parent.

3. The two alleles **segregate** during meiosis, resulting in gametes that carry only one allele for any given inherited trait.

4. If two alleles in an individual organism are different, only one will be fully expressed, and the other will be silent. The expressed allele is said to be **dominant**, the silent allele, **recessive**. In genetics problems dominant alleles are typically assigned capital letters, and recessive alleles are assigned lowercase letters. Organisms that contain two copies of the same allele are **homozygous** for that trait; organisms that carry two different alleles are **heterozygous**. The dominant allele is expressed in the phenotype. This is known as **Mendel's Law of Dominance**. For example, for the genotypes shown below, Yy and YY will both be yellow:

Genes	Genotype	Phenotype
YY	Homozygous	Yellow
Yy	Heterozygous	Yellow
yy	Homozygous	Green

Monohybrid cross

The principles of Mendelian inheritance can be illustrated in a cross between two true-breeding pea plants, one with purple flowers and the other with white flowers. Because only one trait is being studied in this particular mating, it is referred to as a **monohybrid cross**. The individuals being crossed are the **parental** or **P generation**; the progeny generations are the **filial** or **F generations**, with each generation numbered sequentially (e.g., F1, F2, etc.).

The purple flower parent has the genotype PP (i.e., it has two P alleles) and is homozygous dominant. The white flower parent has the genotype pp and is homozygous recessive. When these individuals are crossed, they produce F1 plants that are 100 percent heterozygous (genotype = Pp). Because purple is dominant to white, all the F1 progeny have the purple flower phenotype.

Punnett square

One way of predicting the genotypes expected from a cross is by drawing a **Punnett square diagram**. The parental genotypes are arranged around a grid. Because the genotype of each progeny will be the sum of the alleles donated by the parental gametes, their genotypes can be determined by looking at the intersections on the grid. A Punnett square indicates all the potential progeny genotypes, and the relative frequencies of the different genotypes and phenotypes can be easily calculated.

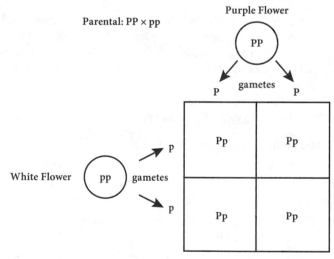

F$_1$ genotypes: 100% Pp (heterozygous)
F$_1$ phenotypes: 100% purple flowers

Figure 15.1

When the F1 generation from our monohybrid cross is self-crossed (i.e., Pp × Pp), the F2 progeny are more genotypically and phenotypically diverse than their parents. Because the F1 plants are heterozygous, they will donate a P allele to half of their descendants and a p allele to the other half. One-fourth (25%) of the F2 plants will have the genotype PP, 50 percent will have the genotype Pp, and 25 percent will have the genotype pp. Because the homozygous dominant and heterozygous genotypes both produce the dominant phenotype purple flowers, 75 percent of the F2 plants will have purple flowers, and 25 percent will have white flowers.

This is a standard pattern of Mendelian inheritance. Its hallmarks are the disappearance of the silent (recessive) phenotype in the F1 generation and its subsequent reappearance in 25 percent of the individuals in the F2 generation. If we were to take a closer look at the physical characteristics of the plants themselves, we would find that the 1:2:1 genotypic ratio produces a 3:1 phenotypic ratio.

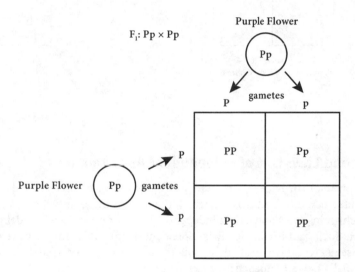

F_2 genotypes: 1:2:1; 1PP: 2Pp:1pp)
F_2 phenotypes: 3:1; 3 purple:1 white

Figure 15.2

Testcross

Mendel also developed the **testcross,** a diagnostic tool used to determine the genotype of an organism. Only with a recessive phenotype can genotype be predicted with 100 percent accuracy. If the dominant phenotype is expressed, the genotype can be either homozygous dominant or heterozygous. Thus, homozygous recessive organisms always breed true. This fact can be used to determine the unknown genotype of an organism with a dominant phenotype, such as when an organism with a dominant phenotype of unknown genotype (Ax) is crossed with a phenotypically recessive organism (genotype aa). Since the recessive parent is homozygous, it can donate only the recessive allele, a, to the progeny. If the dominant parent's genotype is AA, all of its gametes will carry an A, and all of the progeny will have genotype Aa. If the dominant parent's genotype is Aa, half of the progeny will be Aa and express the dominant phenotype, and half will be aa and express the recessive phenotype. In a testcross, the appearance of the recessive phenotype in the progeny indicates that the phenotypically dominant parent is genotypically heterozygous.

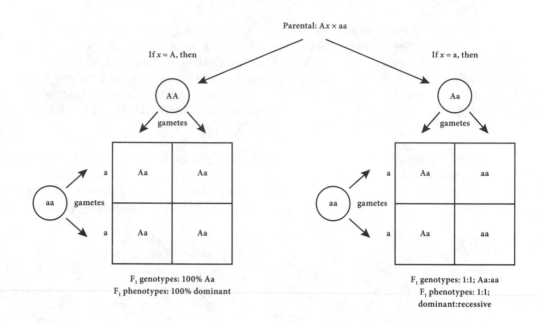

Figure 15.3

Mendel's Second Law: Law of Independent Assortment

The segregation principle provides a satisfactory explanation for the inheritance of a single allele and also can be extended to a dihybrid cross, in which the parents differ in two traits, as long as the genes are on separate chromosomes and assort independently during meiosis. Mendel postulated that the inheritance of one such trait is completely independent of any other. In this way, a plant with purple flowers is no more likely to be a dwarf than a plant with white flowers (see the example below). This is known as **Mendel's Law of Independent Assortment**.

Note that according to modern, non-Mendelian genetics, genes on the same chromosome will not follow this rule and instead will stay together unless **crossing over** occurs (see Chapter 13, Cellular Biology). Nevertheless, crossing over exchanges information between chromosomes and may break the linkage of certain patterns. For example, red hair is usually linked with freckles, but some blondes and brunettes have freckles as well. Generally, the closer the genes are on the chromosome, the more likely they are to be inherited together.

Dihybrid cross

In the following example, a purple-flowered tall pea plant is crossed with a white-flowered dwarf pea plant; both plants are doubly homozygous (tall is dominant to dwarf, T = tall allele, t = dwarf allele; purple is dominant to white, P = purple allele, p = white allele). The purple parent's genotype is TTPP, and it thus produces only TP gametes; the white parent's genotype is ttpp and produces only tp gametes. The F1 progeny will all have the genotype TtPp and will be phenotypically dominant for both traits.

When the F1 generation is self-crossed (TtPp × TtPp), it produces four different phenotypes: tall purple, tall white, dwarf purple, and dwarf white, in the ratio 9:3:3:1, respectively. This is the typical pattern for Mendelian inheritance in a dihybrid cross between heterozygotes with independently assorting traits.

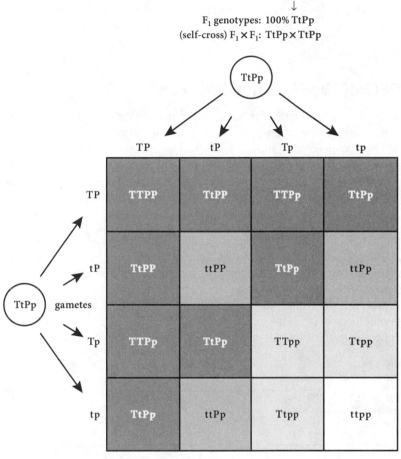

Parental: TTPP × ttpp

↓

F₁ genotypes: 100% TtPp

(self-cross) F₁ × F₁: TtPp × TtPp

F₂ phenotypes: 9:3:3:1
F₂ tall purple:3 tall white:3 dwarf purple:1 dwarf white

Figure 15.4

Drosophila melanogaster

Modern work with the fruit fly (*Drosophila melanogaster*) helped to provide explanations for Mendelian genetic patterns. The fruit fly possesses several advantages for genetic research:

- It reproduces often (short life cycle).
- It reproduces in large numbers (large sample size).
- Its chromosomes (especially in the salivary gland) are large and easily recognizable in size and shape.
- Its chromosomes are few (4 pairs, $2N = 8$).
- Mutations occur relatively frequently.

Through genetic and mutational analyses of *D. melanogaster*, scientists have elucidated the patterns of embryological development, discovering how genes expressed early in development can affect the adult organism.

NON-MENDELIAN INHERITANCE PATTERNS

In most practical applications, inheritance patterns are often more complicated than Mendel would have hoped. One major source of complications is in the relationship between **phenotype** and **genotype**. In theory, 100 percent of individuals with the recessive phenotype have a homozygous recessive genotype, and 100 percent of individuals with the dominant phenotype have either homozygous or heterozygous genotypes. Such clean concordance between genotype and phenotype is not always the case.

Incomplete Dominance

Some progeny phenotypes are apparently **blends** of the parental phenotypes. The classic example is flower color in snapdragons: homozygous dominant red snapdragons, when crossed with homozygous recessive white snapdragons, produce 100 percent pink progeny in the F1 generation. When F1 progeny are self-crossed, they produce red, pink, and white progeny in the ratio of 1:2:1, respectively. The pink color is the result of the combined effects of the red and white genes in heterozygotes. An allele is incompletely dominant if the phenotype of the heterozygote is an intermediate of the phenotypes of the homozygotes.

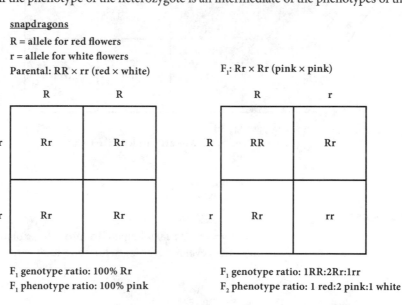

Figure 15.5

Codominance

Codominance occurs when **multiple** alleles exist for a given gene and more than one of them is **dominant**. Each dominant allele is fully dominant when combined with a recessive allele, but when two dominant alleles are present, the phenotype is the result of the expression of both dominant alleles simultaneously.

The classic example of codominance and multiple alleles is the inheritance of **ABO blood groups** in humans. Blood type is determined by three different alleles: I^A, I^B, and i. Only two alleles are present in any single individual, but the population contains all three alleles. I^A and I^B are both dominant to i. Individuals who are homozygous I^A or heterozygous I^Ai have blood type A; individuals who are homozygous I^B or heterozygous I^Bi have blood type B; and individuals who are homozygous ii have blood type O. However, I^A and I^B are codominant; individuals who are heterozygous $I^A I^B$ have a distinct blood type, AB, which combines characteristics of both the A and B blood groups.

Codominance differs from incomplete dominance because in incomplete dominance the phenotype expressed is a blend of both genotypes. In codominance, however, both alleles in the genotype are expressed at the same time without a blending of phenotype.

Sex Determination

The two members of each of the chromosome pairs are identical in shape except for one pair: the sex chromosomes. Different species vary in their systems of sex determination. In sexually differentiated species most chromosomes exist as pairs of homologues called **autosomes**, but sex is determined by a pair of sex chromosomes. All humans have 22 pairs of autosomes; additionally, women have a pair of homologous X chromosomes, and men have a pair of heterologous chromosomes, an X and a Y chromosome. The sex chromosomes pair during meiosis and segregate during the first meiotic division. Since females can produce only gametes containing the X chromosome, the gender of a zygote is determined by the genetic contribution of the male gamete. If the sperm carries a Y chromosome, the zygote will be male; if it carries an X chromosome, the zygote will be female. For every mating, there is a 50 percent chance that the zygote will be male and a 50 percent chance that it will be female.

Genes located on the X or Y chromosome are called **sex-linked**. In humans, most sex-linked genes are located on the X chromosome, although some Y-linked traits have been found (e.g., hair on the outer ear).

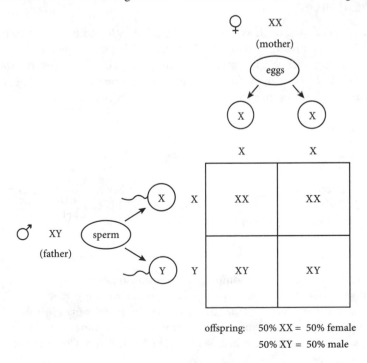

Figure 15.6

Sex Linkage

In humans, women have two X chromosomes and men have only one. As a result, recessive genes carried on the X chromosome will produce the recessive phenotypes whenever they occur in men because no dominant allele is present to mask them. The recessive phenotype will thus be much more frequently found in men. Examples of sex-linked recessives in humans are the genes for **hemophilia** and **color-blindness**.

The pattern of inheritance for a sex-linked recessive is somewhat complicated. Because men pass the X chromosome only to their daughters and the gene is carried only on the X chromosome, affected men cannot pass the trait to their male offspring. Affected men will, however, pass the gene to all of their daughters. Nevertheless, unless the daughter also receives the gene from her mother, she will be a phenotypically normal carrier of the trait. Because all of the daughter's male children will receive their only X chromosome from her, half of her sons will receive the recessive sex-linked allele. Thus, sex-linked recessives generally affect only men; they cannot be passed from father to son, but they can be passed from grandfather to grandson via a daughter who is a carrier, thereby skipping a generation.

Environmental Factors

The environment can often affect the expression of a gene. Interaction between the environment and the genotype produces the phenotype. For example, *Drosophila* with a given set of genes have crooked wings at low temperatures but straight wings at higher temperatures.

Temperature also influences the hair color of the Himalayan hare. The same genes for color result in white hair on the warmer parts of the body and black hair on colder parts. If the naturally warm portions are cooled (e.g., by the application of ice), the hair will grow in black.

Cytoplasmic Inheritance

Heredity systems exist outside the nucleus. For example, DNA is found in mitochondria and other cytoplasmic bodies. These cytoplasmic genes may interact with nuclear genes and are important in determining the characteristics of their organelles. Drug resistance in many microorganisms is regulated by cytoplasmic DNA, known as plasmids, that contain one or more genes. Plasmids can be passed from one bacterial cell to another via transformation (described below).

GENETIC PROBLEMS

Although genetic replication is very accurate, chromosome number and structure can be altered by abnormal cell division during meiosis or by mutagenic agents. This can result in the appearance of abnormal characteristics of the offspring in question.

Nondisjunction

Nondisjunction is either the failure of homologous chromosomes to separate properly during meiosis I or the failure of sister chromatids to separate properly during meiosis II. The resulting **zygote** might either have three copies of that chromosome, called **trisomy** (somatic cells will have $2N + 1$ chromosomes), or a single copy of that chromosome, called **monosomy** (somatic cells will have $2N - 1$ chromosomes). A classic case of trisomy is the birth defect **Down syndrome**, which is caused by trisomy of chromosome 21. Most monosomies and trisomies are lethal, causing the embryo to spontaneously abort early in the pregnancy.

Nondisjunction of the sex chromosomes may also occur, resulting in individuals with extra or missing copies of the X or Y chromosomes.

Chromosomal Breakage

Chromosomal breakage may occur spontaneously or be induced by environmental factors, such as mutagenic agents and X-rays. The chromosome that loses a fragment is said to have a deficiency.

Mutations

Mutations are changes in the genetic information coded in the DNA of a cell. Mutations that occur in **somatic** cells can lead to tumors in the individual. Mutations that occur in the sex cells (**gametes**) will be passed down to the offspring. Most mutations occur in regions of DNA that do not code for proteins and are silent (not expressed in the phenotype). Mutations that do change the sequence of amino acids in proteins are most often recessive and deleterious.

Mutagenic agents

Mutagenic agents induce mutations. These include cosmic rays, X-rays, ultraviolet rays, and radioactivity as well as chemical compounds such as colchicine, which inhibits spindle formation, or mustard gas, which alkylates guanine in DNA. Mutagenic agents are sometimes also **carcinogenic** (cancer-causing).

Mutation types

In a gene mutation, nitrogen bases are **added**, **deleted**, or **substituted**, thus altering the amino acid sequence. Inappropriate amino acids may be inserted into polypeptide chains, and a mutated protein may be produced. Therefore, a mutation is a genetic "error" with the "wrong" base or a missing base in the DNA at any particular position.

In a **point mutation** a nucleic acid is replaced by another nucleic acid. The number of nucleic acids substituted may vary, but generally point mutations involve between one and three nucleotides. There are three possible effects on the **codon**, the sequence of three nucleotides that determines the identity of the amino acid. First, the new codon may code for the same amino acid (a **silent mutation**), and no change in the resulting protein is seen. Second, the new codon may code for a different amino acid (a **missense mutation**). This may or may not lead to a problem with the resulting protein, depending on the role of that amino acid in determining the protein structure. Finally, the new codon may be a stop codon (a **nonsense mutation**). Nonsense mutations are often lethal or severely inhibit the functioning of the protein, which can lead to many different problems depending on the role of that protein in organism function. The length of the genome does not change with any of these mutations, but the primary structure of the proteins formed from an RNA sequence with a nonsense mutation could be much shorter due to the premature stop.

In a **frameshift mutation** nucleic acids are deleted or inserted into the genome sequence. This frequently is lethal. The insertion or deletion of nucleic acids throws off the entire sequence of codons from that point on because the genome is "read" in groups of three nucleic acids. Since nucleic acids are inserted or deleted, the length of the genome changes.

Examples of genetic disorders

- **Phenylketonuria** (PKU) is a molecular disease caused by the inability to produce the proper enzyme for the metabolism of phenylalanine. A degradation product (phenylpyruvic acid) accumulates as a result. The administration of any product that contains phenylalanine, such as aspartame, to an individual with any of the hyperphenylaninemia conditions could be detrimental to his or her general health. Therefore, these individuals are unable to consume products containing aspartame. Hyperphenylaninemia may result from an impaired conversion of phenylalanine to tyrosine. The most common and clinically important impairment is phenylketonuria, which is characterized by an increased concentration of phenylalanine in blood, increased concentration of phenylalanine and its by-products (such as phenylpyruvate, phenylacetate, and phenyllactate) in urine, and mental retardation. Phenylketonuria is caused by a deficiency of phenylalanine hydrolase.

- **Sickle-cell anemia** is a disease in which red blood cells become crescent-shaped because they contain defective hemoglobin. The sickle-cell hemoglobin carries less oxygen. This disease is caused by a substitution of valine (coded by GUA or GUG) for glutamic acid (coded by GAA or GAG) because of a single base-pair substitution in the gene coding for hemoglobin. While the decreased ability to carry oxygen can have negative effects on patients, these individuals do have less severe symptoms of malaria should they become infected, indicating a possible evolutionary advantage in regions where malaria infection is common.

BACTERIAL GENETICS

Bacterial Genome

The bacterial genome consists of a single circular chromosome located in the **nucleoid** region of the cell. Many bacteria also contain smaller circular rings of DNA called **plasmids**, which contain accessory genes. **Episomes** are plasmids that are capable of integration into the bacterial genome.

Replication

Replication of the bacterial chromosome begins at a unique origin of replication and proceeds in both directions simultaneously. DNA is synthesized in the 5′ to 3′ direction.

Genetic Variance

Bacterial cells reproduce by **binary fission** and proliferate very rapidly under favorable conditions. Although binary fission is an **asexual** process, bacteria have three mechanisms for increasing the genetic variance of a population: **transformation**, **conjugation**, and **transduction**.

Transformation

Transformation is the process by which a foreign chromosome fragment (**plasmid**) is incorporated into the bacterial chromosome via recombination, creating new inheritable genetic combinations.

Conjugation

Conjugation can be described as **sexual mating** in bacteria; it is the transfer of genetic material between two bacteria that are temporarily joined. A cytoplasmic conjugation bridge is formed between the two cells, and genetic material is transferred from the donor male (+) type to the recipient female (−) type. Only bacteria containing plasmids called sex factors are capable of conjugating. The best studied sex factor is the **F factor** in *E. coli*. Bacteria possessing this plasmid are termed F$^+$ cells; those without it are called F$^-$ cells. During conjugation between an F$^+$ and an F$^-$ cell, the F$^+$ cell replicates its F factor and donates the copy to the recipient, converting it to an F$^+$ cell. Genes that code for other characteristics, such as **antibody resistance**, may be found on the plasmids and transferred into recipient cells along with these factors.

Sometimes the sex factor becomes integrated into the bacterial genome. During conjugation, the entire bacterial chromosome replicates and begins to move from the donor cell into the recipient cell. The conjugation bridge usually breaks before the entire chromosome is transferred, but the bacterial genes that enter the recipient cell can easily recombine with the genes already present to form novel genetic combinations. These bacteria are called **Hfr** cells, meaning that they have a **high frequency of recombination**.

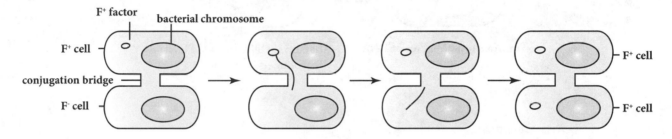

Figure 15.7

Transduction

A **bacteriophage** is a virus that infects its host bacterium by attaching to the bacterium, boring a hole through the bacterial cell wall, and injecting its viral DNA while its protein coat remains attached to the cell wall. Transduction occurs when fragments of the bacterial chromosome become packaged into the viral progeny produced during such a viral infection. These virions may infect other bacteria and introduce new genetic arrangements through recombination with the new host cell's DNA. The closer two genes are to one another on a chromosome, the more likely they will be to transduce together; this fact allows geneticists to map genes to a high degree of precision.

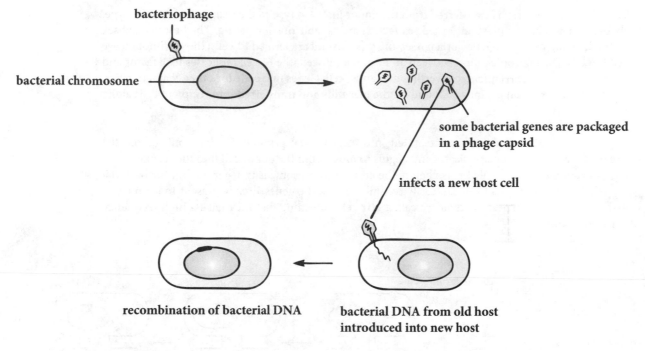

bacteriophage

bacterial chromosome

some bacterial genes are packaged in a phage capsid

infects a new host cell

recombination of bacterial DNA

bacterial DNA from old host introduced into new host

Figure 15.8

Recombination

Recombination occurs when linked genes are separated. It occurs by breakage and rearrangement of adjacent regions of DNA when organisms carrying different genes or alleles for the same traits are crossed.

Gene Regulation

The regulation of **transcription,** one of the steps of gene expression, enables prokaryotes to control their metabolism. Regulation of transcription is based on the accessibility of **RNA polymerase** to the genes being transcribed and is directed by an **operon**, which consists of **structural** genes, an **operator** region, and a **promoter** region on the DNA before the protein coding genes. Structural genes contain sequences of DNA that code for proteins. The operator is the sequence of nontranscribable DNA that is the **repressor** binding site. The promoter is the noncoding sequence of DNA that serves as the initial binding site for RNA polymerase. There is also a **regulator** gene, which codes for the synthesis of a repressor molecule that binds to the operator and blocks RNA polymerase from transcribing the structural genes.

RNA polymerase must also move past the operator to transcribe the structural genes. Regulatory systems function by preventing or permitting the RNA polymerase to pass on to the structural genes. Regulation may be via **inducible systems** or **repressible systems**. Inducible systems are those that require the presence of a substance, called an **inducer**, for transcription to occur. Repressible systems are in a constant state of transcription unless a **corepressor** is present to inhibit transcription.

Inducible systems

In an inducible system the repressor binds to the operator, forming a barrier that prevents RNA polymerase from transcribing the structural genes. For transcription to occur, an inducer must bind to the repressor, forming an **inducer-repressor complex**. This complex cannot bind to the operator, thus removing it as a barrier and permitting transcription. The proteins synthesized are thus said to be inducible. The structural genes typically code for an enzyme, and the inducer is usually the substrate, or a derivative of the substrate, upon which the enzyme normally acts. When the substrate (inducer) is present, enzymes are synthesized; when it is absent, enzyme synthesis is negligible. In this manner, enzymes are transcribed only when they are actually needed.

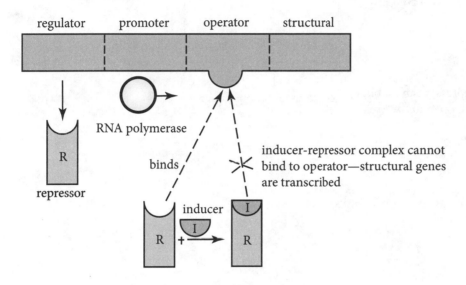

Figure 15.9

Repressible systems

In a repressible system the repressor is inactive until it combines with the corepressor. The repressor can bind to the operator and prevent transcription only when it has formed a repressor-corepressor complex. Corepressors are often the **end products** of the biosynthetic pathways they control. The proteins produced (usually enzymes) are said to be repressible because they are normally being synthesized; transcription and translation occur until the corepressor is synthesized. Operons containing mutations such as deletions or whose regulator genes code for defective repressors are incapable of being turned off; their enzymes, which are always being synthesized, are referred to as **constitutive**.

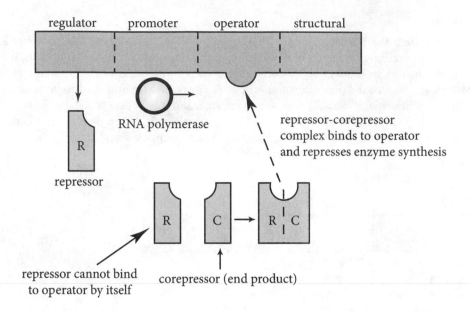

Figure 15.10

REVIEW PROBLEMS

1. A woman with blood genotype I^Ai and a man with blood genotype I^Bi have two children, both type AB. What is the probability that a third child will be blood type AB?

    (A) 25%

    (B) 33%

    (C) 50%

    (D) 66%

2. In humans, the allele for black hair (B) is dominant to the allele to brown hair (b), and the allele for curly hair (C) is dominant to the allele for straight hair (c). When a person of unknown genotype is crossed against a straight- and brown-haired individual, the phenotypic ratio is

    > 25% curly black hair
    >
    > 25% straight black hair
    >
    > 25% curly brown hair
    >
    > 25% straight brown hair

    What is the genotype of the unknown parent?

    (A) BBCC

    (B) BbCC

    (C) bbCc

    (D) BbCc

3. Assuming classical Mendelian inheritance, how can one differentiate between a homozygous dominant individual and one who is heterozygous for the dominant trait?

    (A) By crossing the individuals in question

    (B) By crossing each individual with a known homozygous recessive and examining the offspring

    (C) By crossing each individual with a known heterozygote and examining the offspring

    (D) Both B and C

4. If a male hemophiliac (X^hY) is crossed with a female carrier of both color blindness and hemophilia (X^cX^h), what is the probability that a female child will be phenotypically normal?

    (A) 0%

    (B) 25%

    (C) 50%

    (D) Same as for a male child

5. Explain the concept of Mendel's law of segregation.

6. Why are lethal dominant alleles much less common than lethal recessive alleles?

7. Many point mutations do not have any effect on the gene product. What are two possible explanations for this observation?

SOLUTIONS TO REVIEW PROBLEMS

1. **A** This is a cross between two heterozygotes for a trait that has codominant alleles. The inheritance pattern for human blood groups is not a simple dominant/recessive pattern because the A and B alleles are both phenotypically expressed when the genotype is I^AI^B.

    This is a cross between a woman heterozygous for blood type A and a man heterozygous for blood type B: $I^Ai \times I^Bi$.

F1 genotypes:		phenotypes:	
25% I^AI^B		25% type AB	
25% I^Bi		25% type B	
25% I^Ai		25% type A	
25% ii		25% type O	

    The birth of each child is an independent event. Hence, the fact the first two children this couple had were type AB has no influence whatsoever on the probability that a third child will be AB. So there is a 25 percent chance that any child, not just the third, will be type AB.

2. **D** In this dihybrid problem, a doubly recessive individual is crossed with an individual of unknown genotype—this is known as a testcross. The straight- and brown-haired individual has the genotype bbcc and can thus produce only bc gametes. Looking at the F1 offspring, there is a 1:1:1:1 phenotypic ratio. The fact that both the recessive and dominant traits are present in the offspring means that the unknown parental genotype must contain both recessive alleles (b and c). The unknown parental genotype must therefore be BbCc. If you want to double-check the answer, you can work out the Punnett square for the cross BbCc × bbcc: BbCc can produce four different types of gametes, BC, Bc, bC, and bc, whereas bbcc can produce only bc gametes, as previously mentioned.

    So the unknown parental genotype is BbCc, choice (D).

3. **D** To differentiate between a homozygous dominant and a heterozygous dominant for a trait that exhibits classic dominant/recessive Mendelian inheritance, one must perform a cross that results in offspring that reveal the unknown parental genotype; this is known as a testcross. If we cross the homozygous dominant with a homozygous recessive, we will get 100 percent phenotypically dominant offspring; if we cross the heterozygous dominant with the homozygous recessive, we will get 50 percent phenotypically dominant and 50 percent phenotypically recessive offspring. Thus, using a homozygous recessive as a testcrosser will allow us to distinguish between the two. We can also use a known heterozygote as the testcrosser because when this is crossed with the homozygous dominant, 100 percent phenotypically dominant offspring are produced, and when it is crossed with the heterozygote, the phenotypic ratio of the offspring is 3:1 dominant:recessive. Hence, the correct answer is (D), because both (B) and (C) are viable options. Crossing the individuals in question, as in (A), will result in 100 percent phenotypically dominant offspring and hence will not be helpful.

4. **C** In this problem, we are told that the female in this cross is a carrier of two sex-linked traits: color blindness and hemophilia. We are also told that the genes for these traits are not found on the same X chromosome, as indicated by her genotype, X^cX^h. So of the female offspring, half, or 50 percent, will be phenotypically normal.

5. The chromosomal basis for Mendel's Law of Segregation is as follows: For any given trait, all individuals have two alleles located on separate but homologous chromosomes, one inherited from each parent. During meiosis, or gamete formation, these homologous chromosomes pair and line up along the equatorial plate. As meiosis proceeds, the spindle fibers attached to the homologues move them toward opposite poles of the cell. Because the alleles are on different chromosomes, they segregate and wind up in different gametes. The paired condition of the alleles is restored with the fusion of egg and sperm during fertilization.

6. Lethal dominant alleles are much less common than lethal recessive alleles because a lethal dominant allele kills both heterozygotes and homozygotes, preventing the transmission of the allele to offspring (unless the gene is late acting). Dominant lethals usually appear in an individual as a result of spontaneous mutations and die with that individual. Thus, the frequency with which dominant lethals appear in the gene pool always remains very low. Lethal recessive alleles only kill homozygotes; however, heterozygotes are phenotypically normal and will not die as a result of their single copy of the lethal recessive. Hence, heterozygotes are able to pass on the lethal allele to offspring and thus maintain the frequency of the allele in the gene pool.

7. A point mutation causes the substitution of one base pair for another. Sometimes, as in the case of sickle-cell anemia, it may have a very profound effect on the gene product (hemoglobin) because it changes the message carried by the gene. In some cases, however, a mutated gene codes for the same product. This can be explained by the redundancy of the genetic code: most amino acids have more than one triplet coding for them. The substitution of the third cytosine in the triplet CCC (proline) by any of the remaining bases (G, A, or U) will not change the amino acid sequence because the codons CCG, CCA, and CCU code for proline as well. In eukaryotes, a point mutation may occur in an intron (noncoding region) and thus will not affect the gene product because noncoding regions are excised after transcription.

CHAPTER SIXTEEN

Evolution

The change in the genetic makeup of a population with time is termed **evolution**. Evolution is explained by the constant propagation of new variations in the genes of a species, some of which impart an adaptive advantage. All living things (past and present) are descendents from a single common ancestor. Each of these organisms arose as a direct result of some genetic alteration in the species that lived before them, and this process is called evolution. Most evolutionary changes occur slowly over a long period of time.

THEORIES OF EVOLUTION

Lamarckian Evolution

This discredited theory proposed by Jean-Baptiste Lamarck held that new organs or changes in existing ones arose because of the needs of the organism. The amount of change was thought to be based on the **use or disuse** of the organ. The theory of use and disuse was based upon a fallacious understanding of genetics. Any useful characteristic acquired in one generation was thought to be transmitted to the next. An example of an **acquired characteristic** was the long necks of giraffes. Supposedly, early giraffes permanently stretched their necks to reach for leaves on higher branches of trees. The offspring were believed to inherit the valuable trait of longer necks as a result of this excessive use.

Modern genetics has disproved theories of acquired characteristics. In reality, only changes in the DNA of the sex cells can be inherited. In contrast, changes acquired during an individual's life are changes in somatic cells. August Weismann showed that these changes are not inherited in an experiment in which he cut off the tails of mice for 20 generations (somatic change) only to find that the 21st generation was born with tails.

Darwin's Theory of Natural Selection

In Charles Darwin's theory, pressures in the environment select for the organism most **fit** to survive and reproduce. In the evolutionary sense, **fitness** is the ability to survive and reproduce. Darwin essentially concluded that a member of a particular species that is equipped with beneficial traits, allowing it to cope effectively with the immediate environment, will produce more offspring than individuals with less favorable genetic traits. The genes of parents that are more fit are therefore passed down to more offspring and become increasingly prevalent in the gene pool. Darwin subsequently chose the words **natural selection** to describe his theory because nature selects the best set of parents for the next generation. Darwin outlined a number of basic agents leading to evolutionary change.

Overpopulation

More offspring are produced than can survive. Thus, the food, air, light, and space are insufficient to support the entire population.

Variations

Offspring naturally show differences (variations) in their characteristics compared to those of their parents. Darwin did not know the source of these differences. Hugo de Vries later suggested mutations as the cause of variations. Some mutations are beneficial, although most are harmful.

Competition

The developing population must compete for the necessities of life. Many young must die, and the number of adults in the population generally remains constant from generation to generation.

Natural selection

Some organisms in a species have variations that give them an advantage over other members of the species. In the struggle for existence, these organisms may have adaptations that are advantageous for survival. For example, a giraffe with a variation of a longer neck would be able to get more food from higher branches of a tree and therefore would be more fit. This principle is encapsulated in the phrase "survival of the fittest."

Inheritance of the variations

The individuals that survive (those with the favorable variations) live to adulthood to reproduce and thus **transmit** these favorable variations or adaptations to their offspring. These favored genes gradually dominate the gene pool.

Evolution of new species

Over many generations of natural selection, the favorable changes (adaptations) are perpetuated in the species. The accumulation of these favorable changes eventually results in such significant changes of the gene pool that we can say a new species has evolved. These physical changes in the gene pool were perpetuated or selected for by environmental conditions.

For example, the rapid evolution of DDT-resistant insects illustrates the theory of natural selection and speciation. A change in the environment such as the introduction of DDT (an insecticide) constitutes a favorable change for the DDT-resistant mutant flies. These mutants existed before the environmental change. Now, conditions select for survival of DDT-resistant mutants.

COMPONENTS OF EVOLUTION

Speciation

Speciation is the evolution of new species, which are groups of individuals that can interbreed freely with each other but not with members of other species. Gene flow is impossible between different species.

Different selective pressures act upon the gene pools of each group, causing them to evolve independently. Genetic variation, changes in the environment, migration to new environments, adaptation to new environments, natural selection, genetic drift, and isolation are all factors that can lead to speciation.

Before speciation, small, local populations called **demes** often form within a species. For example, all the beavers along a specific portion of a river form a deme. There may be many demes belonging to a specific species. Members of a deme resemble one another more closely than they resemble members of other demes. They are closely related genetically since mating between members of the same deme occurs more frequently. They are also influenced by similar environmental factors and thus are subject to the same selection processes.

If these demes become **isolated**, speciation may occur. When groups are isolated from each other, there is no gene flow among them. Any difference arising from mutations or new combinations of genes will be maintained in the isolated population. Over time, these genetic differences may become significant enough to make mating impossible. If the gene pools within a species become sufficiently different so that two individuals cannot mate and produce fertile offspring, two different species have developed and one or more new species have formed. Genetic and eventually reproductive isolation often results from the geographic isolation of a population.

Evolutionary History

Biologists seek to understand the evolutionary relationships among species alive today. This evolutionary history is termed **phylogeny**. Evolutionary history may be visualized as a branching tree on which the common ancestor is found at the trunk and the modern species are found at the tips of the branches.

Convergent evolution

Groups among the branches often develop in similar ways when exposed to similar environments. When two species from different ancestors develop similar traits, this is known as **convergent evolution**. For example, sharks and dolphins have come to resemble one another physically despite belonging to different classes of vertebrates (sharks are members of Chondrichthyes, whereas dolphins are members of Mammalia). Despite different recent ancestors, they evolved certain similar features in adapting to the conditions of aquatic life.

Parallel evolution

Parallel evolution is similar to convergent evolution but occurs when a more recent ancestor can be identified. For example, marsupial (pouched) mammals and placental mammals are both in the class Mammalia but diverged due to geographic separation. Descendants of the ancestral marsupial mammal include the pouched wolf, anteater, mouse, and mole. These species have developed parallel to the placental wolf, anteater, mouse, and mole. Despite their geographic separation, the pouched mammals and their placental counterparts faced similar environments; thus, they developed similar adaptations.

Divergent evolution

In contrast, **divergent evolution** occurs when species with a shared ancestor develop differing traits due to dissimilarities between their environments. For example, bears of the family Ursidae within the class Mammalia share many similar traits but have diverged from a common ancestor to adapt to their specific environments. Polar bears have white coats to blend in with their arctic environment, whereas black bears have developed darker fur to blend in with their wet, forest environments. Over time, additional changes accumulated between these bears, resulting in the inability to cross-breed and eventual speciation.

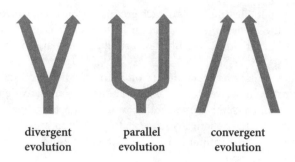

divergent
evolution

parallel
evolution

convergent
evolution

Figure 16.1

Adaptive radiation is the emergence of a number of lineages from a single ancestral species. A single species may diverge into a number of distinct species; the differences between them are those adaptive to a distinct lifestyle, or **niche**. A classic example is Darwin's finches of the Galápagos island chain. Over a comparatively short period of time, a single species of finch underwent adaptive radiation, resulting in 13 separate species of finches, some of them on the same island. Such adaptations minimized competition among the birds, enabling each emerging species to become firmly established in its own environmental niche.

Population Genetics

A **population** includes all members of a particular species inhabiting a given location. The **gene pool** of a population is the sum total of all the alleles for any given trait in the population. **Gene frequency** is the decimal fraction representing the presence of an allele for all members of a population that have this particular gene. In basic Mendelian genetics, only two alleles exist for a given trait: one dominant and one recessive. The letter p is used for the frequency of the dominant allele of a particular gene. The letter q represents the frequency of the recessive allele. Since by definition these are the only two alleles that can be present, for a given gene, $p + q = 1$.

The Hardy-Weinberg principle

Evolution can be viewed as a result of changing gene frequencies within a population. Gene frequency is the relative frequency of a particular allele. When the gene frequencies of a population are not changing, the gene pool is stable and the population is not evolving. However, this is true only in ideal situations in which the following conditions are met:

- The population is very large.
- No mutations affect the gene pool.
- Mating between individuals in the population is random.
- There is no net migration of individuals into or out of the population.
- The genes in the population are all equally successful at reproducing.

Under these idealized conditions, a certain equilibrium will exist among all of the genes in a gene pool, which is described by the **Hardy-Weinberg equation**.

For a gene with only two alleles, T and t, p = the frequency of allele T and q = the frequency of allele t. For that gene, $p + q = 1$ since the combined frequencies of the alleles must total 100 percent. Thus,

$$(p + q)^2 = (1)^2 \text{, and}$$

$$p^2 + 2pq + q^2 = 1$$

where p^2 = frequency of TT (dominant homozygotes)
$2pq$ = frequency of Tt (heterozygotes)
q^2 = frequency of tt (recessive homozygotes)

The Hardy-Weinberg equation may be used to determine gene frequencies in a large population in the absence of microevolutionary change (defined by the five conditions given above).

For example, individuals from a nonevolving population can be randomly crossed to demonstrate that the gene frequencies remain constant from generation to generation. If you know that the gene frequency of the dominant gene for tallness, T, is 0.80 and the gene frequency of the recessive gene for shortness, t, is 0.20, then $p = 0.80$ and $q = 0.20$. In a cross between two heterozygotes, the resulting F1 genotype frequencies will be 64% TT, 16% + 16% = 32% Tt, and 4% tt:

	$p = 0.80$ (T)	$q = 0.20$ (t)
$p = 0.80$ (T)	$(p^2 = 0.64)$ TT = 64%	$(pq = 0.16)$ Tt = 16%
$q = 0.20$ (t)	$(pq = 0.16)$ Tt = 16%	$(q^2 = 0.04)$ tt = 4%

The gene frequencies of the F1 generation can be calculated as follows:

64% TT = 64% T allele   +   0% t allele
32% Tt = 16% T allele   + 16% t allele
4% tt = 0% T allele   +   4% t allele

Gene frequencies = 80% T allele   + 20% t allele

Thus, $p = 0.80$ and $q = 0.20$. These frequencies are the same as those in the parent generation, demonstrating Hardy-Weinberg equilibrium in a nonevolving population.

Microevolution

No population can be represented indefinitely by the Hardy-Weinberg equilibrium because such idealized conditions do not exist in nature. Real populations have **unstable** gene pools and **migrating** populations. The agents of microevolutionary change—natural selection, mutation, assortive mating, genetic drift, and gene flow—are all deviations from the five conditions of a Hardy-Weinberg population.

Natural selection

Genotypes with favorable variations are selected through natural selection, and the frequency of favorable genes increases within the gene pool. Genotypes with low adaptive values tend to disappear.

Mutation

Gene mutations change allele frequencies in a population, shifting gene equilibria by introducing additional alleles. These gene mutations can either be favorable or detrimental for the offspring.

Assortive mating

If mates are not randomly chosen but rather selected according to criteria such as phenotype and proximity (**sexual selection**), the relative genotype ratios will be affected and will depart from the predictions of the Hardy-Weinberg equilibrium.

Genetic drift

Genetic drift refers to changes in the composition of the gene pool due to chance. Genetic drift tends to be more pronounced in small populations or new populations, where it is sometimes called the **founder effect**.

Gene flow

Migration of individuals between populations will result in a loss or gain of genes, thus changing the composition of a population's gene pool.

EVIDENCE OF EVOLUTION

Fossil Record

Fossils are the most direct evidence of evolutionary change. They represent the preserved remains of an organism. Fossils are generally found in sedimentary rocks.

Types of fossils

Many types of fossils can provide information. Paleontologists can find actual remains, including teeth, bones, etc., in rock, tar pits, ice, and **amber** (the fossil resin of trees). **Petrification** is the process in which minerals replace the cells of an organism. **Imprints** are impressions left by an organism (e.g., footprints). **Molds** form hollow spaces in rocks as the organisms within decay. **Casts** are formed by minerals deposited in molds.

Significant fossil discoveries

The trilobite is a primitive arthropod (similar to lobsters and crabs), which was a dominant form of the early Paleozoic era. Dinosaurs were ancient animals related to both reptiles and birds. Various forms lived on all the ancient continents. They were a dominant form of the Mesozoic era. Eohippus, the dawn horse, was a primitive horse the size of a fox with four toes and short teeth with pointed cusps for feeding on soft leaves. Fossil evidence indicates a gradual evolution within the horse lineage to the modern horse, which has one toe (hoof) and two vestigial toes as side splints, flat teeth with ridges for grinding grain and tough prairie grass, and long legs for running. The woolly mammoth was a hairy elephant found in the Siberian ice. Saber-tooth tigers have been preserved in asphalt tar pits. Insects have been discovered preserved in amber. *Archaeopteryx* is the link between reptiles (it has teeth and scales) and birds (it also has feathers).

Comparative Anatomy

Homologous structures

Homologous structures have the same basic anatomical features and evolutionary origins. They demonstrate similar evolutionary patterns with late divergence of form due to differences in exposure to evolutionary forces. Although the origins and anatomical features of these structures are similar, their functions may not be. Examples of homologous structures include the wings of a bat, the flipper of a whale, the forelegs of horses, and the arms of humans.

Analogous structures

Analogous structures have similar functions but may have different evolutionary origins and entirely different patterns of development. The wings of a fly (membranous) and the wings of a bird (bony and covered with feathers) are analogous structures. Analogous organs demonstrate a superficial resemblance that cannot be used as a basis for classification.

Comparative Embryology

The **stages of development** of the embryo resemble the stages in an organism's evolutionary history. The human embryo passes through stages that demonstrate common ancestry with other organisms. The two-layer **gastrula** is similar to the structure of the hydra, a cnidarian. The three-layer gastrula is similar in structure to the flatworm. Gill slits in the embryo indicate a common ancestry with fish. The similarity of these stages suggests a common ancestry and development history.

The earlier the stage at which the development begins to diverge, the more dissimilar the adult organisms will be. For example, it is difficult to differentiate between the embryo of a human and that of a gorilla until relatively late in the development of each embryo.

Embryological development suggests other evidence of evolution from common ancestors. The avian embryo has teeth, suggesting shared ancestry with reptiles. The larvae of some mollusks resemble annelids. Human embryos possess a tail, like most other mammals.

Comparative Biochemistry (Physiology)

Most organisms demonstrate the same basic needs and metabolic processes. They require the same nutrients and contain similar cellular organelles and energy storage forms (ATP). For example, respiratory processes are very similar in most organisms. The similarity of the enzymes involved in these processes suggests that all organisms must contain some DNA sequences in common. The more recently organisms shared a common ancestor, the greater the similarity of their chemical constituents (enzymes, hormones, antibodies, blood) and genetic information. Thus, we can conclude that all organisms are descended from a single common ancestral form. The chemical similarity of the blood of different organisms very closely parallels the evolutionary pattern. A chimpanzee's blood shows close similarity to that of a human but is quite different from that of a rabbit or fish. Thus, the more time that has elapsed since the divergence of two species, the more different their biochemical characteristics.

Vestigial Structures

Vestigial structures have no known current function but apparently had some ancestral function. There are many examples of vestigial structures in humans, other animals, and plants:

- In humans, the appendix is small and useless. In herbivores, it assists in the digestion of cellulose.
- In humans, the tail is reduced to a few useless bones (coccyx) at the base of the spine.
- Splints on the legs of horses are the vestigial remains of the two side toes of more primitive horses.
- Python "legs" are reduced to useless bones embedded in the sides of the adult. The whale has similar hind-limb bones.

Geographic Barriers

Species multiplication is generally accompanied by **migration** to lessen **intraspecific competition**. Separation of a widely distributed population by emerging geographic barriers increases the likelihood of genetic adaptations on either side of the barrier. Each population may evolve specific adaptations to the environment in which it lives in addition to accumulating neutral (random, nonadaptive) changes. These adaptations will remain unique to the population in which they evolve—provided that interbreeding is prevented by the barrier. In time, genetic differences will reach the point where interbreeding becomes impossible between the populations and **reproductive isolation** would be maintained even if the barrier were removed. Following are two examples:

- **Marsupials:** A lineage of pouched mammals (marsupials) paralleling the development of placental mammals developed on the Australian side of a large water barrier. The geographic barrier protected the pouched mammals from competition and hybridization with modern placental mammals. This barrier resulted in the development of uniquely Australian marsupials, such as kangaroos and pouched wolves, as well as other Australian plants and animals such as the eucalyptus tree and duckbilled platypus.
- **Darwin's finches**: Over a comparatively short period of time, a single species of Galápagos finch underwent adaptive radiation to form 13 different species of finches. Slight variations in the beak, for example, favored ground or tree feeding. Such adaptations minimized the competition among the birds, enabling each emerging species to become firmly entrenched in its environmental niche. The evolution of these adaptations was helped by the geographic isolation of some of these species on different islands of the Galápagos island chain.

ORIGIN AND EARLY EVOLUTION OF LIFE

The Heterotroph Hypothesis

The first forms of life lacked the ability to synthesize their own nutrients; they required preformed molecules. These "organisms" were heterotrophs, which depended upon outside sources for food. The primitive seas contained simple inorganic and organic compounds such as salts, methane, ammonia, hydrogen, and water. Energy was present in the form of heat, electricity, solar radiation (including X-rays and ultraviolet light), cosmic rays, and radioactivity.

The presence of these building blocks and energy may have led to the synthesis of simple organic molecules such as sugars, amino acids, purines, and pyrimidines. These molecules dissolved in the "**primordial soup**," and after many years, the simple monomeric molecules combined to form a supply of macromolecules.

Evidence of organic synthesis

In 1953, Stanley L. Miller set out to demonstrate that the application of ultraviolet radiation, heat, or a combination of these to a mixture of methane, hydrogen, ammonia, and water could result in the formation of complex organic compounds. Miller set up an apparatus in which the four gases were continuously circulated past electrical discharges from tungsten electrodes.

After circulating the gases for one week, Miller analyzed the liquid in the apparatus and found that an amazing variety of organic compounds, including urea, hydrogen cyanide, acetic acid, and lactic acid had been synthesized.

Formation of primitive cells

Colloidal protein molecules tend to clump together to form **coacervate droplets** (a cluster of colloidal molecules surrounded by a shell of water). These droplets tend to absorb and incorporate substances from the surrounding environment. In addition, the droplets tend to possess a definite internal structure. It is highly likely that such droplets developed on the early Earth. Although these coacervate droplets were not living, they did possess some properties normally associated with living organisms.

Most of these systems were unstable; however, a few systems may have arisen that were stable enough to survive. A small percentage of the droplets possessing favorable characteristics may have eventually developed into the first primitive cells. These first primitive cells probably possessed nucleic acid polymers and became capable of reproduction.

Development of Autotrophs

The primitive heterotrophs slowly evolved complex **biochemical pathways**, enabling them to use a wider variety of nutrients. They evolved anaerobic respiratory processes to convert nutrients into energy. However, these organisms required nutrients at a faster rate than they were being synthesized. Life would have ceased to exist if autotrophic nutrition had not developed. Autotrophs are able to produce organic compounds, including energy-containing molecules, from substances in their surroundings. The pioneer autotrophs developed primitive photosynthetic pathways, capturing solar energy and using it to synthesize carbohydrates from carbon dioxide and water.

Development of Aerobic Respiration

The primitive autotrophs fixed carbon dioxide during the synthesis of carbohydrates and released molecular oxygen as a waste product. The addition of molecular oxygen to the atmosphere converted the atmosphere from a **reducing** to an **oxidizing** one. Some molecular oxygen was converted to ozone, which functions in the atmosphere to block high-energy radiation. In this way, living organisms destroyed the conditions that made their development possible. Once molecular oxygen became a major component of the Earth's atmosphere, both heterotrophs and autotrophs evolved the biochemical pathways of aerobic respiration. Now equilibrium exists between oxygen-producing and oxygen-consuming organisms.

General Categories of Living Organisms

All living organisms can be divided into four basic categories. The **autotrophic anaerobes** include chemosynthetic bacteria. The **autotrophic aerobes** include the green plants and photoplankton. The **heterotrophic anaerobes** include yeasts. The **heterotrophic aerobes** include amoebas, earthworms, and humans.

REVIEW PROBLEMS

1. Can the muscular strength that a weight lifter gains be inherited by the athlete's children?

2. Which organism has a greater evolutionary fitness: one that lives 70 years and has 5 fertile offspring or one that lives 40 years and has 10 fertile offspring?

3. Homologous structures are
    (A) similar in function but not in origin.
    (B) similar in origin but not necessarily in function.
    (C) completely dissimilar.
    (D) found only in mammals.

4. Will chance variation have a greater effect in a large or a small population? What is this effect called?

5. As the climate got colder during the Ice Age, a particular species of mammal evolved a thicker layer of fur. This is an example of what kind of selection?

6. At what point are two populations descended from the same ancestral stock considered separate species?

7. In a nonevolving population, there are two alleles, R and r, which code for the same trait. The frequency of R is 30 percent. What are the frequencies of all the possible genotypes?

8. As the ocean became saltier, whales and fish independently evolved mechanisms to maintain the concentration of salt in their bodies. This can be explained by
    (A) homologous evolution.
    (B) analogous evolution.
    (C) convergent evolution.
    (D) parallel evolution.

9. In a particular Hardy-Weinberg population, there are only two eye colors: brown and blue. Thirty-six percent of the population has blue eyes, the recessive trait. What percentage of the population is heterozygous for brown eyes?

10. In a certain population, 64 percent of individuals are homozygous for curly hair (CC). The gene for curly hair is dominant to the gene for straight hair, c. Use the Hardy-Weinberg equation to determine what percentage of the population has curly hair.

11. Which of the following was NOT a belief of Darwin's?
    (A) Evolution of species occurs gradually and evenly over time.
    (B) There is a struggle for survival among organisms.
    (C) Genetic mutation and recombination are the driving forces of evolution.
    (D) Those individuals with fitter variants will survive and reproduce.

12. The proposed "primordial soup" was composed of organic precursor molecules formed by interactions between all of the following gases EXCEPT

    (A) oxygen.
    (B) helium.
    (C) nitrogen.
    (D) hydrogen.

SOLUTIONS TO REVIEW PROBLEMS

1. No. The only characteristics that are inherited are those genetically coded for, not those acquired through the use or disuse of body parts. Therefore, the musculature of the weight lifter, an acquired characteristic, cannot be inherited by that athlete's children.

2. The organism that lives 40 years and has 10 fertile offspring has the greater evolutionary fitness because it makes a greater genetic contribution to the next generation. It has twice as many direct descendants as the organism that lives 70 years and has 5 fertile offspring.

3. **B** Homologous structures are similar in origin but not necessarily similar in function. Analogous structures are similar in function but not in origin. Homologous structures are not limited to mammals; e.g., the forelimbs of crocodiles and birds are homologous structures.

4. Chance variation will have a greater effect in a small population because any one variant individual is a greater percentage of the whole population. This effect is called genetic drift.

5. This is an example of natural selection, the phenotypic norm of a particular species shifting to adapt to a selective pressure, such as an increasingly colder environment. Only those individuals with a thick layer of fur were able to survive during the Ice Age, thus that trait led to greater fitness (the production of more offspring, in this case due to living longer).

6. Two populations are considered separate species when they can no longer interbreed and produce viable, fertile offspring.

7. The frequency of R = 30%. Thus, $p = 0.30$. The frequency of recessive gene r = 100% − 30% = 70%. Thus, $q = 0.70$. Frequency of genotypes = $p^2 + 2pq + q^2 = 1$, where p^2 = RR, $2pq$ = Rr, and q^2 = rr.

p^2	=	$(0.3)^2$	=	0.09	=	9% RR
$2pq$	=	$2(0.3)(0.7)$	=	0.42	=	42% Rr
q^2	=	$(0.7)^2$	=	0.49	=	49% rr

8. **C** Whales and fish have similar body structures (streamlined body with fins and tail), although they belong to different classes of vertebrates. When organisms that differ phylogenetically develop in similar ways when exposed to similar environments, the process is known as convergent evolution.

9. The percentage of the population with blue eyes (genotype = bb) = 36% = q^2 = 0.36; therefore, $q = 0.6$. Because $p + q = 1$, $p = 0.4$. The frequency of heterozygous brown eyes is $2pq = 2(0.4)(0.6) = 0.48$. So 48% of the population is heterozygous for brown eyes.

10. The variable p represents the frequency of the dominant allele (C), and q represents the frequency of the recessive allele (c). The CC frequency is 64%, which means that $p^2 = 0.64$, or $p = 0.8$. Because $p + q = 1$, $q = 1 − 0.8 = 0.2$.

    The problem asks for the percentage of the population with curly hair; this includes both homozygotes and heterozygotes (CC and Cc). The genotype frequencies can be found using the equation $p^2 + 2pq + q^2$.

CC	=	p^2	= $(0.8)^2$	=	0.64	=	64% homozygous curly
Cc	=	$2pq$	= $2(0.8)(0.2)$	=	0.32	=	32% heterozygous curly
cc	=	q^2	= $(0.2)^2$	=	0.04	=	4% straight hair

Therefore, the percentage of the population with curly hair is 64% + 32% = 96%.

11. **C** Darwin believed the driving force behind evolution was the fitness of the organism for its particular environment.

12. **B** He, a noble gas, is inert and does not form molecules with other atoms.

CHAPTER SEVENTEEN

Microorganisms

MICROBIOLOGY

Bacteria

Bacteria are **prokaryotes**: one-celled organisms that do not have a true nucleus or membrane-bound organelles. As a result, a bacterium's ribosomes and genetic material are free-floating in the cytoplasm. Bacteria can have specialized structures to help them complete necessary functions, including flagella and cilia, which increase their motility.

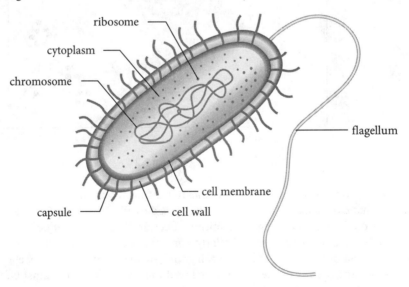

Figure 17.1

Bacteria come in three major shapes:

- **Coccus**: spherical bacteria that can join together to make diplococci (two bacteria joined together), streptococci (chains of spherical bacteria), or staphylococci (clusters of spherical bacteria)

- **Bacillus**: rod-shaped bacteria that can also join together, forming diplobacilli, streptobacilli (chains of rod-shaped bacteria), etc.
- **Spirillum**: spiral shaped bacteria

Another major distinction between types of bacteria is whether they are **Gram positive** or **Gram negative**. This is determined by Gram staining, a technique discovered by Hans Christian Gram. The process begins with the application of crystal violet and iodine, which create a complex that adheres to the outermost layer of bacteria. For Gram positive bacteria, the outermost layer is a thick peptidoglycan cell wall; for Gram negative bacteria, the outermost layer is thin and composed of lipids. When a decolorizer, such as alcohol, is subsequently added, the peptidoglycan wall of a Gram positive bacterium is dehydrated, trapping the stain inside. This results in Gram positive bacteria displaying a purple color under a light microscope. In contrast, when a decolorizer is added to Gram negative bacteria, the entire outer membrane is removed, taking the purple color with it. Treatment with decolorizer is followed by addition of a second, red dye, such as safranin, which restains the Gram negative bacteria. This results in Gram negative bacteria displaying a lighter, pink color under a light microscope.

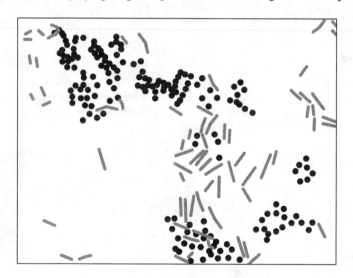

Figure 17.2

Gram staining not only dictates the classification of bacteria but also helps determine the types of antibiotics that can be used to treat infections caused by these bacteria. Certain antibiotics that attack or move through cell walls have mechanisms of action that make them effective only against Gram positive or Gram negative bacteria. Similarly, some types of antibiotics may have activity against both types of bacteria but be more effective against one or the other. For instance, drugs that specifically target the peptidoglycans of the bacterial cell wall may be ineffective against Gram negative bacteria because the drug cannot reach the peptidoglycans behind the bacteria's outer lipid membranes. Knowing whether the bacteria infecting a patient are Gram positive or Gram negative can play a major role in determining the antibiotic of choice to treat an infection.

Unlike many other types of cells, bacteria reproduce **asexually**. This can happen through three primary means: **transformation** (acquiring DNA from the environment), **transduction** (being injected with DNA by a bacteriophage), or **conjugation** (direct DNA transfer via contact between bacterial cells). These methods are discussed in more detail in Chapter 15, Genetics.

Viruses

Viruses cannot reproduce without a host and therefore are not considered to be living particles. Their genetic material, which is either DNA or RNA, is contained with in a protein capsid. Viruses lack most other cellular organelles as they do not need to reproduce or maintain cellular functions. Many shapes of viruses exist, and these shapes are distinguished by electron microscopy.

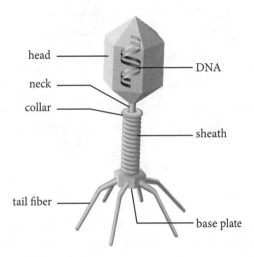

Figure 17.3

When a virus infects a cell it enters the **lytic cycle**. During this time the virus penetrates the cell's membrane and injects its own DNA, taking control of the cell's genetic machinery and inducing the cell to replicate the viral DNA instead of its own DNA. Eventually the cell will lyse and release viral DNA into the extracellular matrix, at which point these viral particles can infect new cells and continue the lytic cycle. Viruses that replicate by the lytic cycle, killing their host cells, are called **virulent**.

If the initial infection takes place on a bacterial **lawn** (a plated culture), then very shortly a **plaque,** or clearing in the lawn, occurs corresponding to the area of lysed bacteria. The physical characteristics of a plaque are useful in identifying mutant phage strains that may arise.

If the bacteriophage does not lyse its host cell, it becomes **integrated** into the bacterial genome in a less harmful form (**provirus**), lying dormant for one or more generations as part of the **lysogenic cycle.** The virus does not spread as quickly during this phase and so it is considered to be a **latent** infection. The virus may stay integrated indefinitely, replicating along with its host's genome. However, either spontaneously or as a result of environmental circumstances (e.g., radiation, ultraviolet light, or chemicals), the provirus can reemerge and enter a lytic cycle. Cells containing proviruses are normally resistant to further infection (**superinfection**) by similar phages. One example of the lysogenic cycle occurs with **human immunodeficiency virus (HIV),** which often stays in the lysogenic cycle for months or even years, during which time the patient is asymptomatic as the virus divides within the host.

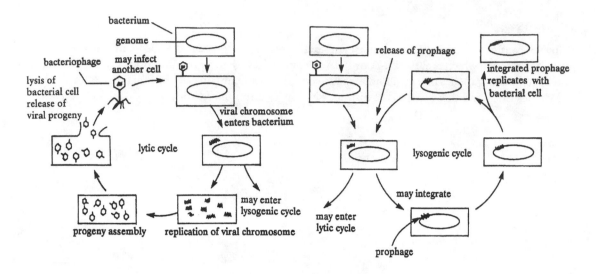

Figure 17.4

Fungi

Fungi are eukaryotic organisms and resemble human cells much more than they resemble bacteria or viruses. Many of their organelles mimic those found in human cells. Unlike human cells, however, fungi have cell walls, similar to plants and bacteria. Fungal cell walls contain chitin, which differentiates them from plants and bacteria. Fungi are unable to produce their own food and so must consume other organisms for energy (again, like humans). As a result, fungi are referred to as heterotrophs.

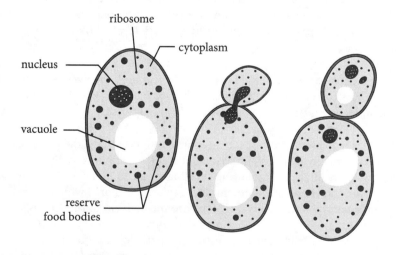

Figure 17.5

Fungi undergo both sexual and asexual reproduction and have both **haploid** and **diploid** phases, making their reproductive cycles more complicated than those of most other organisms. Asexual reproduction in fungi usually occurs via **fission**, where one organism divides into two daughter cells. This is a common means of reproduction among bacteria as well. Sexual reproduction can only occur with diploid cells; during this process the cells undergo meiosis to create four **spores**. These spores are all haploid, meaning they only have one copy of the organism's genetic material, which is how one diploid organism can produce four identical progeny. Spores are far more resilient to hostile conditions than diploid cells, so spore production often occurs when the environment is not sufficiently favorable for fission to take place. Spore production preserves the integrity of the fungus and allows the fungus to survive until the conditions improve and it can divide again.

Parasites

Parasites are organisms that live off of and harm a host that receives no benefit from the presence of the parasite. Parasites include helminths and protozoa.

Helminths: parasitic worms, including tapeworms and roundworms. These are often ingested via contaminated food or water and live off of the food present in the digestive tract of the host.

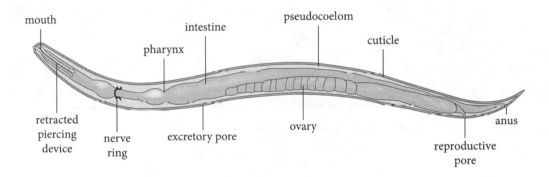

Figure 17.6

Protozoa: unicellular eukaryotes that have many different features, depending on the organism. Many protozoa cause disease, including dysentery.

MICROBIAL ECOLOGY

The **nitrogen cycle**, the **carbon cycle**, and **photosynthesis** are three processes with direct and strong influences on the function of life on Earth, and all three cycles involve microbial organisms. It is important to understand the basics of each of these cycles in terms of their impact on microbiology, but note that general ecology, comparative anatomy and physiology, and plant biology are no longer tested on the PCAT, so be sure to study the following ideas only in the context of microbial ecology.

The Nitrogen Cycle

Bacteria fix free atmospheric nitrogen gas into nitrates and nitrites usable by plants to make proteins. As these plants (and the animals that eat them and one another) produce waste and decompose, ammonia and ammonium ions are released into the environment. Bacteria then break the ammonia back down into nitrite and nitrate, which can replenish stores in plants or be converted to atmospheric nitrogen. This process forms the core of the nitrogen cycle as nitrogen is repeatedly used and recycled.

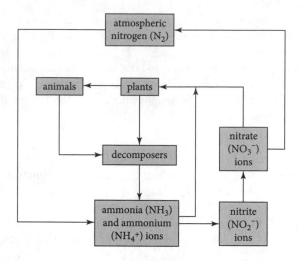

Figure 17.7

The Carbon Cycle

Microbes contribute to the transfer of carbon molecules through the carbon cycle via fermentation, catabolism, and anabolism. The carbon cycle itself involves the transfer of carbon and carbon-containing compounds between plants, animals, the atmosphere, and other environmental components.

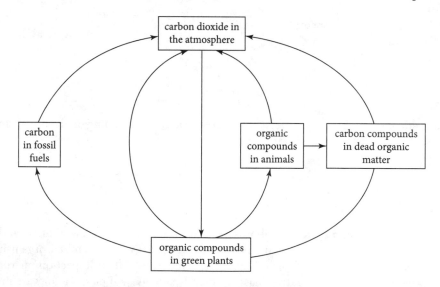

Figure 17.8

Photosynthesis

Cells containing chlorophyll (often plant cells but also some bacterial cells) are capable of undergoing photosynthesis. In this reaction sunlight, carbon dioxide, and water are utilized to produce sugars, which serve as an energy source for the cell. Organisms that produce their own energy in this way are called **autotrophs**. Autotrophs are eaten by **heterotrophs** (organisms that cannot fix carbon) and serve as the base of the food chain.

REVIEW PROBLEMS

1.   Which of the following is true about bacteria?

   (A) They are eukaryotes.

   (B) Their genetic material is contained within a nuclear membrane.

   (C) Some bacteria have special features to increase motility.

   (D) Bacteria only use RNA for genetic material.

2.   Describe the difference between Gram positive and Gram negative bacteria, and explain why this is important in determining which antibiotic to use against a particular infection.

3.   Which of the following is the correct definition of transduction?

   (A) Direct transfer of genetic material between bacterial cells

   (B) Infection with genetic material via a phage

   (C) Acquisition of genetic material from the environment

   (D) Reproduction via binary fission

4.   Explain the differences between the lytic and the lysogenic cycle. How would antiviral treatment options vary depending on the stage of the cycle the virus is in?

5.   Why is it advantageous for a fungus to produce spores?

   (A) Spore production creates two identical daughter cells.

   (B) Spores are created via binary fission, which is a more efficient means of reproduction.

   (C) Spores are diploid, enabling them to divide again if necessary.

   (D) Spores can tolerate more harsh environments than other types of fungal cells.

SOLUTIONS TO REVIEW PROBLEMS

1. **C**   Bacteria are prokaryotes, not eukaryotes, because they lack a membrane-bound nucleus and other membrane-bound organelles. As a result their genetic material is not contained within a nuclear membrane. Bacteria use only DNA for their genetic material, but viruses can use either DNA or RNA for their genetic material.

2.   Gram positive bacteria have a thick peptidoglycan layer surrounding the cell that stains purple when Gram stain is applied. In contrast, Gram negative bacteria have a much thinner peptidoglycan layer and stain pink with Gram stain. This distinction is important because some antibiotics work by attacking the peptidoglycan layer or other structural differences between the types of bacteria. As a result, certain antibiotics will be more effective against Gram positive or Gram negative bacteria. Some antibiotics work on both types of bacteria; this depends on the mechanism of action of the antibiotic. Choosing an antibiotic appropriate for the infecting bacteria helps to decrease resistance in the bacteria and improves the effectiveness of antibiotic therapy.

3. **B**   Direct transfer of genetic material between cells is referred to as conjugation. Acquiring genetic material from the environment is known as transformation. Binary fission occurs when a bacterial cell splits in two and does not involve the transfer of genetic material via transduction.

4.   During the lytic cycle the virus penetrates the cell membrane and injects its DNA. This induces the cell to replicate viral DNA instead of its own DNA. Eventually the cell will lyse and release its contents, including the viral DNA, which can infect other cells. During the lysogenic cycle the virus integrates into the bacterial genome and remains latent within the cell until it becomes activated. It is incredibly difficult to treat viruses that are creating latent infections because the cells show no outward sign of infection and therefore are difficult to target. Targeting cells in the lytic cycle is much easier because the drug can work on blocking any of the stages of the lytic cycle.

5. **D**   Spore formation does not create two identical daughter cells but rather four haploid spores. Binary fission is not used to produce spores because binary fission results in two identical progeny. Spores are haploid, not diploid, and therefore cannot divide again.

CHAPTER EIGHTEEN

Medical Microbiology

The field of medical microbiology relies heavily on contributions from **epidemiology**, which is the study of disease within populations, or groups of people within certain areas. Epidemiology includes the causes of disease (e.g., pathogens), how diseases are spread, patterns that exist in the spread of disease, and effects of these diseases in populations. Epidemiology is an important aspect of public health and explores the role of risk factors, preventative medicine, vaccinations, and even pharmaceuticals. As introduced in Chapter 17, Microorganisms, bacteria, viruses, fungi, and parasites all can contribute to the disease state. The PCAT tests your understanding of how diseases caused by these microorganisms are transmitted and what tools healthcare professionals use to work against the spread of infection.

TRANSMISSION

Transmission, or spread of disease from one host to another, can occur through direct or indirect contact. **Direct contact** involves touching the contaminated person and spreading the disease through physical contact, such as with sexually transmitted infections. **Indirect contact** includes transmission via **droplets** (particles suspended in fluid, such as airborne mucus), **vectors** (intermediary living organisms, such as ticks), soil, food, or water.

Prevention

Transmission of disease via inanimate objects can be reduced by using **sterilization**, which kills all pathogens, or **disinfection**, which kills some but not all microbes present. Methods of sterilization include using extreme heat, radiation, or ethylene gas (an alkylating agent). Methods of disinfection include using microwaves, pasteurization (heating at moderate temperatures), or chemicals such as alcohols, halogens, or hydrogen peroxide. Pathogens on living tissue can also be killed through the use of **antiseptics**, which are similar to disinfectants, but care must be taken not to harm the healthy tissue of the host.

Immunization

After transmission occurs, a strong immune system can sometimes fight off the pathogen before serious damage to body tissues takes place. If memory B and T cells are present, this response can occur even faster. Therefore, experiencing an infection once generally gives the host natural **active immunity** from that pathogen and the host does not experience the disease state again for as long as the memory cells remain in circulation.

However, when viruses are involved, the initial disease state may be too severe or long-lasting for this natural process to be useful. To bypass this process, an **attenuated** (weakened) or dead pathogen, or a fragment of a pathogen, may be injected as a **vaccine**. The injected microbe still causes an immune response, including the formation of memory cells, but the disease state is not required. In this way, the host gains immunity from future infection but does not suffer most of the adverse effects of an actual infection.

Immunity can also be acquired through direct transmission of antibodies from one source to another, establishing **passive immunity**. Passive immunity allows the individual to fight off infection by the pathogen specific to the transferred antibodies. However, any antibody is eventually broken down by the body, and once this happens immunity is lost because no corresponding memory B cells are present to create new antibodies. Passive immunity is most often given by a mother to her fetus through the placenta and to her newborn through breast milk, but it also can be acquired through injection in a clinical setting.

PHARMACEUTICALS

Once a disease has been transmitted, different antimicrobial agents may be used to control or eradicate the disease depending on which type of organism is causing the infection.

Antibacterials

Antibacterial agents work specifically on bacteria. Some agents only work on certain types of bacteria because of the structure of the bacteria (e.g., Gram positive or Gram negative, as discussed in Chapter 17, Microorganisms) or because of the mechanism of action of the drug.

Bactericidal agents kill bacteria; **bacteriostatic** agents stop bacteria from dividing. Bacteriostatic agents depend on the patient having a functioning immune system to eliminate the bacteria after their reproduction is stopped. As a result, these drugs are not commonly used in patients who are immunocompromised or who, for whatever reason, will not be able to eliminate the infection on their own.

Some bacteria have developed **resistance** to certain types of antibacterial agents and as a result these agents are no longer effective against these bacteria. There are many mechanisms that bacteria have developed to increase their resistance to antibacterial agents, including pumping out the antibiotic, producing enzymes that inactivate the antibiotic, and mutating their own DNA to make them immune to the effects of antibiotics. This has dramatically changed how antibacterial agents are used to treat infection. More information on resistance and the consequent changes that are being implemented in healthcare settings can be found later in the chapter.

Antivirals

Antiviral agents work specifically on viruses. Viral infections are much more difficult to treat than bacterial infections because viruses are neither cells nor alive and thus cannot be targeted by typical pharmaceuticals, which interrupt cell functions. Viral infections are also more difficult to treat because viruses are often contained in host cells; to destroy the virus, the host cell must often be damaged or destroyed as well. As a result, prevention of viral infections is much more successful than treating them. For example, at present there is no antiviral treatment for human papilloma virus (HPV). Not only can HPV cause physical symptoms for patients, it also can predispose women to certain types of cervical cancer. Vaccines do exist to help the host develop immunity to infection by this virus. This is an example of a situation in which prevention, rather than treatment, is the best course of action.

However, antiviral agents do exist and often interfere with a virus's ability to penetrate cells or replicate its genetic material. For example, some of the drugs used to treat human immunodeficiency virus (HIV) work by providing faulty nucleotides to the virus (nucleoside reverse transcriptase inhibitors), which interferes with proper DNA replication, or by disabling protease (protease inhibitors). Protease is an enzyme necessary for DNA replication and therefore for viral reproduction. While neither of these drugs is able to eliminate the infection completely, if a proper treatment plan is developed and followed, a patient may be able to keep viral replication to a minimum, effectively holding the HIV infection at bay and decreasing the chance of progressing to acquired immunodeficiency syndrome (AIDS).

Antifungals

Antifungal agents work specifically on fungi. As with antibacterial agents, most antifungal agents capitalize on the differences between a microorganism's cells and eukaryotic human cells. For example, because fungal cells contain cell walls and human cells do not, many antifungals work by destroying cell walls. This works to eliminate the infection while maintaining the integrity of the host's cells.

An example of an antifungal that utilizes these structural differences is the drug fluconazole. This is an antifungal medication that prevents the conversion of an ergosterol precursor to ergosterol itself. Ergosterol is an essential component of the cell membrane of the fungus but is not present in human cells. Without ergosterol, the cell membrane loses its structural integrity, and the fungal cell is destroyed.

Antiparasitics

Antiparasitic agents work specifically on parasites. Because of the wide variety of characteristics among parasitic organisms, these drugs have a number of different mechanisms of action, but all of them work to destroy the parasite without damage to the host.

Resistance

Resistance occurs within microbes after extended exposure to a particular antimicrobial. Some organisms are inherently resistant to certain antimicrobials or have mutations that make them resistant to a particular drug. However, resistance often comes about by natural selection for a strain of an organism that possesses resistance to a particular antimicrobial. For instance, if a particular strain of *Staphylococcus* bacteria is continually exposed to penicillin, eventually all the susceptible individuals of this strain will be eradicated by the antibiotic. This leaves only the bacteria with an inherent mechanism that prevents them from being eliminated by the antibiotic. Therefore, only the bacteria resistant to the antibiotic will continue to replicate, causing all future members of that strain to have resistance.

Over the past several decades, resistance has become an increasingly significant problem due to the increased use of antibiotics. As more antibiotics have been discovered and used, more resistant strains of bacteria have become prominent. Development of new antibiotics has not been able to keep up with the increasing rate of resistance. As a result, many hospitals have implemented antimicrobial stewardship programs. These programs are run by a team of pharmacists, doctors, nurses, and other healthcare professionals and are intended to decrease the unnecessary use of antimicrobial agents in the hospital setting. There is also a focus on using antimicrobial agents specific to the microbe being treated rather than using a **broad-spectrum** antimicrobial (one that treats many different species of microbe rather than a narrow range). When specific rather than general agents are used, the rate of increasing resistance slows because a selective pressure is not being placed on organisms other than the one the drug is intended to treat.

REVIEW PROBLEMS

1. Explain the importance of epidemiology to public health and healthcare in general.

2. What is the difference between bactericidal and bacteriostatic agents?

3. Why are viruses so difficult to treat?

4. One mechanism by which antiviral agents work is

   (A) killing the virus.
   (B) uncoating the viral DNA for destruction by endonucleases.
   (C) stopping viral replication.
   (D) inhibiting formation of the viral cell wall.

5. Explain why microbial resistance to antimicrobial agents is increasing and why it is such a concern for healthcare providers.

SOLUTIONS TO REVIEW PROBLEMS

1. Epidemiology studies disease by exploring the causes and transmission of diseases and identifying which populations are most susceptible to certain infections. Epidemiologists gather information about risk factors, prevalence of disease, prevention of diseases, and outbreaks, as well as track epidemics and pandemics. This information is critical to maintaining a healthy population.

2. Bactericidal drugs actually kill bacteria; bacteriostatic drugs stop the bacteria from reproducing but do not destroy the bacterial cells.

3. Viral infections are difficult to treat because viruses are contained within the host cell for most of their life cycles. As a result, the host cell often must be destroyed to treat the viral infection. In addition, many viral infections are difficult to detect once the virus is contained within the cell because their location makes targeting the virus difficult.

4. **C** Viruses are not technically alive; therefore, antiviral agents cannot kill them. Uncoating the viral DNA for destruction is not a mechanism of antiviral agents. Viruses also do not have cell walls, so antivirals do not inhibit viral cell wall formation.

5. Due to increased use of antibiotics, bacteria with resistance to antibiotics have been proliferating. The development of new antibiotics has not been able to keep up with this pressure. The concern with increased resistance is that, over time, many infections will not be able to be treated with antibiotics. As a result, many hospitals have implemented antimicrobial stewardship programs to cut down on unnecessary antibiotic use.

CHAPTER NINETEEN

Integument and Immune Systems

The body's ability to resist infection is highly dependent on both the integument and immune systems. The integument serves as the initial barrier to infection and prevents a large proportion of environmental microorganisms from entering the body. Should the organisms penetrate the integument, the immune system has several mechanisms to protect the body from infection and destroy the invading organisms.

THE INTEGUMENTARY SYSTEM

The **integument**, which is composed of the skin, hair, and nails, provides a physical barrier to prevent the entrance of pathogens into the body. Many microorganisms live on the surface of human skin and make up the normal skin flora, also known as the **skin microbiome**. These microorganisms often participate in mutualism (relationships that benefit both the microorganisms and the human). By occupying the surface of the skin, these microorganisms prevent other, more harmful organisms from occupying that same space; in return, the microorganisms get a stable environment with access to nutrients. However, some of the normal flora can become pathogenic if they penetrate the integument.

The **skin** itself is also a nonspecific defense mechanism that protects against pathogenic invasion. Sebaceous glands in the skin secrete oil onto the surface of the skin to keep its pH relatively acidic (a range of approximately 4–6), which decreases bacterial growth. These secretions also help keep the skin moist. **Sweat** is secreted from other glands and helps cool the skin by evaporative cooling. Sweat also contains enzymes that help destroy bacterial cell walls as well as pheromones used in chemical communication among humans.

The skin is divided into two different layers, the **dermis** and the **epidermis**, which are connected together by the **basement membrane**. The dermis contains the blood supply to the skin and most of the specialized cells, whereas the epidermis contains mainly keratinocytes, which differentiate into corneocytes: protective, waterproof cells that do not undergo further replication and are routinely sloughed off and replaced.

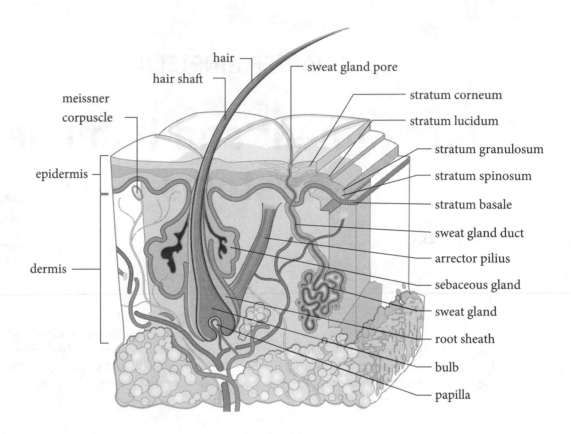

Figure 19.1

Parts of the skin are covered with **hair**, which aids the skin with the above functions. Hair serves to direct sweat and waste away from the skin, helping with evaporative cooling when the body is hot. Conversely, hair also traps heat, preventing the body from becoming too cool. Hair also serves as a sensory organ, allowing the detection of nearby motion.

Other components of the integument help prevent infection as well. **Mucous** secretions in the nose and aqueous secretions in the eyes help prevent foreign organisms from entering the body and resist infection. Similarly, **enzymes** in the mouth and throat break down many entering microorganisms and decrease their pathogenicity. Finally, **nails** protect the tips of the fingers and toes from physical injury and can be used as tools.

THE IMMUNE SYSTEM

In addition to the integument, the **immune system** plays a key role in the destruction of internal pathogens. The body can distinguish between self and nonself and can recognize and remember nonself qualities in other cells (**antigens**). This allows the body to recognize pathogens it has previously encountered and to mount a quicker immune response against these antigens if exposed to them again. The immune system has two major types of immunity: **humoral**, which involves antibody production, and **cell-mediated**, which involves cells that combat fungal and viral infections.

Another nonspecific defense mechanism employed by the immune system is the **inflammatory response**. When white blood cells are activated, they release chemicals, such as **histamine**, that activate the immune response. This response dilates and increases the permeability of blood vessels. These effects together increase the flow of white blood cells and other immune cells to the affected area, allowing the body to more effectively ward off infection. Inflammation is often accompanied by the rise in body temperature termed a **fever**, which in theory increases the ability to fight infection by killing temperature-dependent pathogens and speeding up healing processes. However, whether or not fever is practically beneficial is still a topic of scientific debate.

The **lymphatic system** is another important part of the immune system and is found in the extravascular space of most tissues. **Lymph** flows through the lymphatic vessels from lymph node to lymph node. The **lymph nodes** and **spleen** serve as reservoirs of white blood cells and filters for lymph, removing antigen-presenting cells and foreign matter and activating the immune system when necessary (see Chapter 23, Circulatory System).

Cell-Mediated Immunity

The immune system contains several varieties of white blood cells, or **leukocytes**, each with a specific function.

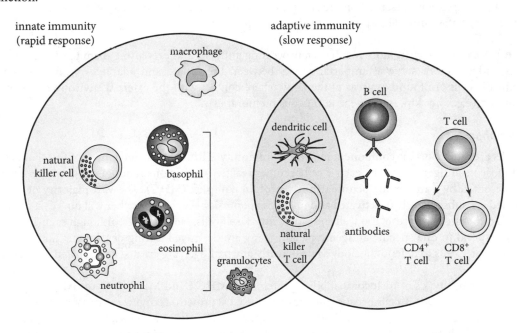

innate immunity
(rapid response)

adaptive immunity
(slow response)

macrophage

natural killer cell

basophil

eosinophil

neutrophil

dendritic cell

natural killer T cell

granulocytes

B cell

T cell

antibodies

CD4⁺ T cell

CD8⁺ T cell

Figure 19.2

Granulocytes

Granulocytes are attracted to the site of injury, where they phagocytize antigens and antigenic material.

Neutrophils, the most common type of granulocyte, are often the first responders to sites of inflammation. These cells are attracted to cytokines and in turn attract additional white blood cells once they arrive at the site of tissue damage. Although they can help moderate various infections and environmental trauma, neutrophils are particularly adapted to attack bacteria. Neutrophil counts are often elevated during the acute stages of inflammation and are the main component of pus.

Eosinophils are much less common and are responsible for immune responses, especially allergic and asthmatic responses. Elevated eosinophil counts on a complete blood count (CBC) often indicate an allergic response or infection by a parasite, including those that live on the surface of the skin (ectoparasites), such as fleas and ticks, and those that live in intercellular spaces (endoparasites), such as the parasitic worms known as helminths.

Basophils and the related **mast cells** are similarly involved in allergic responses and parasite infections and often are responsible for the release of histamine, which stimulates blood vessel dilation as previously described.

Monocytes

Monocytes are large, long-lived immune cells that can differentiate into macrophages and dendritic cells.

The main role of **macrophages** is to phagocytize dead cells and pathogens. If a pathogen is ingested, its antigens are then presented on the surface of the macrophage to stimulate other immune cells to mount a specific immune response to the invading pathogen.

Dendritic cells are even more focused on processing antigens and presenting them to other immune cells and therefore serve as important links between the innate and adaptive immune systems. Dendritic cells are found in areas of the body where contact with the external environment is more common (e.g., the skin, intestine, and mucous membranes).

T lymphocytes

T cells are an important component in specific immunity. Through rearrangement of the chains that compose its antigen receptors, each T cell becomes reactive to only one random antigen type, usually as presented by a **major histocompatibility protein complex (MHC)**. The vast majority of T cells created are subsequently deactivated and undergo apoptosis because they either will not react with the MHC or because they react too well and would attack self cells. Nevertheless, although each T cell can only respond to one specific antigen type and many are destroyed during development, a sufficient number of T cells to defend the body against nearly any pathogen are created and allowed to circulate.

The two major types of histocompatibility proteins are MHC I and MHC II. **Cytotoxic T (T_C) cells** (also known as **CD8$^+$ T cells** because they contain the CD8 protein) recognize and respond to antigens presented by MHC I complexes. These complexes come from cells infected with viruses or developing tumors and signal T_C cells to destroy those cells. In contrast, **T helper (T_H) cells** (also known as CD4$^+$ T cells) recognize and respond to antigens presented by MHC II complexes. Activated T_H cells release cytokines to stimulate the immune response, causing other white blood cells to mature and attack. **Natural killer T (NKT) cells** behave similarly to both T_C and T_H cells but respond to antigens presented by other types of cells.

Once a reaction has occurred, **memory T cells** reactive to the same antigens are formed and remain in circulation for long periods of time, allowing a quicker, more targeted response if the antigen reappears. **Regulatory** or **suppressor T (T_{reg}) cells** have the opposite function, serving to tone down T cell response to self cells or following an infection.

T cells begin their development in the bone marrow, where T lymphocyte precursor cells are formed. They travel via the bloodstream to the **thymus**, where they mature. It is because these cells mature in the thymus that they are referred to as T cells. Once maturation is complete, these cells are released into the lymph to perform their immune function.

T cells are a vital component of the immune system. Patients with acquired immunodeficiency syndrome (AIDS) have very low levels of certain types of T cells and as a result are particularly subject to infection because the immune system is so weakened by this loss.

B lymphocytes

B cells, when stimulated, create and express **antibodies** (also known as **immunoglobulins**) that have a high affinity for the antigen expressed by the stimulating T lymphocyte. Immunoglobulins have a very particular structure (outlined later in this chapter) and utilize the specificity of this structure to aid in the targeted destruction of pathogens. Like T cells, B cells can also stimulate the formation of memory cells.

B lymphocytes, like T cells, begin their development in the bone marrow. However, unlike T cells, their development is completed there; they do not travel to other parts of the body to mature.

The following table outlines the most important cells found in the immune system as well as their functions.

Cell Type	Function
Granulocytes	
Basophil	Least common of all the granulocytes (1%); fight parasites; mediate allergic response
Eosinophil	Much less common than neutrophils (5%); fight parasites; mediate allergic response
Neutrophils	Most common of the granulocytes (94%); phagocytic
Monocytes	
Macrophage	Phagocytic; secrete cytokines; present antigens
Dendritic cells	Present antigens; activate immune system
Lymphocytes	
B cells	Produce antigen-specific antibodies
T cells	Helper T ($CD4^+$) cells activate other immune cells; cytotoxic T ($CD8^+$) cells and natural killer T (NKT) cells destroy cells marked for destruction; memory T cells remain after an infection so a response can be mounted more quickly if infected again

Table 19.1

Humoral Immunity

The immune system also contains components that are not cells. Various chemicals, hormones, and enzymes supplement the action of the cells and serve equally important roles.

Antibodies

Large proteins secreted by B cells known as antibodies or **immunoglobulins** provide specific, targeted responses to a given antigen. Several types of immunoglobulins exist within the immune system, and each plays a unique role in immunity. Nevertheless, the structure of all immunoglobulins is relatively consistent and resembles a "Y," with antigen binding sites at either end of the top of the "Y." Each side of the structure consists of two chains, a light chain and a heavy chain, which are held together with disulfide bonds. The variable portion of the structure is the antigen-binding region.

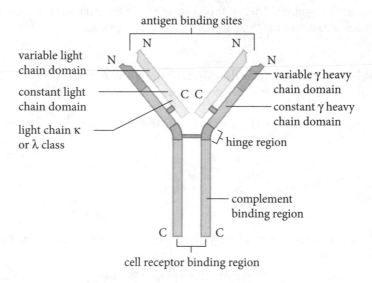

Figure 19.3

The antigen-binding region of the antibody is unique to each antigen and is the reason that specificity for a particular antigen exists. The immune system can generate millions of unique antigen binding sites, which confers the ability to mount an immune response against any number of antigens.

Antibody-mediated immunity includes both active and passive immunity. **Active immunity** occurs as a result of an immune response. This can be due to exposure to a pathogen or antigen, such as during an infection. It can also be the result of **vaccination**, where an individual is deliberately exposed to a weakened, inactivated, or killed form of the antigen. This exposure stimulates the body's immune system to mount an immune response against the antigen presented. The features of this antigen are then stored in the "nonself" memory, allowing the body to mount a similar immune response should the antigen present itself again. This type of immune response, because it requires the development of cells specific to a particular antigen, can take weeks or months to build up.

Passive immunity, in contrast, is acquired by the transfer of antibodies from one individual to another. This can occur during pregnancy, for example, when maternal antibodies cross the placenta and enter fetal circulation. Injections of gamma globulin, which is the fraction of the blood containing antibodies, can also provide passive immunity by transferring antibodies to a particular illness to a given individual. While passive immunity is effective immediately upon transfer of antibodies, once the antibodies are no longer circulating in the immune system the effect of the immunity is lost.

Types of Immunity

While immunity can be characterized by the types of immune components involved, it can also be divided into **innate** and **adaptive immunity** based on how the immunity is acquired. Each of these categories involves components from both cell-mediated and humoral immunity.

Innate immunity

Innate immunity is comprised of the body's initial, generalized defenses against pathogens. This type of immunity does not require the cells of the immune system to be previously exposed to any given antigen to be activated. However, it is not a specific response, and the body is limited in the types of immune response it can mount. Innate immunity includes:

- anatomic features (including the integument, as described above)
- physiologic response (fever, pH change, enzymes)
- phagocytic cells (monocytes, neutrophils, macrophages)
- inflammation

Adaptive immunity

Acquired or **specific** immunity consists of cells capable of recognizing self versus nonself cells—for example, cells that can differentiate invading cells from host cells—and that are specific to a particular antigen. The activity of cells that participate in an adaptive immune response is increased with each exposure. Thus, there are memory components to acquired immunity: Cells recognize antigens they have been exposed to previously, and the immune response mounted against increases in magnitude after each repeat exposure to an antigen. Cells that are involved in adaptive immunity are:

- lymphocytes (B and T cells)
- plasma cells
- antigen-presenting cells (macrophages, B cells)

Innate and acquired immunity work together to protect the host and defend against invading pathogens. Phagocytic cells can stimulate production of specific T lymphocytes to assist in pathogen killing and destruction. T lymphocytes, in turn, can release cytokines, which increase the killing activities of phagocytes. Other examples of this type of cooperation exist, and they work to increase the function and efficacy of the immune system.

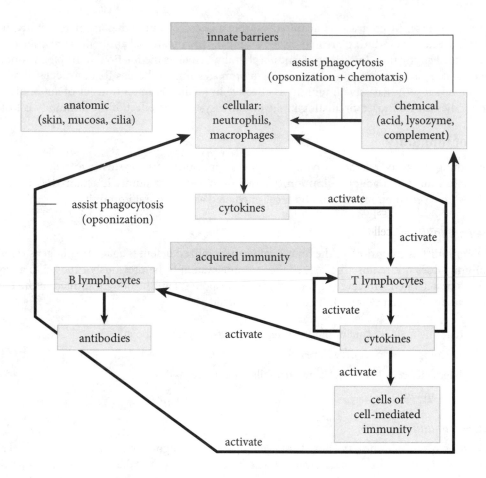

Figure 19.4

Transplant rejection

Transplanted tissues or organs are detected as nonself by the recipient's immune system. This is because the antigens on the donated organ are those of the donor, not of the recipient. As a result, the recipient's immune system attacks the transplanted organ. This attack can lead to rejection of the organ, which can ultimately result in destruction of the organ or death of the patient. As a result, immunosuppressing drugs are used to lower the immune response to transplants and decrease the likelihood of rejection. These work by lowering the body's immune response to antigens; while this decreases the likelihood of rejecting the organ, it also lowers the recipient's overall immune response. The recipient is then referred to as **immunocompromised** because his or her immune system is not functioning at its full capacity.

REVIEW PROBLEMS

1. What is the role of histamine in the immune response?
    (A) To induce a fever
    (B) To reduce inflammation
    (C) To dilate the blood vessels
    (D) To recruit immunoglobulin

2. Describe the roles of the three types of granulocytes (basophils, eosinophils, and neutrophils) and the two types of monocytes (macrophages and dendritic cells).

3. What type of cell responds to activated MHC II complexes?
    (A) Cytotoxic T cell
    (B) Helper T cell
    (C) Natural killer cell
    (D) Plasma cell

4. Which cells produce a memory-driven response to pathogens?
    (A) Neutrophils
    (B) Macrophages
    (C) Cytokines
    (D) B lymphocytes

5. Compare and contrast the maturation process of T lymphocytes and B lymphocytes.

6. Differentiate between active and passive immunity and give examples of each.

7. Where is the antigen-binding region found on the immunoglobulin structure?
    (A) Heavy chain
    (B) Light chain
    (C) N-terminus
    (D) Cytoplasmic tail

SOLUTIONS TO REVIEW PROBLEMS

1. **C** Histamine triggers the inflammatory response and dilates blood vessels, thereby increasing blood flow to an injured area, which increases the number of immune cells that can reach the damaged tissue. In contrast, cytokines trigger the fever response and activate B lymphocytes, which in turn produce immunoglobulin.

2. Neutrophils are the first responders to inflammation and phagocytize pathogens. Eosinophils and basophils are involved in inflammation and the allergic response, and both are involved in combating parasites. Among other actions, basophils specifically stimulate histamine release, while eosinophils release cytokines. Macrophages phagocytize pathogens and dead or damaged cells. Dendritic cells present antigens to allow for a targeted immune response.

3. **B** The major histocompatibility complex (MHC) presents proteins to immune cells. MHC II in particular presents to helper T lymphocytes, and these cells then activate other T cells and B cells. Cytotoxic T cells recognize and attack foreign antigens, natural killer cells similarly destroy tumor cells and cells infected with viruses, and plasma cells release large quantities of antibodies, but none of these types of cells interact with MHC.

4. **D** Macrophages are part of the general immune response and do not exert a targeted effect or retain memory of antigens. Cytokines activate B cells but do not themselves possess a memory for antigens. Neutrophils are phagocytic and also do not have a memory for specific antigens.

5. Both T lymphocytes and B lymphocytes begin development in the bone marrow. Immature T cells are released into the bloodstream, where they travel to the thymus. It is in the thymus that T cells complete the maturation process and develop their permanent characteristics. B cells, however, complete their maturation in the bone marrow. When B cells are released from the bone they are mature and ready to undertake their anti-pathogenic activities.

6. Active immunity is due to exposure to an antigen, for example during infection or vaccination. Passive immunity requires the transfer of antibodies from one individual to another. This can occur, for example, from a pregnant woman to her fetus.

7. **C** The heavy chain, light chain, and cytoplasmic tail are all components of antibody structure, but none of them play a role in binding antigens. It is only the N terminus that binds to antigens and thus determines the specificity of the antibody.

CHAPTER TWENTY

Nervous System

The **nervous system** is responsible for controlling most body functions, enabling organisms to receive and respond to **stimuli** from their external and internal environments. Signals from the nervous system travel quickly, reaching in excess of 100 meters per second in some cases, which results in transmission of information much more rapidly than through the endocrine system (see Chapter 25).

The nervous system is composed of both **neurons** (specialized nervous tissue) and **neuroglia** (cells that support and protect the neurons). These cells work together to form the major organs of the nervous system, which include the brain and spinal cord as well as complex sensory organs, such as the eye and ear. In turn, these organs often involve two divisions: the **central nervous system (CNS)** and the **peripheral nervous system (PNS)**.

NEURON

Structure

Neurons are the functional units of the nervous system and are used to convert stimuli into **electrochemical signals** and conduct them through the nervous system. Each neuron is generally an elongated cell consisting of **dendrites**, a **cell body**, and an **axon**. **Dendrites** are cytoplasmic extensions that receive information and transmit it toward the cell body. The cell body (**soma**) contains the nucleus and controls the metabolic activity of the neuron. The **axon** is a long cellular process that transmits impulses, or **action potentials**, away from the cell body. Most mammalian axons are sheathed by an insulating substance known as **myelin**, which prevents leakage of signal from the axons and allows for faster conduction of impulses. The gaps between segments of myelin, the **nodes of Ranvier**, are where the action potential actually propagates; this occurs through a process known as saltatory ("hopping") conduction. Myelin itself is produced by glial cells known as **oligodendrocytes** in the central nervous system and by **Schwann cells** in the peripheral nervous system. The axons end in swellings known as **synaptic terminals** (also called boutons or knobs). **Neurotransmitters** are released from these terminals into the **synapse** (or synaptic cleft), which is the gap between the axon terminals of one cell and the dendrites of the next cell. Axons may be very long, such as the axon of a neuron traveling from the spinal cord to the tip of the foot.

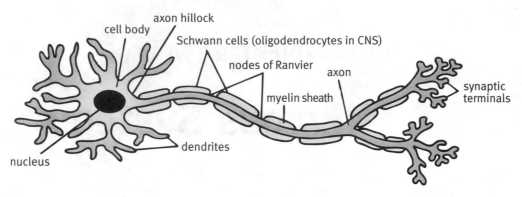

Figure 20.1

The four major types of cells in the CNS and two major types in the PNS are summarized in the following table:

Cells in the CNS and PNS	
Cell Type	**Cell Function**
CNS	
Astrocytes	Maintain the integrity of the blood–brain barrier, regulate nutrient and dissolved gas concentrations, and absorb and recycle neurotransmitters
Oligodendrocytes	Myelinate CNS axons as well as provide structural framework for the CNS
Microglia	Remove cellular debris and pathogens
Ependymal cells	Line the brain ventricles and aid in the production, circulation, and monitoring of cerebral spinal fluid
PNS	
Satellite cells	Surround the neuron cell bodies in the ganglia
Schwann cells	Enclose the axons in the PNS and aid in the myelination of some peripheral axons

Table 20.1

Function

Neurons are specialized to receive signals from sensory receptors or from other neurons in the body. These signals create action potentials, which travel the length of the axon to invade the nerve terminal, thereby causing the release of neurotransmitter into the synapse.

Resting potential

Even at rest, a neuron is **polarized** due to unequal distribution of ions between the inside and outside of the cell. The potential difference at rest between the extracellular space and the intracellular space is called the **resting potential**. A typical resting membrane potential is –70 millivolts (mV), which means the inside of the neuron is more negative than the outside. This difference is caused by selective ionic permeability of the neuronal cell membrane and is maintained by the active transport of ions by the **Na$^+$/K$^+$ pump** (also called the Na$^+$/K$^+$ ATPase), which pumps 3 Na$^+$ out of the cell for every 2 K$^+$ it transports into the cell. This uneven exchange results in one more positive charge leaving the cell than entering it, creating a negative internal environment. Furthermore, the cell membrane is selectively permeable to K$^+$, allowing some of the K$^+$ that was pumped into the cell to move back out through facilitated diffusion, making the internal environment even more negative.

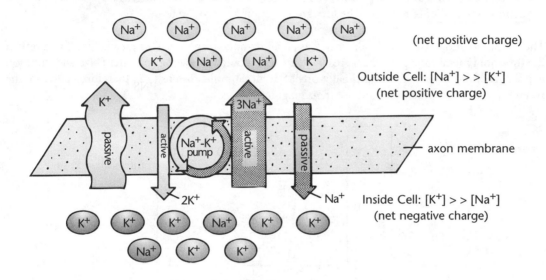

Figure 20.2

Action potential

The nerve cell body receives both excitatory and inhibitory impulses from other cells, often in the form of internal charges. If the cell becomes sufficiently excited and **depolarized** (i.e., the inside of the cell becomes less negative and more positive) to reach the **threshold potential**, then **voltage-gated ion channels** located in the nerve cell membrane open in response. An action potential begins when voltage-gated Na$^+$ channels open in response to depolarization, allowing Na$^+$ to rush down its electrochemical gradient into the cell and causing further, rapid depolarization of that segment of the axon. The Na$^+$ also causes the next portion of the axon toward the terminal to become depolarized, causing voltage-gated Na$^+$ channels to open there as well, continuing the process and moving the action potential toward the terminal. Once the action potential reaches the synaptic terminal, a final voltage-gated channel, this time for calcium, is opened. This allows Ca^{2+} to rush in and trigger the exocytosis of **synaptic vesicles** containing neurotransmitters.

After the signal has been propagated through a segment of the axon, the high voltage there causes voltage-gated K^+ channels to open, allowing K^+ to rush down its electrochemical gradient and out of the cell. Meanwhile, the voltage-gated Na^+ channels also close, and the Na^+/K^+ pump begins to pump Na^+ out of the cell again. Together, these processes return the cell to a negative potential in a process known as **repolarization**. In fact, the neuron's voltage shoots past the resting potential and becomes even more negative inside than normal due to the K^+ still being free to leave the cell; this is called **hyperpolarization**. This results in the **refractory period**, a period of time after an action potential during which new action potentials are very difficult or impossible to initiate immediately. The refractory period allows the neuron time to regenerate neurotransmitter and also helps ensure the action potential only moves in the forward direction, toward the terminal.

The action potential itself can be described as an all-or-none response. This means that if and only if the threshold membrane potential is reached, an action potential with a consistent size and duration is produced; the neuron fires maximally or not at all. Stimulus intensity is therefore coded by the **frequency** of action potentials and not their magnitude.

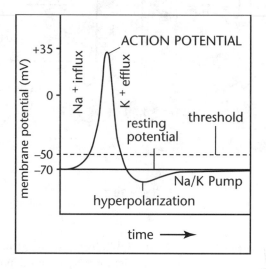

Figure 20.3

Impulse propagation

Although axons can theoretically propagate action potentials bidirectionally, information transfer will occur only in one direction: from dendrite to synaptic terminal. This is because synapses operate only in one direction and because refractory periods make the backward travel of action potentials impossible.

Nevertheless, different axons do propagate action potentials at **different speeds**. The greater the **diameter** of the axon and the more heavily it is **myelinated**, the faster the impulses travel. Myelin increases the conduction velocity by insulating segments of the axon such that the membrane is permeable to ions only in the nodes of Ranvier. In this way, the action potential "hops" from node to node.

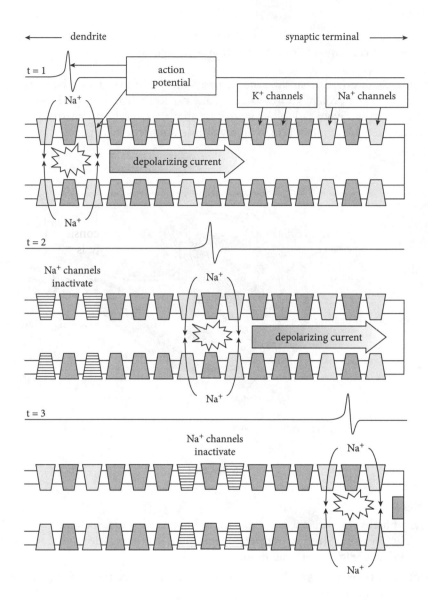

Figure 20.4

Synapse

The synapse is the gap between the axon terminal of one neuron (called the **presynaptic neuron** because it is before the synapse) and the dendrites of another neuron (the **postsynaptic neuron**). Neurons may also communicate with postsynaptic cells other than neurons, such as cells in muscles or glands; these are called **effector cells**.

The nerve terminal contains thousands of membrane-bound vesicles full of chemical messengers known as **neurotransmitters**. When the action potential arrives at the nerve terminal and depolarizes it, the synaptic vesicles fuse with the presynaptic membrane and release neurotransmitter into the synapse. The neurotransmitter diffuses across the synapse and acts on receptor proteins embedded in the postsynaptic membrane. The released neurotransmitter will lead to depolarization of the postsynaptic cell and consequent firing of an action potential.

Neurotransmitter is removed from the synapse in a variety of ways: it may be taken back up into the nerve terminal (via a protein known as an uptake carrier) where it may be reused or degraded; it may be degraded by enzymes located in the synapse (e.g., acetylcholinesterase inactivates the neurotransmitter acetylcholine); or it may simply diffuse out of the synapse.

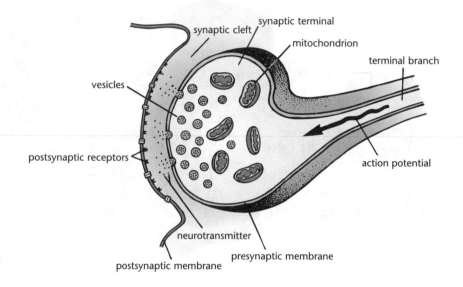

Figure 20.5

Effects of drugs

- **Curare** blocks postsynaptic nicotinic acetylcholine receptors, such as those on muscles, so acetylcholine is unable to interact with them. This leads to muscle relaxation and paralysis by blocking the ability to constrict muscles.

- **Botulinum toxin** prevents the release of acetylcholine from the presynaptic membrane and also results in paralysis.

- **Anticholinesterases** are used as nerve gases and in the insecticide Parathion. As the name implies, these substances inhibit the activity of the acetylcholinesterase enzyme responsible for degrading acetylcholine released into the synapse. As a result, acetylcholine is not degraded and continues to affect the postsynaptic membrane. Therefore, no coordinated muscular contractions can take place.

Neuron Types

Although their general characteristics remain the same, neurons can become specialized to perform specific tasks. Neurons that carry **sensory** information about the external or internal environment to the brain or spinal cord are called **afferent neurons**. Neurons that carry **motor** commands from the brain or spinal cord to various parts of the body (e.g., muscles or glands) are called **efferent neurons**. Some neurons (**interneurons**) participate only in local circuits, linking sensory and motor neurons in the brain and spinal cord; their cell bodies and their nerve terminals are in the same location.

Nerves are essentially bundles of axons covered with connective tissue. A network of nerve fibers is called a **plexus**. Neuronal cell bodies often cluster together: such clusters are called **ganglia** in the periphery; in the central nervous system, they are called **nuclei**.

ORGANIZATION OF THE NERVOUS SYSTEM

The human nervous system can be viewed as having several different divisions, each with unique properties and functions:

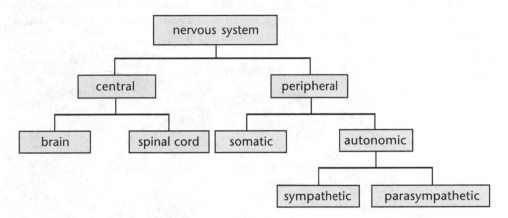

Figure 20.6

Central Nervous System

The central nervous system (CNS) consists of the brain and spinal cord.

Brain

The brain is a mass of neurons that resides in the skull. Its functions include interpreting sensory information, forming motor plans, and cognitive function (thinking). The brain consists of an outer portion of cell bodies called the **gray matter** and an inner portion of myelinated axons called the **white matter**. The brain also can be divided into the forebrain, midbrain, and hindbrain.

Forebrain (Prosencephalon)

- The **forebrain** consists of the **telencephalon** and the **diencephalon**. A major component of the telencephalon is the **cerebral cortex**, which is the highly convoluted gray matter that can be seen on the surface of the brain. The cortex processes and integrates sensory input and motor responses and is important for memory and creative thought. The **olfactory bulb** is the center for reception and integration of olfactory (smell-related) input.

- The diencephalon contains the thalamus and hypothalamus. The **thalamus** is a relay and integration center for the spinal cord and cerebral cortex. The **hypothalamus** controls visceral functions such as hunger, thirst, sex drive, water balance, blood pressure, and temperature regulation. It also plays an important role in the control of the endocrine system.

Midbrain (Mesencephalon)

- The **midbrain** is a relay center for visual and auditory impulses. It also plays an important role in motor control.

Hindbrain (Rhombencephalon)

- The **hindbrain** is the posterior part of the brain and consists of the cerebellum, the pons, and the medulla. The **cerebellum** helps to modulate motor impulses initiated by the cerebral cortex and is important in the maintenance of balance, hand-eye coordination, and the timing of rapid movements. One function of the **pons** is to act as a relay center to allow the cortex to communicate with the cerebellum. The **medulla** (also called the medulla oblongata) controls many vital functions such as breathing, heart rate, and gastrointestinal activity. Together, the midbrain, pons, and medulla constitute the **brainstem**.

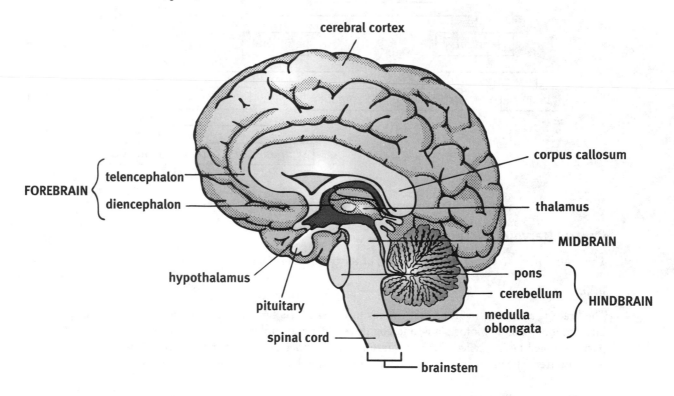

Figure 20.7

Spinal cord

The spinal cord is an elongated extension of the brain that acts as the conduit for sensory information to the brain and motor information from the brain. The spinal cord can also integrate simple motor responses (e.g., **reflexes**) by itself. A cross-section of the spinal cord reveals an outer white matter area containing motor and sensory axons and an inner gray matter area containing nerve cell bodies. Sensory information enters the spinal cord through the **dorsal horn**; the cell bodies of these sensory neurons are located in the dorsal root ganglia. All motor information exits the spinal cord through the **ventral horn**. For simple reflexes like the knee-jerk reflex, sensory fibers (entering through the dorsal root ganglion) synapse directly on ventral horn motor fibers. Other reflexes include interneurons between the sensory and motor fibers that allow for some processing in the spinal cord.

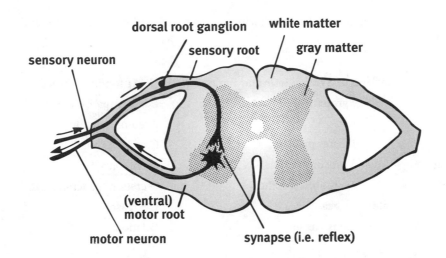

Figure 20.8

Peripheral Nervous System

The peripheral nervous system (PNS) consists of nerves and ganglia. The sensory nerves that enter the CNS and the motor nerves that leave the CNS are part of the peripheral nervous system. The PNS has two primary divisions: the **somatic** and the **autonomic** nervous systems, each of which has both motor and sensory components.

Somatic nervous system

The somatic nervous system (SNS) innervates skeletal muscles and is responsible for voluntary movement as well as reflex arcs (pathways that control motor reflexes).

Autonomic nervous system

The autonomic nervous system (ANS) is sometimes also called the **involuntary nervous system** because it regulates the body's internal environment without the aid of conscious control. The autonomic innervation of the body includes both sensory and motor fibers. The ANS innervates cardiac and smooth muscle. Smooth muscle is located in areas such as blood vessels, the digestive tract, the bladder, and bronchi (see Chapter 21), so the ANS is important in blood pressure control, gastrointestinal motility, excretion, respiration, and reproduction. The ANS is comprised of two subdivisions, the **sympathetic** and the **parasympathetic** nervous systems, which generally act in opposition to one another.

- **Sympathetic nervous system:** The sympathetic division is responsible for the "**flight or fight**" responses that ready the body for action in an emergency situation. It increases blood pressure and heart rate, increases blood flow to skeletal muscles, and decreases gut motility. It also dilates the bronchioles to increase gas exchange. The sympathetic nervous system uses **norepinephrine** as its primary neurotransmitter.

- **Parasympathetic nervous system:** The parasympathetic division acts to conserve energy and restore the body to resting activity levels after exertion ("**rest and digest**"). It acts to lower heart rate and increase gut motility. One very important parasympathetic nerve that innervates many of the thoracic and abdominal viscera is called the **vagus nerve**. It uses **acetylcholine** as its primary neurotransmitter.

Below is a summary table that lists the major functions of the parasympathetic and sympathetic nervous systems.

Comparison of Sympathetic and Parasympathetic Autonomic Functions		
Organ	**Sympathetic Effect**	**Parasympathetic Effect**
Lens	n/a	Accommodation
Iris	Dilates pupil	Constricts pupil
Salivary glands	Vasoconstriction	Secretion
Sweat glands	Secretion (specific)	Secretion (generalized)
Heart (force and rate)	Increases	Decreases
Peripheral blood vessels	Constriction	Dilation
Visceral blood vessels	Constriction	Dilation
Lungs	Vasodilation, bronchoconstriction	Bronchodilation, secretion
Gastrointestinal tract	Decreases peristalsis and secretion	Increases peristalsis and secretion
Rectum and anus	Inhibits smooth muscle in rectum and constricts sphincter	Increases smooth muscle tone and relaxes sphincter
Adrenal medulla	n/a	secretion
Bladder	Relaxation of the detrusor muscle and constriction of internal sphincter	Contraction of the detrusor muscle and inhibition of internal sphincter
Genitalia	Ejaculation	Penile erection / engorgement of clitoris and labia

Table 20.2

SPECIAL SENSES

The human body has a number of organs that are specialized receptors adapted to detect stimuli.

The Eye

The eye detects light energy (photons) and transmits information about intensity, color, and shape to the brain. The eyeball is covered by a thick, opaque layer known as the **sclera**, which is also known as the white of the eye. Beneath the sclera is the **choroid** layer, which helps to supply the retina with blood. The choroid is a dark, pigmented area that reduces reflection in the eye. The innermost layer of the eye is the **retina**, which contains the **photoreceptors** that sense light.

The transparent **cornea** at the front of the eye bends and focuses light rays. The rays then travel through an opening called the **pupil**, whose diameter is controlled by the pigmented, muscular **iris**. The iris responds to the intensity of light in the surroundings (light makes the pupil constrict). The light continues through the lens, which is suspended behind the pupil. The **lens**, the shape and focal length of which is controlled by the **ciliary muscles**, focuses the image onto the retina.

In the retina are **photoreceptors** that transduce light into action potentials. The two main types of photoreceptors are cones and rods. **Cones** respond to high-intensity illumination and are sensitive to color, whereas **rods** detect low-intensity illumination and are important in night vision. Cones and rods contain various pigments that absorb specific wavelengths of light. Cones contain three different pigments that absorb red, green, and blue wavelengths; the rod pigment, **rhodopsin**, only absorbs a single wavelength. The photoreceptor cells synapse onto **bipolar cells**, which in turn synapse onto **ganglion cells**. Axons of the ganglion cells bundle to form the optic nerve, which conducts visual information to the brain. The point at which the optic nerve exits the eye is called the **blind spot** because photoreceptors are not present there. The **fovea**, a small area of the retina above the blind spot, is densely packed with cones and is important for high-acuity vision.

The eye also contains a jelly-like material called **vitreous humor** that helps maintain its shape and optical properties. **Aqueous humor** is a more watery substance that fills the space between the lens and the cornea.

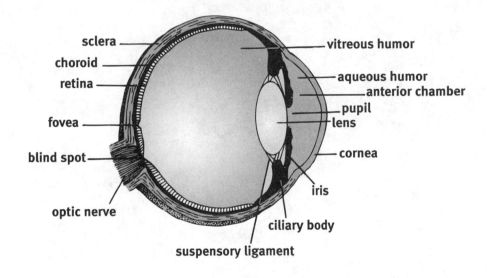

Figure 20.9

Disorders of the eye

- **Myopia (nearsightedness)** occurs when the image is focused in front of the retina.
- **Hyperopia (farsightedness)** occurs when the image is focused behind the retina.
- **Astigmatism** is caused by an irregularly shaped cornea.
- **Cataracts** develop when the lens becomes opaque; light cannot enter the eye, and blindness results.
- **Glaucoma** is an increase of pressure in the eye because of blocking of the outflow of the aqueous humor, which results in optic nerve damage.

THE EAR

The ear transduces sound energy (**pressure waves**) into impulses perceived by the brain as sound. Sound waves pass through three regions as they enter the ear. First, they enter the **outer ear**, which consists of the **auricle** (external ear) and the **auditory canal**. At the end of the auditory canal is the **tympanic membrane** (eardrum) of the middle ear, which vibrates at the same frequency as the incoming sound. Next, the three bones, or **ossicles** (malleus, incus, and stapes or hammer, anvil, and stirrup), of the middle ear amplify the stimulus and transmit it through the oval window, which leads to the fluid-filled inner ear. The inner ear consists of the **cochlea** and the **vestibular apparatus**, which is involved in maintaining equilibrium. Vibration of the ossicles exerts pressure on the fluid in the cochlea, stimulating **hair cells** in the **basilar membrane** to transduce the pressure into action potentials, which travel via the **auditory (cochlear) nerve** to the brain for processing.

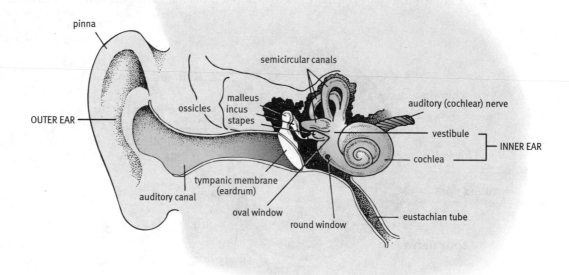

Figure 20.10

REVIEW PROBLEMS

1. Which of the following statements best characterizes an axon?

   (A) It is a long, slender process that fires every time neurotransmitters bind to the postsynaptic membrane.

   (B) It transmits nonelectrical impulses.

   (C) It transmits information from the cell body to the axon terminals.

   (D) None of the above

2. Resting membrane potential depends on

   (A) the differential distribution of ions across the axon membrane.

   (B) active transport.

   (C) selective permeability.

   (D) all of the above.

3. All of the following are associated with the myelin sheath EXCEPT

   (A) faster conduction of nervous impulses.

   (B) nodes of Ranvier forming gaps along the axon.

   (C) increased energy output for nervous impulse conduction.

   (D) saltatory conduction of action potentials.

4. The all-or-none law states that

   (A) all hyperpolarizing stimuli will be carried to the axon terminal without a decrease in size.

   (B) the size of the action potential is proportional to the size of the stimulus that produced it.

   (C) increasing the intensity of the depolarization increases the size of the impulse.

   (D) once an action potential is triggered, an impulse of a given magnitude and speed is produced.

5. Discuss two major differences between the somatic and the autonomic divisions of the peripheral nervous system.

6. By increasing the intensity of the stimulus, the action potential will

   (A) increase in amplitude.

   (B) increase in frequency.

   (C) increase in speed.

   (D) increase in wavelength.

7. Which of the following pairings is correct?

   (A) Sensory nerves–Afferent

   (B) Motor nerves–Afferent

   (C) Sensory nerves–Efferent

   (D) Sensory nerves–Ventral

8. When a sensory receptor receives a threshold stimulus, it will do all of the following EXCEPT

   (A) become depolarized.
   (B) transduce the stimulus to an action potential.
   (C) inhibit the spread of the action potential to sensory neurons.
   (D) cause the sensory neuron to send action potentials to the central nervous system.

9. Which of the following structures is most important for focusing light on the retina?

   (A) Cornea
   (B) Aqueous humor
   (C) Lens
   (D) Sclera

10. When the potential across the axon membrane is more negative than the normal resting potential, the neuron is said to be in a state of

    (A) depolarization.
    (B) hyperpolarization.
    (C) repolarization.
    (D) refraction.

11. Chemical X is found to denature all enzymes in the synaptic cleft. What are the effects on acetylcholine if chemical X is added to the cleft?

    (A) Acetylcholine is not released from the presynaptic membrane.
    (B) Acetylcholine does not bind to the postsynaptic membrane.
    (C) Acetylcholine is not inactivated in the synaptic cleft.
    (D) Acetylcholine is degraded before it acts on the postsynaptic membrane.

12. Which of the following statements concerning the somatic division of the peripheral nervous system is INCORRECT?

    (A) Its pathways innervate skeletal muscles.
    (B) Its pathways are usually voluntary.
    (C) Some of its pathways are referred to as reflex arcs.
    (D) It includes the vagus nerve.

13. In the ear, what structure transduces pressure waves to action potentials?

    (A) Tympanic membrane
    (B) Hair cells
    (C) Oval window
    (D) Semicircular canals

SOLUTIONS TO REVIEW PROBLEMS

1. **C** Axons carry information from the cell body of the neuron to the axon terminal by way of action potentials. From there, the impulse is transmitted to another neuron or to an effector. However, the axon does not fire unless the impulse is strong enough to depolarize the axon membrane to the threshold membrane potential.

2. **D** Resting membrane potential is a result of an unequal distribution of ions between the inside and the outside of the cell, and of the other facets of cell structure listed.

3. **C** Discussed in impulse propagation section of this chapter.

4. **D** Discussed in action potential section of this chapter.

5. First, the somatic nervous system regulates voluntary actions (except in the cases of monosynaptic and polysynaptic reflexes), whereas the autonomic nervous system regulates involuntary actions. Second, the somatic nervous system innervates skeletal muscle, whereas the autonomic nervous system innervates cardiac and smooth muscle.

6. **B** Discussed in action potential section of this chapter.

7. **A** Discussed in vertebrate nervous system section of this chapter.

8. **C** Discussed in vertebrate nervous system section of this chapter.

9. **C** Discussed in special senses section of this chapter.

10. **B** When the neuron goes past the resting potential and becomes even more negative inside than normal, this is termed hyperpolarization.

11. **C** Acetylcholine is inactivated in the synaptic cleft by the enzyme acetycholinesterase after it has acted upon the postsynaptic membrane. If chemical X denatures acetylcholinesterase, acetylcholinesterase will not be able to inactivate acetylcholine and prevent the continuous depolarization of the effector membrane.

12. **D** Discussed in peripheral nervous system section of this chapter.

13. **B** Discussed in special senses section of this chapter.

CHAPTER TWENTY-ONE

Musculoskeletal System

The musculoskeletal system forms the basic internal framework of the vertebrate body. Muscles and bones work in close coordination to produce voluntary movement. In addition, bone and muscle perform a number of other independent functions. Physical support and locomotion are the functions of animal skeletal systems. The muscular system generates force.

SKELETAL SYSTEM

An endoskeleton serves as the framework within all vertebrate organisms. Muscles are attached to the bones, permitting movement. The endoskeleton also provides protection by surrounding delicate vital organs in bone. The rib cage protects the thoracic organs (heart and lungs), whereas the skull and vertebral column protect the brain and spinal cord. The two major components of the skeleton are cartilage and bone.

Structure of the Skeleton

Cartilage

Cartilage is a type of connective tissue that is softer and more flexible than bone. Cartilage is retained in adults in places where firmness and flexibility are needed. For example, in humans, the external ear, nose, walls of the larynx and trachea, and skeletal joints contain cartilage. **Chrondrocytes** are cells responsible for synthesizing cartilage.

Bone

Bone is a specialized type of mineralized connective tissue that has the ability to withstand physical stress. Ideally adapted for body support, bone tissue is hard and strong while at the same time somewhat elastic and lightweight. There are two basic types of bone: compact bone and spongy bone.

1. **Compact bone** is dense bone that does not appear to have any cavities when observed with the naked eye. The bony matrix is deposited in structural units called **osteons** (Haversian systems). Each osteon consists of a central microscopic channel called a **Haversian canal**, surrounded by a number of concentric circles of bony matrix (calcium phosphate) called **lamellae**.

2. **Spongy bone** is much less dense and consists of an interconnecting lattice of bony **spicules** (trabeculae); the cavities between the spicules are filled with yellow or red bone marrow. **Yellow marrow** is inactive and infiltrated by adipose tissue; **red marrow** is involved in blood cell formation.

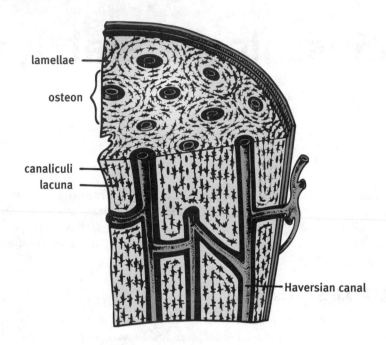

Figure 21.1

Osteocytes

Two other types of cells found in bone tissue are osteoblasts and osteoclasts. **Osteoblasts** synthesize and secrete the organic constituents of the bone matrix; once they have become surrounded by their matrix, they mature into osteocytes. **Osteoclasts** are large, multinucleated cells involved in bone reabsorption, wherein bone is broken down and minerals are released into the blood.

Bone formation

Bone formation occurs by either endochondral ossification or by intramembranous ossification. In **endochondral ossification**, existing cartilage is replaced by bone. Long bones arise primarily through endochondral ossification. In **intramembranous ossification**, mesenchymal (embryonic or undifferentiated) connective tissue is transformed into and replaced by bone.

Organization of the Skeleton

The axial skeleton is the basic framework of the body, consisting of the skull, vertebral column, and rib cage. It is the point of attachment of the appendicular skeleton, which includes the bones of the appendages (limbs) and the pectoral and pelvic girdles.

Bones are held together in a number of ways. Sutures or immovable joints hold the bones of the skull together. Bones that move relative to one another are held together by movable joints and are additionally supported and strengthened by ligaments. Ligaments serve as bone-to bone-connectors. Tendons attach skeletal muscle to bones and bend the skeleton at the movable joints.

The point of attachment of a muscle to a stationary bone (the proximal end in limb muscles) is called the **origin**. The point of attachment of a muscle to the bone that moves (distal end in limb muscles) is called the **insertion**. **Extension** indicates a straightening of a joint, whereas **flexion** refers to a bending of a joint.

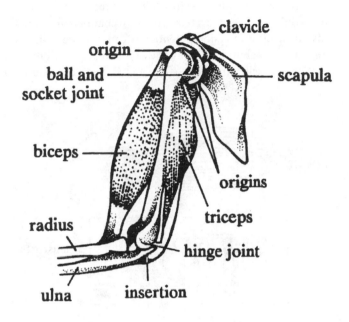

Figure 21.2

MUSCULAR SYSTEM

Muscle tissue consists of bundles of specialized contractile fibers held together by connective tissue. There are three morphologically and functionally distinct types of muscle in mammals: skeletal muscle, smooth muscle, and cardiac muscle.

Nervous control of the muscular system involves the axons of the pyramidal cells of the motor cortex, which descend from the brain to synapse on lower motor neurons in the brain stem and the spinal cord. Because there are no intervening synapses, the **pyramidal system** is able to provide rapid commands to the skeletal muscles and various other organs. Several other centers can issue somatic motor commands as a result of processing performed at the unconscious, involuntary level. These centers and their associated tracts comprise the **extrapyramidal system**. The red nucleus, located in the mesencephalon, is the component of the extrapyramidal system primarily in control of skeletal muscle tone.

Skeletal Muscle

Skeletal muscle is responsible for voluntary movements and is innervated by the somatic nervous system. Each fiber is a multinucleated cell created by the fusion of several mononucleated embryonic cells. Embedded in the fibers are filaments called **myofibrils**, which are further divided into contractile units called **sarcomeres**. The myofibrils are enveloped by a modified endoplasmic reticulum that stores calcium ions and is called the **sarcoplasmic reticulum**. The cytoplasm of a muscle fiber is called sarcoplasm, and the cell membrane is called the sarcolemma. The **sarcolemma** is capable of propagating an action potential and is connected to a system of transverse tubules (T system) oriented perpendicularly to the myofibrils. The **T system** provides channels for ion flow throughout the muscle fibers and can also propagate an action potential. Because of the high-energy requirements of contraction, mitochondria are very abundant in muscle cells and are distributed along the myofibrils. Skeletal muscle has striations of light and dark bands and is therefore also referred to as **striated muscle**.

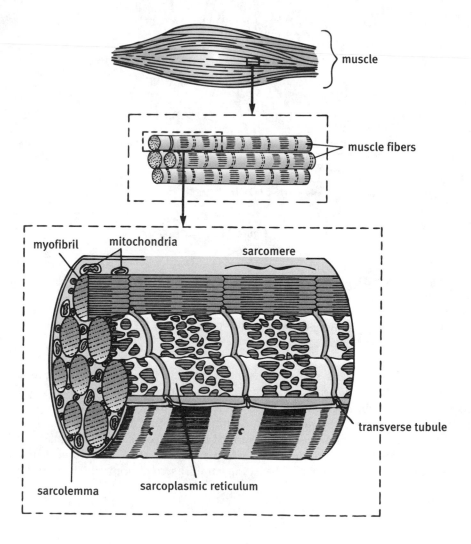

Figure 21.3

Sarcomeres

The sarcomere is composed of thin and thick filaments. The thin filaments are chains of actin molecules. The thick filaments are composed of organized bundles of myosin molecules.

Electron microscopy reveals that the sarcomere is organized as follows. **Z lines** define the boundaries of a single sarcomere and anchor the thin filaments. The **M line** runs down the center of the sarcomere. The **I band** is the region containing thin filaments only. The **H zone** is the region containing thick filaments only. The **A band** spans the entire length of the thick filaments and any overlapping portions of the thin filaments. When the muscles contract, the Z lines move toward each other. Note that during contraction, the A band is not reduced in size, whereas the H zone and I band are.

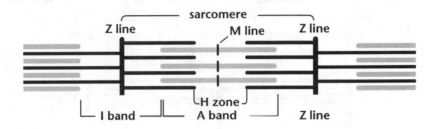

Figure 21.4

Contraction

Muscle contraction is stimulated by a message from the somatic nervous system sent via a motor neuron. The link between the nerve terminal (synaptic bouton) and the sarcolemma of the muscle fiber is called the **neuromuscular junction**. The space between the two is known as the synapse, or synaptic cleft. Depolarization of the motor neuron results in the release of neurotransmitters (e.g., acetylcholine) from the nerve terminal. The neurotransmitter diffuses across the synaptic cleft and binds to special receptor sites on the sarcolemma. If enough of these receptors are stimulated, the permeability of the sarcolemma is altered and an action potential is generated.

Once an action potential is generated, it is conducted along the sarcolemma and the T system and into the interior of the muscle fiber. This causes the sarcoplasmic reticulum to release calcium ions into the sarcoplasm. Calcium ions initiate the contraction of the sarcomere by binding to troponin C on the actin filaments. Allosteric changes occur in the proteins that allow myosin heads to bind to these sites on the actin. Use of energy allows a power stroke to occur, pulling the Z bands closer together. Actin and myosin slide past each other, and the sarcomere contracts.

An interesting point is that several hours after death, all of the muscles in the body go into a state of **rigor mortis**. In this condition, the muscles contract and become rigid, even without action potentials. The rigidity is caused by an absence of adenosine triphosphate (ATP), which is required for the myosin heads to be released from the actin filaments. The muscles typically remain rigid for 12 to 24 hours after death until the muscle proteins degrade.

There are five major types of muscle contraction: isotonic, dynamic, concentric, eccentric, and isometric. An **isotonic** contraction occurs when a muscle shortens against a fixed load while the tension on that muscle remains constant. A **dynamic** contraction includes both concentric and eccentric types of contractions. In general, a dynamic contraction results in the change in length of the muscle with a corresponding change in tension on that muscle. A **concentric** contraction is a type of dynamic contraction where the muscle fibers shorten and the tension on the muscle increases. An **eccentric** contraction is a type of dynamic contraction where the muscle fiber lengthens and the tension on the muscle increases. An **isometric** contraction occurs when both ends of the muscle are fixed and no change in length occurs during the contraction, but the tension increases.

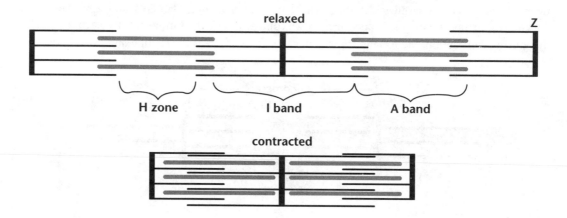

Figure 21.5

Stimulus and muscle response

Individual muscle fibers generally exhibit an all-or-none response; only a stimulus above a minimal value called the threshold value can elicit contraction. The strength of the contraction of a single muscle fiber cannot be increased, regardless of the strength of the stimulus. However, the strength of contraction of the entire muscle can be increased by recruiting more muscle fibers. The different types of muscle responses are summarized as follows:

- A **simple twitch** is the response of a single muscle fiber to a brief stimulus at or above the threshold stimulus and consists of a latent period, a contraction period, and a relaxation period. The latent period is the time between stimulation and the onset of contraction. During this time lag, the action potential spreads along the sarcolemma, and Ca^{2+} ions are released. After the contraction period, there is a brief relaxation period in which the muscle is unresponsive to a stimulus; this period is known as the **absolute refractory period**.

- When the fibers of a muscle are exposed to very frequent stimuli, the muscle cannot fully relax. The contractions begin to combine, becoming stronger and more prolonged. This is known as **temporal summation**. The contractions become continuous when the stimuli are so frequent that the muscle cannot relax. This type of contraction is known as **tetanus** and is stronger than a simple twitch of a single fiber. If tetanus is maintained, the muscle will fatigue, and the contraction will weaken.

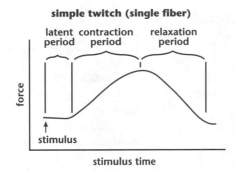
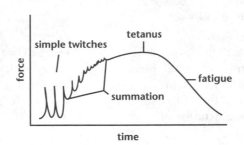

Figure 21.6

- **Tonus** is a state of partial contraction. Muscles are never completely relaxed and maintain a partially contracted state at all times.

During periods of strenuous activity, skeletal muscles convert glucose to pyruvic acid through the process of glycolysis. This process enables skeletal muscles to continue contracting even in the absence of oxygen. Lactic acid is generated when pyruvic acid is reacted with the enzyme lactate dehydrogenase. This process allows the pyruvate to enter the citric acid (or Krebs) cycle.

The purpose of the **Cori cycle** during periods of strenuous activity is to convert lactic acid in the liver to glucose for discharge into the bloodstream. Once the glucose is in the blood, the muscles are then able to use the glucose as an immediate source of energy or rebuild their glycogen reserves. Conversion of glucose into pyruvate in the muscle cells is necessary for the creation of ATP during periods of strenuous exercise and does not involve the Cori cycle. During periods of intense exercise, the production of lactic acid is increased, and glycogen is broken down into glucose; however, that is not by means of the Cori cycle.

Smooth Muscle

Smooth muscle is responsible for involuntary actions and is innervated by the autonomic nervous system. Smooth muscle is found in the digestive tract, bladder, uterus, and blood vessel walls, among other places. Smooth muscle cells possess one centrally located nucleus and lack the striations of skeletal muscle.

Cardiac Muscle

The muscle tissue of the heart is composed of cardiac muscle fibers. These fibers possess characteristics of both skeletal and smooth muscle fibers. As in skeletal muscle, actin and myosin filaments are arranged in sarcomeres, giving cardiac muscle a striated appearance. However, cardiac muscle cells generally have only one or two centrally located nuclei.

Comparison of Different Muscle Types		
Smooth Muscle	**Cardiac Muscle**	**Skeletal Muscle**
• Nonstriated • One nucleus per cell • Involuntary/autonomic nervous system • Smooth, continuous contractions	• Striated • One to two nuclei per cell • Involuntary/autonomic nervous system • Strong, forceful contractions	• Striated • Multinucleated cells • Voluntary/somatic nervous system • Strong, forceful contractions

Table 21.1

Energy Reserves

ATP is the primary source of energy for muscle contraction. Very little ATP is actually stored in the muscles, so other forms of energy must be stored and rapidly converted to ATP.

Creatine phosphate

In vertebrates energy can be temporarily stored in a high-energy compound called creatine phosphate.

Myoglobin

Myoglobin is a hemoglobin-like protein found in muscle tissue. Myoglobin has a high oxygen affinity and maintains the oxygen supply in muscles by binding oxygen tightly.

REVIEW PROBLEMS

Questions 1, 2, and 3 are based on the following diagram:

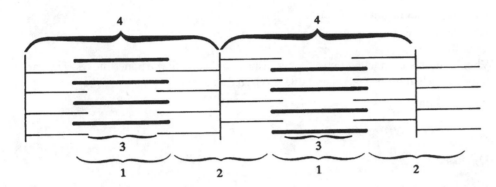

1. During muscle contraction, which of the following regions decrease(s) in length?

    (A) 1 only

    (B) 2 only

    (C) 4 only

    (D) 2, 3, and 4

2. Region 1 refers to

    (A) the thick filaments only.

    (B) the thin filaments only.

    (C) the A band.

    (D) the I band.

3. Which region represents one sarcomere?

    (A) 1

    (B) 2

    (C) 3

    (D) 4

4. Which of the following cells is correctly coupled with its definition?

    (A) Osteoblasts—bone cells involved in the secretion of bone matrix

    (B) Osteoclasts—immature bone cells

    (C) Osteocytes—multinucleated cells actively involved in bone reabsorption

    (D) Chondrocytes—undifferentiated bone marrow cells

5. Describe the microscopic structure of compact bone. Include the following terms in your discussion: bone matrix, osteon, Haversian canal, lamellae, and osteocyte.

6. When a muscle fiber is subjected to very frequent stimuli

    (A) an oxygen debt is incurred.

    (B) a muscle tonus is generated.

    (C) the threshold value is reached.

    (D) a simple twitch is repeatedly generated.

7. When a muscle is attached to two bones, usually only one of the bones moves. The part of the muscle attached to the stationary bone is referred to as

    (A) proximal.

    (B) distal.

    (C) origin.

    (D) insertion.

8. Two processes are involved in bone formation. How do they differ from one another?

Questions 9–11 refer to the following types of muscle:

    I. Cardiac muscle

    II. Skeletal muscle

   III. Smooth muscle

9. Which type of muscle is always multinucleated?

    (A) I only

    (B) II only

    (C) III only

    (D) Both I and II

10. Which type of muscle has strong, forceful contractions?

    (A) I only

    (B) II only

    (C) III only

    (D) Both I and II

11. Which type of muscle lacks sarcomeric striations?

    (A) I only

    (B) II only

    (C) III only

    (D) Both II and III

SOLUTIONS TO REVIEW PROBLEMS

1. **D** Discussed in the sarcomere section in this chapter.

2. **C** Discussed in the sarcomere section in this chapter.

3. **D** Discussed in the sarcomere section in this chapter.

4. **A** Discussed in structure of vertebrate skeleton section in this chapter.

5.   Discussed in structure of vertebrate skeleton section in this chapter.

6. **D** Discussed in summation section of stimulus and muscle response in this chapter.

7. **C** Discussed in muscle/bone interactions section in this chapter.

8.   The processes involved in bone formation are endochondral ossification and intramembranous ossification. In endochrondral ossification, cartilage is replaced with bone. In intramembranous ossification, mesenchyme, or undifferentiated cells, are transformed into bone cells.

9. **B** Discussed in skeletal muscle section in this chapter.

10. **D** Discussed in smooth muscle and cardiac muscle section in this chapter.

11. **C** Discussed in smooth muscle section in this chapter.

CHAPTER TWENTY-TWO

Circulatory and Respiratory Systems

The human cardiovascular system is composed of a muscular, four-chambered heart, a network of blood vessels, and the blood itself. Blood is pumped into the **aorta**, which branches into a series of **arteries**. The arteries branch into **arterioles** and then into microscopic **capillaries**. Exchange of gases, nutrients, and cellular waste products occurs via diffusion across capillary walls. The capillaries then converge into **venules** and eventually into **veins**, conducting deoxygenated blood back toward the heart. From the heart, deoxygenated blood is sent to the **lungs**, where CO_2 is exchanged for O_2, and this oxygenated blood returns to the heart to be pumped throughout the body once more.

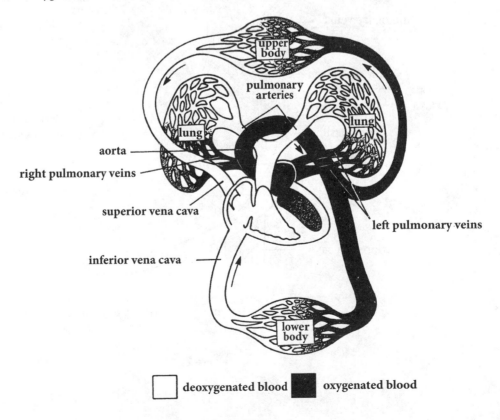

Figure 22.1

THE HEART

The heart is the driving force of the circulatory system. The right and left halves can be viewed as two separate pumps: the right side of the heart pumps **deoxygenated** blood into **pulmonary** circulation (toward the lungs), whereas the left side pumps **oxygenated** blood into **systemic** circulation (throughout the body). The two upper chambers are called **atria**, and the two lower chambers are called **ventricles**. The atria are thin-walled, whereas the ventricles are extremely muscular. The left ventricle is more muscular than the right ventricle because it is responsible for generating the force that propels systemic circulation and because it pumps against a higher resistance. As a result, in patients with increased systemic resistance, the left ventricle can become hypertrophied (enlarged), which over time can lead to congestive heart failure and other cardiovascular diseases.

Blood returning from the body first flows through the right atria, then through the tricuspid valve into the right ventricle, and finally through the pulmonary semilunar valve into the pulmonary arteries to continue to the lungs. Blood returning from the lungs flows through the pulmonary veins into the left atrium, then through the mitral valve into the left ventricle, and finally out through the aortic semilunar valve into systemic circulation.

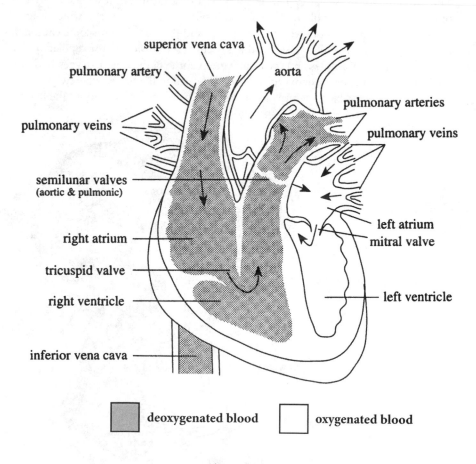

Figure 22.2

Valves

The **atrioventricular valves**, located between the atria and ventricles on both sides of the heart, prevent backflow of blood into the atria. The valve on the right side of the heart has three cusps and is called the **tricuspid valve**. The valve on the left side of the heart has two cusps and is called the **mitral valve**. The **semilunar valves** have three cusps and are located between the left ventricle and the aorta (the aortic valve) and between the right ventricle and the pulmonary artery (the pulmonic valve). The "lub-dub" sound of a heartbeat is made up of the closing of the atrioventricular and semilunar valves, respectively.

Contraction

The heart's pumping cycle is divided into two alternating phases, **systole** and **diastole,** which together make up the **heartbeat.** Systole is the period during which the ventricles contract, forcing blood out of the heart into the lungs and circulatory system. Diastole is the period of cardiac muscle relaxation during which blood drains into all four chambers. This is reflected in physiologic measurements such as blood pressure. Systolic blood pressure measures the pressure in a patient's blood vessels when the ventricles are contracting, and diastolic blood pressure measures the pressure during cardiac relaxation. **Cardiac output** is defined as the total volume of blood the left ventricle pumps out per minute. Cardiac output = **heart rate** (number of beats per minute) × **stroke volume** (volume of blood pumped out of the left ventricle per contraction).

Control of heart rate

Cardiac muscle contracts rhythmically without stimulation from the nervous system, producing impulses that spread through its internal conducting system. An ordinary cardiac contraction originates in, and is regulated by, the **sinoatrial (SA) node** (the **pacemaker**), a small mass of specialized tissue located in the wall of the right atrium. The SA node spreads impulses through both atria, stimulating them to contract simultaneously. The impulse arrives at the **atrioventricular (AV) node**, which slowly conducts impulses to the rest of the heart, allowing enough time for atrial contraction and for the ventricles to fill with blood. The impulse is then carried by the **bundle of His (AV bundle)**, which branches into the right and left bundle branches, and finally through the **Purkinje fibers** in the walls of both ventricles, generating a strong contraction. This contraction forces the blood out of the heart into circulation.

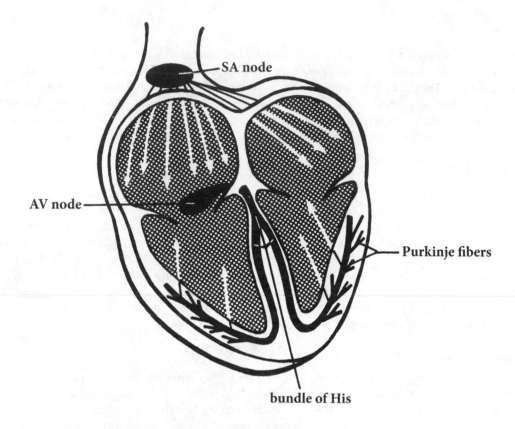

Figure 22.3

The **autonomic nervous system** modifies the rate of heart contraction. The parasympathetic system innervates the heart via the **vagus nerve** and causes a decrease in the heart rate. The sympathetic system innervates the heart via the cervical and upper thoracic ganglia and causes an increase in the heart rate. The adrenal medulla exerts hormonal control via epinephrine (adrenaline) secretion, which causes an increase in heart rate.

BLOOD VESSELS

The three types of blood vessels are arteries, veins, and capillaries. **Arteries** are thick-walled, muscular, elastic vessels that transport oxygenated blood away from the heart—except for the **pulmonary arteries**, which transport deoxygenated blood from the heart to the lungs. **Veins** are relatively thin-walled, inelastic vessels that conduct deoxygenated blood toward the heart—except for the **pulmonary veins**, which carry oxygenated blood from the lungs to the heart. Much of the blood flow in veins depends on their compression by skeletal muscles during movement rather than on the pumping of the heart. Venous circulation is often at odds with gravity; thus, larger veins, especially those in the legs, have valves that prevent backflow. Capillaries have very thin walls composed of a single layer of endothelial cells across which respiratory gases, nutrients, enzymes, hormones, and wastes can readily diffuse. **Capillaries** have the smallest diameter of all three types of vessels; red blood cells must often travel through them single file.

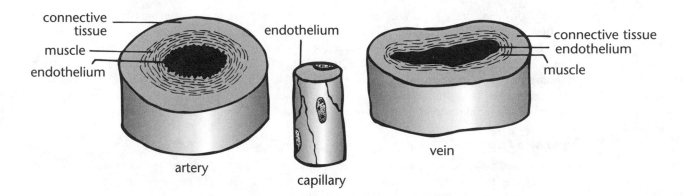

Figure 22.4

Lymph Vessels

The lymphatic system is a secondary circulatory system distinct from the cardiovascular circulation. Its vessels transport excess **interstitial fluid**, called **lymph**, to the cardiovascular system, thereby keeping **fluid** levels in the body constant. The smallest lymphatic vessels (**lacteals**) collect fats in the form of chylomicrons from the villi in the small intestine and deliver them into the bloodstream, bypassing the liver. **Lymph** nodes are swellings along lymph vessels containing phagocytic cells (**lymphocytes**) that filter the lymph, removing and destroying foreign particles and pathogens (see Chapter 19, Integument and Immune Systems).

BLOOD

On the average, the human body contains four to six liters of blood. Blood has both liquid (55 percent) and cellular components (45 percent). **Plasma** is the liquid portion of the blood. It is an aqueous mixture of nutrients, salts, respiratory gases, wastes, hormones, and blood proteins (e.g., immunoglobulins, albumin, and fibrinogen). The cellular components of the blood are erythrocytes, leukocytes, and platelets.

Leukocytes

Leukocytes (known as **white blood cells** or WBCs) are larger than erythrocytes and serve protective functions. White blood cells are discussed further in the context of immunity in Chapter 19.

Platelets

Platelets are cell **fragments** that lack nuclei and are involved in clot formation. Many drugs inhibit platelet formation or adhesion to decrease clot development.

Erythrocytes

Erythrocytes (known as **red blood cells** or RBCs) are the oxygen-carrying components of blood. An erythrocyte contains approximately 250 million molecules of hemoglobin, each of which can bind up to four molecules of oxygen. When hemoglobin binds oxygen it is called **oxyhemoglobin**. This is the primary form of oxygen transport in the blood. Erythrocytes have a distinct biconcave, disk-like shape that gives them both increased surface area for gas exchange and greater flexibility for movement through tiny capillaries. **Erythrocytes** are formed from stem cells in the **bone marrow**; their formation is stimulated by erythropoietin, a hormone made in the kidneys. In the bone marrow, erythrocytes lose their nuclei, mitochondria, and membranous organelles. Once mature, erythrocytes circulate in the blood for about 120 days, after which they are phagocytized by special cells in the spleen and liver. Finding immature erythrocytes circulating in the bloodstream—that is, before they have lost their organelles—can be an indicator for a number of disease states, such as hemolytic anemia, which is caused by the rapid destruction of red blood cells due to an infection or disorder.

ABO blood types

Erythrocytes have characteristic cell-surface proteins (**antigens**). Antigens are macromolecules that are foreign to the host organism and trigger an immune response. The two major groups of red blood cell antigens are the **ABO group** and the **Rh factor**.

Characteristics of Human Blood Types				
Blood Type	**Antigen**	**Antibody**	**Can Donate To**	**Can Receive From**
A	A	anti-B	A and AB	A and O
B	B	anti-A	B and AB	B and O
AB	A and B	none	AB only	all (universal acceptor)
O	none	anti-A and anti-B	all (universal donor)	O only

Table 22.1

It is extremely important during blood transfusions that **donor** and **recipient** blood types be appropriately matched. The aim is to avoid transfusion of red blood cells that will be clumped ("rejected") by antibodies (proteins in the immune system that bind specifically to antigens) present in the recipient's plasma. For example, a person with blood type A has antigens for type A blood and antibodies for type B blood. This means that, if transfused with any blood containing type B antigens (type B or type AB blood), they will mount an immune response, and their anti-B antibodies will clump and "reject" the transfusion. Therefore, to avoid rejection of the transfusion, the recipient must have a natural blood type with the same antigens as the blood type being transfused. If a patient with type O blood, for example, is given blood of any type except type O, then they will reject the transfusion because they do not have type A or type B antigens and as a result have anti-A and anti-B antibodies.

Type AB blood is termed the "**universal recipient**," as it has neither anti-A nor anti-B antibodies and therefore will not reject transfusions of any blood type. **Type O** blood is considered to be the "**universal donor**"; it will not elicit a response from the recipient's immune system because it does not possess any surface antigens.

Rh factor

The Rh factor is another antigen that may be present on the surface of red blood cells. Individuals may be Rh+, possessing the Rh antigen, or Rh−, lacking the Rh antigen. Consideration of the Rh factor is particularly important during **pregnancy**. An Rh− woman can be sensitized by an **Rh+ fetus** if fetal red blood cells (which will have the Rh factor) enter maternal circulation during birth. If this woman subsequently carries another Rh+ fetus, the anti-Rh antibodies she produced when sensitized by the first birth may cross the placenta and destroy fetal red blood cells. This results in a type of severe anemia for the fetus known as **erythroblastosis fetalis**. Erythroblastosis is not caused by ABO blood-type mismatches between mother and fetus because anti-A and anti-B antibodies cannot cross the placenta. Rhogam is a drug comprised of a mixture of antibodies given to mothers who are Rh– to prevent their immune systems from attacking the fetal red blood cells.

Rh factor is also an issue with blood transfusions. If patients who do not possess the Rh antigen (that is, who are Rh–) are given blood that is Rh+, their bodies can mount an immune response and reject the transfusion.

FUNCTIONS OF THE CIRCULATORY SYSTEM

Blood transports nutrients and O_2 to tissue and wastes and CO_2 from tissue. Platelets in the blood are involved in injury repair, and leukocytes in the blood are the main component of the immune system (see Chapter 19).

Transport of Gases

Erythrocytes transport O_2 throughout the circulatory system. The hemoglobin molecules in erythrocytes bind to O_2. Hemoglobin contains iron, and each hemoglobin molecule is capable of binding to four molecules of O_2. Hemoglobin also binds to CO_2, in which case it is referred to as deoxyhemoglobin.

Transport of Nutrients and Waste

Amino acids and **simple sugars** are absorbed into the bloodstream at the intestinal capillaries and, after processing, are transported throughout the body. Throughout the body, metabolic **waste products** (e.g., water, urea, and carbon dioxide) diffuse into capillaries from surrounding cells; these wastes are then delivered to the appropriate excretory organs.

Clotting

When platelets come into contact with the exposed collagen of a damaged vessel, they release a chemical that causes neighboring platelets to adhere to one another, forming a **platelet plug**. Subsequently, both the platelets and the damaged tissue release the clotting factor thromboplastin. **Thromboplastin**, with the aid of its cofactors calcium and vitamin K, converts the inactive plasma protein **prothrombin** to its active form, **thrombin**. Thrombin then converts **fibrinogen** (another plasma protein) into fibrin. Threads of **fibrin** coat the damaged area and trap blood cells to form a clot. Clots prevent extensive blood loss while the damaged vessel heals itself. The fluid left after blood clotting is called **serum**. This complex series of reactions that lead to clotting is called the **clotting cascade**.

Warfarin, a commonly used anticoagulant, works by inhibiting the recycling of vitamin K. Without this essential cofactor, the clotting cycle is inhibited, and patients are less likely to be able to form clots. Other types of anticoagulant medications work at other points along the clotting cascade.

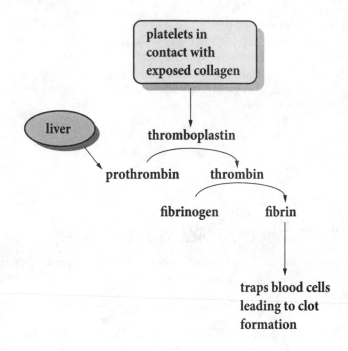

Figure 22.5

THE RESPIRATORY SYSTEM

In the human respiratory system, air enters the **lungs** after traveling through a series of respiratory **airways**. The air passages consist of the nose, pharynx (throat), larynx, trachea, bronchi, bronchioles, and the alveoli. Gas exchange between the lungs and the circulatory system occurs across the very thin walls of the **alveoli,** which are air-filled sacs at the terminals of the airway branches. Three hundred million alveoli provide approximately 100 m^2 of moist respiratory surface for gas exchange. After gas exchange, air rushes back through the respiratory pathway and is exhaled.

The primary function of the respiratory system in humans is to provide the necessary energy for all body functions, including growth, maintenance of homeostasis, defense mechanisms, repair, and reproduction of cells. The respiratory system also provides a very large area for gas exchange, as well as continually moving oxygenated air over this area, protecting the respiratory surface from infection, dehydration, and temperature changes. It moves air over the vocal cords for the production of sound and assists in the regulation of body pH by regulating the rate of carbon dioxide removal from the blood.

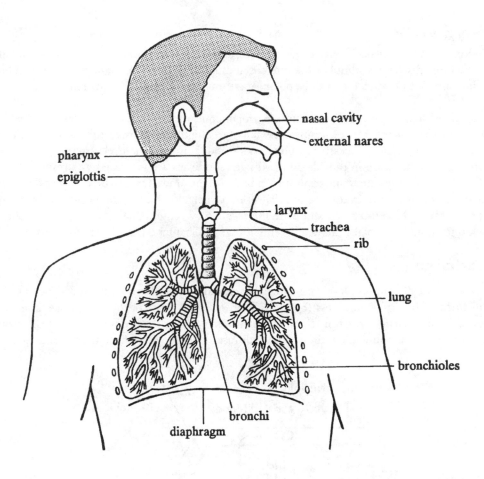

Figure 22.6

Ventilation

Ventilation of the lungs (breathing) is the process by which air is inhaled and exhaled. The purpose of ventilation is to take in oxygen from the atmosphere and eliminate carbon dioxide from the body.

During **inhalation,** the diaphragm contracts and flattens, and the external intercostal muscles contract, pushing the rib cage and chest wall up and out. The phrenic nerve innervates the diaphragm and causes it to contract and flatten. These actions cause the thoracic cavity to increase in volume. This volume increase, in turn, reduces the pressure, causing the lungs to expand and fill with air, thus resulting in inhalation.

Exhalation is generally a passive process. The lungs and chest wall are highly elastic and tend to recoil to their original positions after inhalation. The diaphragm and external intercostal muscles relax, and the chest wall pushes inward. The consequent decrease in thoracic cavity volume causes the pressure to increase. This forces air out of the alveoli, causing the lungs to deflate.

Surfactant is a protein complex excreted by cells in the lungs. Surfactant keeps the lungs from collapsing, decreases surface tension, and assists with lung function. Babies born prematurely do not always produce surfactant and must be given artificial surfactants until they can produce surfactant on their own.

Control of ventilation

Ventilation is regulated by neurons (referred to as **respiratory centers**) located in the **medulla oblongata,** whose rhythmic discharges stimulate the intercostal muscles or the diaphragm to contract. When the partial pressure of CO_2 rises, the medulla oblongata stimulates an increase in the rate of ventilation.

The primary goal of respiration is to maintain proper concentrations of oxygen, carbon dioxide, and hydrogen ions in tissues. Hence, respiratory activity is highly responsive to changes in the blood levels of these compounds. Excessive carbon dioxide and hydrogen ion levels are the primary stimuli for respiration. When carbon dioxide and hydrogen ion levels are increased, the respiratory center stimulates both the inspiratory and expiratory muscles of the lungs. Oxygen blood levels do not have a significant effect on the respiratory center. However, oxygen blood levels are monitored by peripheral **chemoreceptors**, which indirectly stimulate the respiratory center. Changes in acid-base chemistry due to kidney function can also influence ventilation (see Chapter 24, Excretory System).

Gas Exchange

A dense network of minute blood vessels called **pulmonary capillaries** surrounds the alveoli. Gas exchange occurs by diffusion across these capillary walls and those of the alveoli; gases move from regions of higher partial pressure to regions of lower partial pressure. Oxygen diffuses from the alveolar air into the blood while carbon dioxide diffuses from the blood into the lungs to be exhaled.

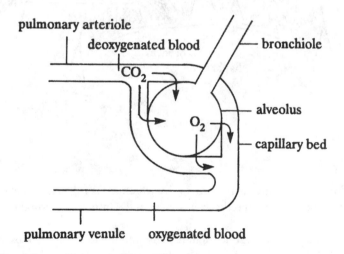

Figure 22.7

Lung Capacities

The volume of air contained by the lungs varies dramatically during inhalation and exhalation. **Total lung capacity** represents the maximum volume of air the lungs can hold. However, at rest, humans only breathe as much as needed, which involves moving a significantly smaller volume of air than the total lung capacity, an amount referred to as the **tidal volume (TV)**. Nevertheless, under stress, significantly more air can be moved through the lungs than the tidal volume; this is called the **vital capacity**. The **inspiratory reserve volume** is the difference between the vital capacity and the upper limit of tidal volume, and the **expiratory reserve volume** is the difference between the vital capacity and the lower limit of tidal reserve volume. Even with heavy breathing, however, the lungs will never normally empty completely since a **residual volume** will always remain (the difference between vital capacity and total lung capacity). Should the residual volume of air somehow be removed, such as if forced out due to extreme water pressures during deep-sea diving, the lung may not be able to re-inflate due to its internal surface tension.

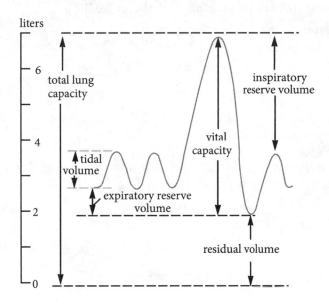

Figure 22.8

REVIEW PROBLEMS

1. Erythrocytes are anaerobic. Why is this advantageous for the organism?

2. The lymphatic system

    (A) transports hormones throughout the body.
    (B) transports absorbed chylomicrons to the circulatory system.
    (C) filters the blood.
    (D) contains vessels that are nearly identical to arteries.

3. Draw the reactions of the clotting process. Include all of the proteins and cofactors involved.

4. What role do the surface proteins on erythrocytes play in blood transfusions?

5. All of the following facilitate gas exchange in the lungs EXCEPT

    (A) thin alveolar surfaces.
    (B) moist alveolar surfaces.
    (C) differences in the partial pressures of O_2 and CO_2.
    (D) active transport.

6. What muscles play a role in ventilation? Compare the muscular motions involved in inhalation with those involved in exhalation.

7. Which is the correct sequence of the passages that air travels through during inhalation?

    (A) Pharynx → Trachea → Bronchioles → Bronchi → Alveoli
    (B) Pharynx → Trachea → Lungs → Bronchi → Alveoli
    (C) Pharynx → Larynx → Bronchi → Trachea → Alveoli
    (D) Pharynx → Larynx → Trachea → Bronchi → Alveoli

8. Which of the following is generally an active process?

    (A) Inhalation
    (B) Exhalation
    (C) Gas exchange
    (D) Diffusion

SOLUTIONS TO REVIEW PROBLEMS

1. If erythrocytes were aerobic, they would use some of the O_2 that they carry for their own energy requirements, thus decreasing the amount of O_2 transported to the rest of the body. Because they are anaerobic, they do not have any O_2 requirements of their own and can deliver all the O_2 they carry to other cells.

2. **B** The main function of the lymphatic system is to collect excess interstitial fluid and return it to the circulatory system, maintaining the balance of body fluids. However, this is not one of the answer choices. A second function of the lymphatic system is to absorb chylomicrons from the small intestine and deliver them to cardiovascular circulation; this is choice (B). The remaining answer choices describe the circulatory system but not the lymphatic system.

3. See Figure 22.5.

4. In a blood transfusion, the donor blood must be carefully matched with the blood of the recipient. If the erythrocytes in the donor blood have a different class of surface proteins (antigens) than the recipient's erythrocytes, the recipient's immune system might "attack" the surface protein of the donor, thus rejecting the donor blood. For example, if the donor blood is type A and the recipient blood is type B, the recipient's anti-A antibodies would attack the donor's erythrocytes, because type A blood has type A antigens.

5. **D** Discussed in gas exchange section of this chapter.

6. The muscles involved in ventilation are the diaphragm, which separates the thoracic cavity from the abdominal cavity, and the intercostal muscles of the rib cage. During inhalation, the diaphragm contracts and flattens while the external intercostals contract, pushing the rib cage up and out. These actions cause an overall increase in the size of the thoracic cavity. During exhalation, both the diaphragm and the external intercostals relax, causing a decrease in the size of the thoracic cavity. In forced expiration, the internal intercostals contract, pulling the rib cage down.

7. **D** Discussed in vertebrate respiratory system section of this chapter.

8. **A** Exhalation is generally a passive process involving elastic recoil of the lungs and relaxation of both the diaphragm and the external intercostal muscles. (However, during vigorous exercise, active muscular contraction assists in expiration.) Gas exchange and diffusion are also passive processes and involve molecules moving down their partial pressure gradients. Inhalation is an active process requiring contraction of the diaphragm and the external intercostals.

CHAPTER TWENTY-THREE

Digestive System

Humans are **heterotrophic** and thus unable to synthesize all of their own nutrients. Instead, food provides the raw material for energy, repair, and growth of tissues. This food must first be **ingested** (eaten), after which **digestion** (breakdown) occurs. **Digestion** consists of the degradation of large molecules into smaller molecules that can be **absorbed** into the bloodstream and used directly by cells. **Intracellular** digestion occurs within the cell, usually in membrane-bound vesicles. **Extracellular** digestion refers to a digestive process that occurs outside of the cell, within a lumen or tract.

DIGESTIVE TRACT

The human digestive tract begins with the **oral cavity** and continues with the **pharynx**, **esophagus**, **stomach**, **small intestine**, **large intestine**, and anus. Accessory organs, such as the salivary glands, pancreas, liver, and gallbladder, also play essential roles in digestion.

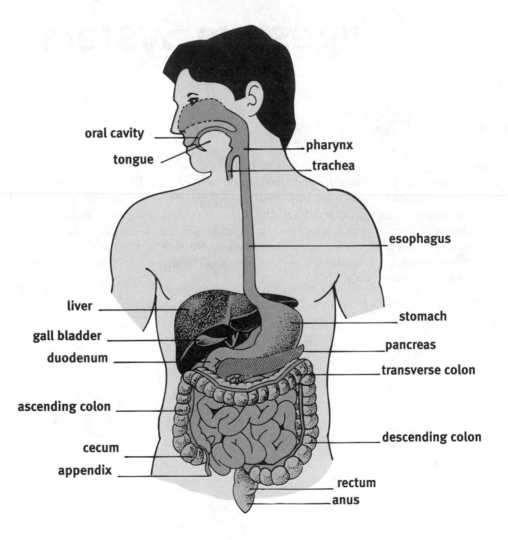

Figure 23.1

Oral Cavity

The oral cavity (the mouth) is where **mechanical** and **chemical** digestion of food begins. Mechanical digestion is the breakdown of large food particles into smaller particles through physical actions, such as the biting and chewing action of teeth (**mastication**) or the churning motion of the stomach. Chemical digestion refers to the enzymatic breakdown of macromolecules into smaller molecules and begins in the mouth when the salivary glands secrete **saliva**. Saliva **lubricates** food to facilitate swallowing and provides a solvent for food particles. Saliva is secreted in response to a nervous reflex triggered by the presence of food in the oral cavity. Saliva contains the enzyme **salivary amylase (ptyalin)**, which hydrolyzes starch to maltose (a disaccharide). Food that has been sufficiently moistened and broken down to be swallowed down the esophagus is called a **bolus**.

Esophagus

The esophagus is the muscular tube leading from the mouth to the stomach. Food is moved down the esophagus by rhythmic waves of involuntary muscular contractions called **peristalsis**. The esophagus is closed off from the stomach by contraction of a muscular structure called the **lower esophageal (cardiac) sphincter**.

The body of the esophagus lies within the thoracic cavity, which is negatively pressured relative to the environment on inhalation. The abdominal cavity has a relative positive pressure. Therefore, without normal defense mechanisms, the pressure gradients favor a continual reflux of gastric (stomach) materials into the esophagus, resulting in a pathological condition known as gastroesophageal reflux disease (GERD). The pathophysiology of gastroesophageal reflux is as follows:

- Reflux can occur after spontaneous transient lower esophageal sphincter relaxations not associated with swallowing.
- Patients with GERD usually have a decreased lower esophageal sphincter pressure (5–10 mmHg above gastric baseline pressure), leading to an increased passage of stomach contents into the esophagus.
- Resting pressures of the lower esophageal sphincter normally range from 15–35 mmHg above gastric baseline pressure.

Stomach

The stomach, a large, muscular organ located in the upper abdomen, stores and partially digests food. The walls of the stomach are lined by the gastric mucosa, a mucous membrane that contains the gastric glands. Mucous cells in gastric pits along the membrane secrete **mucus** to protect the stomach lining from the harshly acidic juices (pH = 2) present in the stomach. Chief cells found within the gastric glands synthesize pepsinogen, which is converted to **pepsin** upon contact with stomach acid and breaks down proteins. Parietal cells, also present within gastric glands, synthesize and release hydrochloric acid (HCl), which alters the pH of the stomach and kills bacteria, and intrinsic factor, which is necessary for the absorption of vitamin B_{12}. The churning of the stomach (mechanical digestion), combined with this enzymatic activity (chemical digestion), produces an acidic, semifluid mixture of partially digested food known as **chyme**. The chyme passes into the first segment of the small intestine, the **duodenum**, through the pyloric sphincter.

Small Intestine

Chemical digestion is completed in the small intestine. The small intestine is divided into three sections: the **duodenum**, the **jejunum**, and the **ileum**. The small intestine is highly adapted to **absorption**. To maximize the surface area available for digestion and absorption, the intestine is extremely long (greater than six meters in length) and highly coiled. In addition, numerous finger-like projections called **villi** extend out of the intestinal wall. Villi contain capillaries and lacteals (vessels of the lymphatic system). Amino acids and monosaccharides pass through the villi walls into the capillary system. Blood from the digestive tract enters the hepatic portal system of the liver, where it is detoxified and stripped of some of its nutrients. Large fatty acids and glycerol pass into the lacteals and are then reconverted into fats (fatty acid + glycerol). Note that some nutrients, such as glucose and amino acids, are actively absorbed (i.e., requiring energy), whereas others are passively absorbed.

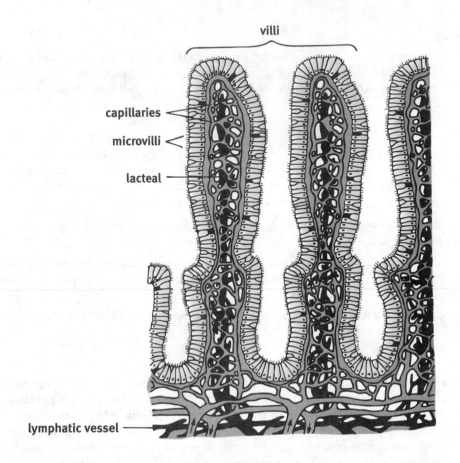

Figure 23.2

Most digestion in the small intestine occurs in the duodenum, where the secretions of the intestinal glands, pancreas, liver, and gallbladder mix together with the acidic chyme entering from the stomach. The intestinal mucosa secretes **lipases** (for fat digestion), **aminopeptidases** (for polypeptide digestion), and **disaccharidases** (for maltose, lactose, and sucrose digestion). For example, the disaccharidase **lactase** breaks down lactose (milk sugar). This enzyme is most often present in infants, but many adults lack the enzyme and are **lactose-intolerant**. In these people, lactose in the small intestine cannot be digested and is metabolized by bacteria, producing intestinal discomfort.

Digestion Hormones

The activity of the digestive system is regulated by several hormones, which allow for optimum flow of materials through the digestive tract and help regulate the hunger and satiation mechanisms. These hormones include:

- **Gastrin**: produced in the G cells of the duodenum, gastrin primarily functions to stimulate histamine and pepsinogen secretion as well as increase gastric blood flow. Gastrin also stimulates the parietal cells to produce HCl, which denatures proteins and activates digestive enzymes.

- **Intrinsic factor**: a secretion of the parietal cells that facilitates the absorption of vitamin B_{12} across the intestinal lining.

- **Cholecystokinin (CCK):** produced and stored in the I cells of the duodenal and jejunal mucosa. It is involved in stimulation of pancreatic enzyme and somatostatin secretion as well as gallbladder contraction. CCK also acts as a hunger suppressant.
- **Secretin:** synthesized and stored in the S cells of the upper intestine. It stimulates the secretion of bicarbonate-containing substances from the pancreas and inhibits gastric emptying and gastric acid production.

Liver

The liver produces **bile** that is stored in the **gallbladder** before release into the small intestine. Bile contains no enzymes; it **emulsifies** fats, breaking down large globules into small droplets. Emulsification of fats exposes a greater surface area of the fat to the action of pancreatic lipase. In the absence of bile, fats cannot be digested. The liver's functions also include storage of glycogen, conversion of ammonia to urea, protein synthesis, detoxification, and cholesterol metabolism.

Pancreas

The pancreas produces enzymes such as **amylase** for carbohydrate digestion, **trypsin** for protein digestion, and **lipase** for fat digestion. When the pancreas releases chymotrypsin and enterokinase, enterokinase cleaves trypsinogen to trypsin. Trypsin then cleaves and activates the other zymogens (enzyme precursors). The pancreas secretes a bicarbonate-rich juice that neutralizes the acidic chyme arriving from the stomach in the duodenum. The pancreatic enzymes operate optimally at this higher pH.

Large Intestine

The large intestine is approximately 1.5 m long and absorbs salts and any water not already absorbed by the small intestine. The **rectum** provides for transient storage of feces before elimination through the anus.

REVIEW PROBLEMS

1. Define extracellular digestion. How is the stomach specialized for extracellular digestion?

2. Where are proteins digested?

   (A) Mouth and stomach
   (B) Stomach and large intestine
   (C) Small intestine and large intestine
   (D) Stomach and small intestine

3. All of the following processes occur in the mouth EXCEPT

   (A) mechanical digestion.
   (B) moistening of food.
   (C) bolus formation.
   (D) chemical digestion of proteins.

4. The graphs below show the relative activities of pepsin and chymotrypsin in solutions of varying pH. Which graph refers to which enzyme?

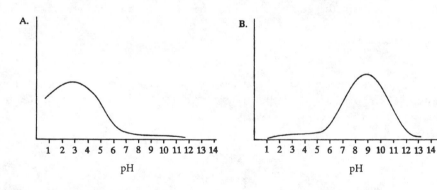

5. Outline the digestion of a piece of bread.

6. Why is pancreatic juice alkaline, and what would happen if its alkaline components were removed?

7. Starch is hydrolyzed into maltose by

   (A) salivary amylase.
   (B) maltase.
   (C) pancreatic amylase.
   (D) both A and C.

8. The intestinal capillaries transport nutrients from the intestines to the

   (A) large intestine.
   (B) liver.
   (C) kidney.
   (D) heart.

SOLUTIONS TO REVIEW PROBLEMS

1.　Digestion refers to a mechanical or chemical process whereby macromolecules are converted into smaller molecules that are more readily absorbed and used by cells. Extracellular digestion describes a process in which molecules are broken down outside of the cell. The stomach is a cavity perfectly adapted for extracellular digestion. Macromolecules are digested in an environment confined by the lower esophageal and pyloric sphincters. The cells lining the stomach walls are specialized for HCl and pepsinogen secretion by their ability to withstand acidic conditions. Muscular contractions aid in digestion by churning and crushing food. Little absorption occurs in the stomach; chyme is propelled into the small intestine, where further digestion and absorption occur.

2.　**D**　Protein digestion begins in the stomach with pepsin and continues in the small intestine.

3.　**D**　Chewing, the mechanical digestion of food, occurs in the mouth, as does moistening of food by saliva and bolus formation. In addition, salivary amylase begins digestion of complex carbohydrates.

4.　Graph A refers to pepsin, whereas graph B refers to chymotrypsin. Pepsin is a gastric enzyme; it works best under the highly acidic conditions of the stomach. Chymotrypsin is an enzyme of the small intestine and thus operates optimally in alkaline environments.

5.　In the mouth, teeth chew the bread into smaller particles, and salivary amylase digests some of the starch (the major component of bread) into maltose. The bread enters the stomach, where there is mechanical digestion of the bread into semiliquid chyme but no chemical digestion of starch. Chyme then enters the small intestine. In the small intestine, pancreatic amylase hydrolyzes starch into maltose while maltase, sucrase, and lactase hydrolyze various disaccharides into their respective monosaccharides. Most of the monosaccharides (e.g., glucose, fructose, and galactose) are absorbed into the circulatory system through the intestinal wall.

6.　Pancreatic juice is an alkaline (basic) fluid that helps neutralize the acidity of the chyme entering the small intestine from the stomach. This is necessary because the small intestine enzymes work optimally at a neutral or alkaline pH. Also, the walls (mucosa) of the small intestine are not specialized for protection against acidic conditions. Therefore, without alkaline pancreatic juice, the intestinal enzymes would not function, and the intestinal walls would be destroyed.

7.　**D**　Amylase, whether it is produced in the mouth or the pancreas, digests starch into maltose, a disaccharide.

8.　**B**　Intestinal capillaries transport amino acids and monosaccharides to the liver, where initial processing of many nutrients begins.

CHAPTER TWENTY-FOUR

Excretory System

Excretion refers to the removal of **metabolic wastes** produced in the body. Most of the body's activities produce metabolic wastes, including mineral salts, that must be removed. **Aerobic respiration** leads to the production of **carbon dioxide** and water. **Deamination** of amino acids in the liver leads to the production of **nitrogenous wastes** such as urea and ammonia. Excretion is distinguished from **elimination**, the removal of indigestible material, such as dietary fiber.

The principal organs of excretion in humans are the lungs, liver, skin, and kidneys. In the **lungs**, carbon dioxide and water vapor diffuse from the blood and are continually exhaled. Sweat glands in the **skin** excrete water and dissolved salts (and a small quantity of urea). Perspiration serves to regulate body temperature, since the evaporation of sweat produces cooling. The **liver** processes nitrogenous wastes, hemoglobin, and other chemicals for excretion. Urea is produced by the deamination of amino acids in the liver and diffuses into the blood for ultimate excretion in the **kidneys**. Bile salts are excreted as bile and pass out with the feces. The kidneys function to maintain the osmolarity of the blood, excrete numerous waste products and toxic chemicals, and conserve glucose, salt, and water.

KIDNEYS

The kidneys regulate the concentration of salt and water in the blood through the formation and excretion of urine. The kidneys are bean-shaped and are located behind the stomach and liver. Each kidney is composed of approximately one million units called **nephrons**.

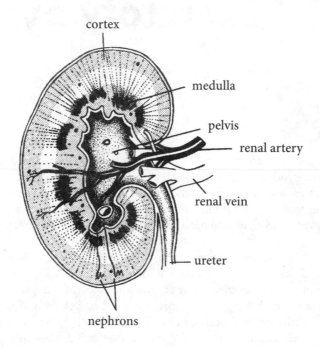

Figure 24.1

Structure

The kidney is divided into three regions: the outer **cortex**, the inner **medulla**, and the renal **pelvis**. A **nephron** consists of a bulb called **Bowman's capsule**, which embraces a special capillary bed called a **glomerulus**. Bowman's capsule leads into a long, coiled tubule divided into functionally distinct units: the **proximal convoluted tubule**, the **loop of Henle**, the **distal convoluted tubule**, and the **collecting duct**. The nephron is positioned such that the loop of Henle and collecting duct run through the medulla, while the convoluted tubules and Bowman's capsule are in the cortex. Concentrated urine in the collecting tubules flows into the pelvis of the kidney, a funnel-like region that opens directly into the **ureter**. The ureters from the kidneys empty into the **urinary bladder**, where urine collects until expelled via the **urethra**. Most of the nephron is surrounded by a complex **peritubular capillary** network that facilitates reabsorption of amino acids, glucose, salts, and water.

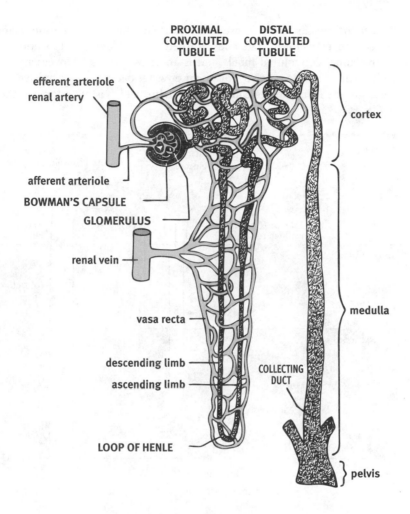

Figure 24.2

Urine Formation

Filtration, secretion, and reabsorption are the three processes that lead to urine formation.

- **Filtration**: Blood pressure forces 20 percent of the blood plasma entering the glomerulus through its capillary walls and into the surrounding Bowman's capsule via diffusion. The fluid and small solutes entering the nephron are called the **filtrate**. The filtrate is isotonic with blood plasma. Particles too large to filter through the glomerulus, such as blood cells and albumin, remain in the circulatory system. Filtration is a passive process driven by the hydrostatic pressure of the blood. As a result, having increased blood pressure can lead to kidney damage over time since the increased hydrostatic pressure exerts extra pressure on the kidney tissues.

- **Secretion**: The nephron secretes waste substances such as acids, ions, and other metabolites from the interstitial fluid into the filtrate by both **passive** and **active** transport. Materials are secreted from the peritubular capillaries into the nephron tubule.

- **Reabsorption**: Essential substances (**glucose**, **salts**, and **amino acids**) and water are reabsorbed from the filtrate and returned to the blood. Reabsorption occurs primarily in the proximal convoluted tubule and is an active process. Movement of these molecules is accompanied by the passive movement of water because water passively follows solute. This results in the formation of **concentrated urine**, which is hypertonic to the blood.

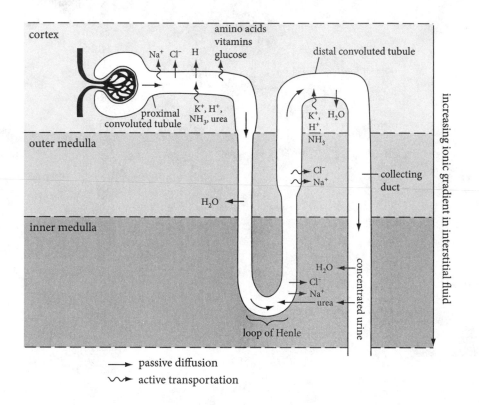

Figure 24.3

Nephron Function

Through the **selective permeability** of its walls and the maintenance of an **osmolarity gradient**, the nephron reabsorbs nutrients, salts, and water from the filtrate and returns them to the body, thus maintaining the bloodstream's solute concentration.

The primary function of the nephron is to clean the blood plasma of unwanted substances as the filtrate passes through the kidney. Because blood plasma contains both wanted and unwanted substances, the nephron will selectively reabsorb wanted substances back into the plasma, while the remaining substances are excreted in the urine. The primary site of nutrient reabsorption in the nephron is the proximal convoluted tubule. The ascending loop of Henle, collecting duct, and descending loop of Henle are the primary sites that regulate water, sodium, and potassium loss in the nephron. The distal convoluted tubule is the primary site for secretion of substances into the filtrate.

Each part of the loop of Henle plays a distinct role in regulating water absorption and electrolyte concentrations. The descending loop of Henle is very permeable to water but not to ions or urea. The thin ascending limb of the loop of Henle, however, is impermeable to water but is permeable to ions, allowing for passive diffusion of ions. In the thick ascending limb of the loop of Henle, sodium, potassium, and chloride are actively reabsorbed from the urine.

The selective permeability of the tubules establishes an osmolarity gradient in the surrounding interstitial fluid. By exiting and then re-entering at different segments of the nephron, solutes create an osmolarity gradient, with tissue osmolarity increasing from the **cortex** to the **inner medulla**. The solutes that contribute to the maintenance of the gradient are urea and sodium chloride (Na^+ and Cl^-). The osmolarity of urine (determined by the concentration of dissolved particles) is established in the renal tubule by means of this **counter-current-multiplier system**: a system in which energy is used to create a concentration gradient. Here, the anatomic arrangement of the loop of Henle within the kidney permits the establishment of the concentration gradient that enables the reabsorption of 99 percent of the filtrate in the renal tubules. This makes the production of concentrated urine possible.

The counter-current multiplier system causes the interstitial space in the medulla of the kidney to be **hyperosmolar** with respect to the dilute filtrate flowing through the renal tubule. As the filtrate flowing in the collecting ducts passes through this region of the kidney, on its way to the pelvis and ureter, water flows out of the collecting ducts by **osmosis**. This water is removed by capillaries present in the medulla. The reabsorption of water in this zone of the kidney, which permits the concentration of urine, depends on the permeability of the collecting ducts to water. Regulation of the permeability of the distal convoluted tubule and collecting ducts to water is accomplished by the hormone **ADH (vasopressin)**. ADH increases the permeability of the collecting duct to water, allowing more water to be absorbed and more concentrated urine to be formed. In some disease states people have excess secretion of ADH, which causes those individuals to retain too much fluid.

Aldosterone is a steroid hormone that causes increased transport of sodium and potassium ions along the distal convoluted tubule and collecting duct, resulting in decreased excretion of sodium ions and increased excretion of potassium ions in the urine. Since water flows to the area of higher solute concentration through osmosis, this also causes additional water reabsorption. Furthermore, aldosterone does not affect renal blood flow.

Antidiuretic hormone (ADH), also known as vasopressin, is a peptide hormone with the same net effect of increased water reabsorption as aldosterone. However, as discussed previously, ADH directly affects water absorption by the distal convoluted tubule and collecting ducts, opening additional **aquaporins** (water channels) in these structures to allow water to be reasborbed more readily. Both hormones cause a decrease in urine output and a corresponding increase in blood pressure, allowing the human body to compensate for periods of dehydration or other causes of low blood pressure.

Diuretics, drugs that increase urine production, can target different parts of the kidneys to cause the same net effect. For example, loop diuretics inhibit sodium reabsorption in the ascending loop of the nephron, whereas thiazide diuretics inhibit the sodium-chloride transporter in the distal convoluted tubule. Both have the net effect of increasing the amount of water present in the urine and therefore increase urine excretion.

Maintenance of pH

Body fluid **pH** remains relatively constant at 7.4; this consistency is attained by the removal of carbon dioxide by the lungs and hydrogen ions by the kidneys. pH is assessed via the following laboratory tests:

- arterial pH
- arterial partial pressure of carbon dioxide (Pco_2)
- plasma bicarbonate (HCO_3^-)

There are two types of acid-base disorders:

1. **Respiratory disorders**: affect the blood acidity by causing changes in the P_{CO_2}
2. **Metabolic disorders**: affect the blood acidity by causing changes in the HCO_3^-

Below is a summary of acid-base disorders and compensatory mechanisms by the human body.

Condition		Defect	Blood pH	Compensation
Respiratory	Acidosis	Increased P_{CO_2}	Decreased	Increased HCO_3^-
	Alkalosis	Decreased P_{CO_2}	Increased	Decreased HCO_3^-
Metabolic	Acidosis	Decreased HCO_3^-	Decreased	Decreased P_{CO_2}
	Alkalosis	Increased HCO_3^-	Increased	Increased P_{CO_2}

Table 24.1

Compensation mechanisms that affect P_{CO_2} are performed by the respiratory system and can affect change quite quickly. However, compensation mechanisms that affect HCO_3^- are performed by the kidneys, and therefore the compensatory effect can take longer to manifest. These changes in acid-base chemistry within the body, as well as the cause of the change (respiratory or metabolic), dictate how a patient will be treated medically. For example, a change in pH due to a change in respiratory rate or function may be the result of airway obstruction or chronic obstructive pulmonary disease (COPD), whereas metabolic acidosis may be due to kidney dysfunction or volume loss, so these disorders must be treated accordingly.

REVIEW PROBLEMS

1. Which of the following would most likely filter through the glomerulus into Bowman's capsule?

    (A) Erythrocytes
    (B) Monosaccharides
    (C) Leukocytes
    (D) Platelets

2. Draw a nephron and label all of its segments.

3. Which region of the kidney has the lowest solute concentration?

    (A) Nephron
    (B) Cortex
    (C) Medulla
    (D) Pelvis

4. In the nephron, amino acids enter the peritubular capillaries via

    (A) filtration.
    (B) secretion.
    (C) reabsorption.
    (D) osmoregulation.

5. Glucose reabsorption in the nephron occurs in the

    (A) loop of Henle.
    (B) distal tubule.
    (C) proximal tubule.
    (D) collecting duct.

6. Urine is

    (A) hypotonic to the blood.
    (B) hypertonic to the blood.
    (C) hypertonic to the filtrate.
    (D) hypotonic to the vasa recta.

SOLUTIONS TO REVIEW PROBLEMS

1. **B** Monosaccharides would most likely filter through the glomerulus. Cells, cell fragments, and proteins remain on the circulatory side.

2. See Figure 24.2.

3. **B** Discussed in nephron function section in this chapter.

4. **C** Discussed in osmoregulation section in this chapter.

5. **C** Discussed in function of nephron section in this chapter.

6. **B** Discussed in function of nephron section in this chapter.

CHAPTER TWENTY-FIVE

Endocrine System

The endocrine system acts as a means of internal communication, coordinating the activities of the organ systems. **Endocrine glands** synthesize and secrete chemical substances called **hormones** directly into the circulatory system. In contrast, **exocrine glands**, such as the gallbladder, secrete substances transported by ducts.

ENDOCRINE GLANDS

Glands or organs that synthesize or secrete hormones include the pituitary, hypothalamus, thyroid, parathyroids, adrenals, pancreas, testes, ovaries, pineal gland, kidneys, gastrointestinal glands, heart, and thymus. Some hormones regulate a single type of cell or organ, whereas others have more widespread actions. The specificity of hormonal action is usually determined by the presence of specific receptors on or in the target cells.

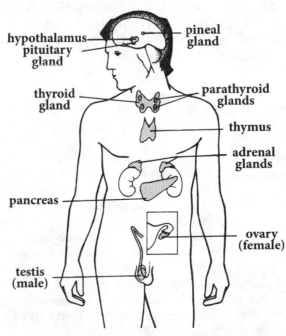

Figure 25.1

Adrenal Glands

The adrenal glands are situated on top of the kidneys and consist of the adrenal cortex and the adrenal medulla.

Adrenal cortex

In response to stress, adrenocorticotropic hormone (ACTH), which is produced by the anterior pituitary, stimulates the adrenal cortex to produce more than two dozen different steroid hormones, collectively known as **adrenocortical steroids**, or simply **corticosteroids**. In the bloodstream, these corticosteroids are bound to transport proteins called **transcortins**. Corticosteroids exert their mechanism of action by determining which genes are transcribed in the nuclei of their target cells and at what rate. The subsequent changes in the nature and concentration of the enzymes produced in the target cells will affect cellular metabolism. The three major classes of corticosteroids are described below:

- **Glucocorticoids:** Glucocorticoids, such as **cortisol** and **cortisone**, are involved in glucose regulation and protein metabolism. Glucocorticoids raise blood glucose levels by promoting protein breakdown and **gluconeogenesis** and decreasing protein synthesis. Glucocorticoids increase the plasma glucose levels and are antagonistic to the effects of insulin. Glucocorticoids release amino acids from skeletal muscle as well as lipids from adipose tissue. They also promote peripheral use of lipids and have anti-inflammatory effects.

- **Mineralocorticoids:** Mineralocorticoids, particularly **aldosterone**, regulate plasma levels of sodium and potassium and, consequently, the total extracellular water volume. Aldosterone causes active reabsorption of sodium and passive reabsorption of water in the **nephron** of the kidney. This results in an increase in both blood volume and blood pressure. Excess production of aldosterone results in excess retention of water with resulting hypertension (high blood pressure). The mineralocorticoids are stimulated by angiotensin II and inhibited by ANP (atrial natriuretic peptide). See Chapter 24, Excretory System, for more information on the action of aldosterone.

- **Cortical sex hormones:** The adrenal cortex secretes small quantities of **androgens** (male sex hormones) like androstenedione and dehydroepiandrosterone in both men and women. In men, most of the androgens are produced by the **testes**, so the physiologic effect of the adrenal androgens is quite small. In women, however, overproduction of the adrenal androgens may have masculinizing effects, such as excessive facial hair.

Adrenal medulla

The adrenal medulla produces **epinephrine** (adrenaline) and **norepinephrine** (noradrenaline), both of which belong to a class of amino acid–derived compounds called **catecholamines**.

Epinephrine increases the conversion of glycogen to glucose in liver and muscle tissue, causing an increase in blood glucose levels and an increase in the basal metabolic rate. Both epinephrine and norepinephrine increase the rate and strength of the heartbeat and dilate and constrict blood vessels in such a way as to increase the blood supply to the skeletal muscles, heart, and brain, while decreasing the blood supply to the kidneys, skin, and digestive tract. Both epinephrine and norepinephrine will also promote the release of lipids by adipose tissue. These effects are known as the "fight or flight response" and are elicited by sympathetic nervous stimulation in response to stress.

Epinephrine will inhibit certain vegetative functions, such as digestion, which are not immediately important for survival. Both of these hormones are also **neurotransmitters**, proteins used by neurons to transmit signals. The release of these hormones is stimulated during sympathetic activation by sympathetic preganglionic fibers.

Pituitary Gland

The pituitary (**hypophysis**) is a small, trilobed gland at the base of the brain. The two main lobes, anterior and posterior, are functionally distinct. (In humans, the third lobe, the intermediate lobe, is rudimentary.) Specifically, the pituitary gland hangs below the hypothalamus and is connected to it by a slender cord known as the **infundibulum**.

Anterior pituitary

The anterior pituitary synthesizes both direct hormones, which directly stimulate their target organs, and tropic hormones, which stimulate other endocrine glands to release hormones. The hormonal secretions of the anterior pituitary are regulated by hypothalamic secretions called releasing/inhibiting hormones or factors.

The **direct hormones** of the anterior pituitary include:

- **Growth hormone (GH, somatotropin):** GH promotes bone and muscle growth. GH also promotes protein synthesis and lipid mobilization and catabolism. In children, a GH deficiency can lead to stunted growth (**dwarfism**), while overproduction of GH results in **gigantism**. Overproduction of GH in adults causes **acromegaly**, a disorder characterized by a disproportionate overgrowth of bone, localized especially in the skull, jaw, feet, and hands.
- **Prolactin:** Prolactin stimulates milk production and secretion in female mammary glands.

The **tropic hormones** of the anterior pituitary include:

- **Adrenocorticotropic hormone (ACTH):** ACTH stimulates the adrenal cortex to synthesize and secrete glucocorticoids and is regulated by the releasing hormone corticotropin-releasing factor (CRF).
- **Thyroid-stimulating hormone (TSH):** TSH stimulates the thyroid gland to synthesize and release thyroid hormones, including thyroxine.
- **Luteinizing hormone (LH):** In women, LH stimulates ovulation and formation of the **corpus luteum**. LH is also responsible for regulating progesterone secretion in women. In men, LH stimulates the interstitial cells of the testes to synthesize testosterone.
- **Follicle-stimulating hormone (FSH):** In women, FSH causes maturation of ovarian follicles that begin secreting estrogen; in men, FSH stimulates maturation of the seminiferous tubules and sperm production.
- **Melanocyte-stimulating hormone (MSH):** MSH is secreted by the intermediate lobe of the pituitary. In mammals, the function of MSH is unclear, but in frogs, MSH causes darkening of the skin via induced dispersion of molecules of pigment in melanophore cells.
- **Endorphins:** These are neurotransmitters that have pain-relieving properties.

Posterior pituitary

The posterior pituitary (**neurohypophysis**) does not synthesize hormones; it stores and releases the peptide hormones **oxytocin** and **antidiuretic hormone**, which are produced by the neurosecretory cells of the hypothalamus. Hormone secretion is stimulated by action potentials descending from the hypothalamus. These hormones are described in further detail below:

- **Oxytocin:** Oxytocin, which is secreted during childbirth, increases the strength and frequency of uterine muscle contractions. Oxytocin secretion is also induced by suckling; oxytocin stimulates milk secretion in the mammary glands.

- **Antidiuretic hormone (ADH; vasopressin):** ADH increases the permeability of the nephron's **collecting duct** to water, thereby promoting water reabsorption and increasing blood volume, which subsequently increases blood pressure. ADH is secreted when plasma osmolarity increases, as sensed by osmoreceptors in the hypothalamus, or when blood volume decreases, as sensed by baroreceptors in the circulatory system.

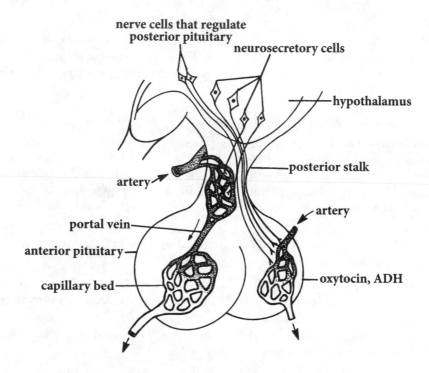

Figure 25.2

Hypothalamus

The hypothalamus is part of the forebrain and is located directly above the pituitary gland. The hypothalamus receives neural transmissions from other parts of the brain and from peripheral nerves that trigger specific responses from its **neurosecretory cells**. The neurosecretory cells regulate pituitary gland secretions via negative feedback mechanisms and through the actions of inhibiting and releasing hormones.

Interactions with the anterior pituitary

Hypothalamic-releasing hormones stimulate or inhibit the secretions of the anterior pituitary. For example, GnRH stimulates the anterior pituitary to secrete FSH and LH. Releasing hormones are secreted into the hypothalamic-hypophyseal portal system. In this circulatory pathway, blood from the capillary bed in the hypothalamus flows through a portal vein into the anterior pituitary, where it diverges into a second capillary network. In this way, releasing hormones can immediately reach the anterior pituitary.

A complicated feedback system regulates the secretions of the endocrine system. For example, when the plasma levels of adrenal cortical hormones drop, hypothalamic cells (via a negative feedback mechanism) release ACTH-releasing factor (ACTH-RF) into the portal system. When the plasma concentration of corticosteroids exceeds the normal plasma level, the steroids themselves exert an inhibitory effect on the hypothalamus.

Interactions with the posterior pituitary

Neurosecretory cells in the hypothalamus synthesize both oxytocin and ADH and transport them via their axons into the posterior pituitary for storage and secretion.

Thyroid

Thyroid hormones affect the function of nearly every organ system in the body. In children, thyroid hormones are essential for growth and neurological development; in adults, thyroid hormones are essential for maintenance of metabolic stability. They increase the rate of metabolism throughout the body.

Thyroid hormones (thyroxine and triiodothyronine)

The thyroid hormones, **thyroxine (T4)** and **triiodothyronine (T3)**, are formed from the glycoprotein **thyroglobulin**, which is synthesized in thyroid cells. Because of the specific tertiary structure of this glycoprotein, iodinated tyrosine residues present in thyroglobulin are able to bind together to form active thyroid hormones. The thyroid hormones possess the following characteristics:

- T3 is five times more potent than T4.
- T4 and T3 are transported via plasma proteins. Approximately 99.5% of these hormones are bound to proteins, but only an unbound hormone is able to enter a cell and elicit a cellular response.
- All of the T4 in the body is formed and secreted by the thyroid gland; however, only 20% of T3 is produced by the thyroid gland.
- The majority of T3 is produced by the conversion of T4 to T3 by the enzyme 5'-monodeiodase, found primarily in the peripheral tissues.

In **hypothyroidism**, thyroid hormones are undersecreted or not secreted at all. Common symptoms of hypothyroidism include a slowed heart rate and respiratory rate, fatigue, cold intolerance, and weight gain. Hypothyroidism in newborn infants, called **cretinism**, is characterized by mental retardation and short stature. In **hyperthyroidism**, the thyroid is overstimulated, resulting in the oversecretion of thyroid hormones. Symptoms often include increased metabolic rate, feelings of excessive warmth, profuse sweating, palpitations, weight loss, and protruding eyes. In both disorders, the thyroid often enlarges, forming a bulge in the neck called a goiter.

Hypothyroidism is often treated with supplementation of thyroid hormones via synthetic or animal-derived products. Hyperthyroidism can be treated by antithyroid medications that suppress the thyroid's release of excess hormone or ablation of the thyroid with radiotherapy. After ablation the thyroid no longer produces thyroid hormone, and the patient must take thyroid supplementation for the rest of his or her life.

Calcitonin

Calcitonin decreases plasma Ca^{2+} concentration by inhibiting the release of Ca^{2+} from bone. Calcitonin secretion is regulated by plasma Ca^{2+} levels. Calcitonin is antagonistic to parathyroid hormone.

Pancreas

The pancreas is both an **exocrine** organ and an **endocrine** organ. The exocrine function is performed by the cells that secrete digestive enzymes into the small intestine via a series of ducts. The endocrine function is performed by small glandular structures called the **islets of Langerhans**, which are composed of alpha and beta cells. Alpha cells produce and secrete glucagon; beta cells produce and secrete insulin. The endocrine hormones secreted by the pancreas include the following:

- **Glucagon:** Glucagon stimulates protein and fat degradation, the conversion of glycogen to glucose, and gluconeogenesis, all of which serve to increase blood glucose levels. Glucagon's actions are largely antagonistic to those of insulin.

- **Insulin:** Insulin is a protein hormone secreted in response to a high blood glucose concentration. It stimulates the uptake of glucose by muscle and adipose cells and the storage of glucose as glycogen in muscle and liver cells, thus lowering blood glucose levels. It also stimulates the synthesis of fats from glucose and the uptake of amino acids. Insulin's actions are antagonistic to those of **glucagon** and the **glucocorticoids**. Underproduction of insulin, or insensitivity to insulin, leads to **diabetes mellitus**, which is characterized by hyperglycemia (high blood glucose levels). Diabetes is the most common endocrine disorder and, if improperly managed, is characterized by long-term complications involving the eyes, nerves, kidneys, and blood vessels. Table 25.1 identifies the distinguishing characteristics of Type I and Type II diabetes.

Distinguishing Characteristics	Type I	Type II
% diabetics	10	90
Age of onset	Usually <30 years	Usually >30 years
Pathogenesis	Presence of islet cell antibodies Autoimmune Decreased insulin secretion	Resistance to insulin Hepatic glucose production
Plasma insulin	Usually none	Low, normal, or high Etiology dependent
Family history	Usually none	Strong
Obesity	Uncommon	Common

Table 25.1

Parathyroid Glands

The parathyroid glands are four small, pea-shaped structures embedded in the posterior surface of the thyroid. These glands synthesize and secrete **parathyroid hormone (PTH)**, which regulates plasma Ca^{2+} concentration. PTH raises the Ca^{2+} concentration in the blood by stimulating Ca^{2+} release from the bone and decreasing Ca^{2+} excretion in the kidneys. Calcium in bone is bonded to phosphate, and breakdown of the bone releases phosphate as well as calcium. Parathyroid hormone compensates for this by stimulating excretion of phosphate by the kidneys.

Kidneys

When blood volume falls, the kidneys produce **renin**—an enzyme that converts the plasma protein angiotensinogen to angiotensin I. Angiotensin I is converted to angiotensin II, which stimulates the adrenal cortex to secrete **aldosterone**. Aldosterone helps restore blood volume by increasing sodium reabsorption at the kidney, leading to an increase in water. This removes the initial stimulus for renin production. The kidneys also produce **erythropoietin (EPO)**. EPO is a glycoprotein that stimulates red blood cell production; it is normally produced in the kidneys. This hormone causes the following:

- stimulation of the stem cells to differentiate into rubriblasts (least mature erythrocytes)
- increased rate of mitosis
- increased release of reticulocytes from the bone marrow
- increased hemoglobin (HgB) formation, which creates the critical HgB concentration necessary for maturity to be reached at a more rapid rate

Gastrointestinal Hormones

Ingested food stimulates the stomach to release the hormone gastrin. **Gastrin** is carried to the gastric glands and stimulates the glands to secrete HCl in response to food in the stomach. Secretion of pancreatic juice, the exocrine product of the pancreas, is also under hormonal control; the hormone **secretin** is released by the small intestine when acidic food material enters from the stomach. Secretin stimulates the secretion of an alkaline bicarbonate solution from the pancreas that neutralizes the acidity of the **chyme** (partially digested food coming from the stomach). The hormone **cholecystokinin** is released from the small intestine in response to the presence of fats and causes the contraction of the gallbladder and release of bile into the small intestine. **Bile,** which is not a hormone, is involved in the emulsification and digestion of fats.

Pineal Gland

The pineal gland is a tiny structure at the base of the brain that secretes the hormone **melatonin**. The role of melatonin in humans is unclear, but it is believed to play a role in the regulation of **circadian rhythms**—physiological cycles lasting approximately 24 hours. Melatonin secretion is regulated by light and dark cycles in the environment. In primitive vertebrates, melatonin lightens the skin by concentrating pigment granules in melanophores (melatonin is an antagonist to MSH).

MECHANISM OF HORMONE ACTION

Hormones are classified on the basis of their chemical structure into two major groups: peptide hormones and steroid hormones. There are two ways in which hormones affect the activities of their target cells: via extracellular receptors or intracellular receptors.

Peptides

Peptide hormones range from simple short peptides (amino acid chains), such as ADH, to complex polypeptides, such as insulin. Peptide hormones act as first messengers. When they bind to **specific receptors** on the surface of their target cells, they trigger a series of enzymatic reactions within each cell, the first of which may be the conversion of ATP to cyclic adenosine monophosphate (cyclic AMP); this reaction is catalyzed by the membrane-bound enzyme adenylate cyclase. **Cyclic AMP** acts as a **second messenger**, relaying messages from the extracellular peptide hormone to cytoplasmic enzymes and initiating a series of successive reactions in the cell. This is an example of a **cascade effect**; with each step, the hormone's effects are amplified. Cyclic AMP activity is inactivated by the cytoplasmic enzyme phosphodiesterase.

Steroids

Steroid hormones, such as estrogen and aldosterone, belong to a class of lipid-derived molecules with a characteristic ring structure. They are produced by the testes, ovaries, placenta, and adrenal cortex. Because they are lipid soluble, steroid hormones cross the phospholipid bilayer and enter their target cells directly in order to bind to specific receptor proteins in the cytoplasm. This receptor-hormone complex enters the nucleus and directly activates the expression of specific genes by binding to receptors on the chromatin. This induces a change in mRNA transcription and protein synthesis.

REVIEW PROBLEMS

1. Name the different parts of the adrenal gland and the hormones secreted from each.

2. Discuss the relationship between the hypothalamus and the pituitary gland.

3. Increased activity of the parathyroid gland leads to
   (A) a decrease in blood glucose levels.
   (B) an increase in metabolic rate.
   (C) a decrease in body temperature.
   (D) an increase in blood Ca^{2+} concentrations.

4. Which of the following statements concerning growth hormone is NOT true?
   (A) Overproduction of growth hormone in children results in gigantism.
   (B) Overproduction of growth hormone in adults results in acromegaly.
   (C) A deficiency of growth hormone results in dwarfism.
   (D) Growth hormone is secreted by the hypothalamus.

5. Describe the regulation of plasma Ca^{2+} concentration. Include all of the hormones and organs involved.

6. Thyroid hormone deficiency may result in
   (A) acromegaly.
   (B) cretinism.
   (C) gigantism.
   (D) hyperthyroidism.

7. Match the following hormones with their respective functions.
   (A) Growth hormone
   (B) ACTH
   (C) Oxytocin
   (D) Progesterone
   (E) Aldosterone
   (F) Glucagon
   (G) Thyroxine

   1. Promotes growth of muscle
   2. Stimulates the release of glucose into the blood
   3. Prepares the uterus for implantation of a fertilized egg
   4. Stimulates the secretion of glucocorticoids
   5. Increases the rate of metabolism
   6. Induces water reabsorption in the kidneys
   7. Increases uterine contractions during childbirth

8. What is negative feedback?

9. Why is the level of blood glucose so important? What hormones are involved in the regulation of blood glucose levels?

10. Destruction of all beta cells in the pancreas would cause

    (A) glucagon secretion to stop and a decrease in blood glucose.
    (B) glucagon secretion to stop and an increase in blood glucose.
    (C) insulin secretion to stop and an increase in blood glucose.
    (D) insulin secretion to stop and a decrease in blood glucose.

11. A man trapped for three days underneath the ruins of a collapsed building was rescued and rushed to the nearest hospital. He suffered from internal bleeding and was very dehydrated. Why was a high level of aldosterone found in his blood?

12. Oxytocin and vasopressin are

    (A) produced and released by the hypothalamus.
    (B) produced and released by the pituitary.
    (C) produced by the hypothalamus and released by the pituitary.
    (D) produced by the pituitary and released by the hypothalamus.

SOLUTIONS TO REVIEW PROBLEMS

1. The adrenal gland is divided into the adrenal cortex and the adrenal medulla. The adrenal cortex secretes steroid hormones called mineralocorticoids (e.g., aldosterone) as well as glucocorticoids (e.g., cortisol) and sex hormones (e.g., androstenedione). The adrenal medulla secretes the catecholamines norepinephrine and epinephrine, which are amino acid derivatives.

2. The posterior pituitary stores and secretes hormones produced by the neurosecretory cells of the hypothalamus. In contrast, the anterior pituitary produces hormones whose secretions are regulated by hypothalamic releasing hormones. Hypothalamic releasing hormones stimulate the anterior pituitary to secrete a particular hormone, whereas hypothalamic inhibiting hormones inhibit anterior pituitary secretions. The releasing and inhibiting hormones are secreted into a circulatory pathway known as the hypothalamic-hypophyseal portal system, which allows for high, localized concentrations of the various stimulating and inhibitory hormones and rapid, direct transport of these hormones to the pituitary.

3. **D** Discussed in section on parathyroid glands in this chapter.

4. **D** Discussed in section on hormones of the anterior pituitary in this chapter.

5. Calcium levels in the blood are regulated by two hormones: calcitonin and parathyroid hormone (PTH). Calcitonin is secreted by the thyroid gland when plasma Ca^{2+} levels are high and decreases the plasma Ca^{2+} concentration by inhibiting bone resorption (which releases Ca^{2+} into the blood). When plasma Ca^{2+} levels are low, PTH is secreted by the parathyroid glands. PTH increases plasma Ca^{2+} concentration by increasing bone resorption, increasing Ca^{2+} reabsorption in the kidney (thus reducing the amount of Ca^{2+} excreted in the urine), and stimulating the conversion of vitamin D into its active form (1,25-dihydroxycholecalciferol), which increases intestinal absorption of Ca^{2+}.

6. **B** Discussed in section on thyroid gland in this chapter.

7. **A** 1
    B 4
    C 7
    D 3
    E 6
    F 2
    G 5

8. Negative feedback is a means of regulation whereby an end-product inhibits one or more of the earlier steps that lead to its production or secretion. For example, high plasma levels of thyroxine inhibit the pituitary gland from secreting TSH, thus removing the stimulus on the thyroid to secrete more thyroxine. Negative feedback mechanisms are also used by the body to regulate enzyme production and activity.

9. Glucose is the primary source of energy used by cells during aerobic respiration, so blood glucose levels determine the amount of energy available for cellular activity. Many

hormones involved in the regulation of blood glucose levels do so by stimulating the liver either to store or release glucose. When glucose levels are low, the adrenal medulla secretes epinephrine, which stimulates the liver to convert glycogen stores into glucose and release it into the blood. Epinephrine also acts on muscles, transforming their glycogen stores into lactic acid, which is transported to the liver and converted to glucose. The pancreas secretes glucagon, which also stimulates the liver to convert glycogen to glucose. When additional glucose is needed, the adrenal cortex secretes glucocorticoids, which stimulate the liver to synthesize glucose from noncarbohydrates in a process called gluconeogenesis. Insulin is antagonistic to glucagon, epinephrine, and glucocorticoids; it lowers blood glucose levels by stimulating the uptake of glucose by adipose and muscle tissue and by promoting the conversion of glucose into glycogen in liver and muscle cells.

10. **C**   Discussed in section on endocrine functions of the pancreas in this chapter.

11.   Internal bleeding leads to a decrease in the volume of blood in the circulatory system. When blood volume falls, the kidney produces renin, which leads to an increase in aldosterone. Aldosterone causes increased water reabsorption in the nephrons, leading to an increase in blood volume. Thus, the man's body responded to the blood loss by secreting aldosterone.

12. **C**   Discussed in section on anterior pituitary in this chapter.

CHAPTER TWENTY-SIX

Reproductive System

Reproduction in animals is a complex process involving the formation and fertilization of gametes and regulation of these processes by both parents. Once fertilization occurs, an embryo is formed, and that embryo matures into a fetus through rapid division and differentiation.

SEXUAL REPRODUCTION

Sexual reproduction differs from asexual reproduction in that there are two parents involved and the end result is a genetically unique offspring. Sexual reproduction occurs via the fusion of two gametes, specialized sex cells produced by each parent. Sexual reproduction requires the following:

- The production of **functional sex cells** or **gametes** by adult organisms
- The union of these cells (**fertilization** or **conjugation**) to form a zygote
- The development of the zygote into another adult, completing the cycle

Gonads

The gametes are produced in specialized organs called the **gonads**. The male gonads, called **testes**, produce **sperm** in the tightly coiled seminiferous tubules. The female gonads, called **ovaries**, produce **oocytes** (eggs). Some species are **hermaphrodites**, which have both functional male and female gonads. These include the hydra and the earthworm.

Gametogenesis

The production of functional sex cells is called **gametogenesis**. In males, the process is more specifically called **spermatogenesis**, or sperm production, and occurs in the seminiferous tubules of the testes. In females, the process is more specifically called **oogenesis**, or egg production, and occurs in the ovaries. Spermatogenesis and oogenesis will be discussed in more detail in the sections on the male and female reproductive systems, respectively.

Fertilization

Fertilization is the union of the egg and sperm nuclei to form a zygote with a diploid number of chromosomes. **Internal fertilization** is practiced by terrestrial vertebrates and provides a direct route for sperm to reach the egg cell. This increases the chance for fertilization success, and females produce fewer eggs. The number of eggs produced is affected by other factors as well. If the early development of the offspring occurs outside of the mother's body, more eggs will be laid to increase the chances of offspring survival. The amount of parental care after birth is also related to the number of eggs produced. Species that care for their young produce fewer eggs.

MALE REPRODUCTIVE SYSTEM

The **testes** are located in an external pouch called the **scrotum** that maintains the testes' temperature at 2°C to 4°C lower than body temperature, a condition essential for sperm survival. Sperm pass from the testes through the **vas deferens** to the **ejaculatory duct** and then to the **urethra**. The urethra passes through the penis and opens to the outside at its tip. In males, the urethra is a common passageway for both the reproductive and excretory systems. The testes are also the sites of production of testosterone. **Testosterone** regulates secondary male sex characteristics including facial and pubic hair and voice changes.

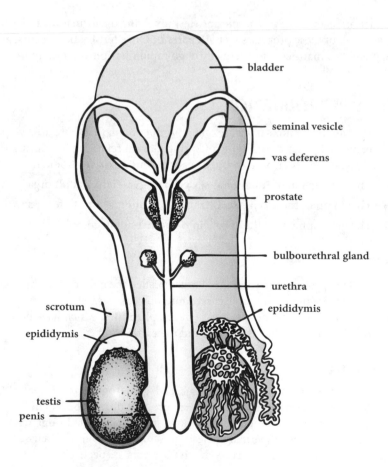

Figure 26.1

Spermatogenesis

Spermatogenesis, or sperm production, occurs in the seminiferous tubules. Diploid cells called **spermatogonia** differentiate into diploid cells called **primary spermatocytes**, which undergo the first meiotic division to yield two haploid **secondary spermatocytes** of equal size; the second meiotic division produces four haploid **spermatids** of equal size. After meiosis the spermatids undergo a series of changes leading to the production of mature sperm, or **spermatozoa**, which are specialized for transporting the sperm nucleus to the egg, or **ovum**. The mature sperm is an elongated cell with a head, neck, body, and tail. The head consists almost entirely of the nucleus. The tail (flagellum) propels the sperm, while mitochondria in the neck and body provide energy for locomotion. A caplike structure called the **acrosome**, derived from the Golgi apparatus, develops over the anterior half of the head. The acrosome contains enzymes needed to penetrate the tough outer covering of the ovum. After a male has reached sexual maturity, approximately 3 million primary spermatocytes begin to undergo spermatogenesis per day, the maturation process taking a total of 65–75 days.

FEMALE REPRODUCTIVE SYSTEM

The **ovaries** are found in the abdominal cavity below the digestive system. The ovaries consist of thousands of follicles; a **follicle** is a multilayered sac of cells that contains, nourishes, and protects an immature ovum. It is actually the follicle cells that produce estrogen. Approximately once a month, an immature ovum is released from the ovary into the abdominal cavity and drawn by cilia into the nearby **oviduct**. The oviducts are also known as fallopian tubes. Each fallopian tube opens into the upper end of a muscular chamber called the **uterus**, the site of fetal development. The lower, narrow end of the uterus is called the **cervix**. The cervix connects with the vaginal canal, which is the site of sperm deposition during intercourse and is also the passageway through which a baby is expelled during childbirth.

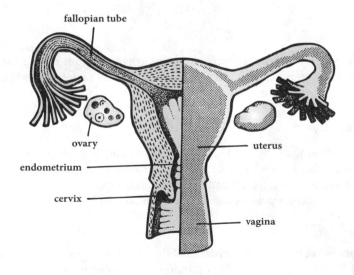

Figure 26.2

Oogenesis

Oogenesis, the production of female gametes, occurs in the ovarian follicles. At birth, most of the immature ova, known as **primary oocytes,** that a female will produce during her lifetime are already in her ovaries. Primary oocytes are diploid cells that form by mitosis in the ovary. After menarche (the first time a female menstruates), one primary oocyte per month completes meiosis I, yielding two daughter cells of unequal size—a **secondary oocyte** and a small cell known as a **polar body.** The secondary oocyte is expelled from the follicle during ovulation. Meiosis II does not occur until fertilization. The oocyte cell membrane is surrounded by two layers of cells; the inner layer is the **zona pellucida**, and the outer layer is the **corona radiata**. Meiosis II is triggered when these layers are penetrated by a sperm cell, yielding two haploid cells—a mature ovum and another polar body. The first polar body may also undergo meiosis II; either way, the polar bodies rapidly degenerate. The mature ovum is a large cell containing the cytoplasm, RNA, organelles, and nutrients needed by the developing embryo. When the polar bodies are formed, they lack these resources, having given them to the developing oocyte.

Female Sex Hormones

The ovaries synthesize and secrete the female sex hormones, including estrogens and progesterone. The secretion of both estrogens and progesterone is regulated by **luteinizing hormone (LH)** and **follicle stimulating hormone (FSH)**, which, in turn, are regulated by gonadotropin-releasing hormone (GnRH).

Estrogens

Estrogens are steroid hormones necessary for normal female maturation. They stimulate the development of the female reproductive tract and contribute to the development of secondary sexual characteristics and sex drive. Estrogens are also responsible for the thickening of the endometrium (the inner lining of the uterine wall). Estrogens are secreted by the ovarian follicles and the corpus luteum.

Progesterone

Progesterone is a steroid hormone secreted by the corpus luteum during the luteal phase of the menstrual cycle. Progesterone stimulates the development and maintenance of the endometrial walls in preparation for implantation.

The Menstrual Cycle

The hormonal secretions of the ovaries, hypothalamus, and anterior pituitary play important roles in the female reproductive cycle. From puberty through menopause, interactions between these hormones result in a monthly cyclical pattern known as the menstrual cycle. The menstrual cycle may be divided into the follicular phase, ovulation, luteal phase, and menstruation.

Follicular phase

The follicular phase begins with the cessation of the menstrual flow from the previous cycle. During this phase, FSH from the anterior pituitary promotes the development of the follicle, which grows and begins secreting estrogen.

Ovulation

Midway through the cycle, ovulation occurs—a mature ovarian follicle bursts and releases an ovum. Ovulation is caused by a surge in LH that is preceded and in part caused by a peak in estrogen levels.

Women ovulate approximately once every four weeks (except during pregnancy and, usually, lactation) until menopause, which typically occurs between the ages of 45 and 50. During menopause the ovaries become less sensitive to the hormones that stimulate follicle development (FSH and LH) and eventually atrophy. The remaining follicles disappear, estrogen and progesterone levels greatly decline, and ovulation stops. The profound changes in hormone levels are often accompanied by physiological and psychological changes that persist until a new balance is reached.

Luteal phase

After ovulation, LH induces the ruptured follicle to develop into the **corpus luteum**, which secretes estrogen and progesterone. **Progesterone** causes the glands of the endometrium to mature and produce secretions that prepare it for the implantation of an embryo. Progesterone and estrogen are essential for the maintenance of the endometrium.

Menstruation

If the ovum is not fertilized, the corpus luteum atrophies. The resulting drop in progesterone and estrogen levels causes the endometrium (with its superficial blood vessels) to slough off, giving rise to the menstrual flow (**menses**).

If fertilization occurs, the developing placenta produces **hCG** (human chorionic gonadotropin), maintaining the corpus luteum and thus the supply of estrogen and progesterone that maintains the uterus. Eventually the placenta takes over production of these hormones and hCG is no longer produced.

Fertilization

An egg can be fertilized during the 12–24 hours after ovulation. Fertilization occurs in the lateral, widest portion of the fallopian tube. Sperm must travel through the vaginal canal, cervix, uterus, and into the fallopian tubes to reach the ovum. Sperm remain viable and capable of fertilization for 1–2 days after intercourse.

The first barrier that the sperm must penetrate is the corona radiata. Enzymes secreted by the sperm aid in penetration of the corona radiata. The acrosome is responsible for penetrating the zona pellucida; it releases enzymes that digest this layer, thereby allowing the sperm to come into direct contact with the ovum cell membrane. Once in contact with the membrane, the sperm forms a tubelike structure called the **acrosomal process,** which extends to the cell membrane and penetrates it, fusing the sperm cell membrane with that of the ovum. The sperm nucleus now enters the ovum's cytoplasm. It is at this stage of fertilization that the ovum completes meiosis II.

The acrosomal reaction triggers a **cortical reaction** in the ovum, causing calcium ions to be released into the cytoplasm; this, in turn, initiates a series of reactions that result in the formation of the **fertilization membrane**. The fertilization membrane is a hard layer that surrounds the ovum cell membrane and prevents multiple fertilizations. The release of Ca^{2+} also stimulates metabolic changes within the ovum, greatly increasing its metabolic rate. This is followed by the fusion of the sperm nucleus with the ovum nucleus to form a diploid zygote. The first mitotic division of the zygote soon follows.

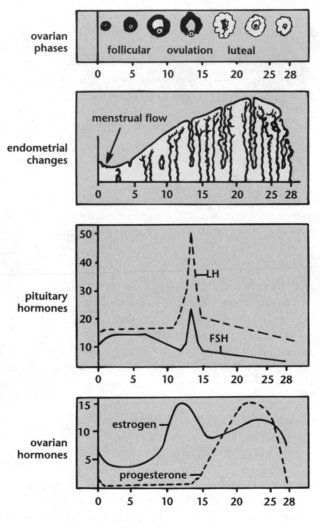

Figure 17.3

Multiple Births

Monozygotic (identical) twins

Monozygotic twins result when a single zygote splits into two embryos. If the splitting occurs at the two-cell stage of development, the embryos will have separate chorions and separate placentas; if it occurs at the blastula stage, then the embryos will have only one chorionic sac and will therefore share a placenta and possibly an amnion. Occasionally the division is incomplete, resulting in the birth of "Siamese" (conjoined) twins, which are attached at some point on the body, often sharing limbs or organs. Monozygotic twins are genetically identical because they develop from the same zygote. Monozygotic twins are therefore of the same sex, blood type, and so on.

Dizygotic (fraternal) twins

Dizygotic twins result when two ova are released in one ovarian cycle and are fertilized by two different sperm. The two embryos implant in the uterine wall individually, and each develops its own placenta, amnion, and chorion (although the placentas may fuse if the embryos implant very close to each other). Fraternal twins share no more characteristics than any other siblings because they develop from two distinct zygotes.

EMBRYOLOGY

Embryology is the study of the development of a unicellular zygote into a complete, multicellular organism. In the course of nine months, a unicellular human zygote undergoes cell division, cellular differentiation, and morphogenesis in preparation for life outside the uterus.

Early Developmental Stages

Fertilization

In mammals, an egg can be fertilized within 12–24 hours after ovulation. Fertilization occurs in the lateral, widest portion of the oviduct where sperm traveling from the vagina encounter an egg. If more than one egg is fertilized, **fraternal (dizygotic) twins** may be conceived. **Identical (monozygotic) twins**, in contrast, occur when one zygote divides into two separate embryos (see Cleavage below).

Cleavage

Early embryonic development is characterized by a series of rapid mitotic divisions known as **cleavage**. These divisions lead to an increase in cell number without a corresponding growth in cell protoplasm (i.e., the total volume of cytoplasm remains constant). Thus, cleavage results in progressively smaller cells with an increasing ratio of nuclei to cytoplasm. Cleavage also increases the surface-to-volume ratio of each cell, thereby improving gas and nutrient exchange.

The first complete cleavage of the zygote occurs approximately 32 hours after fertilization. The second cleavage occurs after 60 hours, and the third cleavage after approximately 72 hours, at which point the eight-celled embryo reaches the uterus. As cell division continues, a solid ball of embryonic cells, known as the **morula**, is formed. **Blastulation** begins when the morula develops a fluid-filled cavity called the **blastocoel**, which by the fourth day becomes a hollow sphere of cells called the **blastula**. The blastula is the stage of the embryo that implants in the uterus. Emergency contraception works partially by inhibiting implantation of the blastula in the uterus, which is why it is most effective if taken within 72 hours of the time of potential fertilization.

In a normal pregnancy the blastula implants in the uterus. In an ectopic pregnancy, the embryo implants outside the uterus, for example, in the fallopian tube. An embryo cannot be maintained for long outside of the uterus; it will abort spontaneously, and hemorrhaging will follow. Ectopic pregnancies can be fatal if not caught in time and managed appropriately.

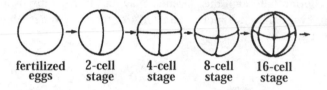

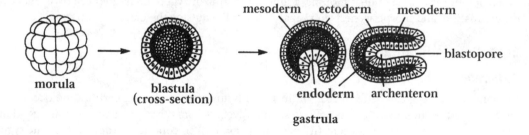

Figure 26.4

Gastrulation

After week two, the embryo is fully implanted in the uterus and cell migrations transform the single cell layer of the blastula into a three-layered structure called a gastrula. These three primary germ layers, listed below, are responsible for the differential development of the tissues, organs, and systems of the body at later stages of growth:

1. **Ectoderm:** gives rise to the integument (including the epidermis, hair, nails, and epithelium of the nose, mouth, and anal canal), the lens of the eye, the retina, and the nervous system

2. **Endoderm:** gives rise to the epithelial linings of the digestive and respiratory tracts (including the lungs) and parts of the liver, pancreas, thyroid, and bladder lining

3. **Mesoderm:** gives rise to the musculoskeletal system, circulatory system, excretory system, gonads, connective tissue throughout the body, and portions of digestive and respiratory organs

Neurulation

By the end of gastrulation, regions of the germ layers begin to develop into a rudimentary nervous system; this process is known as **neurulation** and starts before week three. A rod of mesodermal cells called the **notochord** develops along the longitudinal axis of the embryo just under the dorsal layer of ectoderm. The notochord has an inductive effect on the overlying ectoderm, causing it to bend inward and form a groove along the dorsal surface of the embryo. The dorsal ectoderm folds on either side of the groove; these neural folds grow upward and finally fuse, forming a closed tube. This is the neural tube, which gives rise to the brain and spinal cord (central nervous system). Once the neural tube is formed, it detaches from the surface ectoderm.

The cells at the tip of each neural fold are called the **neural crest cells**. These cells migrate laterally and give rise to many components of the peripheral nervous system, including the **sensory ganglia**, **autonomic ganglia**, **adrenal medulla**, and **Schwann cells**.

Sometimes during development the neural tube does not close properly, resulting in a condition in humans called spina bifida. This opening can be corrected surgically, but most patients have neurological impairments for the rest of their lives. The incidence of spina bifida can be decreased dramatically if the mother takes folic acid supplements during pregnancy.

Development

The final developmental processes can be divided into three different components that continue even after gestation (described below):

- **Organogenesis:** The body organs begin to form. In this process, the cells interact, differentiate, change physical shape, proliferate, and migrate.
- **Growth:** The organs increase in size, which is a continual process from infancy to childhood to adulthood.
- **Gametogenesis:** Eggs develop in women and sperm develop in men, which permits reproduction to occur.

Placental development

The growing fetus receives oxygen directly from its mother through a specialized circulatory system. This system not only supplies oxygen and nutrients to the fetus but removes carbon dioxide and metabolic wastes as well. The two components of this system are the **placenta** and the **umbilical cord**, which both develop in the first few weeks after fertilization.

The placenta and the umbilical cord are outgrowths of the four extra-embryonic membranes formed during development: the **amnion, chorion, allantois,** and **yolk sac**. The **amnion** is a thin, tough membrane containing a watery fluid called amniotic fluid. Amniotic fluid acts as a shock absorber of external pressure during gestation and localized pressure from uterine contractions during labor. Placenta formation begins with the **chorion**, a membrane that completely surrounds the amnion. The chorion assists with transfer of nutrients from the mother to the fetus. A third membrane, the **allantois**, develops as an outpocketing of the gut. The blood vessels of the allantoic wall enlarge and become the umbilical vessels, which will connect the fetus to the developing placenta. The **yolk sac**, the site of early development of blood vessels, becomes associated with the umbilical vessels.

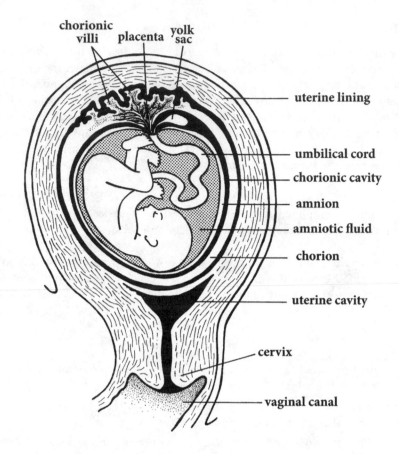

Figure 26.5

Gestation

Human pregnancy, or gestation, is approximately nine months (266 days) long and can be subdivided into three **trimesters**. The primary developments that occur during each trimester are described below.

First trimester

During the first weeks, the major organs begin to develop. The heart begins to beat at approximately 22 days, and soon afterward the eyes, gonads, limbs, and liver start to form. By five weeks the embryo is 10 mm in length; by six weeks the embryo has grown to 15 mm. The cartilaginous skeleton begins to turn into bone by the seventh week. By the end of eight weeks, most of the organs have formed, the brain is fairly developed, and the embryo is referred to as a fetus. At the end of the third month, the fetus is about 9 cm long.

Second trimester

During the second trimester, the fetus does a tremendous amount of growing. It begins to move around in the amniotic fluid, its face appears human, and its toes and fingers elongate. By the end of the sixth month, the fetus is 30–36 cm long.

Third trimester

The seventh and eighth months are characterized by continued rapid growth and further brain development. During the ninth month, antibodies are transported by highly selective active transport from the mother to the fetus for protection against foreign matter. The growth rate slows and the fetus becomes less active as it has less room to move about.

Birth and maturation

Childbirth is accomplished by **labor**, a series of strong uterine contractions. Labor can be divided into three distinct stages. In the first stage, the **cervix** thins and dilates, and the amniotic sac ruptures, releasing its fluids. During this time contractions are relatively mild. The second stage is characterized by rapid contractions, resulting in the birth of the baby (the umbilical cord is usually cut after this stage). During the final stage, the uterus contracts, expelling the placenta and the umbilical cord.

The embryo develops into the adult through the process of maturation, which involves cell division, growth, and differentiation. Differentiation of cells is complete when all organs reach adult form.

REVIEW PROBLEMS

1. Which of the following developmental stages has the greatest nuclear-to-cytoplasmic material ratio?

   (A) Four-celled zygote

   (B) Eight-celled zygote

   (C) Morula

   (D) Blastula

2. Name the three embryonic germ layers. Identify the embryological origin of the following structures: nails, thyroid, lens, testes, aorta, peripheral nerves, and lung epithelium.

3. Describe the structure of a blastula.

4. What is cleavage? When does the embryo first differentiate into germ layers?

5. Upon ovulation, the oocyte is released into the

   (A) fallopian tube.

   (B) ovary.

   (C) follicle.

   (D) abdominal cavity.

6. Describe three ways in which sexual reproduction promotes genetic variability. How does genetic variability benefit a species?

SOLUTIONS TO REVIEW PROBLEMS

1. **D** Discussed in early development section of this chapter.

2. The three embryonic germ layers are the endoderm, mesoderm, and ectoderm. The thyroid and lung epithelium are of endodermal origin. The testes and the aorta are of mesodermal origin. The nails, lens, and peripheral nerves are of ectodermal origin.

3. The name *blastula* refers to an early stage of development in which the embryo consists of a hollow ball of cells surrounding a cavity called the blastocoel.

4. Cleavage is the rapid division of cells early in the embryo's development. A determinate cleavage results in cells whose differentiation pathways are clearly defined; these cells are incapable of individually developing into complete organisms. The appearance of the three primary germ layers—the endoderm, mesoderm, and ectoderm—from such processes occurs during gastrulation.

5. **D** This subtle point about ovulation eludes most people and remains hard to believe until the organs are examined in anatomy class. The ruptured ovarian follicle releases an oocyte into the abdominal cavity, close to the entrance of the fallopian tube. With the aid of beating cilia, the oocyte is drawn into the fallopian tube, through which it travels until it reaches the uterus. If it is fertilized (in the fallopian tube), it will implant in the uterine wall; if it is not fertilized, it will be expelled along with the uterine lining during menstruation.

6. Sexual reproduction promotes genetic variability through the independent assortment of homologous chromosomes, the crossing over between homologous chromosomes during meiosis, and the random fertilization of an egg by a sperm.

   The independent assortment of chromosomes during gametogenesis allows for tremendous genetic variability by creating numerous possible combinations of chromosomes in a given gamete. During metaphase I, homologous chromosomes pair and randomly align at the metaphase plate. The random positioning of the homologous pairs determines which chromosomes are pulled toward each pole of the cell during anaphase. Thus, each resultant daughter cell has a random assortment of chromosomes, some of maternal origin and some of paternal origin.

   In addition to independent assortment, a random exchange of genes between chromosomes can occur via recombination. This allows for greater genetic variability by creating new combinations of genes on each chromosome. Recombination occurs during prophase I of meiosis, when homologous pairs of chromosomes align themselves side by side and exchange genetic information in a process called crossing over.

   Genetic variability is further enhanced by fertilization. An egg cell containing one of the millions of possible gene combinations fuses with a sperm cell containing another of the millions of possible combinations of different genes to create a zygote with a unique assortment of maternal and paternal genes.

   Genetic variability benefits a species because it increases the chances that the offspring will be able to adapt to a myriad of potential environmental stresses and conditions, and promotes evolution over many generations.

Section V

GENERAL CHEMISTRY

CHAPTER TWENTY-SEVEN

Atomic Structure

Chemistry is the study of the nature and behavior of matter. The **atom** is the basic building block of matter, representing the smallest unit of a chemical element. An atom in turn is composed of subatomic particles called **protons**, **neutrons**, and **electrons**. The protons and neutrons in an atom form the **nucleus**, the core of the atom. The electrons exist outside the nucleus in characteristic regions of space called **orbitals**. All atoms of an **element** show similar chemical properties and cannot be further broken down by chemical means.

SUBATOMIC PARTICLES

In the early 1800s, an English scientist by the name of John Dalton formulated a specific theory of invisible building blocks of matter that are now called atoms. Dalton's atomic theory marks the beginning of the modern era of chemistry. Below is a summary of the key points of his hypotheses:

- All **elements** are composed of very small particles called atoms. All atoms of a given element are identical in size, mass, and chemical properties (although we now know **isotopes**, atoms of the same element with different masses due to different numbers of protons, also exist). The atoms of one element are different from atoms of all other elements.

- All **compounds** are composed of atoms of more than one element. For any given compound, the ratio of the numbers of atoms of any two of the elements present is either an integer or a simple fraction.

- A given **chemical reaction** involves only the separation, combination, or rearrangement of atoms; it does NOT result in the creation or destruction of atoms.

Protons

Protons carry a single positive charge and have a mass of approximately one **unified atomic mass unit** (**amu** or **u**), which is equivalent to one **dalton (Da)**. The **atomic number (Z)** of an element is equal to the number of protons found in an atom of that element. All atoms of a given element have the same atomic number. These positively charged particles carry the same quantity of charge as an electron; however, they have a mass that is approximately 1,840 times greater than that of an electron. Although the mass of the nucleus of an atom therefore comprises almost the entire weight of an atom, it occupies only 10^{-13} of the volume of the atom. Putting this in perspective, if the entire atom was the size of a football stadium that seats 100,000 people, the volume of the actual nucleus would be that of a small marble.

Neutrons

Neutrons carry no charge and have a mass only slightly larger than that of protons so can still be considered to have a mass of approximately 1 u. Different **isotopes** of one element have different numbers of neutrons but the same number of protons.

Electrons

Electrons carry a charge equal in magnitude but opposite in sign to that of protons. An electron has a very small mass, approximately 1/1,837 the mass of a proton or neutron, which is negligible for the purposes of the PCAT. The electrons in the electron shell farthest from the nucleus are known as **valence electrons**. The farther the valence electrons are from the nucleus, the weaker the attractive force of the positively charged nucleus and the more likely the valence electrons are to be influenced by other atoms. Generally, the valence electrons and their activity determine the reactivity of an atom. In a neutral atom, the numbers of protons and electrons are equal. Therefore, the atomic number indicates the number of electrons in a neutral atom. A positive or negative charge on an atom is due to a loss or gain of electrons; the result is called an **ion**. Note that a (+) charge indicates a *loss* of negative electrons, whereas a (−) charges indicates a *gain* of electrons.

Some basic features of the three subatomic particles are shown in the table below.

Subatomic Particle	Symbol	Relative Mass	Charge	Location
Proton	$_{1}^{1}H^{+}$	1	+1	Nucleus
Neutron	$_{0}^{1}n$	1	0	Nucleus
Electron	e^{-}	0	−1	Electron orbitals

Table 24.1

Example: Determine the number of protons, neutrons, and electrons in a nickel-58 atom and in a nickel-60^{2+} cation.

Solution: ^{58}Ni has an atomic number of 28 and a mass number of 58. Therefore, ^{58}Ni has 28 protons, 28 electrons, and (58 − 28), or 30, neutrons.

In the $^{60}Ni^{2+}$ species, the number of protons is the same as in the neutral ^{58}Ni atom (28 protons). However, $^{60}Ni^{2+}$ has a positive charge because it has lost 2 electrons, so Ni^{2+} has 26 electrons (as opposed to the 28 electrons in ^{58}Ni). Also, the mass number is two units higher than for the ^{58}Ni atom, and this difference in mass must be due to 2 extra neutrons; thus, it has a total of 32 neutrons (as opposed to 30 neutrons in ^{58}Ni).

MASS NUMBER AND ISOTOPES

Mass Number

The atomic **mass number** (*A*) of an atom is equal to the total number of nucleons (protons and neutrons). The convention $^A_Z X$ is used to show both the atomic number and mass number of an X atom, where *Z* is the atomic number and *A* is the mass number such that:

$$\text{mass number } (A) = \text{number of protons} + \text{number of neutrons}$$

On a larger scale, the **molecular weight** is the weight in grams per one mole (mol) of a given element (g/mol). A **mole** is a unit used to count particles and is represented by **Avogadro's number**, 6.02×10^{23} particles/mol, which is how many atoms of carbon are in 12.0 g of carbon-12. Avogadro's number is the conversion factor between amu and g such that, if one atom of nitrogen has a mass of 14 u, then one mole of nitrogen has a mass of 14 g (see Chapter 30, Stoichiometry).

Isotopes

For a given element, multiple species of atoms with the same number of protons (same atomic number, *Z*) but different numbers of neutrons (different mass numbers, *A*) exist; these are called **isotopes** of the element. Isotopes are referred to either by the convention described above or, more commonly, by the name of the element followed by the mass number. For example, carbon-12 $\left(^{12}_6 C\right)$ is a carbon atom with 6 protons and 6 neutrons, while carbon-14 $\left(^{14}_6 C\right)$ is a carbon atom with 6 protons and 8 neutrons. Since isotopes have the same number of protons and electrons, they generally exhibit the same chemical properties.

In nature, almost all elements exist as a collection of two or more isotopes, and these isotopes are usually present in the same proportions in any sample of a naturally occurring element. Therefore, another common convention used to define the mass of an atom is **standard atomic weight**, which is a weighted average of all the isotopes of an element found naturally on Earth. The periodic table lists the atomic weight for the different elements, which accounts for the relative abundance of the various isotopes. The presence of these isotopes accounts for the fact that the accepted atomic weight for most elements is not a whole number. For example, nitrogen has two stable isotopes, ^{14}N and ^{15}N, but ^{14}N is much more common (99.6%), so the weighted average of the two is 14.007.

Example: Element Q consists of three different isotopes, A, B, and C. Isotope A has an atomic mass of 40 u and accounts for 60% of naturally occurring Q. The atomic mass of isotope B is 44 u and accounts for 25% of Q. Finally, isotope C has an atomic mass of 41 u and a natural abundance of 15%. What is the atomic weight of element Q?

Solution: $0.60(40 \text{ u}) + 0.25(44 \text{ u}) + 0.15(41 \text{ u}) = 24 \text{ u} + 11 \text{ u} + 6.15 \text{ u} = 41.15 \text{ u}$

The atomic weight of element Q is 41.15 g/mol.

BOHR'S MODEL OF THE HYDROGEN ATOM

In 1911, Ernest Rutherford provided experimental evidence that an atom has a dense, positively charged nucleus that accounts for only a small portion of the volume of the atom. In 1900, Max Planck developed the first **quantum theory**, proposing that energy emitted as electromagnetic radiation from matter comes in discrete bundles called **quanta**. The energy value of a quantum is given by the equation $E = hf$, where h is a proportionality constant known as **Planck's constant**, equal to 6.626×10^{-34} J·s, and f (sometimes designated v) is the **frequency** of the radiation.

The Bohr Model

In 1913, Niels Bohr used the work of Rutherford and Planck to develop his model of the electronic structure of the hydrogen atom. Starting from Rutherford's findings, Bohr assumed that the hydrogen atom consisted of a central proton around which an electron traveled in a circular orbit, and that the centripetal force acting on the electron as it revolved around the nucleus was the electrical force between the positively charged proton and the negatively charged electron.

Bohr's model used the quantum theory of Planck in conjunction with concepts from classical physics. In classical mechanics, an object, such as an electron, revolving in a circle may assume an infinite number of values for its radius and velocity. Therefore, the **angular momentum** ($L = mvr$) and **kinetic energy** $\left(KE = \dfrac{mv^2}{2} \right)$ can take on any value. However, by incorporating Planck's quantum theory into his model, Bohr placed conditions on the value of the angular momentum. Like Planck's energy, the angular momentum (L) of an electron is quantized according to the following equation:

$$L = \frac{nh}{2\pi}$$

where h is Planck's constant and n is the principal quantum number, which can be any positive integer. Since h, 2, and π are constants, the angular momentum changes only in discrete amounts with respect to n.

Bohr then equated the allowed values of the angular momentum to the energy of the electron. He obtained the following equation:

$$E = -\frac{Ry}{n^2}$$

where Ry is an experimentally determined constant (known as the **Rydberg energy** and representing the product of three different constants: R_H, h, and c) equal to 2.18×10^{-18} J/electron. Therefore, like angular momentum, the energy of the electron changes in discrete amounts with respect to n.

A value of zero energy was assigned to the state in which the proton and electron were separated completely, meaning that there was no attractive force between them. Therefore, the electron in any of its quantized states in the atom would have a negative energy as a result of the attractive forces between the electron and proton. This explains the negative sign in the above equation for energy.

Applications of the Bohr Model

In his model of the structure of hydrogen, Bohr postulated that an electron can exist only in certain fixed-energy states. In terms of quantum theory, the energy of an electron is **quantized**. Using this model, certain generalizations concerning the characteristics of electrons can be made. The energy of the electron is related to its **orbital radius**: the smaller the radius, the lower the energy state of the electron. The smallest orbit (radius) an electron can have corresponds to $n = 1$, which is the ground state of the hydrogen electron. At the **ground state** level, the electron is in its lowest energy state. The Bohr model is also used to explain the atomic emission spectrum and atomic absorption spectrum of hydrogen, and it is helpful in interpretation of the spectra of other atoms.

Atomic emission spectra

At room temperature, the majority of atoms in a sample are in the ground state. However, electrons can be excited to higher energy levels by heat (or other) energy to yield the excited state of the atom. Because the lifetime of the excited state is brief, the electrons will return rapidly to the ground state while emitting energy in the form of photons. The electromagnetic energy of these photons may be determined using the following equation:

$$E = \frac{hc}{\lambda}$$

where h is Planck's constant, c is the velocity of light in a vacuum (3.00×10^8 m/s), and λ is the wavelength of the radiation.

The different electrons in an atom will be excited to different energy levels. When these electrons return to their ground states, each will emit a photon with a wavelength characteristic of the specific transition it undergoes. The quantized energies of light emitted under these conditions do not produce a continuous spectrum (as expected from classical physics). Rather, the spectrum is composed of light at specific frequencies and is thus known as a **line spectrum**, where each line on the emission spectrum corresponds to a specific electronic transition. Because each element can have its electrons excited to different distinct energy levels, each element possesses a unique **atomic emission spectrum**, which can be used as a fingerprint. One particular application of atomic emissions spectroscopy is in the analysis of stars; although physical samples of the stars cannot be taken, the light from a star can be resolved into its component wavelengths, which are then matched to the known line spectra of the elements.

The Bohr model of the hydrogen atom explained the atomic emission spectrum of hydrogen, which is the simplest emission spectrum among all the elements. The group of hydrogen emission lines corresponding to transitions from upper levels $n > 2$ to $n = 2$ is known as the **Balmer series** (four wavelengths in the visible region), while the group corresponding to transitions between upper levels $n > 1$ to $n = 1$ is known as the **Lyman series** (higher energy transitions in the UV region). Below is a summary of various series in the hydrogen atomic emission spectrum where n_f and n_i are the final and initial states, respectively.

Series	n_f	n_i	Spectrum region
Lyman	1	2, 3, 4 . . .	Ultraviolet
Balmer	2	3, 4, 5 . . .	Visible and Ultraviolet
Paschen	3	4, 5, 6 . . .	Infrared

Table 24.2

When the energy of each frequency of light observed in the emission spectrum of hydrogen was calculated according to Planck's quantum theory, the values obtained closely matched those expected from energy-level transitions in the Bohr model. That is, the energy associated with a change in the quantum number from an initial value n_i to a final value n_f is equal to the energy of Planck's emitted photon. Thus:

$$E = \frac{hc}{\lambda} = -Ry\left(\frac{1}{n_i^2} - \frac{1}{n_f^2}\right)$$

and the energy of the emitted photon corresponds to the precise difference in energy between the higher-energy initial state and the lower-energy final state.

Atomic absorption spectra

When an electron is excited to a higher energy level, it must absorb energy. The energy absorbed as an electron jumps from an orbital of low energy to one of higher energy is characteristic of that transition. This means that the excitation of electrons in a particular element results in energy absorptions at specific wavelengths. Thus, in addition to an emission spectrum, every element possesses a characteristic **absorption spectrum**. Not surprisingly, the wavelengths of absorption correspond directly to the wavelengths of emission since the energy difference between levels remains unchanged. Absorption spectra can thus be used in the identification of elements present in a gas phase sample.

QUANTUM MECHANICAL MODEL OF ATOMS

While the concepts put forth by Bohr offered a reasonable explanation for the structure of the hydrogen atom and ions containing only one electron (such as He^{1+} and Li^{2+}), they did not explain the structures of atoms containing more than one electron. This is because Bohr's model does not take into consideration the repulsion between multiple electrons surrounding one nucleus. Modern quantum mechanics has led to a more rigorous and generalized study of the electronic structure of atoms. The most important difference between the Bohr model and modern quantum mechanical models is that Bohr's assumption that electrons follow a circular orbit at a fixed distance from the nucleus is no longer considered valid. Rather, electrons are described as being in a state of rapid motion within regions of space around the nucleus called **orbitals**. An orbital is a representation of the probability of finding an electron within a given region. In the current quantum mechanical description of electrons, pinpointing both the exact location and momentum of an electron at any given point in time is impossible. This idea is best described by the **Heisenberg uncertainty principle**, which states that it is impossible to simultaneously determine, with perfect accuracy, the momentum (defined as mass times velocity) and the position of an electron. This means that if the momentum of the electron is being measured accurately, its position will not be certain, and vice versa.

Quantum Numbers

Modern atomic theory states that any electron in an atom can be completely described by four **quantum numbers**: n, ℓ, m_ℓ, and m_s. Furthermore, according to the **Pauli exclusion principle**, no two electrons in a given atom can possess the same set of four quantum numbers. The position and energy of an electron described by its quantum numbers is known as its **energy state**. The value of n limits the values of ℓ, which in turn limit the values of m_ℓ. The values of three of the quantum numbers qualitatively give information about the orbitals: n about the size, ℓ about the shape, and m_ℓ about the orientation of the orbital. All four quantum numbers are discussed below.

Principal quantum number

The first quantum number is commonly known as the **principal quantum number** and is denoted by the letter n. This is the quantum number used in Bohr's model that can theoretically take on any positive integer value and represents the **shell** where an electron is present in an atom. The maximum n that can be used to describe the electrons of an element at its ground state corresponds with that element's period (row) in the periodic table. For example, nitrogen is in period 2, so neutral N in its ground state has electrons with n values of 1 and 2. The larger the integer value of n, the higher the energy level and radius of the electron's orbit. The maximum number of electrons in an electron shell n is $2n^2$.

The difference in energy between adjacent shells decreases as the distance from the nucleus increases because the difference is related to the expression $\frac{1}{n_2^2} - \frac{1}{n_1^2}$. For example, the energy difference between the third and fourth shells ($n = 3$ and $n = 4$) is less than that between the second and third shells ($n = 2$ and $n = 3$).

Azimuthal quantum number

The second quantum number is called the **azimuthal (angular momentum) quantum number** and is designated by the letter ℓ. This number tells us the shape of the orbitals and refers to the **subshells** or **sublevels** that occur within each principal energy level. For any given n, the value of ℓ can be any integer in the range of 0 to $n - 1$. The four subshells corresponding to $\ell = 0$, 1, 2, and 3 are known as the sharp, principal, diffuse, and fundamental subshells, or s, p, d, and f subshells, respectively. The maximum number of electrons that can exist within a subshell is given by the equation $4\ell + 2$. The greater the value of ℓ, the greater the energy of the subshell. However, the energies of subshells from different principal energy levels may overlap. For example, the 4*s* subshell will have a lower energy than the 3d subshell because its average distance from the nucleus is smaller.

Magnetic quantum number

The third quantum number is the **magnetic quantum number** and is designated m_ℓ. This number describes the orientation of the **orbital** in space. An orbital is a specific region within a subshell that may contain no more than two electrons. The magnetic quantum number specifies the particular orbital within a subshell where an electron is highly likely to be found at a given point in time. The possible values of m_ℓ are all integers from ℓ to $-\ell$ including 0. Therefore, the s subshell ($\ell = 0$), has only one possible value of m_ℓ (0) and will contain one orbital; in contrast, the p subshell ($\ell = 1$) has three possible m_ℓ values (-1, 0, $+1$) and three orbitals. The d subshell ($\ell = 2$) has five possible m_ℓ values (-2, -1, 0, $+1$, $+2$) and five orbitals; the f subshell ($\ell = 3$) has seven possible m_ℓ values (-3, -2, -1, 0, $+1$, $+2$, $+3$) and contains seven orbitals. The shape and energy of each orbital are dependent upon the subshell in which the orbital is found. For example, a p subshell with its three possible m_ℓ values (-1, 0, $+1$) has three dumbbell-shaped orbitals that are oriented in space around the nucleus along the *x*, *y*, and *z* axes. These 3 orbitals are often referred to as p_x, p_y, and p_z.

Spin quantum number

The fourth quantum number is also called the **spin quantum number** and is denoted by m_s. The spin of a particle is its intrinsic angular momentum and is a characteristic of a particle. The two spin orientations are designated $+\frac{1}{2}$ and $-\frac{1}{2}$. Whenever two electrons are in the same orbital, they must have opposite spins. Electrons in different orbitals (different m_ℓ values) with the same m_s values are said to have **parallel** spins. Electrons with opposite spins (different m_s values) in the same orbital (same m_ℓ value) are often referred to as **paired**.

The following table is an example that shows all of the possible quantum numbers for the eight electrons in the second shell ($n = 2$). The numbers in parentheses represent the number of electrons in the region limited by the coresponding quantum number. Thus, all eight electrons in the second shell have $n = 2$, two electrons have $\ell = 0$, six electrons have $\ell = 1$, and so on. Note that the numbers in parentheses for each row must add up to eight, the total number of electrons in the shell.

n	2 (8)						
ℓ	0 (2)		1 (6)				
m_ℓ	0 (2)		−1 (2)		0 (2)		+1 (2)
m_s	$+\frac{1}{2}(1)$	$-\frac{1}{2}(1)$	$+\frac{1}{2}(1)$	$-\frac{1}{2}(1)$	$+\frac{1}{2}(1)$	$-\frac{1}{2}(1)$	$+\frac{1}{2}(1)$

Table 27.3

Electron Configuration and Orbital Filling

For a given atom or ion, the pattern by which subshells are filled and the number of electrons within each principal level and subshell are designated by an **electron configuration**. In electron configuration notation, the first number denotes the principal energy level, the letter designates the subshell, and the superscript gives the number of electrons in that subshell. For example, $2p^4$ indicates that there are four electrons in the second subshell (p) of the second principal energy level ($n = 2$). Note that the third and fourth quantum numbers (m_ℓ and m_s) are not indicated in the electron configuration but can be determined for a given electron using the rules from earlier in this chapter if necessary.

When writing the electron configuration of an atom, it is necessary to remember the order in which subshells are filled. According to the **Aufbau principle**, subshells are filled from lowest to highest energy, and each subshell will fill completely before electrons begin to enter the next one. The $(n + \ell)$ **rule** is used to rank subshells by increasing energy. This rule states that the lower the sum of the first and second quantum numbers, the lower the energy of the subshell. If two subshells possess the same $(n + \ell)$ value, the subshell with the lower n value has a lower energy and will fill first. The order in which the subshells fill is shown in the following chart.

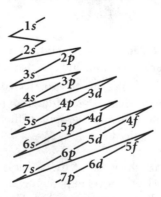

Figure 27.1

Example: Which will fill first, the 3d subshell or the 4s subshell?

Solution: For 3d, $n = 3$ and $\ell = 2$, so $(n + \ell) = 5$. For 4s, $n = 4$ and $\ell = 0$, so $(n + \ell) = 4$. Therefore, the 4s subshell has a lower energy and will fill first. This can also be determined from examining Figure 27.1.

To determine which subshells are filled, you must know the number of electrons in the atom. In the case of uncharged atoms, the number of electrons equals the atomic number. If the atom is charged, the number of electrons is equal to the atomic number plus the extra electrons if the atom is negative or the atomic number minus the missing electrons if the atom is positive.

In subshells that contain more than one orbital, such as the 2p subshell with its three orbitals, the orbitals will fill according to **Hund's Rule**. Hund's Rule states that, within a given subshell, orbitals are filled such that there are a maximum number of half-filled orbitals with parallel spins. Electrons "prefer" empty orbitals to half-filled ones because a pairing energy must be overcome for two electrons carrying repulsive negative charges to exist in the same orbital.

Example:　　What are the written electron configurations for nitrogen (N) and iron (Fe) according to Hund's Rule?

Solution:　　Nitrogen has an atomic number of 7, thus its electron configuration is $1s^2 \, 2s^2 \, 2p^3$. According to Hund's Rule, the two s orbitals will fill completely, while the three p orbitals will each contain one electron, all with parallel spins.

$$\underset{1s^2}{\underline{\uparrow\downarrow}} \quad \underset{2s^2}{\underline{\uparrow\downarrow}} \quad \underset{2p^3}{\underline{\uparrow}\;\underline{\uparrow}\;\underline{\uparrow}}$$

Iron has an atomic number of 26, and its 4s subshell fills before the 3d. Using Hund's Rule, the electron configuration will be:

$$\underset{1s^2}{\underline{\uparrow\downarrow}} \qquad \underset{2s^2}{\underline{\uparrow\downarrow}} \quad \underset{2p^6}{\underline{\uparrow\downarrow}\;\underline{\uparrow\downarrow}\;\underline{\uparrow\downarrow}} \quad \underset{3s^2}{\underline{\uparrow\downarrow}} \quad \underset{3p^6}{\underline{\uparrow\downarrow}\;\underline{\uparrow\downarrow}\;\underline{\uparrow\downarrow}} \quad \underset{3d^6}{\underline{\uparrow\downarrow}\;\underline{\uparrow}\;\underline{\uparrow}\;\underline{\uparrow}\;\underline{\uparrow}} \quad \underset{4s^2}{\underline{\uparrow\downarrow}}$$

Iron's electron configuration is written as $1s^2 \, 2s^2 \, 2p^6 \, 3s^2 \, 3p^6 \, 3d^6 \, 4s^2$. Subshells may be listed either in the order in which they fill (e.g., 4s before 3d) or with subshells of the same principal quantum number grouped together, as shown here. Both methods are correct.

The presence of paired or unpaired electrons affects the chemical and magnetic properties of an atom or molecule. If the material has unpaired electrons, a magnetic field will align the spins of these electrons and weakly attract the atom to the field. These materials are said to be **paramagnetic**. Materials that have no unpaired electrons and are slightly repelled by a magnetic field are said to be **diamagnetic**.

Valence Electrons

The valence electrons of an atom are those electrons that are in its outer energy shell or that are available for chemical bonding. For elements in Groups IA and IIA, only the outermost s electrons are valence electrons. For elements in Groups IIIA through VIIIA, the outermost s and p electrons in the highest energy shell are valence electrons. For transition elements, the valence electrons are those in the outermost s subshell and in the d subshell of the next-to-outermost energy shell. For the inner transition elements (the lanthanide and actinide series), the valence electrons are those in the s subshell of the outermost energy shell, the d subshell of the next-to-outermost energy shell, and the f subshell of the energy shell two levels below the outermost shell.

Group IIIA–VIIA elements beyond Period 2 might, under some circumstances, accept electrons into their empty d subshells, which gives them more than eight valence electrons.

Example: Which are the valence electrons of elemental iron, elemental selenium, and the sulfur atom in a sulfate ion?

Solution: Iron has 8 valence electrons: 2 in its 4s subshell and 6 in its 3d subshell.

Selenium has 6 valence electrons: 2 in its 4s subshell and 4 in its 4p subshell. Selenium's 3d electrons are not part of its valence shell.

Sulfur in a sulfate ion has 12 valence electrons: its original 6 plus 6 more from the oxygen to which it is bonded. Sulfur's 3s and 3p subshells can only contain 8 of these 12 electrons; the other 4 electrons have entered the sulfur atom's 3d subshell, which in elemental sulfur is empty.

REVIEW PROBLEMS

1. The Mg^{2+} ion has how many electrons?

   (A) 12
   (B) 10
   (C) 14
   (D) 24

2. It can be shown using mass spectrometry that the ratio of naturally occurring chlorine-35 to its isotope chlorine-37 is 3:1. Assuming no other isotopes exist, what is the standard atomic weight of chlorine?

3. A student represents electrons within the same orbital as having parallel spins. This goes against which of the following principles?

   (A) Bohr's model of the hydrogen atom
   (B) Pauli exclusion principle
   (C) Heisenberg's uncertainty principle
   (D) Planck's quantum theory

4. What are the four quantum numbers? Discuss how they are related and to what each refers.

5. The maximum number of electrons in a shell with a principal quantum number of 4 is

   (A) 2.
   (B) 10.
   (C) 16.
   (D) 32.

6. In Bohr's model of the hydrogen atom, the energy of an electron is directly dependent on

   (A) the spin quantum number (m_s).
   (B) Planck's constant (h).
   (C) the principal quantum number (n).
   (D) the angular momentum quantum number (ℓ).

7. Which of the following describes the excitation exhibited when an electron jumps from its ground state to a higher energy level?

   (A) Balmer series
   (B) Atomic absorption spectrum
   (C) Lyman series
   (D) Atomic emission spectrum

8. The Pauli exclusion principle states that

   (A) no two electrons can have the same four quantum numbers.
   (B) it is impossible to determine simultaneously the momentum and the position of an electron.
   (C) energy is emitted from matter as quantized units.
   (D) an electron will enter an empty orbital in a subshell before entering half-filled orbitals.

9. Atoms with the same atomic numbers but with different mass numbers are known as
   - (A) elements.
   - (B) isomers.
   - (C) ions.
   - (D) isotopes.

10. If the principal quantum number of a shell is equal to 2, what types of orbitals will be present?
    - (A) s
    - (B) s and p
    - (C) s, p, and d
    - (D) s, p, d, and f

11. What quantity of energy is emitted when a hydrogen electron relaxes from $n = 3$ to $n = 2$? ($R_H = 2.18 \times 10^{-18}$ J)

12. What wavelength (in nm) corresponds to the energy calculated in Question 11? ($c = 3 \times 10^8$ m/s)

13. What is the total number of electrons that could be held in a subshell with an angular momentum number equal to 2?
    - (A) 2
    - (B) 6
    - (C) 8
    - (D) 10

14. An element with an atomic number of 26 has how many electrons in the $3d$ subshell?
    - (A) 0
    - (B) 2
    - (C) 6
    - (D) 8

15. An energy value of -328 kJ/mol corresponds to the energy of an electron in which principal energy level? ($R_H = 1{,}312$ kJ/mol)
    - (A) 1
    - (B) 2
    - (C) 3
    - (D) 4

16. In going from $1s^2\, 2s^2\, 2p^6\, 3s^2\, 3p^6\, 4s^1$ to $1s^2\, 2s^2\, 2p^6\, 3s^2\, 3p^5\, 4s^2$, an electron would
    - (A) absorb energy.
    - (B) emit energy.
    - (C) relax to the ground state.
    - (D) bind to another atom.

17. The values of the spin quantum number are directly related to

    (A) the principal quantum number.

    (B) the angular momentum quantum number.

    (C) the magnetic quantum number.

    (D) none of the above.

18. Which of the following orbitals has the lowest energy?

    (A) 2p

    (B) 3s

    (C) 3d

    (D) 4s

19. Which of the following correctly represents the excited state of scandium?

    (A) $1s^2\ 2s^2\ 2p^6\ 3s^2\ 3p^6\ 3d^1\ 4s^2$

    (B) $1s^2\ 2s^3\ 2p^5\ 3s^2\ 3p^6\ 3d^1\ 4s^2$

    (C) $1s^2\ 2s^2\ 2p^6\ 3s^2\ 3p^6\ 3d^2\ 4s^1$

    (D) $1s^2\ 2s^2\ 2p^6\ 3s^2\ 3p^6\ 3d^2\ 4s^2$

20. The photon frequency of red light is $4.51 \times 10^{14}\ s^{-1}$. If $Ry = 2.18 \times 10^{-18}$, what is the energy of the photon? Is this enough energy to cause a hydrogen electron to be excited from $n = 1$ to $n = 3$?

SOLUTIONS TO REVIEW PROBLEMS

1. **B** Magnesium has an atomic number of 12, meaning that it has 12 protons and 12 electrons. However, the Mg^{2+} ion has a positive charge because it has lost 2 electrons. Therefore, the Mg^{2+} ion has 10 electrons.

2. **35.5**

   Mass spectrometry shows that three out of every four chlorine atoms are Cl-35 and one is Cl-37. Thus, 75% of all chlorine atoms are Cl-35, and 25% are Cl-37. Using this information and the atomic weights of the isotopes (Cl-35 = 35 g/mol, Cl-37 = 37 g/mol), the atomic weight of chlorine can be determined as follows:

   $(0.75)(35 \text{ g/mol}) + (0.25)(37 \text{ g/mol})$

   $= (26.25 + 9.25) \text{ g/mol}$

   $= 35.5 \text{ g/mol}$

3. **B** Discussed in the section on quantum numbers in this chapter.

4. Discussed in the section on quantum numbers in this chapter.

5. **D** The maximum number of electrons within a principal energy level is given by the equation $2n^2$. Therefore, a shell with a principal quantum number equal to 4 will hold a maximum of 32 electrons.

6. **C** In the Bohr model for hydrogen, the energy of the electron is given by the equation $E = -\dfrac{Ry}{n^2}$ where R_H is a theoretically determined constant. Therefore, the energy of the electron is dependent only on n, the principal quantum number.

7. **B** For electrons to jump from ground state to higher energy levels, they must absorb energy. Therefore, the movements from ground state to excited state are characterized by an atomic absorption spectrum.

8. **A** Discussed in the section on quantum numbers in this chapter.

9. **D** Atomic weight equals the number of protons (atomic number) plus the number of neutrons. If two atoms have the same atomic number but different atomic weights, then the number of neutrons must be different. This is the definition of an isotope.

10. **B** When the principal quantum number is equal to 2, then the angular momentum quantum number will have values of $\ell = 0$ and 1. When $\ell = 0$, the subshell is an s subshell, and, when $\ell = 1$, the subshell is a p subshell. Therefore, the second principal energy level contains an s subshell and a p subshell.

11.   **3.03×10^{-19} J**

To calculate the energy emitted when a hydrogen electron relaxes from $n = 3$ to $n = 2$, the equation $E = -R_H\left(\dfrac{1}{n_i^2} - \dfrac{1}{n_f^2}\right)$ is used, where $R_H = 2.18 \times 10^{-18}$ J and n_i and n_f are equal to 3 and 2, respectively. The calculation is performed as follows:

$$E = -2.18 \times 10^{-18} \text{ J}\left(\frac{1}{3^2} - \frac{1}{2^2}\right)$$

$$E = -2.18 \times 10^{-18} \text{ J}\left(\frac{1}{9} - \frac{1}{4}\right)$$

$$E = -2.18 \times 10^{-18} \text{ J}\left(\frac{4}{36} - \frac{9}{36}\right)$$

$$E = -2.18 \times 10^{-18} \text{ J}\left(-\frac{5}{36}\right)$$

$$E = 3.03 \times 10^{-19} \text{ J}$$

The value of the energy is positive because energy is released when an electron falls from an excited state back to the ground state.

12.   **656 nm**

The wavelength in nm of a photon that carries the 3.03×10^{-19} J of energy found in Question 11 can be determined as follows:

$$E = \frac{hc}{\lambda}, \text{ thus, by rearrangement, } \lambda = \frac{hc}{E}.$$

$$\lambda = \frac{\left(6.626 \times 10^{-34} \text{ J} \cdot \text{s}\right)\left(3 \times 10^8 \text{m/s}\right)}{3.03 \times 10^{-19} \text{ J}}$$

$$= 656 \text{ nm}$$

13. **D**   The angular momentum number 2 corresponds to the d subshell, and d is capable of holding a maximum of $4(2) + 2 = 10$ electrons.

14. **C**   An element with an atomic number of 26 will have 6 electrons in its 3d subshell. This can be determined by writing the electron configuration for the element: $1s^2\ 2s^2\ 2p^6\ 3s^2\ 3p^6\ 3d^6\ 4s^2$. The number of electrons must equal 26; recall that the $4s$ subshell must be filled before the 3d because it has the lower energy. Thus, 3d will carry 6 electrons.

15. **B**   To determine which of the principal energy levels has an energy of -328 kJ/mol, the equation $E = -\dfrac{R_H}{n^2}$ is used ($R_H = 1{,}312$ kJ/mol). Solving for n:

$$-328 \text{ kJ/mol} = -\frac{1{,}312 \text{ kJ/mol}}{n^2}$$

$$n^2 = 4$$

$$n = 2$$

Therefore, the second principal energy level has an energy of -328 kJ/mol.

16. **A** The difference between the first and second electron configurations is that in the second configuration one electron has moved from the 3p subshell to the 4s subshell. Although the 3p and 4s subshells have the same $(n + \ell)$ value, the 3p subshell fills first because it is slightly lower in energy. For an electron to move from the 3p subshell to the 4s subshell, it must absorb energy.

17. **D** The spin quantum number is the intrinsic angular momentum of an electron in an orbital. The spin number can be either $+\frac{1}{2}$ or $-\frac{1}{2}$. These numbers are arbitrary and are not dependent on the other three quantum numbers.

18. **A** To determine which subshell has the lowest energy, the $(n + \ell)$ rule must be used. The values of the first and second quantum numbers are added together, and the subshell with the lowest $(n + \ell)$ value has the lowest energy. The sums of the five choices are $(2 + 1) = 3$, $(3 + 0) = 3$, $(3 + 2) = 5$, $(4 + 0) = 4$, $(3 + 1) = 4$. Choices (A) and (B) have the same $(n + \ell)$ value, so the subshell with the lower principal quantum number has the lower energy. This is the 2p subshell.

19. **C** Scandium has 21 electrons. Its ground-state electron configuration is $1s^2\ 2s^2\ 2p^6\ 3s^2\ 3p^6\ 3d^1\ 4s^2$. When it is in its excited state, one or more of the electrons will be present in a subshell with a higher energy than the one in which it is usually located. The number of electrons and ordering of subshells will not vary from the ground-state electron configuration of scandium. Choice (C) has one of the 4s electrons present in the 3d orbital. This represents an excited state because energy is required to cause an electron to jump from 4s to 3d.

20. **2.988×10^{-19} J; No**

    To determine the energy of a photon with a frequency (v) of 4.51×10^{14} s^{-1}, the following calculations are performed:

    $E = hv$

    $E = (6.626 \times 10^{-34}\ \text{J} \cdot \text{s})\ (4.51 \times 10^{14}\ \text{s}^{-1})$

    $E = 2.988 \times 10^{-19}\ \text{J}$

    The energy from red light will not be sufficient to excite a hydrogen electron from $n = 1$ to $n = 3$. This is because the energy necessary to perform that excitation is:

    $$\Delta E = -Ry \times \left(\frac{1}{n_i^2} - \frac{1}{n_f^2} \right)$$

    $$\Delta E = -2.18 \times 10^{-18}\ \text{J} \left(\frac{1}{1^2} - \frac{1}{3^2} \right)$$

    $$\Delta E = -2.18 \times 10^{-18}\ \text{J} \left(\frac{8}{9} \right)$$

    $$\Delta E = -1.937 \times 10^{-18}\ \text{J}$$

    The magnitude of this energy is greater than the energy of red light.

CHAPTER TWENTY-EIGHT

The Periodic Table

In 1869, the Russian chemist Dmitri Mendeleev published the first version of his periodic table, in which he showed that ordering the elements according to atomic weight produced a pattern where similar properties periodically recurred. This table was later revised, using the work of the physicist Henry Moseley, to organize the elements on the basis of increasing atomic number. Using this revised table, the properties of certain elements that had not yet been discovered were predicted: A number of these predictions were later borne out by experimentation. The substance of this work is summarized in the **periodic law**, which states that the chemical properties of the elements are dependent, in a systematic way, upon their atomic numbers.

In the periodic table used today, the elements are arranged in **periods** (rows) and **groups** (columns). There are seven periods, representing the principal quantum numbers $n = 1$ to $n = 7$, and each period is filled sequentially. Groups represent elements that have the same electronic configuration in their **valence**, or outermost, shell and share similar chemical properties. The electrons in the outermost shell are called **valence electrons**. They are involved in chemical bonding and determine the chemical reactivity and properties of the element. The Roman numeral above each group represents the number of valence electrons. There are two sets of groups, designated A and B. The A elements are the **representative elements**, which have either s or p sublevels as their outermost orbitals. These representative elements are those in Groups IA through VIIA, all of which have incompletely filled s or p subshells of the highest principal number. The B elements are the **nonrepresentative elements**, including the **transition elements**, which have partly filled d sublevels, and the **lanthanide** and **actinide** series, which have partly filled f sublevels. The electron configuration for the valence electrons is indicated by the Roman numeral and letter designations. For example, an element in Group VA has a valence electron configuration of s^2p^3 ($2 + 3 = 5$ valence electrons).

PERIODIC PROPERTIES OF THE ELEMENTS

The properties of the elements exhibit certain trends that can be explained in terms of the position of the element in the periodic table or in terms of the electron configuration of the element. All elements seek to gain or lose valence electrons so as to achieve the stable, fully filled formations possessed by the **inert** or **noble gases** of Group VIIIA. Two other important trends exist within the periodic table. First, from left to right across a period, protons are added one at a time and the electrons of the outermost shell experience an increasing amount of nuclear attraction, becoming closer and more tightly bound to the nucleus. This net positive charge from the nucleus, as felt by an electron, is called the **effective nuclear charge** (Z_{eff}). Second, from top to bottom down a given column, the outermost electrons become less tightly bound to the nucleus. This is because the number of filled principal energy levels (which shield the outermost electrons from attraction by the nucleus) increases downward within each group. Taken together, these trends show that Z_{eff} is at a maximum for elements in the top-right of the table and at a minimum for those in the bottom-left and help explain elemental properties such as atomic radius, ionization potential, electron affinity, and electronegativity.

Atomic Radii

The atomic radius of an element is equal to one-half the distance between the centers of two atoms of that element that are just barely touching each other. For example, the atomic radius of a metal is one-half the distance between the two nuclei in two adjacent atoms. In general, the atomic radius decreases across a period from left to right and increases down a given group; the atoms with the largest atomic radii will be located at the bottom of groups and toward the left of the table (Group IA).

As discussed in Chapter 27, Atomic Structure, the electron cloud occupies the majority of the volume of an atom, whereas the nucleus takes up relatively little space. Therefore, something that affects the size of the electron cloud will change the radius of an atom, but altering the size of the nucleus will not directly affect the size of the atom.

From left to right across a period, electrons are added one at a time to the outer energy shell. Electrons within the same shell do not shield one another from the attractive pull of protons. Therefore, since the number of protons is also increasing from left to right across a period, the effective nuclear charge (Z_{eff}) increases as well. The greater the positive charge experienced by the valence electrons (the larger the Z_{eff}), the closer those electrons are pulled toward the nucleus and the smaller the atomic radius.

From top to bottom down a group, the number of electrons and filled electron shells increase. Although the number of valence electrons within a group remains the same, these valence electrons will be found farther from the nucleus as they are in progressively larger energy shells. Z_{eff} will become smaller with distance, so valence electrons in higher energy shells will feel less pull from the nucleus. Also, with more electrons comes increased repulsion from the additional negative ($-$) charges. Thus, the atomic radii will increase.

The **ionic radius** is the radius of a cation or an anion. The ionic radius will affect the physical and chemical properties of an ionic compound. In most situations, cations (positive ions) will be smaller than corresponding neutral atoms since possessing fewer electrons leads to less repulsion among the remaining electrons. Likewise, most anions (negative ions) will be larger than corresponding neutral atoms because having a greater number of electrons causes more repulsion, resulting in a greater distance between electrons and a larger atomic radius.

Ionization Energy

The ionization energy (IE) is the energy required to remove an electron completely from a gaseous atom or ion. Removing an electron from an atom always requires an input of energy and is endothermic. The closer and more tightly bound an electron is to the nucleus, the more difficult it will be to remove and the higher the ionization energy. The **first ionization energy** is the energy required to remove one valence electron from the parent atom, the **second ionization energy** is the energy needed to remove a second valence electron from the univalent ion to form the divalent ion, and so on. Successive ionization energies grow increasingly larger; i.e., the second ionization energy is always greater than the first ionization energy.

For example:

$$Mg(g) \rightarrow Mg^+(g) + e^- \quad \text{First Ionization Energy} = 7.646\,eV$$
$$Mg^+(g) \rightarrow Mg^{2+}(g) + e^- \quad \text{Second Ionization Energy} = 15.035\,eV$$

Ionization energy increases from left to right across a period as Z_{eff} increases. Moving down a group, the ionization energy decreases as Z_{eff} decreases. Group IA elements have low ionization energies because the loss of an electron results in the formation of a stable, noble-gas configuration.

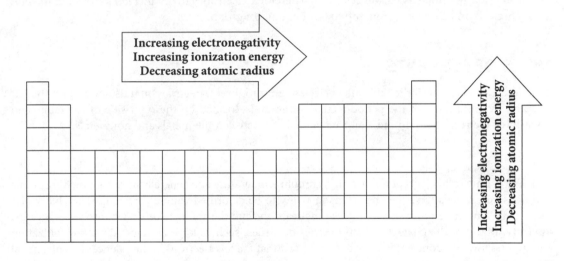

Figure 28.1

Electron Affinity

Electron affinity (EA) is the energy change that occurs when an electron is added to a gaseous atom, and it represents the ease with which the atom can accept an electron. The higher the Z_{eff}, the greater the electron affinity will be. In discussing electron affinities, two sign conventions are used. The more common one states that a positive electron affinity value represents energy release when an electron is added to an atom; the other states that a negative electron affinity represents a release of energy. In this discussion, the first convention will be used.

Electron affinity can be best represented by the following equation, where X is an atom of a given element in the gaseous state (g):

$$X(g) + e^- \rightarrow X^-(g)$$

Generalizations can be made about the electron affinities of particular groups in the periodic table. For example, the Group IIA elements, or **alkaline earth metals**, have low electron affinity values. These elements are relatively stable because their s subshell is filled. Group VIIA elements, or **halogens**, have high electron affinities because the addition of an electron to the atom results in a completely filled shell, which represents a stable electron configuration. Achieving the stable octet involves a release of energy, and the strong attraction of the nucleus for the electron leads to a high change in energy. The Group VIIIA elements (**noble gases**) have electron affinities on the order of zero because they already possess full shells and cannot readily accept electrons. Elements of other groups generally have low values of electron affinity.

Electronegativity

Electronegativity is a measure of the attraction an atom has for electrons in a chemical bond. The greater an atom's electronegativity, the greater its attraction for bonding electrons. Electronegativity values are not determined directly. The most common electronegativity scale is the **Pauling electronegativity scale** where the values range from 0.7 for the most electropositive elements, like cesium, to 4.0 for the most electronegative element, fluorine. Electronegativities are related to effective nuclear charge: Elements with low Z_{eff} will have low electronegativities because their nuclei do not attract electrons strongly, while elements with high Z_{eff} will have high electronegativities because of the strong pull the nucleus has on electrons. Therefore, electronegativity increases from left to right across periods and decreases from top to bottom down a group.

TYPES OF ELEMENTS

The elements of the periodic table may be classified into three categories: **metals**, located on the left side and in the middle of the periodic table; **nonmetals**, located on the right side of the table; and **metalloids** (**semimetals**), found along a diagonal line between the metals and nonmetals.

Metals

Metals are shiny solids (except for mercury) at room temperature and generally have high melting points and densities. Metals have the characteristic ability to be deformed without breaking. The ability of a metal to be hammered into shapes is called **malleability**, and the ability to be drawn into wires is called **ductility**. Many of the characteristic properties of metals, such as large atomic radius, low ionization energy, and low electronegativity, are due to the fact that the few electrons in the valence shell of a metal atom can easily be removed. Because the valence electrons can move freely, metals are good conductors of heat and electricity. Groups IA and IIA represent the most reactive metals and will be discussed below. The transition elements, also discussed later, are metals that have partially filled d orbitals.

Nonmetals

Nonmetals are generally brittle in the solid state and show little or no metallic luster. They have high ionization energies and electronegativities and are usually poor conductors of heat and electricity. Most nonmetals share the ability to gain electrons easily but otherwise display a wide range of chemical behaviors and reactivities. The nonmetals are located on the upper right side of the periodic table and are separated from the metals by a line cutting diagonally through the region of the periodic table containing elements with partially filled p orbitals.

Metalloids

The metalloids or semimetals are found along the line between the metals and nonmetals in the periodic table, and their properties vary considerably. Their densities, boiling points, and melting points fluctuate widely. The electronegativities and ionization energies of metalloids lie between those of metals and nonmetals; therefore, these elements possess characteristics of both those classes. For example, silicon (Si) has a metallic luster, yet it is brittle and is not an efficient conductor. The reactivity of metalloids is dependent upon the element with which they are reacting. For example, boron (B) behaves as a nonmetal when reacting with sodium (Na) and as a metal when reacting with fluorine (F). The elements classified as metalloids are boron (B), silicon (Si), germanium (Ge), arsenic (As), antimony (Sb), and tellurium (Te).

IONS

Ionic solutions are of particular interest to chemists because certain important types of chemical interactions occur in them. For instance, acid-base reactions and oxidation-reduction reactions occur in ionic solutions. Ions and their properties in solution will be introduced here; the chemical reactions mentioned are discussed in detail in Chapter 32, Reaction Types, and Chapter 37, Acids and Bases.

Cations and Anions

Ionic compounds are made up of cations and anions, where a cation is a positive ion and an anion is a negative ion. The nomenclature of ionic compounds is based on the names of the component ions.

- For elements that can form more than one positive ion (usually transition metals), the charge is indicated by a Roman numeral in parentheses following the name of the element.

    Fe^{2+} Iron (II) Cu^+ Copper (I)
    Fe^{3+} Iron (III) Cu^{2+} Copper (II)

- An older, but still commonly used, method is to add the ending -ous or -ic to the root of the Latin name of the element to represent the ions with lesser or greater charge, respectively.

    Fe^+ Ferrous Cu^+ Cuprous
    Fe^{3+} Ferric Cu^{2+} Cupric

- Monatomic anions are named by dropping the ending of the elemental name and adding -ide.

    H^- Hydride S^{2-} Sulfide
    F^- Fluoride N^{3-} Nitride
    O^{2-} Oxide P^{3-} Phosphide

- Many polyatomic anions contain oxygen and are therefore called **oxanions**. When an element forms two oxanions, the name of the one with less oxygen ends in -ite and the one with more oxygen ends in -ate.

    NO_2^- Nitrite SO_3^{2-} Sulfite
    NO_3^- Nitrate SO_4^{2-} Sulfate

- When the series of oxanions contains four oxanions, prefixes are also used. **Hypo-** and **per-** are used to indicate less oxygen and more oxygen, respectively.

    ClO^- Hypochlorite
    ClO_2^- Chlorite
    ClO_3^- Chlorate
    ClO_4^- Perchlorate

- Polyatomic anions often gain one or more H^+ ions to form anions of lower charge. The resulting ions are named by adding the word hydrogen or dihydrogen to the front of the anion's name. An older method uses the prefix bi- to indicate the addition of a single hydrogen ion.

HCO_3^- Hydrogen carbonate or bicarbonate

HSO_4^- Hydrogen sulfate or bisulfate

$H_2PO_4^-$ Dihydrogen phosphate

Ion Charges

Metals, which are found in the left part of the periodic table, generally form positive ions, whereas nonmetals, which are found in the right part of the periodic table, generally form negative ions. Note, however, that anions that contain metallic elements do exist; e.g., MnO_4^- (permanganate) and CrO_4^{2-} (chromate). All elements in a given group tend to form monatomic ions with the same charge. Thus, the alkali metals (Group IA) usually form cations with a single positive charge, the alkaline earth metals (Group IIA) form cations with a double positive charge, and the halogens (Group VIIA) form anions (halides) with a single negative charge. Though other main group elements follow this trend, the intermediate electronegativity of such elements (which makes them less likely to form ionic compounds) and the transition from metallic to nonmetallic character complicates the picture.

THE CHEMISTRY OF GROUPS

Hydrogen

There is no suitable place for hydrogen in the periodic table. Hydrogen does resemble alkali metals because it has a single s valence electron and forms the H^+ ion, which is hydrated in solution. However, it can also form the hydride ion (H^-), which is far too reactive to exist in water. In this respect, hydrogen resembles the halogens in that it only requires one additional electron to reach the next noble gas configuration.

Alkali Metals

The alkali metals are the elements of **Group IA**. They possess most of the physical properties common to metals, yet their densities are lower than those of other metals. The alkali metals have only one loosely bound electron in their outermost shell, giving them the largest atomic radii of all the elements in their respective periods. Their metallic properties and high reactivity are due to their low ionization energies; they easily lose their valence electron to form univalent cations, allowing them to easily form +1 cations. Alkali metals have low electronegativities and react very readily with nonmetals, especially halogens.

Alkaline Earth Metals

The alkaline earth metals are the elements of **Group IIA** and also possess many characteristically metallic properties. Like the alkali metals, these properties are dependent on the ease with which they lose electrons. The alkaline earth metals have two electrons in their outer shell and have smaller atomic radii than the alkali metals. However, the two valence electrons are not held very tightly by the nucleus, so they can be removed to form divalent cations. Therefore, alkaline earth metals commonly form +2 cations. Alkaline earths have low electronegativities and positive electron affinities.

Carbon Group

The family containing carbon, **Group IVA**, exhibits a wide range of characteristics and includes a nonmetal (C), metalloids (Si and Ge), and metals (Sn and Pb). Although these elements do not share many physical properties, they do all have 2 electrons in their outermost p subshells, leading to a configuration that is distant from that of a noble gas. This explains why carbon tends not to form ions (which would need to be +4 or −4 to reach noble gas configuration) but rather participates in electron sharing; it usually is most stable with four covalent bonds (discussed further in Chapter 29, Chemical Bonding).

Pnictogens

Nitrogen and the elements below it in **Group VA** also display a wide variety of properties and include a mixture of nonmetals (N and P), metalloids (As and Sb), and a metal (Bi). Similar to carbon, nitrogen often forms covalent bonds but most commonly forms three per atom instead of carbon's four. Nitrogen also commonly holds a positive charge in organic reactions, making several nitrogen-containing compounds good bases.

Chalcogens

Group IVA, which contains oxygen, is characterized by elements requiring two additional valence electrons to complete their outermost shells. These elements therefore tend to be fairly electronegative and to form −2 anions, but they can also participate in covalent bonds, preferring to have two shared electron pairs and two nonbonded pairs.

Halogens

The halogens, **Group VIIA**, are highly reactive nonmetals with one valence electron less than the closest noble gas. Halogens therefore commonly form −1 anions. Halogens are otherwise highly variable in their physical properties. For instance, the halogens range from gaseous (F_2 and Cl_2) to liquid (Br_2) to solid (I_2) at room temperature. Their chemical properties are more uniform: The electronegativities of halogens are very high, and they are particularly reactive toward alkali metals and alkaline earths, which "want" to donate electrons to the halogens to form stable ionic crystals. Fluorine (F) has the highest electronegativity of all the elements.

Noble Gases

The noble gases, also called the **inert gases**, are found in **Group VIIIA** (also called Group 0). For the purposes of the PCAT, they are completely nonreactive because they each have a complete valence shell, which is an energetically favored arrangement. This gives them no tendency to gain or lose electrons, high ionization energies, and no electronegativities. They possess low boiling points and are gases at room temperature.

Transition Elements

The transition elements, **Groups IB to VIIIB**, are all considered metals; hence, they are also called the **transition metals**. These elements are very hard and have high melting points and boiling points. From left to right across a period, the five d orbitals become progressively more filled. The d electrons are held only loosely by the nucleus and are relatively mobile, contributing to the malleability and high electrical conductivity of these elements. Chemically, transition elements have low ionization energies and may exist in a variety of positively charged forms or **oxidation states**. This is because transition elements are capable of losing various numbers of electrons from the s and d orbitals of their valence shell. Theoretically, the transition metals in Group VIIIB could have eight different oxidation states, from +1 to +8; however, they typically do not exhibit so many. For instance, copper (Cu), in Group IB, can exist in either the +1 or the +2 oxidation state, and manganese (Mn), in Group VIIB, occurs in the +2, +3, +4, +6, or +7 state. Because of this ability to attain positive oxidation states, transition metals form many different ionic and partially ionic compounds. The dissolved ions can form **complex ions** either with molecules of water (**hydration complexes**) or with nonmetals, forming highly colored solutions and compounds (e.g., $CuSO_4 \bullet 5H_2O$, chalcanthite). This complexation may also enhance the relatively low solubility of certain compounds (e.g., AgCl is insoluble in water but quite soluble in aqueous ammonia due to the formation of the complex ion $[Ag(NH_3)_2]^+$). The formation of complexes causes the d orbitals to be split into two energy sublevels. This enables many of the complexes to absorb certain frequencies of light—those containing the precise amount of energy required to raise electrons from the lower to the higher d sublevel. The frequencies not absorbed—known as the **subtraction frequencies**—give the complexes their characteristic colors.

REVIEW PROBLEMS

1. Elements in a given period have the same
    - **(A)** atomic weight.
    - **(B)** maximum azimuthal quantum number.
    - **(C)** maximum principal quantum number.
    - **(D)** valence electron structure.

2. Arrange the following species in terms of increasing atomic (or ionic) radius: Sr, P, Mg, Mg^{2+}.

3. The Ca^{2+} species is electronically similar to the elements in
    - **(A)** Group IIA.
    - **(B)** Group IA.
    - **(C)** Group IVB.
    - **(D)** Group 0.

4. What is the electron configuration for the outermost electrons of elements found in Group IVB?
    - **(A)** $s^2 p^6 d^4$
    - **(B)** $s^2 d^2$
    - **(C)** $s^2 d^4$
    - **(D)** $s^2 p^4$

5. Which of the following elements has the lowest electronegativity?
    - **(A)** Cesium
    - **(B)** Strontium
    - **(C)** Calcium
    - **(D)** Barium

6. Arrange the following calcium species in terms of increasing size: Ca, Ca^+, Ca^{2+}, Ca^{3+}, Ca^-, Ca^{2-}.

7. The order of the elements in the periodic table is based on the
    - **(A)** number of neutrons.
    - **(B)** radius of the atom.
    - **(C)** atomic number.
    - **(D)** atomic weight.

8. The elements within each column of the periodic table
    - **(A)** have similar valence electron configurations.
    - **(B)** have similar atomic radii.
    - **(C)** have the same principal quantum number.
    - **(D)** will react to form stable elements.

9. Discuss the properties of nonmetals and give four examples of nonmetallic elements.

10. Arrange the following elements in terms of increasing first ionization energy: Ga, Ba, Ru, F, N.

11. Explain why the Group 0 elements are so unreactive.

12. Arrange the following elements in terms of decreasing electronegativity: Ca, Cl, Fr, P, Zn.

13. Which group contains an element with an electron configuration of $1s^2\ 2s^2\ 2p^6\ 3s^2\ 3p^6\ 4s^2\ 3d^{10}$ $4p^6\ 4d^5\ 5s^2$?
    - **(A)** VA
    - **(B)** VIIA
    - **(C)** VB
    - **(D)** VIIB

14. Discuss the trends in the atomic radii of different elements. How does the atomic number affect the atomic radius of an element?

15. Which element has the greatest electronegativity?
    - **(A)** Chlorine
    - **(B)** Oxygen
    - **(C)** Sulfur
    - **(D)** Fluorine

16. The change in energy that occurs when an electron is added to an atom is known as the
    - **(A)** electronegativity.
    - **(B)** metallic character.
    - **(C)** electron affinity.
    - **(D)** ionization energy.

17. Discuss the properties of metalloids and give three examples of elements exhibiting metalloid behavior.

18. Which of the following elements is most electronegative?
    - **(A)** S
    - **(B)** Cl
    - **(C)** Na
    - **(D)** Mg

19. Transition metal compounds generally exhibit bright colors because the
    - **(A)** electrons in the partially filled *d* orbitals are easily promoted to excited states.
    - **(B)** metals become complexed in water.
    - **(C)** metals conduct electricity, producing colored light.
    - **(D)** electrons in the d orbitals emit energy as they relax.

20. Discuss the properties of metals and give four examples of metallic elements.

21. Identify the following elements as metal, nonmetal, or semimetal:

    (A) Fr

    (B) Pd

    (C) I

    (D) B

    (E) Sc

    (F) Si

    (G) S

SOLUTIONS TO REVIEW PROBLEMS

1. **C** Discussed in the introduction to this chapter.

2. $\text{Mg}^{2+} < \text{P} < \text{Mg} < \text{Sr}$

The trends in atomic radii are as follows. Going from left to right across a period, the atomic radii decrease because the atomic number increases. The increasing number of protons in the nucleus will have a stronger attraction for the outermost electrons, causing them to be held closer and more tightly to the nucleus. Going down a group, the atomic radius will increase because more filled principal energy levels separate the nucleus and the outermost electrons, shielding the attractive force between them. P has a small radius because it lies far to the right and high in a group. The magnesium species will have smaller radii than the strontium species because they are higher in Group IIA. Finally, positive ions have smaller atomic radii than the corresponding neutral molecules because the loss of electrons leads to a decrease in electron-electron repulsion within the atom, which in turn allows the electrons to move in closer to the nucleus. Therefore, Mg^{2+} will be smaller than Mg. Mg^{2+} has a smaller radius than P because Mg^{2+} has no electrons in orbitals of the third principal energy level.

3. **D** The Ca^{2+} ion is electronically similar to atoms in Group 0 because its outermost valence shell is a complete octet. It is isoelectronic to argon.

4. **B** The electron configuration of the different groups can be written as long as a few basic rules are applied. First, the Roman numeral represents the number of electrons that will lie outside of the noble gas core configuration. Second, the letters A and B tell whether the atom is a representative or a nonrepresentative element. Representative elements will successively fill the s and p orbitals, while the nonrepresentative elements will successively fill the s, d, and maybe f orbitals. Thus, elements in Group IVB are nonrepresentative elements and will have four electrons outside their respective rare gas cores. The correct standard electron configuration for Group IVB elements is thus $s^2 d^2$.

Using G to represent any noble gas, the full electron configuration of a nonspecified group IVB element can be abbreviated as $[G](n-1)d^2 ns^2$, where n is the principal quantum number.

5. **A** The least electronegative elements are located at the bottom left of the periodic table. Cesium has the lowest Z_{eff}, so it is the least electronegative. Note that francium (Fr) would be lower still, but it is not a stable, naturally occurring element.

6. $\text{Ca}^{3+}, \text{Ca}^{2+}, \text{Ca}^+, \text{Ca}, \text{Ca}^-, \text{Ca}^{2-}$

Positive ions will have smaller radii than the corresponding neutral atoms, and, the greater the positive charge, the smaller the ionic radius. Negative ions will have larger radii than the corresponding neutral atoms, and the greater the negative charge, the larger the ionic radius (see answer to Question 2, above).

7. **C** Discussed in the introduction to this chapter.

8. **A** Discussed in the introduction to this chapter.

9.   Nonmetals are brittle, lusterless elements possessing high ionization energies and high electronegativities. They tend to gain electrons to form negative ions. They are poor conductors of heat and electricity. The nonmetals are located on the upper right side of the periodic table.

10.   **Ba < Ru < Ga < N < F**

Two common trends should be remembered when ordering atoms according to their ionization energies. First, the ionization energy increases toward the right across a period because the elements are less willing to give up an electron as the attractive pull (Z_{eff}) of the nucleus increases. Second, the ionization energy decreases down a group because the distance separating the valence electrons from the nucleus increases. Therefore, to order the elements according to their first ionization energy, it is necessary to go from the bottom left of the periodic table, where the lowest values are, across to the top right of the periodic table, where the highest values are.

11.   Group 0 elements are also known as the noble, rare, or inert gases. They are very unreactive because their outermost shells contain complete, stable formations. There is no reason for these elements to attempt to gain or lose electrons to other atoms because they are electronically stable on their own.

12.   **Cl > P > Zn > Ca > Fr**

The two trends to remember with electronegativity are that it increases across a period and decreases down a group. Therefore, chlorine, which is farthest to the top and right, will have the highest value. Francium lies farthest to the left and bottom, so it will have the lowest electronegativity.

13. **D**   This element has seven electrons in its outermost shell, so its Roman numeral designation is VII; because the d orbital is being filled, it is a nonrepresentative, or B, element. Thus, it is found in Group VIIB.

14.   There are two major trends concerning the atomic radii of elements. The first of these is that the atomic radius decreases across a period. This can be explained by the fact that the atomic number (i.e., the number of protons within the nucleus) increases. Thus, the electrostatic force between the valence electrons and the nucleus increases, and the outermost electrons will be pulled closer to the nucleus, making the atom smaller. The second trend concerning atomic radii is that the atomic radius increases down a group. This can be explained by the fact that with every subsequent element down a group, a filled principal energy level has been added. This increases the distance between the nucleus and the valence electrons because orbital size increases with increasing principal quantum number.

15. **D**   The most electronegative elements are located at the top right of the periodic table.

16. **C**   Discussed in the section on periodic properties in this chapter.

17.   Metalloids are elements that possess characteristics of both metals and nonmetals. Their electronic characteristics, such as ionization energies and electronegativities, lie between those of the metals and nonmetals. When undergoing reactions, the metalloids may act as either

metals or nonmetals depending upon the species with which they are reacting. The elements classified as metalloids are boron, silicon, germanium, arsenic, antimony, and tellurium.

18. **B** Chlorine has the greatest electronegativity because, out of all the choices, it lies farthest to the right and top of the periodic table. Chlorine has a great attraction for electrons in a chemical bond because it needs only one more electron to complete a stable octet formation. Therefore, it has a high electronegativity.

19. **A** The closely spaced d orbitals allow for relatively low energy transitions; these transitions often occur in the visible region of the electromagnetic spectrum, as do other electronic transitions from the transition metal d subshell to other nearby, empty subshells.

20. Metals are shiny, lustrous solids that have high melting points and densities. The ease with which metals lose electrons contributes to their high thermal and electrical conductivities, their malleability and ductility, and the ease with which they form compounds with reactive nonmetals. All of the elements on the left side of the periodic table (except H) and all of the transition elements are metals.

21. **A** Fr: metal
    B Pd: metal
    C I: nonmetal
    D B: semimetal
    E Sc: metal
    F Si: semimetal
    G S: nonmetal

CHAPTER TWENTY-NINE

Chemical Bonding

The atoms of many elements can combine to form **molecules**. The atoms in most molecules are held together by attractive forces called **chemical bonds**. These bonds are formed via the interaction of the valence electrons of the combining atoms. Strong chemical bonds known as **intramolecular bonds** hold atoms together as molecules and include ionic and covalent bonds. The chemical and physical properties of the resulting molecules are often very different from those of their constituent elements. In addition to the very strong forces within a molecule, there are weaker **intermolecular forces** between molecules. Intermolecular forces, although weaker than the intramolecular chemical bonds, are of considerable importance in understanding the physical properties of many substances.

BONDING

Many molecules contain atoms bonded according to the **octet rule**, which states that an atom tends to bond with other atoms until it has eight electrons in its outermost shell, thereby forming a stable electron configuration similar to that of the noble gas neon. Exceptions to this rule are as follows: hydrogen (H) and helium (He), which can have only two valence electrons; lithium (Li) and beryllium (Be), which bond to attain two and four valence electrons, respectively; boron (B), which bonds to attain six; and elements beyond the second row, such as phosphorus (P) and sulfur (S), which can expand their octets to include more than eight electrons by incorporating d orbitals.

When classifying strong chemical bonds, it is helpful to introduce two distinct types: ionic bonds and covalent bonds. In **ionic bonding**, one or more electrons from an atom with a smaller ionization energy are transferred to an atom with a greater electron affinity, and the resulting ions are held together by electrostatic forces. In **covalent bonding**, an electron pair is shared between two atoms. In many cases, the bond is partially covalent and partially ionic; we call such bonds **polar covalent bonds**.

IONIC BONDS

When two atoms with large differences in electronegativity react, there is a complete transfer of electrons from the less electronegative atom to the more electronegative atom. The atom that loses electrons becomes a positively charged ion, or **cation**, and the atom that gains electrons becomes a negatively charged ion, or **anion**. For this transfer to occur, the difference in electronegativity must be greater than 1.7 on the Pauling scale. In general, the elements of Groups IA and IIA (low electronegativities) bond ionically to elements of Group VIIA (high electronegativities). Elements of Groups IA and IIA give up their electrons to achieve a noble gas configuration, while Group VIIA elements gain an electron to achieve the noble gas configuration. For example, Na + Cl → Na$^+$Cl$^-$ (sodium chloride). The electrostatic force of attraction between the charged ions is called an **ionic bond**.

Ionic compounds have characteristic physical properties. They form crystal lattices consisting of arrays of positive and negative ions in which the attractive forces between ions of opposite charge are maximized, while the repulsive forces between ions of like charge are minimized. They therefore have high melting and boiling points due to the strong electrostatic forces between the ions. They also can conduct electricity in the liquid and aqueous states, though not in the solid state.

COVALENT BONDS

When two or more atoms with similar electronegativities interact, the energy required to form ions is greater than the energy that would be released upon the formation of an ionic bond (i.e., the process is not energetically favorable). Since a complete transfer of electrons cannot occur, such atoms achieve a noble gas electron configuration by **sharing** electrons in a covalent bond. The binding force between the two atoms results from the attraction that each electron of the shared pair has for the two positive nuclei.

Covalent compounds generally contain discrete molecular units with weak intermolecular forces. Consequently, they have low melting points and do not conduct electricity in the liquid or aqueous states.

Properties of Covalent Bonds

Atoms can share more than one pair of electrons. Two atoms sharing one, two, or three electron pairs are said to be joined by a **single**, **double**, or **triple covalent bond**, respectively. The number of shared electron pairs between two atoms is called the **bond order**; hence, a single bond has a bond order of one, a double bond has a bond order of two, and a triple bond has a bond order of three.

Two key features characterize covalent bonds: bond length and bond energy.

Bond length

Bond length is the average distance between the two nuclei of the atoms involved in the bond. As the number of shared electron pairs increases, the two atoms are pulled closer together, leading to a decrease in bond length. Thus, for a given pair of atoms, a triple bond is shorter than a double bond, which is shorter than a single bond.

Bond energy

Bond energy is the energy required to separate two bonded atoms. For a given pair of atoms, the strength of a bond (and therefore the bond energy) increases as the number of shared electron pairs increases.

Covalent Bond Notation

The shared valence electrons of a covalent bond are called the **bonding electrons**. The valence electrons not involved in the covalent bond are called **nonbonding electrons**. These unshared electron pairs can also be called **lone electron pairs**. A convenient notation, called a **Lewis structure**, is used to represent the bonding and nonbonding electrons in a molecule, facilitating chemical "bookkeeping." The number of valence electrons attributed to a particular atom in the Lewis structure of a molecule is not necessarily the same as the number would be in the isolated atom, and the difference accounts for what is referred to as the **formal charge** of that atom. Often, more than one Lewis structure can be drawn for a molecule; this phenomenon is called **resonance**. Lewis structures, formal charge, and resonance are discussed in detail below.

Lewis structures

When different atoms interact to form a bond, only their outermost regions come in contact. Hence, only the valence electrons are involved. One of the easiest ways to follow the valence electrons in a chemical reaction is with **Lewis dot symbols**. A Lewis dot symbol contains the symbol of an element and one "dot" for each valence electron in an atom. Magnesium, for example, belongs to Group IIA and has two valence electrons (:Mg). Note: Because the transitional-metal lanthanide and actinides all have incompletely filled inner shells, Lewis dot symbols are not written for these elements.

·Li	Lithium	$\ddot{N}$	Nitrogen
·Be·	Beryllium	·$\ddot{O}$:	Oxygen
·$\dot{B}$·	Boron	:$\ddot{F}$:	Fluorine
·$\dot{C}$·	Carbon	:$\ddot{Ne}$:	Neon

Just as a Lewis symbol is used to represent the distribution of valence electrons in an atom, one can also be used to represent the distribution of valence electrons in a molecule. For example, the Lewis symbol of an F ion is : $\ddot{F}$:⁻; the Lewis structure of an F_2 molecule is :$\ddot{F}$——$\ddot{F}$:

Certain steps must be followed in assigning a Lewis structure to a molecule. These steps are outlined below, using hydrogen cyanide (HCN) as an example.

1. Count all the valence electrons of the atoms. The number of valence electrons of the molecule is the sum of the valence electrons of all atoms present:

> H has 1 valence electron;
> C has 4 valence electrons;
> N has 5 valence electrons; therefore,
> HCN has a total of 10 valence electrons.

2. Write the skeletal structure of the compound (i.e., the arrangement of atoms). In general, the least electronegative atom is the central atom. Hydrogen (always) and the halogens F, Cl, Br, and I (usually)

occupy the end positions. Draw single bonds between the central atom and the atoms surrounding it, placing an electron pair in each bond (bonding electron pair).

In HCN, H must occupy a terminal position. Of the remaining two atoms, C is the less electronegative and therefore occupies the central position. The skeletal structure is as follows:

H:C:N

Each bond has 2 electrons, so $10 - 4 = 6$ valence electrons remain.

3. Complete the octets (8 valence electrons) of all atoms bonded to the central atom, using the remaining valence electrons still to be assigned. (Recall that H is an exception to the octet rule since it can have only 2 valence electrons.) In this example H already has 2 valence electrons in its bond with C.

H:C:N̈:

4. Place any extra electrons on the central atom. If the central atom has less than an octet, try to write double or triple bonds between the central and surrounding atoms using the nonbonding, unshared lone electron pairs. The HCN structure above does not satisfy the octet rule for C because C possesses only 4 valence electrons. Therefore, 2 lone electron pairs from the N atom must be moved to form two more bonds with C, creating a triple bond between C and N.

H:C:::N:

5. Finally, bonds are drawn as lines rather than pairs of dots.

$H - C \equiv N$

Now, the octet rule is satisfied for all three atoms because C and N have 8 valence electrons and H has 2 valence electrons.

Formal charges

The number of electrons officially assigned to an atom in a Lewis structure does not always equal the number of valence electrons of the free atom. The difference between these two numbers is the **formal charge** of the atom. Formal charge can be calculated using the following formula:

$$\text{Formal charge} = V - \frac{1}{2}N_{bonding} - N_{nonbonding}$$

where V is the number of valence electrons in the free atom, $N_{bonding}$ is the number of bonding electrons, and $N_{nonbonding}$ is the number of nonbonding electrons. Using a Lewis dot structure, where 2 bonding electrons are represented by a stick and each nonbonding electron is represented with a dot, the formal charge is also represented by:

$$\text{Formal charge} = V - (\text{\# of sticks} + \text{\# of dots})$$

The formal charge of an ion or molecule is equal to the sum of the formal charges of the individual atoms comprising it.

Example: Calculate the formal charge on the central N atom of $[NH_4]^+$.

Solution: The Lewis structure of $[NH_4]^+$ is

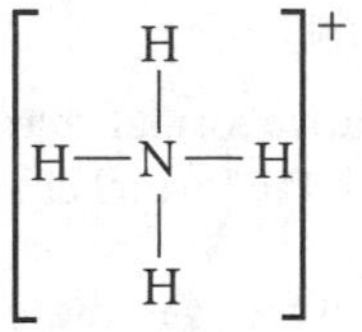

$$
\left[\begin{array}{c} H \\ | \\ H-N-H \\ | \\ H \end{array} \right]^{+}
$$

Nitrogen is in Group VA; thus, it has 5 valence electrons. In $[NH_4]^+$, N has 4 bonds (i.e., 8 bonding electrons and no nonbonding electrons).

So $V = 5$; $N_{bonding} = 8$; $N_{nonbonding} = 0$

Formal charge $= 5 - \frac{1}{2}(8) - 0 = +1$

Likewise, there are 4 "sticks" and 0 "dots" in the Lewis structure, so formal charge (FC) could be calculated like this too:

$$
\begin{aligned}
FC &= V - (\text{\# of sticks} + \text{\# of dots}) \\
FC &= 5 - (4 + 0) = 1
\end{aligned}
$$

Thus, the formal charge on the N atom in $[NH_4]^+$ is +1.

Resonance

For some molecules, two or more non-identical Lewis structures can be drawn; these arrangements are called **resonance structures**. A resonance structure is one of two or more Lewis structures for a single molecule unable to be described fully with only one Lewis structure. The molecule doesn't actually exist as either one of the resonance structures but is rather a composite, or hybrid, of the two.

For example, SO_2 has three resonance structures, two of which are minor: $O=S-O$ and $O-S=O$. The actual molecule is a hybrid of these three structures (spectral data indicate that the two S–O bonds are identical). This phenomenon is known as resonance, and the actual structure of the molecule is called the **resonance hybrid**. Resonance structures are expressed with a double-headed arrow between them:

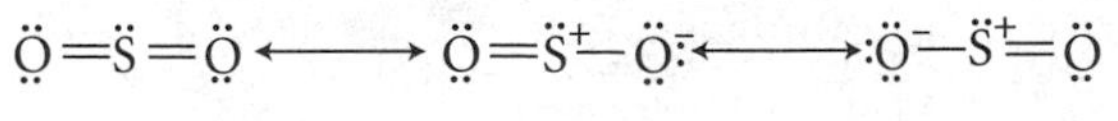

$$
\ddot{O}=\ddot{S}=\ddot{O} \longleftrightarrow \ddot{O}=\overset{+}{\ddot{S}}-\ddot{\ddot{O}}\!\!: \longleftrightarrow :\!\ddot{\ddot{O}}^{-}\!-\overset{+}{\ddot{S}}=\ddot{O}
$$

The last two resonance structures of sulfur dioxide (shown above) have equivalent energy or stability. Often, nonequivalent resonance structures may be written for a molecule. In these cases, the more stable the structure, the more that structure contributes to the character of the resonance hybrid. Conversely, the less stable the resonance structure, the less that structure contributes to the resonance hybrid. The structure on the left of the diagram is the most stable. In this case, the most stable structure has no formal charge on any of the component atoms. Sulfur has more than 8 valence electrons (10 in this case), but that is acceptable because sulfur has a d subshell that can serve to expand the octet. More exceptions to the octet rule are discussed below.

Therefore, formal charges are often useful for qualitatively assessing the stability of a particular resonance structure, and the following guidelines are used.

- A Lewis structure with small or no formal charges is preferred over a Lewis structure with large formal charges.
- A Lewis structure in which negative formal charges are placed on more electronegative atoms is more stable than one in which the formal charges are placed on less electronegative atoms.

Example: Write the resonance structures for the cyanate anion (which contains one nitrogen atom, one oxygen atom, one carbon atom and an overall charge of negative one).

Solution: First, tally the total number of valence electrons:

N has 5 valence electrons;

C has 4 valence electrons;

O has 6 valence electrons; and the species itself has one negative charge (meaning one additional electron).

Total valence electrons $= 5 + 4 + 6 + 1 = 16$

C is the least electronegative of the three given atoms, N, C, and O. Therefore, the C atom occupies the central position in the skeletal structure of $[NCO]^-$. Draw single bonds between the central C atom and the surrounding atoms, N and O, and place a pair of electrons in each bond.

$$N{:}C{:}O$$

Complete the octets of N and O with the remaining $(16 - 4) = 12$ electrons.

$$:\ddot{N}{:}C{:}\ddot{O}:$$

The C octet is incomplete. There are three ways in which double and triple bonds can be formed to complete the C octet. Two lone pairs from the O atom can be used to form a triple bond between the C and O atoms:

$$:\ddot{N}-C\equiv O:$$

Or one lone electron pair can be taken from both the O and the N atoms to form two double bonds, one between N and C and the other between O and C:

$$:\ddot{N}=C=\ddot{O}:$$

Or two lone electron pairs can be taken from the N atom to form a triple bond between the C and N atoms:

$$:N\equiv C-\ddot{O}:$$

These three are all resonance structures of $[NCO]^-$.

Assign formal charges to each atom of each resonance structure: In the first structure, the N has a formal charge of -2, and the O has a charge of $+1$. In the second structure the N has a formal charge of -1, and in the third structure the O has a charge of -1.

The most stable structure is therefore:

$$:N\equiv C-\ddot{\underset{..}{O}}:$$

since the negative formal charge is on the most electronegative atom, O.

Exceptions to the octet rule

Atoms found in or beyond the third period can have more than eight valence electrons, since some of the valence electrons may occupy d orbitals. These atoms can be assigned more than four bonds in Lewis structures.

The Lewis structure of the sulfate ion, SO_4^{2-}, for example, can be drawn in six resonance forms by alternating the placement of pi electrons. Giving the sulfur 12 valence electrons permits three of the five atoms to be assigned a formal charge of zero, which is most favorable energetically.

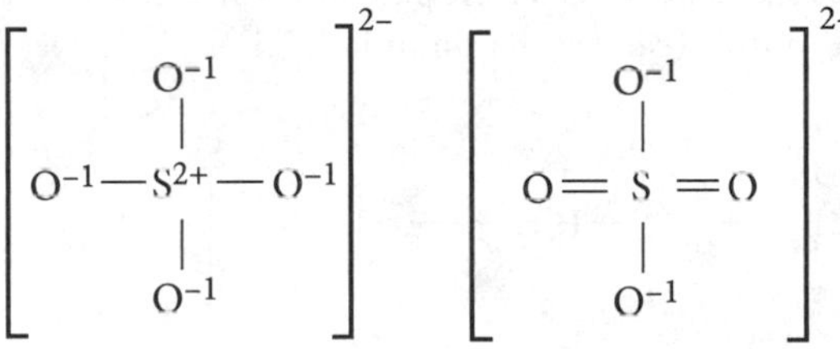

Figure 29.1

Types of Covalent Bonding

The nature of a covalent bond depends on the relative electronegativities of the atoms sharing the electron pairs. Covalent bonds are considered to be polar or nonpolar depending on the difference in electronegativities between the atoms.

Polar covalent bond

Polar covalent bonding occurs between atoms with small differences in electronegativity, generally in the range of 0.4 to 1.7 Pauling units. The bonding electron pair is not shared equally but is pulled more toward the element with the higher electronegativity. As a result, the more electronegative atom acquires a partial negative charge, $\delta-$, and the less electronegative atom acquires a partial positive charge, $\delta+$, giving the molecule a partially ionic character. For instance, the covalent bond in HCl is polar because the two atoms have a small difference in electronegativity (approx. 0.9). Chlorine, the more electronegative atom, attains a partial negative charge, and hydrogen attains a partial positive charge. This difference in charge between the atoms is indicated by an arrow crossed (like a plus sign) at the positive end and pointing to the negative end, as shown below.

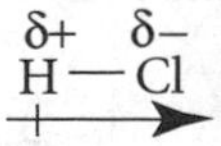

Figure 29.2

A molecule that has such a separation of positive and negative charges is called a **polar molecule**. The **dipole moment** itself is a vector quantity μ, measured in **Debye** units (coulomb-meters) and defined as the product of the charge magnitude (q) and the distance between the two partial charges (r):

$$\mu = qr$$

Nonpolar covalent bond

Nonpolar covalent bonding occurs between atoms that have the same electronegativities. The bonding electron pair is shared equally such that there is no separation of charge across the bond. Nonpolar covalent bonds occur in diatomic molecules such as H_2, Cl_2, O_2, and N_2.

Coordinate covalent bond

In a coordinate covalent bond, the shared electron pair comes from the lone pair of one of the atoms in the molecule. Once such a bond forms, it is indistinguishable from any other covalent bond, so identifying such a bond is useful only in keeping track of the valence electrons and formal charges.

Coordinate bonds are typically found in Lewis acid-base compounds (see Chapter 37, Acids and Bases). A **Lewis acid** is a compound that can accept an electron pair to form a covalent bond; a **Lewis base** is a compound that can donate an electron pair to form a covalent bond. For example, in the reaction between boron trifluoride (BF_3) and ammonia (NH_3):

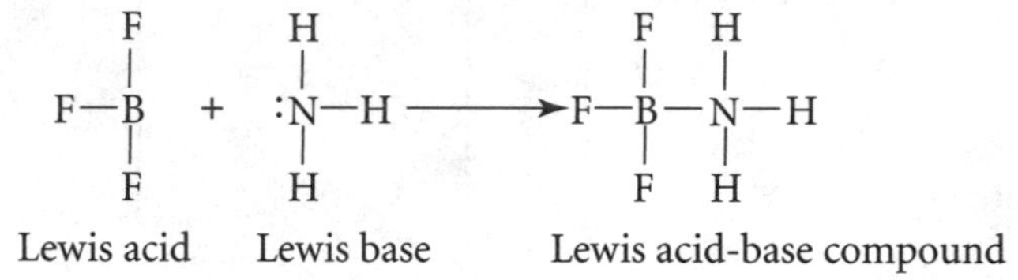

$$
\underset{\text{Lewis acid}}{\overset{\displaystyle \overset{\textstyle F}{\underset{\textstyle F}{|}}}{F-B}}
\quad + \quad
\underset{\text{Lewis base}}{\overset{\displaystyle \overset{\textstyle H}{|}}{\underset{\textstyle H}{|}} :N-H}
\quad \longrightarrow \quad
\underset{\text{Lewis acid-base compound}}{F-B-N-H}
$$

Figure 29.3

NH_3 donates a pair of electrons to form a coordinate covalent bond; thus, it acts as a Lewis base. BF_3 accepts this pair of electrons to form the coordinate covalent bond; thus, it acts as a Lewis acid.

Geometry and Polarity of Covalent Molecules

Molecular geometry

The **valence shell electron-pair repulsion (VSEPR)** theory uses Lewis structures to predict the molecular geometry of covalently bonded molecules. It states that the three-dimensional arrangement of atoms surrounding a central atom is determined by the repulsions between the bonding and the nonbonding electron pairs in the valence shell of the central atom. These electron pairs arrange themselves as far apart as possible, thereby minimizing repulsion.

The following steps are used to predict the geometric structure of a molecule using the VSEPR theory:

1. Draw the Lewis structure of the molecule.
2. Count the total number of bonding and nonbonding electron pairs in the valence shell of the central atom.
3. Arrange the electron pairs around the central atom so that they are as far apart from each other as possible.

4. Determine the bond angle, accounting for the additional repulsion due to nonbonding electrons, which pushes any bonding pairs slightly closer together.

For example, the compound AX_2 has the Lewis structure (X : A : X). A has two bonding electron pairs in its valence shell. To make these electron pairs as far apart as possible, their geometric structure should be linear:

$$X - A - X$$

Valence electron arrangements are summarized in the following table.

Electron Pairs	Nonbonding Pairs	Example	Geometric Arrangement	Shape	Angles
2	0	$BeCl_2$	X —— A —— X	Linear	180°
3	0	BH_3		Trigonal Planar	120°
4	0	CH_4		Tetrahedral	109.5°
4	1	NH_3		Trigonal Pyramidal	107°
4	2	H_2O		Bent	104.5°
5	0	PCl_5		Trigonal Bipyramidal	90°, 120°, 180°
6	0	SF_6		Octahedral	90°, 180°

Example: Predict the geometry of NH_3.

Solution: The Lewis structure of NH_3 is:

$$
\begin{array}{c}
H \\
| \\
H - \underset{\cdot\cdot}{N} - H
\end{array}
$$

The central atom, N, has three bonding electron pairs and one nonbonding electron pair for a total of four electron pairs.

The four electron pairs will be farthest apart when they occupy the corners of a tetrahedron. Since one of the four electron pairs is a lone pair, the observed geometry is trigonal pyramidal.

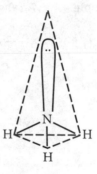

Figure 29.4

In describing the shape of a molecule, only the arrangement of atoms (not electrons) is considered. Even though the electron pairs are arranged in a tetrahedron, the shape of NH_3 is pyramidal. It is not trigonal planar because the lone pair repels the three bonding electron pairs, causing them to move as far away as possible.

Example: Predict the geometry of CO_2.

Solution: The Lewis structure of CO_2 is $:\!O::C::O\!:$.

The double bond behaves just like a single bond for purposes of predicting molecular shape. This compound has two groups of electrons around the carbon. According to the VSEPR theory, the two sets of electrons will orient themselves 180° apart, on opposite sides of the carbon atom, to minimize electron repulsion. Therefore, the molecular structure of CO_2 is linear.

Polarity of molecules

A molecule with a net dipole moment is called polar, as previously mentioned, because it has positive and negative poles. The polarity of a molecule depends on the polarity of the constituent bonds and on the shape of the molecule. A molecule with nonpolar bonds is always nonpolar; a molecule with polar bonds may be polar or nonpolar depending on the orientation of the bond dipoles.

A molecule of two atoms bound by a polar bond must have a net dipole moment and therefore be polar. The two equal and opposite partial charges are localized at the ends of the molecule on the two atoms. A molecule consisting of more than two atoms bound with polar bonds may be either polar or nonpolar since the overall dipole moment of a molecule is the vector sum of the individual bond dipole moments. If the molecule has a particular shape such that the bond dipole moments cancel each other (i.e., if the vector sum is zero), then the result is a nonpolar molecule. For instance, CCl_4 has four polar C—Cl bonds. According to the VSEPR theory, the shape of CCl_4 is tetrahedral. The four bond dipoles point to the vertices of the tetrahedron and cancel each other, resulting in a nonpolar molecule:

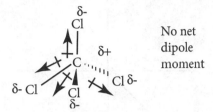

No net
dipole
moment

Figure 29.5

However, if the orientation of the bond dipoles are such that they do not cancel out, the molecules will have a net dipole moment and therefore be polar. For instance, H_2O has two polar O—H bonds. According to the VSEPR model, its shape is angular. The two dipoles add together to give a net dipole moment to the molecule, making the H_2O molecule polar:

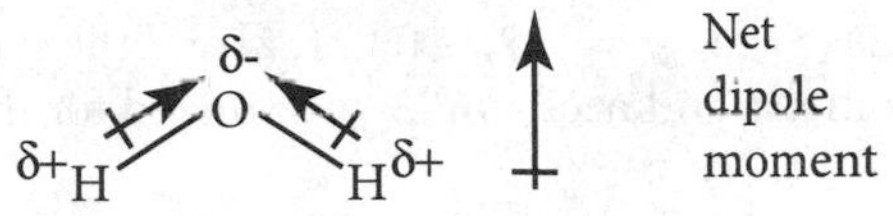

Net
dipole
moment

Figure 29.6

Atomic and Molecular Orbitals

A description of the quantum numbers has already been given in Chapter 27, Atomic Structure. The azimuthal quantum number (ℓ) describes the orbitals of each n shell. The shapes of these orbitals represent the probability of finding an electron at any given instant. $\ell = 0$ represents an s orbital, and s orbitals are spherically symmetric. The 1s orbital ($n = 1$, $\ell = 0$) is plotted below.

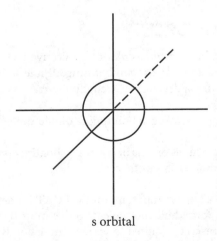

s orbital

Figure 29.7

When $\ell = 1$ there are three possible orbitals (since the magnetic quantum number, m_ℓ, may equal -1, 0, or $+1$). These are called p orbitals and have dumbbell shapes. The three p orbitals, designated p_x, p_y, and p_z are oriented at right angles to each other; the p_x orbital is plotted below.

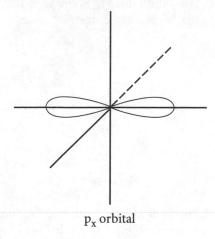

p_x orbital

Figure 29.8

The shapes of the five d orbitals ($\ell = 2$, $m_\ell = -2, -1, 0, 1, 2$) and the seven f orbitals ($\ell = 3$, $m_\ell = -3, -2, -1, 0, 1, 2, 3$) are more complex and need not be memorized for the PCAT.

When two atoms bond to form a molecule, the atomic orbitals interact to form a molecular orbital that describes the probability of finding the bonding electrons. Molecular orbitals are obtained by adding the wave functions of the atomic orbitals. Qualitatively, this is described by the overlap of two atomic orbitals. If the signs of the two atomic orbitals are the same, a **bonding orbital** is formed. If the signs are different, an **antibonding orbital** is formed. When two orbitals of different atoms overlap head-to-head, the resulting bond is called a **sigma (σ) bond**. When parallel p orbitals interact, a **pi (π) bond** is formed.

THE INTERMOLECULAR FORCES

The attractive forces that exist between molecules are collectively known as intermolecular forces. These include **dipole-ion interactions**, **hydrogen bonding**, **dipole-dipole interactions**, and **London dispersion forces (LDF)**. In order of decreasing strength, these are as follows:

$$\text{dipole-ion} > \text{hydrogen bonding} > \text{dipole-dipole} > \text{LDF}$$

Those forces not due to the interactions of ions or hydrogen bonding (i.e., dipole-dipole and LDF) are also collectively referred to as **van der Waals forces**.

Evaluating intermolecular forces is most important on the PCAT for determining melting and boiling points. Stronger intermolecular forces hold molecules together more tightly, so more energy (generally represented by higher temperatures) is required to weaken those bonds to allow for phase changes.

Dipole-Dipole Interactions

Polar molecules tend to orient themselves such that the positive region of one molecule is close to the negative region of another molecule. This arrangement is energetically favorable because an attractive dipole force is formed between the two molecules.

Dipole-dipole interactions are present in the solid and liquid phases but become negligible in the gas phase because the molecules are generally much farther apart. Polar species tend to have higher boiling points than nonpolar species of comparable molecular weight.

Hydrogen Bonding

Hydrogen bonding is a specific, particularly strong form of dipole-dipole interaction. When hydrogen is bound to either fluorine, oxygen, or nitrogen, the hydrogen atom carries little of the electron density of the covalent bond. This positively charged hydrogen atom interacts with the partial negative charge located on the electronegative atoms of nearby molecules. This interaction between the δ^+ on the H and the δ^- on the nearby molecule is the hydrogen bond. On the PCAT, a hydrogen can only hydrogen bond to adjacent molecules if that H is covalently bound to either F, O, or N. Substances that display hydrogen bonding tend to have unusually high boiling points compared with compounds of similar molecular weight that do not hydrogen bond. Hydrogen bonding is particularly important in the behavior of water, alcohols, amines, and carboxylic acids.

Dispersion Forces

The bonding electrons in covalent bonds may appear to be shared equally between two atoms, but, at any particular point in time, they will be located randomly throughout the orbital. This permits unequal sharing of electrons, causing rapid polarization and counterpolarization of the electron cloud and formation of short-lived dipoles. These dipoles interact with the electron clouds of neighboring molecules, inducing the formation of more dipoles. The attractive interactions of these short-lived dipoles are called London dispersion forces (LDF).

Dispersion forces are generally weaker than other intermolecular forces. They do not extend over long distances and are therefore most important when molecules are close together. The strength of these interactions within a given substance depends directly on how easily the electrons in the molecules can move (i.e., be polarized). Large molecules in which the electrons are far from the nucleus are relatively easy to polarize and therefore possess greater dispersion forces. If not for dispersion forces, the noble gases would not liquefy at any temperature since no other intermolecular forces exist between the noble gas atoms. The low temperature at which the noble gases liquefy is to some extent indicative of the magnitude of dispersion forces between the atoms.

Carbon-Carbon Bonding

Carbon-carbon bonds can be categorized based on length and energy level as well as hybridization. In Chapter 39, Structural Formulas, we will review the hybridization of carbon-carbon bonds. The table below compares the bond length and energy levels of the different carbon-carbon bonds.

	Bond Length	Bond Energy
C−C	longest	lowest
C=C	middle	middle
C≡C	shortest	highest

Table 29.1

REVIEW PROBLEMS

1. Is Cl^- an anion or a cation?

2. Consider the following reaction:
    $$H_2\ (g) + F_2\ (g) \longrightarrow HF\ (g)$$
    Is the HF bond more or less polar than an H−H bond?

3. Arrange the following compounds in terms of increasing polarity:
    $$HCN,\ NaCl,\ Cl_2$$

4. **(A)** Which has a greater C−C bond distance, C_2H_4 or C_2H_2?
    (B) Which has a greater C−C bond energy?

5. Which of the following compounds would you expect to be weakly drawn into a magnetic field?
    $$H_2,\ NaCl,\ NO,\ NO_2,\ BF_3,\ PCl_5,\ SO_2$$

6. Which represents the proper Lewis structure of:
    (A) $CHCl_3$?

    1. 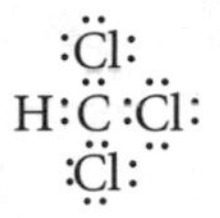
        ```
            ••
           :Cl:
            ••   ••
         H:C:Cl:
            ••   ••
           :Cl:
            ••
        ```

    2. 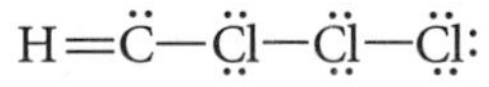
        ```
              ••    ••    ••
         H══C─Cl─Cl─Cl:
              ••    ••    ••
        ```

    3. 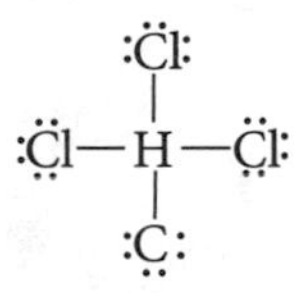
        ```
            ••
           :Cl:
            |
         ••          ••
        :Cl─H─Cl:
         ••   |      ••
            :C:
            ••
        ```

    4. 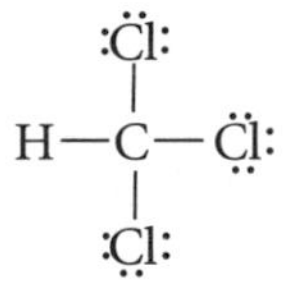
        ```
            ••
           :Cl:
            |        ••
         H─C─Cl:
            |        ••
           :Cl:
            ••
        ```

    (B) N_2?

    1. 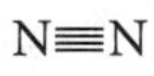 N≡N

    2. 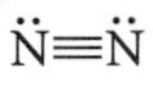 Ṅ≡Ṅ

    3. 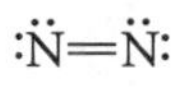 :N̈══N̈:

    4. 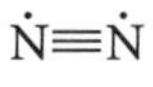 Ṅ≡Ṅ

(C) $[ClO_4]^-$?

1. 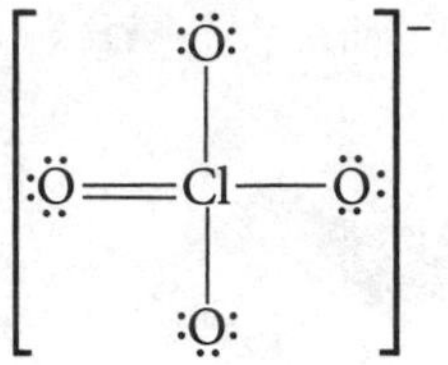

2. 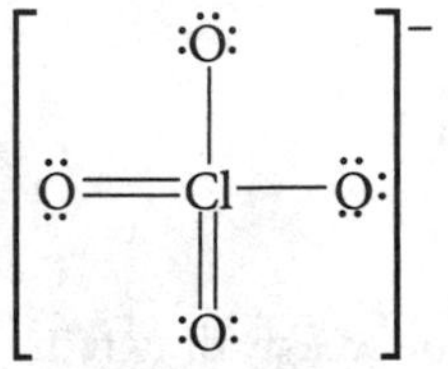

3. 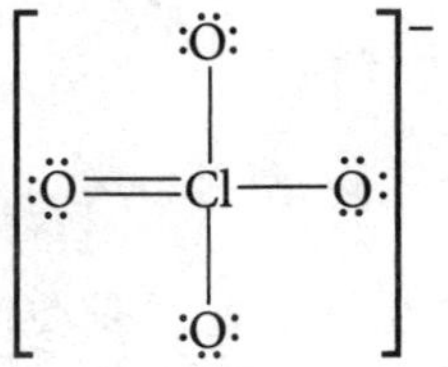

4. 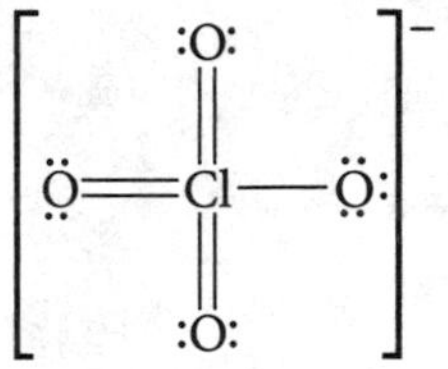

7. Which is not a resonance form of:

(A) 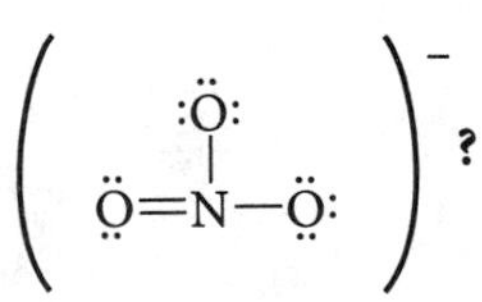 **?**

1. 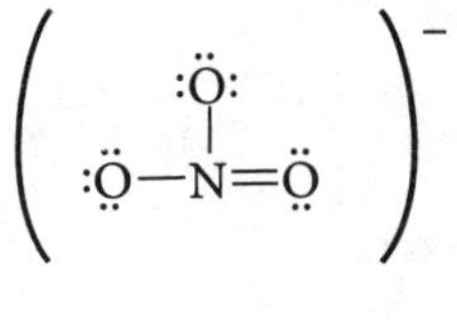

2. 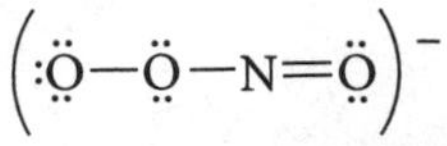

3. 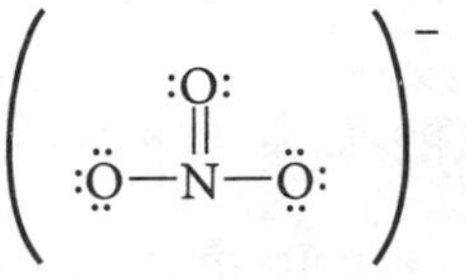 $\left(\begin{array}{c} :\ddot{O}: \\ \| \\ :\ddot{O}-N-\ddot{O}: \end{array} \right)^{-}$

(B) $\left(\ddot{N}\equiv N-\ddot{N}: \right)^{-}$?

1. $\left(:\ddot{N}-N\equiv N \right)^{-}$

2. 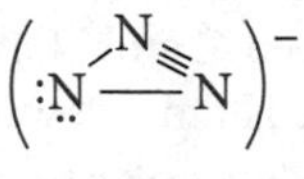 $\left(:\ddot{N}\overset{N}{\underset{}{\text{—}}}N \right)^{-}$

3. $\left(:\ddot{N}=N=\ddot{N}: \right)^{-}$

8. Using formal charges, predict which is the most likely resonance structure for N_2O.

(A) $:N\equiv N=\ddot{O}:$

(B) $:\ddot{N}=O=\ddot{N}:$

(C) $:\ddot{N}=N=\ddot{O}:$

(D) $:N\equiv N-\ddot{O}:$

9. Draw Lewis structures of the most likely ions of the elements from Na to Ca (atomic numbers 11 to 20).

10. Draw Lewis structures for each of the following:
    (A) Nitrate ion ($[NO_3]^-$)
    (B) Phosphoric acid (H_3PO_4)
    (C) Aluminum chloride ($AlCl_3$)
    (D) Sodium phosphate (Na_3PO_4)

11. A hydride is a compound containing the hydride ion, H^-. Predict two elements whose hydrides would contain incomplete octets.

12. Which of the following sets of molecules contains only nonpolar species?
    (A) BH_3, NH_3, AlH_3
    (B) NO_2, CO_2, ClO_2
    (C) HCl, HNO_2, $HClO_3$
    (D) BeH_2, BH_3, CH_4

13. Arrange the following compounds in order of increasing boiling point: C_2H_6, CH_3OH, LiF, HCl.

SOLUTIONS TO REVIEW PROBLEMS

1. Cl^- is an anion. Negative ions are called anions, and positive ions are called cations.

2. The HF bond is more polar than an H–H bond. *Polar* denotes unequal sharing of electrons; H–H must have equal sharing because the two atoms are the same. H and F are different atoms, with different electronegativities, and so the electrons are unequally shared.

3. **Cl_2 < HCN < NaCl**

    Cl_2 is the least polar because it contains two identical atoms that must share electrons equally. HCN is a linear molecule with a triple bond between C and N; it has a dipole moment pointing from the relatively electropositive H atom toward the rather electronegative N atom. Still, we should expect HCN to be less polar than NaCl; the bond between Na and Cl, a metal and a nonmetal whose electronegativities differ greatly, is completely ionic.

4. **A** C_2H_4 has greater bond distance because it is a double bond and is therefore held less closely than C_2H_2, which is a triple bond.

    B C_2H_2 has a greater bond energy because it is a triple bond and more energy is needed to break it.

5. NO and NO_2 would be weakly drawn into a magnetic field because they are paramagnetic. All paramagnetic molecules are weakly drawn into a magnetic field, and any compound with an odd number of valence electrons is paramagnetic. Thus:

    H_2: H has 1 valence electron; $1 + 1 = 2$, so H_2 is not paramagnetic.

    NaCl: Na has 1 valence electron, Cl has 7; $1 + 7 = 8$, so NaCl is not paramagnetic.

    NO: N has 5 valence electrons, O has 6; $6 + 5 = 11$, so NO is paramagnetic.

    NO_2: $5 + (2)(6) = 17$, so NO_2 is paramagnetic.

    BF_3: B has 3 valence electrons, F has 7; $3 + 3(7) = 24$, so BF_3 is not paramagnetic.
    PCl_5: P has 5 valence electrons, Cl has 7; $5 + 5(7) = 40$, so PCl_5 is not paramagnetic.
    SO_2: S has 6 valence electrons, O has 6; $6 + 2(6) = 18$, so SO_2 is not paramagnetic.

6. **A 4**

    Choice 4 is correct. Choice 1 is incorrect because covalent bonds are not marked with lines. Choice 2 has an impossible configuration; H can never be double-bonded to anything since the maximum number of electrons it may possess is 2. Choice 3 is also impossible since having four bonds around H would imply 8 electrons are present, which again would mean that H would have more than its maximum of 2 electrons.

    B 2

    Choices 1 and 3 must be incorrect because, although they satisfy the octet rule, they have the wrong total number of electrons; choice 1 has 8 valence electrons, whereas choice 3 has 12. Given two N atoms, there can be only $(2)(5) = 10$ valence electrons, as in correct choice 2. (Choice 1 is also incorrect because quadruple bonding is impossible due to orbital geometries.) Choice 4 is doubly incorrect because, in addition to only having 8 total electrons, the octet rule is not satisfied as each nucleus has 7, not 8, valence electrons.

C 4

Choice 4 is the preferred structure because four of the five atoms have a formal charge of zero. Since Cl is in the third period, its number of valence electrons can exceed 8.

7. **A 2**

In resonance forms, only the electrons change place; atoms are not rearranged. Choices 1 and 3 are both resonance structures. Choice 2 requires rearrangement of the atoms.

B 2

By the same reasoning as above.

8. **D**   There is no formal charge on the structure of choice A; therefore, this structure might be the most likely resonance structure. However, the expanded octet on N makes the structure impossible since N is in period 2, and $n = 2$ and does not have d orbitals. Choice C is incorrect because the negative formal charge is on N, which is not the most electronegative atom. Choice B is incorrect because O, which is the most electronegative atom, has a formal charge of $+2$. Choice D is most likely because the negative formal charge is on O, the more electronegative element.

9. Na^+ Mg^{2+} Al^{3+} Si^{4+} $:\ddot{P}:^{3-}$ $:\ddot{S}:^{2-}$ $:\ddot{C}l:^-$ **(Ar has none)**
    K^+ Ca^{2+}

Note that a correct ionic Lewis structure must always show the charge on the ion.

10. **A** $[NO_3]^-$

	has	needs
charge:	1 electron	
N:	5 electrons	8 electrons
3 O:	18 electrons	24 electrons
	24 electrons	32 electrons

$(32 - 24)$ electrons $= 8$ electrons $= 4$ bonds

Place N at the center:

(N and O both have a formal charge.)

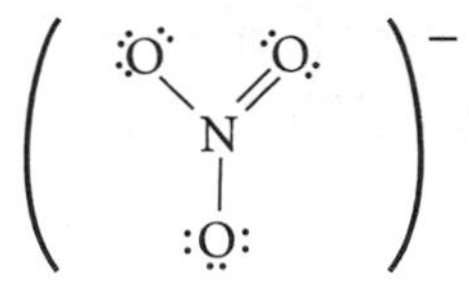

They cannot be reduced because the N octet cannot be expanded. However, since resonance will be present, a better version might be:

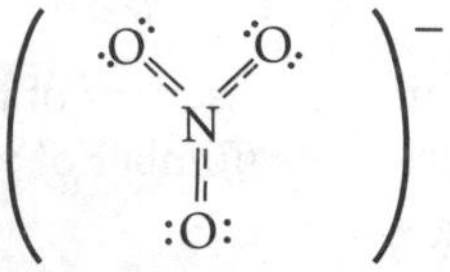

$$\left(\begin{array}{c} \ddot{O} = N = \ddot{O} \\ \| \\ \ddot{O} \end{array} \right)^{-}$$

B H₃PO₄

	has	needs
3 H	3 electrons	$3(2) = 6$ electrons
P	5 electrons	8 electrons (at least)
4 O	24 electrons	32 electrons
	32 electrons	46 electrons

$(46 - 32)$ electrons $= 14$ electrons $= 7$ bonds (at least).

Place the P at the center, the 4 O around it, and H on 3 of the O with single bonds between them; this will use all 7 bonds.

Now check the formal charges:

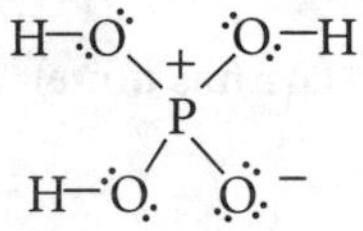

$$\begin{array}{ccc} H-\ddot{O} & & \ddot{O}-H \\ & \searrow + \swarrow & \\ & P & \\ & \swarrow \quad \searrow & \\ H-\ddot{O} & & \ddot{O}- \end{array}$$

The P has a formal charge of $+1$, and the O has a formal charge of -1. These can be eliminated by moving a pair of electrons around from the O into a double bond:

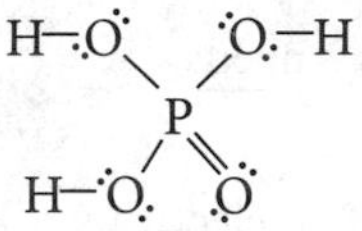

$$\begin{array}{ccc} H-\ddot{O} & & \ddot{O}-H \\ & \searrow \swarrow & \\ & P & \\ & \swarrow \quad \parallel & \\ H-\ddot{O} & & \ddot{O} \end{array}$$

C Both aluminum chloride and sodium phosphate are ionic.

AlCl₃

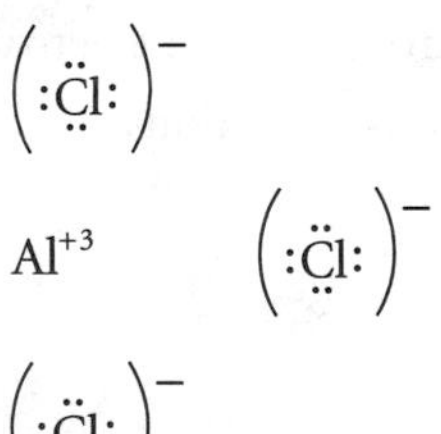

$$\left(:\ddot{\underset{..}{Cl}}: \right)^{-}$$

$$Al^{+3} \qquad \left(:\ddot{\underset{..}{Cl}}: \right)^{-}$$

$$\left(:\ddot{\underset{..}{Cl}}: \right)^{-}$$

D Na_3PO_4

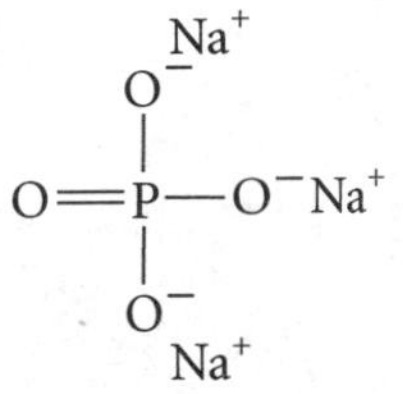

$$O=\overset{\overset{\displaystyle O^- Na^+}{|}}{\underset{\underset{\displaystyle Na^+}{\overset{|}{O^-}}}{P}}-O^- Na^+$$

11.   Be and B, because they can join to only two or three H, respectively, since they have fewer than 4 valence electrons. The elements Mg and Al may also do this, as could Na, Ca, and the other active metals of Groups IA and IIA.

12. **D**

    A. NH_3 is polar (positive end at base of pyramid, negative end at N).

    B. NO_2 and ClO_2 are both angular molecules; therefore, they are polar.

    C.   All three are polar.

13. $C_2H_6 < HCl < CH_3OH < LiF$

For each compound, the following intermolecular forces are present:

C_2H_6: London dispersion forces

HCl: dipole-dipole

CH_3OH: H-bonding

LiF: ionic

CHAPTER THIRTY

Stoichiometry

A **compound** is a pure substance composed of two or more elements in a fixed proportion. Compounds can be broken down chemically to produce their constituent elements or other compounds. All elements, except for some of the noble gases, can react with other elements or compounds to form new compounds. These new compounds can react further to form yet different compounds.

MOLECULES AND MOLES

A molecule is a combination of two or more atoms held together by covalent bonds and is the smallest unit of a compound that still displays the properties of that compound. Molecules may contain two atoms of the same element, as in N_2 and O_2, or may be comprised of two or more different atoms, as in CO_2 and $SOCl_2$. Molecules are usually discussed in terms of **molecular mass** and **moles**.

Ionic compounds do not form true molecules. In the solid state, they can be considered to be a nearly infinite, three-dimensional array of the charged particles of which the compound is composed. Because no actual molecule exists, molecular mass becomes meaningless, and the term **formula mass** is used in its place.

Molecular Mass

Like atoms, molecules can be characterized by their mass. The molecular mass (also known as **molecular weight**) is the sum of the atomic masses of the atoms in the molecule. Similarly, the formula mass of an ionic compound is found by adding up the atomic masses of each constituent atom according to the empirical formula of the substance.

Example: What is the molecular mass of $SOCl_2$?

Solution: To find the molecular mass of $SOCl_2$, add together the atomic masses of each of the atoms:

$$1\ S\ =\ 1 \times 32\ \text{amu}\quad =\ 32\ \text{amu}$$
$$1\ O\ =\ 1 \times 16\ \text{amu}\quad =\ 16\ \text{amu}$$
$$2\ Cl\ =\ 2 \times 35.5\ \text{amu}\ =\ \underline{71\ \text{amu}}$$
$$\text{molecular mass}\ =\ 119\ \text{amu}$$

Mole

A mole is defined as the amount of a substance that contains the same number of particles found in a 12.000 g sample of carbon-12. This quantity, **Avogadro's number,** is equal to 6.022×10^{23}. One mole of a compound has a mass in grams equal to the molecular mass of that compound in amu and contains 6.022×10^{23} molecules of the compound. For example, 62 g of H_2CO_3 represents one mole of carbonic acid and contains 6.022×10^{23} H_2CO_3 molecules. The mass of 1 mole of a compound is called its **molar mass** or **molar weight** and is usually expressed as g/mol. Therefore, the molar mass of H_2CO_3 is 62 g/mol.

The following formula is used to determine the number of moles present in a sample:

$$\text{mol} = \frac{\text{Weight of Sample (g)}}{\text{Molar Weight (g/mol)}}$$

Example: How many moles are in 9.52 g of $MgCl_2$?

Solution: First find the molar mass of $MgCl_2$:

$1(24.31\ \text{g/mol}) + 2(35.45\ \text{g/mol}) = 95.21\ \text{g/mol}$

Now solve for the number of moles:

$$\frac{9.52\ \text{g}}{95.21\ \text{g/mol}} = 0.10\ \text{mol of } MgCl_2$$

Gram Equivalents

For some substances it is useful to define a measure of reactive capacity. This expresses the fact that some molecules are more potent than others in performing certain reactions. An example of this is the ability of different acids to donate protons (H^+ ions) in solution (see Chapter 37, Acids and Bases). For instance, 1 mole of HCl can donate 1 mole of hydrogen ions, while 1 mole of H_2SO_4 can donate 2 moles of hydrogen ions. This difference is expressed using the term **equivalent**: 1 mole of HCl contains 1 equivalent of hydrogen ions, while 1 mole of H_2SO_4 contains 2 equivalents of hydrogen ions. To determine the number of equivalents a compound contains, a new measure of weight, called **gram-equivalent weight (GEW)**, was developed such that:

$$\text{equivalents} = \frac{\text{weight of compound}}{\text{gram equivalent weight}}$$

and

$$\text{gram equivalent weight} = \frac{\text{molar mass}}{n}$$

where *n* is usually either the number of **hydrogen** ions an Arrhenius or Brønsted-Lowry acid could donate per molecule or the number of **hydroxyl groups** an Arrhenius base could donate (or number of hydrogen ions a Brønsted-Lowry base could accept) in a reaction. Gram equivalent weight is dependent on reaction conditions and is determined experimentally; however, on the PCAT, gram equivalent weight can be estimated from the molecular structure. By using equivalents, it is possible to say one equivalent of acid will neutralize one equivalent of base, a statement that is not necessarily true when dealing in moles.

REPRESENTATION OF COMPOUNDS

Law of Constant Composition

The law of constant composition states that all samples of a given compound will contain the same elements in identical mass ratios. For instance, every sample of H_2O will contain two atoms of hydrogen for every atom of oxygen and therefore one gram of hydrogen for every eight grams of oxygen.

Empirical and Molecular Formulas

There are two ways to express a formula for a compound. The **empirical formula** gives the simplest whole number ratio of the elements in the compound. The **molecular formula** gives the exact number of atoms of each element in the compound and is a multiple of the empirical formula. For example, the empirical formula for benzene is CH, whereas the molecular formula is C_6H_6. For some compounds, the empirical and molecular formulas are the same, as in the case of H_2O. An ionic compound, such as NaCl or $CaCO_3$, will have only an empirical formula.

Note that, given a molecular formula, the empirical formula for that molecule can be calculated by simplifying the ratio of the subscripts next to each component. However, given only an empirical formula, the molecular formula of a specific molecule cannot be determined without more information since several different molecules could share the same empirical formula. For example, the empirical formula CH_2 is shared by ethylene (C_2H_4), butane (C_4H_8), and cyclohexane (C_6H_{12})

Percent Composition

The percent composition by mass of an element is the mass percent of the element in a specific compound. To determine the percent composition of an element X in a compound, the following formula is used:

$$\% \text{ composition} = \frac{\text{Mass of X in Formula}}{\text{Formula Weight of Compound}} \times \mathbf{100\%}$$

The percent composition of an element may be determined using either the empirical or molecular formula. If the percent compositions are known, the empirical formula can be derived. It is possible to determine the molecular formula if both the percent compositions and molecular mass of the compound are known.

Example: What is the percent composition of chromium in $K_2Cr_2O_7$ (potassium's molecular mass is 39 g/mol, chromium's is 52 g/mol, and oxygen's is 16 g/mol)?

Solution: The formula mass of $K_2Cr_2O_7$ is: $2(39 \text{ g/mol}) + 2(52 \text{ g/mol}) + 7(16 \text{ g/mol}) = 294$ g/mol

$$\% \text{ composition of } Cr = \frac{2(52\text{g/mol})}{294 \text{ g/mol}} \times 100\%$$

$$= 0.354 \times 100\%$$

$$= 35.4\%$$

Example: What are the empirical and molecular formulas of a compound that contains 40.9% carbon, 4.58% hydrogen, and 54.52% oxygen by mass and has a molecular mass of 264 g/mol (carbon's molar mass is 12 g/mol, hydrogen's is 1 g/mol, and oxygen's is 16 g/mol)?

Method One: First, determine the number of moles of each element in the compound by assuming a 100-gram sample; this converts the percentage of each element present directly into grams of that element. Then convert grams to moles:

$$\# \text{ mol of C} = \frac{40.9 \text{ g}}{12 \text{ g/mol}} = 3.41 \text{ mol}$$

$$\# \text{ mol of H} = \frac{4.58 \text{ g}}{1 \text{ g/mol}} = 4.58 \text{ mol}$$

$$\# \text{ mol of O} = \frac{54.52 \text{ g}}{16 \text{ g/mol}} = 3.41 \text{ mol}$$

Next, find the simplest whole number ratio of the elements by dividing the number of moles of each element by the smallest number obtained in the previous step:

$$C: \frac{3.41}{3.41} = 1.0 \qquad\qquad H: \frac{4.58}{3.41} = 1.3 \qquad\qquad O: \frac{3.41}{3.41} = 1.0$$

Finally, the empirical formula is obtained by converting the numbers obtained into whole numbers (multiplying them by an integer value).

$$C_1H_{1.3}O_1 \times 3 = C_3H_4O_3$$

Multiplying all the subscripts by 3 to obtain all whole numbers for the subscripts shows that $C_3H_4O_3$ is the empirical formula.

To determine the molecular formula, divide the molecular mass by the mass represented by the empirical formula. The resulting value is the number of empirical formula units in the molecular formula.

The empirical formula mass of $C_3H_4O_3$ is:

$3(12 \text{ g/mol}) + 4(1 \text{ g/mol}) + 3(16 \text{ g/mol}) = 88 \text{ g/mol}$

$$\frac{264 \text{ g/mol}}{88 \text{ g/mol}} = 3$$

$C_3H_4O_3 \times 3 = C_9H_{12}O_9$ is the molecular formula.

Method Two: When the molecular mass is given, it can be faster to find the molecular formula first. This is accomplished by multiplying the molecular mass by the given percentages to find the grams of each element present in one mole of compound, then dividing by the respective atomic masses to find the mole ratio of the elements:

$$\# \text{ mol of C} = \frac{(0.409)(264 \text{ g})}{12 \text{ g/mol}} = 9 \text{ mol}$$

$$\# \text{ mol of H} = \frac{(0.0458)(264 \text{ g})}{1 \text{ g/mol}} = 12 \text{ mol}$$

$$\# \text{ mol of O} = \frac{(0.5452)(264 \text{ g})}{16 \text{ g/mol}} = 9 \text{ mol}$$

Thus, the molecular formula, $C_9H_{12}O_9$, is the direct result. The empirical formula can now be found by reducing the subscript ratio to the simplest integral values.

BALANCING EQUATIONS

Chemical equations express how much and what type of reactants must be used to obtain a given quantity of product. From the **law of conservation of mass**, the mass of the reactants in a reaction must be equal to the mass of the products. More specifically, chemical equations must be balanced so that there are the same number of atoms of each element in the products as there are in the reactants. **Stoichiometric coefficients** are used to indicate the number of moles of a given species involved in the reaction. For example, the reaction for the formation of water is:

$$2 \text{ H}_2 \ (g) + \text{O}_2 \ (g) \rightarrow 2 \text{ H}_2\text{O} \ (g)$$

The coefficients indicate that two moles of H_2 gas must be reacted with one mole of O_2 gas to produce two moles of water. In general, stoichiometric coefficients are given as whole numbers.

Example: Balance the following reaction:

$$C_4H_{10} \ (l) + O_2 \ (g) \rightarrow CO_2 \ (g) + H_2O \ (l)$$

Solution: First, balance the carbon in reactants and products.

$$C_4H_{10} + O_2 \rightarrow 4 \, CO_2 + H_2O$$

Second, balance the hydrogen in reactants and products.

$$C_4H_{10} + O_2 \rightarrow 4 \, CO_2 + 5 \, H_2O$$

Third, balance the oxygen in reactants and products.

$$C_4H_{10} + 6.5 \, O_2 \rightarrow 4 \, CO_2 + 5 \, H_2O$$

Stoichiometric coefficients are typically written as integers, so double everything to remove the decimal.

$$2 \, C_4H_{10} + 13 \, O_2 \rightarrow 8 \, CO_2 + 10 \, H_2O$$

Finally, check that all of the elements and the total charge are balanced correctly. If there is a difference in total charge between the reactants and products, then the charge will also have to be balanced. Instructions for balancing charge are found in Chapter 32 in the context of redox reactions.

Applications of Stoichiometry

Once an equation has been balanced, the ratio of moles of reactant to moles of products is known, and that information can be used to solve many types of stoichiometry problems. It is important to use proper units when solving such problems. When performing these calculations, the units should cancel out such that the units obtained in the answer represent those asked for in the problem.

Example: How many grams of calcium chloride are needed to prepare 72 g of silver chloride according to the following equation (calcium's molar mass is 40 g/mol, chlorine's is 35.5 g/mol, and silver's is 108 g/mol)?

$$CaCl_2 \ (aq) + 2 \, AgNO_3 \ (aq) \rightarrow Ca(NO_3)_2 \ (aq) + 2 \, AgCl \ (s)$$

Solution: First, note that the equation is balanced. Then, identify that one mole of $CaCl_2$ yields two moles of AgCl when reacted with two moles of $AgNO_3$. The molar mass of $CaCl_2$ is 110 g/mol, and the molar mass of AgCl is approximately 144 g/mol. Starting with the goal mass of AgCl, convert to moles, find the number of moles of $CaCl_2$ required, and then convert into g of $CaCl_2$ (as grams are the units that the question specifies).

$$72 \text{ g AgCl} \times \frac{1 \text{ mol AgCl}}{144 \text{ g AgCl}} \times \frac{1 \text{ mol CaCl}_2}{2 \text{ mol AgCl}} \times \frac{110 \text{ g CaCl}_2}{1 \text{ mol CaCl}_2} = 27.5 \text{ g of CaCl}_2$$

Thus, 27.5 g of $CaCl_2$ are needed to produce 72 g of AgCl.

Limiting reactant

When reactants are mixed, they are seldom added in the exact stoichiometric proportions as shown in the balanced equation. Therefore, in most reactions, one of the reactants will be consumed first. This reactant is known as the limiting reactant or **limiting reagent** because it limits the amount of product that can be formed in the reaction. The reactant(s) that remains after all of the limiting reactant is used up is called the **excess reactant**.

Example: If 28 g of Fe are reacted with 24 g of S to produce FeS, what is the limiting reactant? How many grams of excess reactant are present in the vessel at the end of the reaction?

The balanced equation is: $Fe + S \xrightarrow{\Delta} FeS$

Solution: First, the number of moles for each reactant must be determined.

$$28 \text{ g Fe} \times \frac{1 \text{ mol Fe}}{56 \text{ g}} = 0.5 \text{ mol Fe}$$

$$24 \text{ g S} \times \frac{1 \text{ mol S}}{32 \text{ g}} = 0.75 \text{ mol S}$$

Since one mole of Fe is needed to react with one mole of S, and there are 0.5 moles of Fe for every 0.75 moles of S, the limiting reagent is Fe. Thus, 0.5 moles of Fe will react with 0.5 moles of S, leaving an excess of 0.25 moles of S in the vessel. The mass of the excess reactant will be:

$$\text{mass of S} = (0.25 \text{ mol S})\frac{32 \text{ g}}{1 \text{ mol S}} = 8 \text{ g of S}$$

Yields

The yield of a reaction, which is the amount of product predicted or obtained when the reaction is carried out, can be predicted from the balanced equation. There are three distinct ways of reporting yields. The **theoretical yield** is the amount of product that can be predicted from a balanced equation, assuming that all of the limiting reagent has been used, no competing side reactions have occurred, and all of the product has been collected. However, the theoretical yield is seldom obtained in real-world conditions; therefore, chemists speak of the **actual yield,** which is the amount of product isolated from the reaction experimentally. There are a variety of reasons why the actual yield is less than the theoretical yield. For example, many reactions are **reversible** (i.e., do not proceed 100 percent from left to right) or use reactants that interact with one another to produce additional end products.

The term **percent yield** is used to express the relationship between the actual yield and the theoretical yield and is given by the following equation:

$$\text{Percent yield} = \frac{\text{Actual yield}}{\text{Theoretical yield}} \times 100\%$$

Example: What is the percent yield for a reaction in which 27 g of Cu is produced by reacting 32.5 g of Zn in excess $CuSO_4$ solution (copper's molar mass is 63.5 g/mol, zinc's is 65 g/mol, sulfur's is 32 g/mol, and oxygen's is 16 g/mol)?

Solution: The balanced equation is as follows:

$$Zn\ (s) + CuSO_4\ (aq) \rightarrow Cu\ (s) + ZnSO_4\ (aq)$$

Calculate the theoretical yield for Cu.

$$32.5\ g\ Zn \times \frac{1\ mol\ Zn}{65\ g} = 0.5\ mol\ Zn$$

$$0.5\ mol\ Zn \times \frac{1\ mol\ Cu}{1\ mol\ Zn} = 0.5\ mol\ Cu$$

$$0.5\ mol\ Cu \times \frac{64g}{1\ mol\ Cu} = 32\ g\ Cu\ (theoretical\ yield)$$

Finally, determine the percent yield.

$$Percent\ yield = \frac{Actual\ yield}{Theoretical\ yield} \times 100\% = \frac{27\ g}{32\ g} \times 100\% = 84\%$$

REVIEW PROBLEMS

1. What is the sum of the coefficients of the following equation when it is balanced?

    $$C_6H_{12}O_6 + O_2 \rightarrow CO_2 + H_2O$$

    (A) 19
    (B) 20
    (C) 21
    (D) 38

2. Determine the molecular formula and calculate the percent composition of each element present in nicotine, which has an empirical formula of C_5H_7N and a molecular mass of 162 g/mol.

3. Acetylene, used as a fuel in welding torches, is produced in a reaction between calcium carbide and water:

    $$CaC_2 + 2\ H_2O \rightarrow Ca(OH)_2 + C_2H_2$$

    How many grams of C_2H_2 are formed from 0.400 moles of CaC_2?

    (A) 0.400
    (B) 0.800
    (C) 4.00
    (D) 10.4

4. Aspirin ($C_9H_8O_4$) is prepared by reacting salicylic acid ($C_7H_6O_3$) and acetic anhydride ($C_4H_6O_3$).

    $$C_7H_6O_3 + C_4H_6O_3 \rightarrow C_9H_8O_4 + C_2H_4O_2$$

    How many moles of salicylic acid should be used to prepare six 5-grain aspirin tablets? (1 g = 15.5 grains)

    (A) 0.01
    (B) 0.10
    (C) 1.00
    (D) 2.00

5. The percent composition of an unknown element X in CH_3X is 32 percent. Which of the following is element X?

    (A) H
    (B) F
    (C) Cl
    (D) Li

6. Twenty-seven grams of silver was reacted with excess sulfur, according to the following equation:

$$2\,Ag + S \rightarrow Ag_2S$$

25.0 g of silver sulfide was collected. What are the theoretical yield, actual yield, and percent yield?

7. What is the mass in grams of a single chlorine atom? Of a single molecule of O_2?

The following reaction will be used to answer questions 8–10.

$$Ag(NH_3)_2{}^+ \rightarrow Ag^+ + 2\,NH_3$$

8. How many moles of $Ag(NH_3)_2{}^+$ are required for the production of 11 moles of ammonia?

9. If 5.80 g of $Ag(NH_3)_2{}^+$ yields 1.40 g of ammonia, how many moles of silver are produced?
    (A) 0.041
    (B) 0.054
    (C) 4.40
    (D) 5.80

10. What are the percent compositions of Ag, N, and H in $Ag(NH_3)_2{}^+$?

11. A hydrocarbon (which by definition contains only C and H atoms) is heated in an excess of oxygen to produce 58.67 g of CO_2 and 27 g of H_2O. What is the empirical formula of the hydrocarbon?

12. Balance the following reaction:

$$NF_3 + H_2O \rightarrow HF + NO + NO_2$$

How many grams of HF are expected to form if 1.5 kg of a 5.2% NF_3 sample is used?

13. Balance the following reactions:
    (A) $I_2 + Cl_2 + H_2O \rightarrow HIO_3 + HCl$
    (B) $MnO_2 + HCl \rightarrow H_2O + MnCl_2 + Cl_2$
    (C) $BCl_3 + P_4 + H_2 \rightarrow BP + HCl$
    (D) $C_3H_5(NO_3)_3 \rightarrow CO_2 + H_2O + N_2 + O_2$
    (E) $HCl + Ba(OH)_2 \rightarrow BaCl_2 + H_2O$

SOLUTIONS TO REVIEW PROBLEMS

1. **A** To answer this question, the equation must first be balanced. Starting with carbon, it can be seen that there are 6 carbons on the reactant side and only one on the product side, so a coefficient of 6 should be placed in front of the carbon dioxide. For the hydrogen, there are 12 atoms on the left and only 2 on the right; thus, a coefficient of 6 should go in front of water. Now, for oxygen, there are 8 atoms on the left and 18 on the right. To balance the oxygen, 10 more atoms of oxygen must be added to the left side. The best way to do this is to put a coefficient of 6 in front of oxygen, since putting a stoichiometric coefficient in front of the glucose molecule would unbalance the equation in terms of carbon and hydrogen. Therefore, the final balanced equation is:

$$C_6H_{12}O_6 + 6\,O_2 \rightarrow 6\,CO_2 + 6\,H_2O$$

Remember that $C_6H_{12}O_6$ has a coefficient of 1, and this must be added to the total number. So $1 + 6 + 6 + 6 = 19$.

2. $C_{10}H_{14}N_2$; 74.1% C, 8.6% H, 17.3% N

To determine the molecular formula of nicotine, the empirical mass of the compound must be calculated.

$5(C) + 7(H) + 1(N) = $ empirical mass

$5(12 \text{ g/mol}) + 7(1 \text{ g/mol}) + 14 \text{ g/mol} = 81 \text{ g/mol}$

The empirical mass (81 g/mol) is then divided into the molecular mass (162 g/mol) to determine the number by which each subscript in the empirical formula must be multiplied to obtain the molecular formula.

$$\frac{162 \text{g/mol}}{81 \text{g/mol}} = 2$$

$2(C_5H_7N) = C_{10}H_{14}N_2 = $ molecular formula

To find the percent composition of each element, divide the molar mass of each element by the molecular mass of nicotine:

$$\% \text{ C} = \frac{120}{162} \times 100\% = 74.1\%$$

$$\% \text{ H} = \frac{14}{162} \times 100\% = 8.6\%$$

$$\% \text{ N} = \frac{28}{162} \times 100\% = 17.3\%$$

The same percentages would be obtained if we used the empirical formula for this calculation.

3. **D** According to the balanced equation, one mole of CaC_2 yields one mole of C_2H_2. Therefore, if 0.400 mol of CaC2 were used, 0.400 mol of C_2H_2 would be produced. Now the number of moles must be converted to grams using the following formula:

$$\text{mol} = \frac{\text{Weight in g}}{\text{Molecular weight}}$$

The molecular mass of C_2H_2 is
$2(12 \text{ g/mol}) + 2(1 \text{ g/mol}) = 26 \text{ g/mol}$

Substituting into the above equation:

$$0.400 \text{ mol} = \frac{x}{26 \text{g/mol}}$$
$$x = 10.4 \text{ g}$$

4. **A** According to the balanced equation, one mole of salicylic acid will yield one mole of aspirin. Therefore, to solve this question, the number of moles of aspirin in six 5-grain tablets, or 30 grains of aspirin, must be determined using the following relationship.

$$\frac{1 \text{ g}}{15.5 \text{ grains}} = \frac{x}{30 \text{ grains}}$$
$$x \approx 2 \text{ g}$$

Therefore, the mass of the aspirin produced is about 2 grams, which must be converted to moles. The molecular mass of aspirin is:
$9(C) + 8(H) + 4(O) = 9(12 \text{ g/mol}) + 8(1 \text{ g/mol}) + 4(16 \text{ g/mol}) = 180 \text{ g/mol}$
Then, the number of moles in two grams of aspirin is calculated.

$$\frac{2 \text{ g}}{180 \text{g/mol}} = 0.01 \text{ mol}$$

5. **D** The easiest way to solve this problem, short of trying every choice, is to work through the problem with slightly backward logic. Because we know that element X comprises 32% of the compound, CH_3 must comprise 68% (100% – 32%). We must calculate the formula mass of CH_3 (12 + 3 = 15 g). The fact that 15 g = 68% of the total mass can be restated as the equation 15 g = 0.68 × total mass; we can solve this to show that the total molecular mass must be 22 g. The mass of X = total mass – 15 g = 7 g. Choice (D), Li, has an atomic mass of 7 g/mol.

6. **31 g, 25 g, 81%**

   According to the balanced equation, two moles of silver react with one mole of sulfur to form one mole of silver sulfide. The theoretical yield is the amount of product that would be collected if all of the limiting reagent reacts. Using a stoichiometric calculation, the theoretical yield of silver sulfide if 27.0 g of silver is used would be as follows:

   $$27.0 \text{ g Ag} \times \frac{1 \text{ mol Ag}}{108 \text{ g Ag}} \times \frac{1 \text{ mol Ag}_2\text{S}}{2 \text{ mol Ag}} \times \frac{248 \text{ g Ag}_2\text{S}}{1 \text{ mol Ag}_2\text{S}} = 31.0 \text{ g Ag}_2\text{S}$$

   The actual yield is the amount of product that is obtained from the experiment. It is usually less than the theoretical yield since the reagents may not react completely and the product may be difficult to collect. In this experiment, the actual yield is given to be 25.0 g of silver sulfide. The percent yield represents the percentage of product actually collected in reference to the theoretical yield. Thus, the percent yield for this experiment would be:

$$\frac{25.0 \text{ g}}{31.0 \text{ g}} \times 100\% = 81\%$$

7. **5.81×10^{-23} g/atom Cl; 5.31×10^{-23} g/molecule O_2**

The mass of a single atom is determined by dividing the atomic mass by Avogadro's number. Therefore, the mass of a chlorine atom is

$$\frac{35.5 \text{ g/mol}}{6.022 \times 10^{23} \text{ atoms/mol}} = 5.89 \times 10^{-23} \text{ g/atom}$$

The mass of an oxygen molecule (O_2) is similarly determined by dividing the molecular mass of oxygen by Avogadro's number.

$$\frac{32 \text{ g/mol}}{6.022 \times 10^{23} \text{ molecules/mol}} = 5.31 \times 10^{-23} \text{ g/molecule}$$

8. **5.5 mol**

From the balanced equation, it can be seen that the ratio between $Ag(NH_3)_2^+$ and NH_3 is 1:2. Thus, to form 11 mol of ammonia, the following calculation must be performed.

$$\frac{1 \text{ mol Ag}(NH_3)_2^+}{2 \text{ mol NH}_3} = \frac{x \text{ mol Ag}(NH_3)_2^+}{11 \text{ mol NH}_3}$$

$$x = 5.5 \text{ mol Ag}(NH_3)_2^+$$

9. **A** To answer this question, the law of conservation of mass, which says that the mass of the products must be equal to the mass of the reactants, is used. Therefore, if 5.8 g of $Ag(NH_3)_2^+$ are allowed to dissociate to form 1.4 g of ammonia, 5.8 g − 1.4 g = 4.4 g of silver must be formed. The following calculation is used to determine the number of moles of silver formed.

$$x \text{ mol} = \frac{4.4 \text{ g}}{108 \text{ g/mol}}$$

$$x = 0.041 \text{ mol}$$

10. **76.1% Ag, 19.7% N, 4.2% H**

The percent composition of elements in a compound or formula is determined by dividing the mass of the element by the total formula mass of the compound. Therefore, in the complex ion $Ag(NH_3)_2^+$, which has a formula mass of 142 g/mol, the percent compositions of Ag, N, and H are as follows:

$$\%Ag = \frac{108 \text{ g/mol}}{142 \text{ g/mol}} \times 100\% = 76.1\%$$

$$\%N = \frac{2(14 \text{ g/mol})}{142 \text{ g/mol}} \times 100\% = 19.7\%$$

$$\%H = \frac{6(1 \text{ g/mol})}{142 \text{ g/mol}} \times 100\% = 4.2\%$$

11. **C_4H_9**

    To answer this problem, several calculations must be performed. First, the number of moles of carbon and hydrogen present in the hydrocarbon must be determined using the assumption that the number of moles of atoms on the reactant side is equal to the number of moles of atoms on the product side. From this information, the empirical formula can be determined.

    First, the moles of carbon and hydrogen are calculated.

    $$\frac{58.67 \text{ g CO}_2}{44 \text{ g/mol}} = 1.33 \text{ mol CO}_2$$

    Since each mole of CO_2 contains 1 mole of carbon, 1.33 moles of CO_2 contains 1.33 moles of carbon. Therefore, the hydrocarbon contains 1.33 moles of carbon.

    $$\frac{27 \text{ g H}_2\text{O}}{18 \text{g/mol H}_2\text{O}} = 1.5 \text{ mol H}_2\text{O}$$

    Since one mole of H_2O contains 2 moles of hydrogen atoms, 1.5 moles of H_2O contains 3.0 moles of hydrogen. Therefore, the hydrocarbon contains 3 moles of hydrogen.

    Using these calculations, the simplest formula that can be written is $C_{1.33}H_3$. However, molecular formulas are not expressed with decimals or fractions, so these coefficients should be multiplied by 3 to give an empirical formula of C_4H_9.

12. **66 g**

    The balanced equation will be:

    $$2 \text{ NF}_3 + 3 \text{ H}_2\text{O} \rightarrow 6 \text{ HF} + \text{NO} + \text{NO}_2$$

    According to the balanced equation, 2 moles of NF_3 is needed to produce 6 moles of HF. To determine the number of grams of HF that will be formed, the amount of NF_3 used must first be calculated.

    $$1{,}500 \text{ g} \times 0.052 = 78 \text{ g NF}_3 \text{ used}$$

    Then a stoichiometric calculation can be set up to see what the theoretical yield of HF would be.

    $$78 \text{ g NF}_3 \times \frac{1 \text{ mol NF}_3}{71 \text{ g NF}_3} \times \frac{6 \text{ mol HF}}{2 \text{ mol NF}_3} \times \frac{20 \text{ g HF}}{1 \text{ mol HF}} = 66 \text{ g HF}$$

    Thus, 66 g of HF would be produced.

13. The following are the correct balanced equations:
    - **(A)** $I_2 + 5 \text{ Cl}_2 + 6 \text{ H}_2\text{O} \rightarrow 2 \text{ HIO}_3 + 10 \text{ HCl}$
    - **(B)** $MnO_2 + 4 \text{ HCl} \rightarrow 2 \text{ H}_2\text{O} + MnCl_2 + Cl_2$
    - **(C)** $4 \text{ BCl}_3 + P_4 + 6 \text{ H}_2 \rightarrow 4 \text{ BP} + 12 \text{ HCl}$
    - **(D)** $4 \text{ C}_3\text{H}_5(\text{NO}_3)_3 \rightarrow 12 \text{ CO}_2 + 10 \text{ H}_2\text{O} + 6 \text{ N}_2 + O_2$
    - **(E)** $2 \text{ HCl} + Ba(OH)_2 \rightarrow BaCl_2 + 2 \text{ H}_2\text{O}$

CHAPTER THIRTY-ONE

Solutions

Solutions are **homogeneous** (uniform in composition) mixtures of substances that combine to form a single phase, generally the liquid phase. Many important chemical reactions, both in the laboratory and in nature, take place in solution.

NATURE OF SOLUTIONS

A solution consists of a solute (e.g., NaCl, NH$_3$, or C$_{12}$H$_{22}$O$_{11}$) dispersed (**dissolved**) in a solvent (e.g., H$_2$O or benzene). The solvent is the component of the solution whose phase remains the same after mixing. If the two substances are already in the same phase, the solvent is the component present in greater quantity. Solute molecules move about freely in the solvent and can interact with other molecules or ions; consequently, chemical reactions occur easily in solution.

Solvation

The interaction between solute and solvent molecules is known as solvation or **dissolution**; when water is the solvent, it is called **hydration**, and the resulting solution is known as an **aqueous solution**. Solvation is possible when the attractive forces between solute and solvent are stronger than those between the solute particles. For example, when NaCl dissolves in water, its component ions dissociate from one another and become surrounded by water molecules. Because water is polar, ion-dipole interactions can occur between the Na$^+$ and Cl$^-$ ions and the water molecules, which are stronger and more favorable than the hydrogen-bonding found between H$_2$O molecules in pure water. For nonionic solutes, solvation involves van der Waals forces between the solute and solvent molecules. The general rule is that like dissolves like: Ionic and polar solutes are soluble in polar solvents, and nonpolar solutes are soluble in nonpolar solvents.

Solubility

The solubility of a substance is the maximum amount of that substance that can be dissolved in a particular solvent at a particular temperature. When this maximum amount of solute has been added, the solution is saturated; if more solute is added, it will not dissolve. For example, at 18°C, a maximum of 83 g of glucose (C$_6$H$_{12}$O$_6$) will dissolve in 100 mL of H$_2$O. Thus, the solubility of glucose is 83 g/100 mL. If more glucose is added, it will remain in solid form, precipitating to the bottom of the container. A solution in which the proportion of solute to solvent is small is said to be **dilute,** and one in which the proportion is large is said to be **concentrated**.

When a dissolved solute comes out of solution and forms crystals, this process is known as **crystallization.** It is also important to note that some substances can form **supersaturated** solutions, which are solutions that contain more solute than found in a saturated solution. Supersaturated solutions are formed by manipulating temperature or pressure. In a supersaturated solution, the addition of more solute will cause the excess solute in the supersaturated solution to separate, and a saturated solution with a precipitate will subsequently form.

Electrolytes

The electrical conductivity of aqueous solutions is governed by the presence and concentration of ions in solution. Therefore, pure water does not conduct an electrical current well since the concentrations of hydrogen and hydroxide ions are very small. Solutes that make conductive solutions are called electrolytes. A solute is considered a strong electrolyte if it dissociates completely into its constituent ions. Examples of **strong electrolytes** include ionic compounds, such as NaCl and KI, and molecular compounds with highly polar covalent bonds that dissociate into ions when dissolved, such as HCl in water. A **weak electrolyte,** on the other hand, ionizes or hydrolyzes incompletely in aqueous solution, and only some of the solute is present in ionic form. Examples include acetic acid and other weak acids, ammonia and other weak bases, and $HgCl_2$. Many compounds do not ionize at all in aqueous solution, retaining their molecular structure in solution, which usually limits their solubility. These compounds are called **nonelectrolytes** and include many nonpolar gases and organic compounds, such as oxygen and sugar.

CONCENTRATION

Units of Concentration

Concentration denotes the amount of solute dissolved in a solvent. The concentration of a solution is most commonly expressed as **percent composition by mass, mole fraction (X), molarity (M), molality (m),** or **normality (N).**

Percent composition by mass

The percent composition by mass (%) of a solute is the mass of the solute divided by the mass of the solution (solute plus solvent) and multiplied by 100.

Example: What is the percent composition by mass of NaCl of a saltwater solution if 100 g of the solution contains 20 g of NaCl?

Solution: $\dfrac{20 \text{ g NaCl}}{100 \text{ g}} \times 100\% = 20\%$ NaCl solution

Mole fraction

The mole fraction (X) of a compound is equal to the number of moles of the compound divided by the total number of moles of all species within the system. The sum of all the mole fractions in a system will always equal 1.

The mole fraction can be calculated with the following equation:

$$X_B = \frac{\text{moles of B}}{\text{sum of moles of all components}}$$

where X_B is the mole fraction of component B.

Example: If 92 g of glycerol is mixed with 90 g of water, what will be the mole fractions of the two components (the molecular mass of $H_2O = 18$ g/mol and the molecular mass of $C_3H_8O_3 = 92$ g/mol)?

Solution:

$$90 \text{ g water} = 90 \text{ g} \times \frac{1 \text{ mol}}{18 \text{ g}} = 5 \text{ mol}$$

$$92 \text{ g glycerol} = 92 \text{ g} \times \frac{1 \text{ mol}}{92 \text{ g}} = 1 \text{ mol}$$

$$\text{Total mol} = 5 + 1 = 6 \text{ mol}$$

$$X_{\text{water}} = \frac{5 \text{ mol}}{6 \text{ mol}} = 0.833$$

$$X_{\text{glycerol}} = \frac{1 \text{ mol}}{6 \text{ mol}} = 0.167$$

As a check, note that the sum of X_{water} and X_{glycerol} is 1:

$$X_{\text{water}} + X_{\text{glycerol}} = 0.833 + 0.167 = 1.000$$

Molarity

The molarity (M) of a solution is the number of moles of solute per liter of solution. Solution concentrations are usually expressed in terms of molarity. Molarity depends on the total volume of the solution, not on the volume of solvent used to prepare the solution.

Example: If enough water is added to 11 g of $CaCl_2$ to make 100 mL of solution, what is the molarity of the solution (the molecular mass of $CaCl_2$ is 110 g/mol)?

Solution:

$$\frac{11 \text{ g CaCl}_2}{110 \text{ g/mol CaCl}_2} = 0.10 \text{ mol CaCl}_2$$

$$100 \text{ mL} \times \frac{1 \text{ L}}{1{,}000 \text{ mL}} = 0.10 \text{ L}$$

$$\text{Molarity} = \frac{\text{mol solute}}{\text{L solution}} = \frac{0.10 \text{ mol CaCl}_2}{0.10 \text{ L solution}} = 1.0 \text{ M CaCl}_2$$

Molality

The molality (m) of a solution is the number of moles of solute per kilogram of solvent. For dilute aqueous solutions at 25°C, the molality is approximately equal to the molarity because the density of water at this temperature is 1 kilogram per liter, but note that this is an approximation and true only for dilute aqueous solutions.

Example: If 10 g of NaOH are dissolved in 500 g of water, what is the molality of the solution (the molecular mass of NaOH is 40 g/mol)?

Solution:

$$\frac{10 \text{ g NaOH}}{40 \text{ g/mol NaOH}} = 0.25 \text{ mol NaOH}$$

$$500 \text{ g H}_2\text{O} \times \frac{1 \text{ kg}}{1{,}000 \text{ g}} = 0.50 \text{ kg H}_2\text{O}$$

$$\text{Molality} = \frac{\text{mol solute}}{\text{kg solvent}} = \frac{0.25 \text{ mol NaOH}}{0.50 \text{ kg H}_2\text{O}} = 0.50 \text{ m NaOH}$$

Normality

The normality (N) of a solution is equal to the number of gram equivalent weights of solute per liter of solution. A gram equivalent weight, or **equivalent**, is a measure of the reactive capacity of a molecule (see Chapter 30, Stoichiometry).

To calculate the normality of a solution, we must know for what purpose the solution is being used because it is the concentration of the reactive species with which we are concerned. Normality is unique among concentration units in that it is reaction dependent. For example, each mole of sulfuric acid contributes 2 equivalents for acid-base reactions (because each mole of sulfuric acid provides 2 moles of H^+ ions) but contributes only 1 equivalent for a sulfate precipitation reaction (because each mole of sulfuric acid provides only 1 mole of sulfate ions). You can calculate normality by multiplying the molarity (M) of a solution by the number of equivalents per mol:

$$N = \text{Molarity} \times \frac{\text{equivalents}}{\text{mol}} = \frac{\text{mol}}{\text{L}} \times \frac{\text{equivalents}}{\text{mol}} = \frac{\text{equivalents}}{\text{L}}$$

Therefore, a 3 M solution of H_2SO_4 would be 6 N in acid-base reactions (3 M × 2 equivalents/mol = 6 N) and 3 N in sulfate precipitation reactions (3 M × 1 equivalents/mol = 3 N).

Dilution

A solution is **diluted** when solvent is added to a solution of higher concentration to produce a solution of lower concentration. The concentration of a solution after dilution can be conveniently determined using the equation below:

$$M_i V_i = M_f V_f$$

where M is molarity, V is volume, and the subscripts i and f refer to initial and final values, respectively.

Example: How many mL of a 5.5 M NaOH solution must be used to prepare 300 mL of a 1.2 M NaOH solution?

Solution:

$$5.5\,M \times V_i = 1.2\,M \times 300 \text{ mL}$$
$$V_i = \frac{1.2\,M \times 300 \text{ mL}}{5.5\,M}$$
$$V_i = 65 \text{ mL}$$

Factors Affecting Solubility

The solubility of a substance varies depending on the temperature of the solution, the solvent, and, in the case of a gas-phase solute, the pressure. Solubility is also affected by the addition of other substances to the solution.

Aqueous Solutions

The most common class of solutions is aqueous solutions (in which the solvent is water). The aqueous state is denoted by the symbol (*aq*). When discussing the chemistry of aqueous solutions and answering questions on the PCAT, it is useful to know how soluble various salts are in water; this information is given by the solubility rules below.

Soluble salts (with exceptions):

- All salts of alkali metal ions (e.g., Li^+, Na^+, K^+, Rb^+, Cs^+, Fr^+) are water soluble.
- All salts of the ammonium ion (NH_4^+) are water soluble.
- All salts with chloride (Cl^-), bromide (Br^-), and iodide (I^-) ions are water soluble, with the exception of salts containing Ag^+, Pb^{2+}, and Hg_2^{2+}.
- All salts of the sulfate ion (SO_4^{2-}) are water soluble, with the exception of those containing Ca^{2+}, Sr^{2+}, Ba^{2+}, and Pb^{2+}.

Insoluble salts (with exceptions):

- All metal oxides (a metal combined with oxygen) are insoluble, with the exception of alkali metal oxides and CaO^-, SrO^-, and BaO, all of which hydrolyze to form solutions of the corresponding metal hydroxides.
- All hydroxides (containing OH^-) are insoluble, with the exception of the alkali metal hydroxides and $Ca(OH)_2$, $Sr(OH)_2$, and $Ba(OH)_2$.
- All salts with carbonates (CO_3^{2-}), phosphates (PO_4^{3-}), sulfides (S^{2-}), and sulfites (SO_3^{2-}) are insoluble, with the exception of those that contain alkali metals or ammonium.

REVIEW PROBLEMS

1. Which of the following choices correctly describes the solubility behavior of potassium chloride (KCl)?

    (A) Solubility in CCl_4 > Solubility in CH_3CH_2OH > Solubility in H_2O
    (B) Solubility in H_2O > Solubility in CH_3CH_2OH > Solubility in CCl_4
    (C) Solubility in CH_3CH_2OH > Solubility in CCl_4 > Solubility in H_2O
    (D) Solubility in H_2O > Solubility in CCl_4 > Solubility in CH_3CH_2OH

2. A simple cake icing can be made by dissolving a large quantity of sugar (sucrose) in boiling water, cooling the mixture, and applying it to the cake before it reaches room temperature. The mixture hardens as it cools because the

    (A) sugar molecules freeze from liquid to solid.
    (B) common ion effect limits the dissolution of sucrose.
    (C) K_{sp} of sucrose increases as the solution cools.
    (D) sugar concentration increases as water boils off, and the solubility of sugar in water decreases as the solution cools.

3. How much NaOH must be added to 200 mL of water to make a 1.0 M NaOH solution?

    (A) 8.0 g
    (B) 16 g
    (C) 40 g
    (D) 80 g

4. To what volume must 10.0 mL of 5.00 M of HCl be diluted to make a 0.500 M HCl solution?

    (A) 1.00 mL
    (B) 50.0 mL
    (C) 100 mL
    (D) 500 mL

5. What is the normality of a 2.0 M solution of phosphoric acid, H_3PO_4, for an acid-base titration?

    (A) 0.67
    (B) 2.0
    (C) 3.0
    (D) 6.0

6. Given that the molecular mass of ethyl alcohol, CH_3CH_2OH, is 46 g/mol and that of water is 18 g/mol, how many grams of ethyl alcohol must be mixed with 100 mL of water for the mole fraction (X) of ethyl alcohol to be 0.2?

7. Name the following ionic compounds:

   (A) $NaClO_4$

   (B) $NaClO$

   (C) $NaNO_3$

   (D) KNO_2

   (E) Li_2SO_4

   (F) $MgSO_3$

8. Which of the following will be the most electrically conductive?

   (A) Sugar dissolved in water

   (B) Saltwater

   (C) Salt dissolved in an organic solvent

   (D) An oil and water mixture

SOLUTIONS TO REVIEW PROBLEMS

1. **B** KCl is an ionic salt and, therefore, is soluble in polar solvents and insoluble in nonpolar solvents. Water, H_2O, is a highly polar liquid. The carbon atom in carbon tetrachloride, CCl_4, is bonded to four atoms, so the molecule is tetrahedral. This geometry means that the individual dipole moments of the bonds cancel and CCl_4 is nonpolar. Ethanol (CH_3CH_2OH) has two carbon atoms in tetrahedral arrangements; most of the dipole moments associated with the bonds are the same, but the C—C and C—OH bonds are different, so ethanol is somewhat polar. Thus, the polarities of the three solvents decrease in the following sequence: $H_2O > CH_3CH_2OH > CCl_4$, with the solubility of KCl decreasing along that sequence as well.

2. **D** The sugar-water solution hardens because it becomes supersaturated as it cools since the solubility (K_{sp}) of sucrose in water decreases significantly with temperature. Evaporation of water during boiling also contributes to the solution's supersaturated state by reducing the amount of solvent present. Choice (A) is incorrect: in this example the sugar is dissolved, not melted (sucrose melts at 185°C, well above the boiling point of even sucrose-saturated water).

3. **A** To answer this question, first find the formula mass of NaOH from the periodic table. Rounding to whole numbers, the atomic mass of Na is 23 g/mol, the atomic mass of O is 16 g/mol, and the atomic mass of H is 1 g/mol, so the formula mass of NaOH is 40 g/mol. Thus, 40 g of NaOH is 1 mol, and 40 g of NaOH dissolved in 1 L of water is a 1 M solution of NaOH. To determine how much of the solute is needed to make 200 mL of such a solution, set up the following ratio:

$$\frac{x}{200 \text{ mL}} = \frac{40 \text{ g}}{1 \text{ L}} \times \frac{1 \text{ L}}{1{,}000 \text{ mL}}$$

$$\frac{x}{200 \text{ mL}} = \frac{40 \text{ g}}{1{,}000 \text{ mL}}$$

$$x = \frac{(40 \text{ g})(200 \text{ mL})}{1{,}000 \text{ mL}} = 8 \text{ g}$$

4. **C** When a solution is diluted, more solvent is added, yet the number of moles of solute remains the same. To solve a dilution problem, the following equation is used:

$$M_i V_i = M_f V_f$$

where i represents the initial conditions and f represents the final conditions. Therefore, the calculation to solve for the final volume is:

$$(5.0 \text{ M})(10 \text{ mL}) = (0.50 \text{ M})(V_f)$$

$$V_f = 100 \text{ mL}$$

and the correct answer is (C).

5. **D** Each mole of H_3PO_4 contains 3 moles of hydrogen and (since this is an acid) three mole equivalents. A 2 M solution of this acid is thus:

$$2\,M \times \frac{3\,N}{1\,M} = 6\,N$$

6. **64.4 g**

The number of moles of water is found by estimating the density of water to be 1 g/mL.

$$mol\,H_2O = \frac{(100\,mL\,H_2O)(1\,g/mL)}{18\,g/mol} = 5.6\,mol$$

If the mole fraction of ethyl alcohol is to be 0.2, then the mole fraction of water must be 0.8. If n equals the total number of moles:

$$5.6\,mol = 0.8n$$

$$n = 7\,mol$$

Then:

mol ethyl alcohol $= (0.2)(7\,mol) = 1.4\,mol$

and:

grams ethyl alcohol $= (1.4\,mol\,ethyl\,alcohol)(46\,g/mol) = 64.4\,g$ ethyl alcohol.

7. (Oxidation numbers—discussed in detail in Chapter 32, Reaction Types—have been placed in parentheses for additional practice.)
   (A) Sodium perchlorate (Cl: $+7$)
   (B) Sodium hypochlorite (C: $+11$)
   (C) Sodium nitrate (N: $+5$)
   (D) Potassium nitrite (N: $+3$)
   (E) Lithium sulfate (S: $+6$)
   (F) Magnesium sulfite (S: $+4$)

8. **B** Only ionic compounds (electrolytes) dissolved in polar solvents will conduct electricity. Sugar is a covalent solid and therefore is not an electrolyte even when dissolved in water. Answers (C) and (D) are incorrect because salt will not dissolve appreciably in an organic solvent and oil and water are immiscible. NaCl is an ionic compound, so (B) is correct.

CHAPTER THIRTY-TWO

Reaction Types

TYPES OF CHEMICAL REACTIONS

Elements and compounds can react to form other species in many ways, and memorizing every reaction would be impossible as well as unnecessary. However, nearly every inorganic reaction can be classified into at least one of five general categories.

Combination Reactions

Combination reactions are reactions in which two or more **reactants** form one **product**. The formation of sulfur dioxide by burning sulfur in air is an example of a combination reaction:

$$S\ (s) + O_2\ (g) \rightarrow SO_2\ (g)$$

Combination reactions can also occur when two compounds react to form a new compound. For example, in the equation below, gaseous ammonia is reacted with gaseous hydrogen chloride and forms ammonium chloride:

$$NH_3\ (g) + HCl\ (g) \rightarrow NH_4Cl\ (s)$$

Decomposition Reactions

A decomposition reaction is defined as one in which a compound breaks down into two or more substances, usually as a result of heating or electrolysis. For example, when compounds that contain oxygen are heated, most will decompose to form molecular oxygen. **Electrolysis** is a specific process that causes the decomposition of a compound by passing an electric current through the reactant. Another example of a decomposition reaction is the breakdown of mercury (II) oxide (the sign Δ represents the addition of heat):

$$2\ HgO\ (s) \xrightarrow{\Delta} 2\ Hg\ (l) + O_2\ (g)$$

Single Displacement Reactions

Single displacement reactions occur when an atom (or ion) of one compound is replaced by an atom of another element. For example, zinc metal will displace copper ions in a copper sulfate solution to form zinc sulfate:

$$Zn\ (s) + CuSO_4\ (aq) \rightarrow Cu\ (s) + ZnSO_4\ (aq)$$

Single displacement reactions are often further classified as **redox** reactions, discussed below.

Net ionic equations

Because many reactions, including some displacements, involve ions in solution, their net equations can also be written in ionic form. In the example where zinc is reacted with copper sulfate, the **ionic equation** is:

$$Zn\ (s) + Cu^{2+}\ (aq) + SO_4^{2-}\ (aq) \rightarrow Cu\ (s) + Zn^{2+}\ (aq) + SO_4^{2-}\ (aq)$$

When displacement reactions occur, there are usually **spectator ions** that do not take part in the overall reaction but simply remain in solution throughout. The spectator ion in the equation above is sulfate, which does not undergo any transformation during the reaction. A **net ionic reaction** can be written showing only the species that actually participate in the reaction:

$$Zn\ (s) + Cu^{2+}\ (aq) \rightarrow Cu\ (s) + Zn^{2+}\ (aq)$$

Net ionic equations are important for demonstrating the actual reaction that occurs during a displacement reaction.

Double Displacement Reactions

In double displacement reactions, also called **metathesis reactions**, elements from two different compounds displace each other to form two new compounds. This type of reaction occurs when one of the products is removed from the solution as a precipitate or gas, or when two of the original species combine to form a weak electrolyte that remains undissociated in solution. For example, when solutions of calcium chloride and silver nitrate are combined, insoluble silver chloride forms in a solution of calcium nitrate:

$$CaCl_2\ (aq) + 2\ AgNO_3\ (aq) \rightarrow Ca(NO_3)_2\ (aq) + 2\ AgCl\ (s)$$

Neutralization reactions

Neutralization reactions are a specific type of double displacement that occurs when an acid reacts with a base to produce a solution of a salt and water. For example, hydrochloric acid and sodium hydroxide will react to form sodium chloride and water.

$$HCl\ (aq) + NaOH\ (aq) \rightarrow NaCl\ (aq) + H_2O\ (l)$$

This type of reaction will be discussed further in Chapter 37, Acids and Bases.

Oxidation-Reduction Reactions

A reaction that involves the transfer of electrons from one species to another is an oxidation-reduction (redox) reaction. This type of reaction can be divided into two half reactions, **oxidation** (loss of electrons) and **reduction** (gain of electrons). The law of conservation of charge states that an electrical charge can be neither created nor destroyed. Thus, an isolated loss or gain of electrons cannot occur; oxidation and reduction must occur simultaneously, resulting in an electron transfer called a **redox reaction**. An **oxidizing agent** causes another atom in a redox reaction to undergo oxidation, and itself is reduced. A **reducing agent** causes the other atom to be reduced, and itself is oxidized.

Assigning oxidation numbers

It is important to know which atom is oxidized and which is reduced. **Oxidation numbers** are assigned to atoms to keep track of the redistribution of electrons during a chemical reaction. From the oxidation numbers of the reactants and products, it is possible to determine how many electrons are gained or lost by each atom. The oxidation number is the number of charges an atom would have in a molecule if electrons were completely transferred in the direction indicated by the difference in electronegativity. Along the same lines, an element is said to be oxidized (loses electrons) if its oxidation number increases in a given reaction, and an element is said to be reduced (gains electrons) if the oxidation number of the element decreases in a given reaction. The oxidation number of an atom in a compound is assigned according to the following rules:

- The oxidation number of a free element (an element in its elemental state) is zero, irrespective of how complex the molecule is.
- The oxidation number for a monatomic ion is equal to the charge of the ion. For example, the oxidation numbers for Na^+, Cu^{2+}, Fe^{3+}, Cl^-, and N^{3-} are $+1$, $+2$, $+3$, -1, and -3, respectively.
- The oxidation number of each Group IA element in a compound is $+1$. The oxidation number of each Group IIA element in a compound is $+2$.
- The oxidation number of each Group VIIA element in a compound is -1, except when combined with an element of higher electronegativity. For example, in HCl, the oxidation number of Cl is -1; in HOCl, however, the oxidation number of Cl is $+1$ because oxygen is more electronegative and has an oxidation state of -2 (oxygen is discussed further below).
- The oxidation number of hydrogen is generally $+1$. However, the oxidation number can be -1 when H is placed with less electronegative elements (Groups IA and IIA). Examples of hydrogen's oxidation state being -1 occur with NaH and CaH_2. Nevertheless, the most common oxidation number of hydrogen is $+1$.
- In most compounds, the oxidation number of oxygen is -2. This is not the case, however, in molecules such as OF_2. Here, because F is more electronegative and has an oxidation state of -1, the oxidation number of oxygen is $+2$. Also, in peroxides such as BaO_2, the oxidation number of O is -1 instead of -2 because of the structure of the peroxide ion, $[O-O]^{2-}$ (for confirmation, note that Ba, a Group IIA element, cannot be a $+4$ cation).
- The sum of the oxidation numbers of all the atoms present in a neutral compound is zero. The sum of the oxidation numbers of the atoms present in a polyatomic ion is equal to the charge of the ion. Thus, for SO_4^{2-}, the sum of the oxidation numbers must be -2.
- Fluorine has an oxidation number of -1 in all compounds because it has the highest electronegativity of all the elements.
- Metallic elements have only positive oxidation numbers; however, nonmetallic elements may have a positive or negative oxidation number.

Example: Assign oxidation numbers to the atoms in the following reaction to determine the oxidized and reduced species and the oxidizing and reducing agents:

$$SnCl_2 + PbCl_4 \rightarrow SnCl_4 + PbCl_2$$

Solution: All these species are neutral, so the oxidation numbers of each compound must add up to zero. In $SnCl_2$, since there are two chlorines present and chlorine has an oxidation number of -1, Sn must have an oxidation number of $+2$. Similarly, the oxidation number of Sn in $SnCl_4$ is $+4$; the oxidation number of Pb is $+4$ in $PbCl_4$ and $+2$ in $PbCl_2$. Notice that the oxidation number of Sn increases from $+2$ to $+4$; it loses electrons and thus is oxidized, making it the reducing agent. Since the oxidation number of Pb has decreased from $+4$ to $+2$, it has gained electrons and been reduced. Pb is the oxidizing agent. The sum of the charges on both sides of the reaction is equal to zero, so charge has been conserved.

Balancing redox reactions

Balancing any reaction requires not only stoichiometric balance but also charge balance. Because redox reactions involve the transfer of electrons (and therefore of charge) between different elements, balancing redox reactions introduces an additional level of complexity. However, with a straightforward, stepwise method, balancing chemical reactions on the PCAT becomes more manageable.

By assigning oxidation numbers to the reactants and products, one can determine how many moles of each species are required for conservation of charge and mass, which is necessary to balance the equation. To balance a redox reaction, both the net charge and the number of atoms must be equal on both sides of the equation. The most common method for balancing redox equations is the **half-reaction method**, also known as the **ion-electron method**, in which the equation is separated into two half reactions—the oxidation part and the reduction part. Each half reaction is balanced separately, and they are then added to give a balanced overall reaction.

Example: Balance the redox reaction between MnO_4 and I in an acidic solution:

$$MnO_4^- + I^- \rightarrow I_2 + Mn^{2+}$$

Solution: Note how the oxidation numbers for I and Mn change (I changes from an oxidation state of -1 to 0, and Mn changes from $+7$ to $+2$) and that the reaction is not balanced. So, use the 5-step method to balance redox reactions.

Step 1:   *Separate the two half reactions.*

$$I^- \rightarrow I_2$$
$$MnO_4^- \rightarrow Mn^{2+}$$

Step 2:   *Balance the atoms of each half reaction.* First, balance all atoms except H and O. Next, add H_2O to balance the O atoms and then add H^+ to balance the H atoms.

To balance the iodine atoms, place a coefficient of two before the I^- ion:

$$2\,I^- \rightarrow I_2$$

For the permanganate half reaction, Mn is already balanced. Balance the oxygen atoms by adding $4\,H_2O$ to the right side:

$$MnO_4^- \rightarrow Mn^{2+} + 4\,H_2O$$

Finally, add H^+ to the left side to balance the 4 H_2Os. These two half reactions are now balanced:

$$MnO_4^- + 8\ H^+ \rightarrow Mn^{2+} + 4\ H_2O$$

Step 3:   *Balance the electrons of each half reaction.* Each half reaction must have the same net charge on the left and right sides, and the only species that can be used to balance charges are electrons, each with a -1 charge. Additionally, the reduction half reaction must consume the same number of electrons as supplied by the oxidation half.

For the oxidation reaction, the left side has a charge of -2, and the right side has a charge of 0. Add 2 electrons to the right side of the reaction to balance both sides to be -2:

$$2\ I^- \rightarrow I_2 + 2\ e^-$$

For the reduction reaction, there is a charge of $+7$ on the left and $+2$ on the right. By adding 5 electrons to the left side, the charges on both sides become $+2$, balancing the half reaction:

$$MnO_4^- + 8\ H^+ + 5\ e^- \rightarrow Mn^{2+} + 4\ H_2O$$

Next, both half reactions must have the same number of electrons so that, when the half reactions are combined, the electrons cancel. Therefore, multiply the oxidation half by 5 and the reduction half by 2.

$$5(2\ I^- \rightarrow I_2 + 2\ e^-)$$
$$2(MnO_4^- + 8\ H^+ + 5\ e^- \rightarrow Mn^{2+} + 4\ H_2O)$$

Step 4:   *Combine the half reactions.*

$$10\ I^- \rightarrow 5\ I_2 + 10\ e^-$$
$$2\ MnO_4^- + 10\ e^- + 16\ H^+ \rightarrow 2\ Mn^{2+} + 8\ H_2O$$

The sum of the two equations is:

$$10\ I^- + 10\ e^- + 16\ H^+ + 2\ MnO_4^- \rightarrow 5\ I_2 + 10\ e^- + 2\ Mn^{2+} + 8\ H_2O$$

To find the final equation, cancel out the electrons and anything that appears on both sides of the equation:

$$10\ I^- + 16\ H^+ + 2\ MnO_4^- \rightarrow 5\ I_2 + 2\ Mn^{2+} + 8\ H_2O$$

Step 5:   *Confirm that mass and charge are balanced.* Here, there is a $+4$ net charge on each side of the reaction equation, and the atoms are stoichiometrically balanced.

For redox reactions in a basic (instead of acidic) solution, an additional step is required because H^+ will not be readily available and should not appear as a reactant. Use the same initial steps 1–4, but then add enough hydroxide (OH^-) to both sides to completely combine with the free H^+, forming water. Then, remove any species that appears on both sides and complete step 5 as usual to confirm everything is still balanced.

For example, in order to balance the same redox reaction of MnO_4 and I in a basic solution (instead of acidic), start by completing the same steps 1–3. Recall that during Step 4, you combined the half reactions:

Step 4: *Combine the half reactions in basic solution.*

$$10 \, I^- + 10 \, e^- + 16 \, H^+ + 2 \, MnO_4^- \rightarrow 5 \, I_2 + 10 \, e^- + 2 \, Mn^{2+} + 8 \, H_2O$$

Then, add 16 OH^- to both sides to neutralize the H^+:

$$10 \, I^- + 10 \, e^- + 16 \, H^+ + 16 \, OH^- + 2 \, MnO_4^- \rightarrow 5 \, I_2 + 10 \, e^- + 2 \, Mn^{2+} + 8 \, H_2O + 16 \, OH^-$$

Combine the H^+ and OH^- into water:

$$10 \, I^- + 10 \, e^- + 16 \, H_2O + 2 \, MnO_4^- \rightarrow 5 \, I_2 + 10 \, e^- + 2 \, Mn^{2+} + 8 \, H_2O + 16 \, OH^-$$

Cancel out any species (here, e^- and H_2O) that appear on both sides to find the balanced redox reaction in a basic solution:

$$10 \, I^- + 8 \, H_2O + 2 \, MnO_4^- \rightarrow 5 \, I_2 + 2 \, Mn^{2+} + 16 \, OH^-$$

Step 5: Finally, confirm that mass and charge are balanced. Here, there is a -12 net charge on each side of the reaction equation, and the atoms are stoichiometrically balanced.

Redox reaction examples

Redox reactions can occur as variations of the major types of reactions above: combination, decomposition, and displacement.

1. **Combination reactions**: These types of reactions occur with one or more free elements.

Example:	Equation	$N_2 \, (g) + 3 \, H_2 \, (g) \rightarrow 2 \, NH_3 \, (g)$
	Oxidation #s	0 0 $-3 \, +1$

2. **Decomposition reactions**: These types of reactions lead to the production of one or more free elements.

Example:	Equation	$2 \, H_2O \, (l) \rightarrow H_2 \, (g) + O_2 \, (g)$
	Oxidation #s	$+1 \, -2$ 0 0

3. **Displacement reactions**: In this type of reaction, an atom or an ion of one element is displaced from a given compound by an atom from a totally different element.

Example:	Equation	$2 \, Na \, (s) + 2 \, H_2O \, (l) \rightarrow 2 \, NaOH + H_2 \, (g)$
	Oxidation #s	0 $+1 \, -2$ $+1 \, -2 \, +1$ 0

REVIEW PROBLEMS

1. The reaction below is best classified as which type of reaction?

$$CH_3CO_2Na + HClO_4 \rightarrow CH_3CO_2H + NaClO_4$$

   (A) Double-displacement reaction

   (B) Combination reaction

   (C) Decomposition reaction

   (D) Single-displacement and decomposition reaction

2. Which of the following represents the net ionic equation for the reaction given?

$$AgNO_3\ (aq) + Cu\ (s) \rightarrow CuNO_3\ (aq) + Ag\ (s)$$

   (A) $AgNO_3\ (aq) + Cu\ (s) \rightarrow CuNO_3\ (aq) + Ag\ (s)$

   (B) $Ag^+\ (aq) + Cu\ (s) \rightarrow Cu^+\ (aq) + Ag\ (s)$

   (C) $AgNO_3\ (aq) + Cu\ (s) \rightarrow Cu^+\ (aq) + NO_3^-\ (aq) + Ag\ (s)$

   (D) $Ag^+\ (aq) + NO_3^-\ (aq) + Cu\ (s) \rightarrow CuNO_3\ (aq) + Ag\ (s)$

3. Assign oxidation numbers to each atom of the following reaction equation:

$$2\ Fe\ (s) + O_2\ (g) + 2\ H_2O\ (l) \rightarrow 2\ Fe(OH)_2\ (s)$$

4. Using the ion-electron method, balance the following equation of a reaction taking place in an acidic solution:

$$ClO_3^- + AsO_2^- \rightarrow AsO_4^{3-} + Cl^-$$

SOLUTIONS TO REVIEW PROBLEMS

1. A Because the only change is that the Na from CH_3CO_2Na exchanges with the H from $HClO_4$, this is a double displacement reaction. Alternately, this reaction could be classified as a neutralization, since it is a reaction between an acid and a base.

1. B In displacement reactions, there are often ionic species that do not play a role in the overall reaction. Instead, they remain in solution throughout the entire reaction. Thus, displacement reactions can be written in terms of net ionic equations, which express the reactions of the participating species. In the reaction between aqueous silver nitrate and copper metal to form aqueous copper (I) nitrate and metallic silver, the nitrate ion does not participate in the reaction; thus, it is a spectator ion. Therefore, the only species that are involved in the reaction are copper metal and the Ag^+ ion, which react to form the Cu^+ ion and silver metal.

3. Fe (*s*): Fe 0;

O$_2$ (*g*): O 0;

H_2O (*l*): H +1, O −2;

$Fe(OH)_2$ (*s*): Fe +2, O −2, H +1

To assign oxidation numbers, use the rules given in the text. Fe (*s*) and O$_2$ (*g*) have oxidation numbers of zero because they are free elements. Hydrogen in H_2O (*l*) has an oxidation number of +1 because oxygen is more electronegative than hydrogen; likewise, oxygen in H_2O (*l*) has an oxidation number of −2. Oxygen and hydrogen in $Fe(OH)_2$ (*s*) have the same oxidation numbers as in H_2O (*l*). Each OH group contributes a charge of −1 to $Fe(OH)_2$, and since there are 2 OH groups, their overall contribution to the compound is −2. Since $Fe(OH)_2$ (*s*) is a neutral compound and thus has no overall charge, the sum of all the oxidation numbers of the atoms in this compound is zero. Consequently, the Fe in $Fe(OH)_2$ (*s*) must possess a charge of +2 to make the overall charge on the compound zero.

4. The balanced equation is:

$$ClO_3^- + 3\ H_2O + 3\ AsO_2^- \rightarrow 3\ AsO_4^{3-} + Cl^- + 6\ H^+$$

CHAPTER THIRTY-THREE

Chemical Kinetics

When studying a chemical reaction, it is important to consider not only the chemical properties of the reactants but also the **conditions** under which the reaction occurs, the **mechanism** by which it takes place, the **rate** at which it occurs, and the **equilibrium** toward which it proceeds.

REACTION MECHANISMS

The **mechanism** of a chemical reaction is the actual series of steps through which it occurs. Knowing the accepted mechanism of a reaction often helps to explain the reaction's rate, position of equilibrium, and thermodynamic characteristics. Consider the reaction below:

$$A_2 + 2\,B \rightarrow 2\,AB$$

This equation seems to imply a mechanism in which two molecules of B collide with one molecule of A_2 to form two molecules of AB. But suppose instead that the reaction actually takes place in two steps.

Step 1: $A_2 + B \rightarrow A_2B$ (slow)

Step 2: $A_2B + B \rightarrow 2\,AB$ (fast)

Note that these two steps add up to the overall (net) reaction. A_2B, which does not appear in the overall reaction because it is neither a reactant nor a product, is called an **intermediate**. Reaction intermediates are often difficult to detect, but a proposed mechanism can be supported through experiments.

The slowest step in a proposed mechanism is called the **rate-determining step**, because the overall reaction cannot proceed faster than that step.

REACTION RATES

Chemical kinetics is the study of the rates (or speed) of reactions. The **reaction rate** is the change of concentration of reactant or finished product with respect to time. Any given chemical reaction can be represented by the following equation:

$$\text{Reactants} \rightarrow \text{Products}$$

This equation indicates that reactant molecules are decreasing or being consumed and the product molecules are increasing or being formed. The process of chemical kinetics is concerned with how "fast" the reactants are being transformed into products.

Definition of Rate

Consider a reaction $2A + B \rightarrow C$, in which one mole of C is produced from every two moles of A and one mole of B. The rate of this reaction may be described in terms of either the disappearance of reactants over time or the appearance of products over time.

$$\text{rate} = \frac{\text{decrease in concentration of reactants}}{\text{time}} = \frac{\text{increase in concentration of products}}{\text{time}}$$

Because the concentration of a reactant decreases during the reaction, a minus sign is placed before a rate that is expressed in terms of reactants. For the reaction above, the rate of reaction with respect to A is $-\frac{\Delta[A]}{\Delta t}$, with respect to B is $-\frac{\Delta[B]}{\Delta t}$, and with respect to C is $\frac{\Delta[C]}{\Delta t}$.

Rate is expressed in the units of moles per liter per second (mol/[L × s]) or molarity per second (molarity/s).

Rate Law

For nearly all forward, irreversible reactions, the rate is proportional to the product of the concentrations of the reactants, each raised to some power. For the general reaction

$$aA + bB \rightarrow cC + dD$$

the rate is proportional to $[A]^x[B]^y$, that is:

$$\text{rate} = k[A]^x[B]^y$$

This expression is the **rate law** for the general reaction above, where k is the **rate constant**. The rate constant is defined as a constant of proportionality between the chemical reaction rate and the concentration of the reactants. Multiplying the units of k by the concentration factors raised to the appropriate powers gives the rate in units of concentration/time. The exponents x and y are called the **orders of reaction**; x is the order with respect to A, and y is the order with respect to B. These exponents may be integers (including 0) or fractions and must be determined experimentally.

It is important to note that the exponents of the rate law are **not** necessarily equal to the stoichiometric coefficients in the overall reaction equation. The exponents **are** equal to the stoichiometric coefficients of the rate-determining step. If one of the reactants or products in the rate-determining step is an intermediate not included in the overall reaction, then calculating the rate law in terms of the original reactants is more complex.

The **overall order of a reaction** (or the **reaction order**) is defined as the sum of the exponents, here equal to $x + y$.

Experimental determination of rate law

The values of k, x, and y in the rate law equation (rate $= k[A]^x[B]^y$) must be determined experimentally for a given reaction at a given temperature. The rate is usually measured as a function of the initial concentrations of the reactants, A and B.

Example: Given the data below, find the rate law for the following reaction at 300 K.

$$A + B \rightarrow C + D$$

Solution: First, look for two trials in which the concentrations of all but one of the substances are held constant.

Trial	$[A]_{initial}$ (M)	$[B]_{initial}$ (M)	$r_{initial}$ (M/s)
1	1.00	1.00	2.0
2	1.00	2.00	8.1
3	2.00	2.00	15.9

a) In trials 1 and 2, the concentration of A is kept constant while the concentration of B is doubled. The rate increases by a factor of 8.1/2.0, or approximately 4. Write down the rate expression for each of the two trials.

Trial 1: $\qquad\qquad\qquad r_1 = k[A]^x [B]^y = k(1.00)^x (1.00)^y$
Trial 2: $\qquad\qquad\qquad r_2 = k[A]^x [B]^y = k(1.00)^x (2.00)^y$

Divide the second equation by the first:

$$\frac{r_2}{r_1} = \frac{8.1}{2.0} = \frac{k(1.00)^x(2.00)^y}{k(1.00)^x(1.00)^y} = (2.00)^y$$

$$4 = (2.00)^y$$

$$y = 2$$

b) In trials 2 and 3, the concentration of B is kept constant while the concentration of A is doubled; the rate is increased by a factor of 15.9/8.1, or approximately 2. The rate expressions of the two trials are:

Trial 2: $\qquad\qquad\qquad r_2 = k(1.00)^x (2.00)^y$
Trial 3: $\qquad\qquad\qquad r_3 = k(2.00)^x (2.00)^y$

Divide the second equation by the first:

$$\frac{r_3}{r_2} = \frac{15.9}{8.1} = \frac{k(2.00)^x(2.00)^y}{k(1.00)^x(2.00)^y} = (2.00)^x$$

$$2 = (2.00)^x$$

$$x = 1$$

So $r = k[A][B]^2$.

The order of the reaction with respect to A is 1 and with respect to B is 2; the overall reaction order is $1 + 2 = 3$.

To calculate k, substitute the values from any one of the above trials into the rate law. For example:

2.0 M/s $= k \times 1.00$ M $\times (1.00$ M$)^2$

$k = 2.0$ M^{-2} s^{-1}

Therefore, the rate law is $r = (2.0$ M^{-2} s$^{-1}) [A][B]^2$.

Reaction Orders

Chemical reactions are often classified on the basis of kinetics as zero-order, first-order, second-order, mixed-order, or higher-order reactions. The general reaction $aA + bB \rightarrow cC + dD$ will be used in the discussion below.

Zero-order reactions

A zero-order reaction has a constant rate, which is independent of the reactants' concentrations. Thus, the rate law is:

rate $= k$, where k has units of M·s^{-1}

With respect to the administration of a medication, a zero-order reaction is one in which the amount of drug administered/eliminated per unit time remains constant. For example, 25 mg of a drug are administered/eliminated each hour.

Plasma Drug Concentration vs. Time Plot

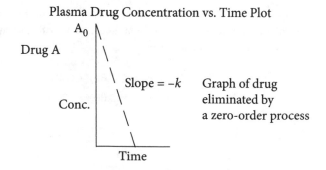

Graph of drug eliminated by a zero-order process

The concentration of Drug A can be calculated at any given time with the equation:

$$[A] = [A_0] - (k_0)(t)$$

Where: A_0 = initial concentration of Drug A in the body
k_0 = zero-order rate constant
t = time

The zero-order half-life changes with time and is proportional to the initial drug concentration. It is inversely proportional to the zero-order rate constant and can be represented with the following equation:

$$\text{half-life} = \frac{1}{2}\frac{A_0}{k_0}$$

First-order reactions

A first-order reaction (order = 1) has a rate proportional to the concentration of one reactant.

$$\text{rate} = k[A] \text{ or rate} = k[B]$$

First-order rate constants have units of s^{-1}.

The classic example of a first-order reaction is the process of radioactive decay. The concentration of radioactive substance A at any time t can be expressed mathematically as:

$$[A_t] = [A_0]\, e^{-kt}$$

where $[A_0]$ = initial concentration of A
$[A_t]$ = concentration of A at time t
k = rate constant
t = elapsed time

The half-life ($t_{1/2}$) of a reaction is the time needed for the concentration of the radioactive substance to decrease to one-half of its original value. Half-lives can be calculated from the rate law as follows:

$$t_{1/2} = \frac{\ln 2}{k} = \frac{0.693}{k}$$

where k is the first-order rate constant.

With respect to medicine, a first-order reaction is one in which the percentage of drug administered/eliminated per unit time remains constant. In other words, the amount of drug administered/eliminated is proportional to the amount of drug remaining. For example, 25 percent of the drug is eliminated each hour.

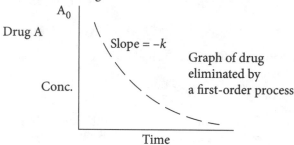

Plasma Drug Concentration vs. Time Plot

The concentration of Drug A can be calculated at any given time with the equation:

$$\ln [A] = \ln [A_0] - k_e(t)$$

Remember: $\ln x = (\log x)(2.3)$

Where $[A_0]$ = initial concentration of Drug A in the body
k_e = first-order elimination rate constant
t = time

Regarding the first-order half-life, the time to reduce the remaining portion of the drug in the body by one-half remains constant irrespective of the drug's concentration in the blood. The first-order half-life = $\frac{0.693}{k}$.

Now you can see how these chemical reaction equations can be related to the practice of pharmacy!

Second-order reactions

A second-order reaction (order = 2) has a rate proportional to the product of the concentration of two reactants or to the square of the concentration of a single reactant. For example, rate = $k[A]^2$, rate = $k[B]^2$, or rate = $k[A][B]$. The units of second-order rate constants are $M^{-1} s^{-1}$.

Higher-order reactions

A higher-order reaction has an order greater than 2.

Mixed-order reactions

A mixed-order reaction has a fractional order; e.g., rate = $k[A]^{1/3}$.

Efficiency of Reactions

Collision theory of chemical kinetics

For a reaction to occur, molecules must collide with each other. The collision theory of chemical kinetics states that the rate of a reaction is proportional to the **number of collisions per second** between the reacting molecules. It is important to note that reaction rates almost always increase with increasing temperatures. On the other hand, reaction rates decrease with decreasing temperatures.

Not all collisions, however, result in a chemical reaction. An **effective collision** (one that leads to the formation of products) occurs only if the molecules collide with the correct orientation and sufficient force to break the existing bonds and form new ones. The minimum energy of collision necessary for a reaction to take place is called the **activation energy**, E_a, or the **energy barrier**. Only a fraction of colliding particles have enough kinetic energy to exceed the activation energy. This means that only a fraction of all collisions are effective. The rate of a reaction can therefore be expressed as:

$$\text{rate} = fZ$$

where Z is the total number of collisions occurring per second and f is the fraction of collisions that are effective.

Transition state theory

When molecules collide with sufficient energy, they form a **transition state** in which the old bonds are weakened and the new bonds are beginning to form. The transition state then dissociates into products, and the new bonds are fully formed. For a reaction $A_2 + B_2 \rightarrow 2AB$, the change along the **reaction coordinate** (a measure of the extent to which the reaction has progressed from reactants to products; see below) can be represented as follows:

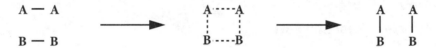

Figure 33.1

The **transition state**, also called the **activated complex**, has greater energy than either the reactants or the products and is denoted by the symbol ‡. The activation energy is required to bring the reactants to this particular energy level. Once an activated complex is formed, it can either dissociate into the products or revert to reactants without any additional energy input. Transition states are distinguished from intermediates in that, existing as they do at energy maxima, transition states do not have a finite lifetime.

A **potential energy diagram** illustrates the relationship between the activation energy, the heats of reaction, and the potential energy of the system before and after the reaction. The most important factors in such diagrams are the **relative** energies of the products and reactants. The **enthalpy change** of the reaction (ΔH) is the difference between the potential energy of the products and the potential energy of the reactants. A negative enthalpy change indicates an **exothermic reaction** (where heat is given off), and a positive enthalpy change indicates an **endothermic reaction** (where heat is absorbed).

The activated complex exists at the top of the energy barrier. The difference in potential energies between the activated complex and the reactants is the activation energy of the forward reaction; the difference in potential energies between the activated complex and the products is the activation energy of the reverse reaction.

For example, consider the formation of HCl from H_2 and Cl_2.

$$H_2 + Cl_2 \rightleftharpoons 2\,HCl$$

The following figure gives the energy profile of the reaction. It shows that the reaction is exothermic. The potential energy of the products is less than the potential energy of the reactants; heat is evolved, and the heat of reaction is negative.

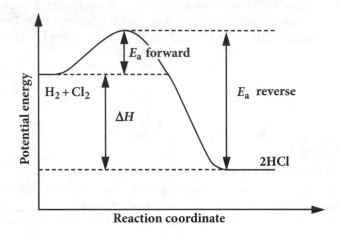

Figure 33.2

Factors Affecting Reaction Rate

The rate of a chemical reaction depends on the individual species undergoing reaction and on the reaction environment. The rate of reaction will increase if there is an increase in the number of effective collisions or a stabilization of the activated complex compared to the reactants.

Reactant concentrations

The greater the concentrations of the reactants (the more particles per unit volume), the greater the number of effective collisions per unit time, so the reaction rate will increase as reactant concentrations increase for all but zero-order reactions. For reactions occurring in the gaseous state, the partial pressures of the reactants can serve as measures of concentration.

Temperature

For nearly all reactions, the reaction rate will increase as the temperature of the system increases. Since the temperature of a substance is a measure of the particles' average kinetic energy, increasing the temperature increases the average kinetic energy of the molecules. Consequently, the proportion of molecules having energies greater than E_a (and thus capable of undergoing reaction) increases with higher temperature.

Medium

The rate of a reaction may also be affected by the medium in which it takes place. Due to differences in intermolecular forces and other stabilizing factors, certain reactions proceed more rapidly in aqueous solution, whereas other reactions proceed more rapidly in benzene. The state of the medium (liquid, solid, or gas) can also have a significant effect.

Catalysts

Catalysts are substances that increase reaction rate without themselves being consumed; they do this by lowering the activation energy. Catalysts are important in biological systems and in industrial chemistry; **enzymes** are biological catalysts. Catalysts may increase the frequency of collision between the reactants, change the relative orientation of the reactants to make a higher percentage of collisions effective, donate electron density to the reactants, or reduce intramolecular bonding within reactant molecules. The following figure compares the energy profiles of catalyzed and uncatalyzed reactions.

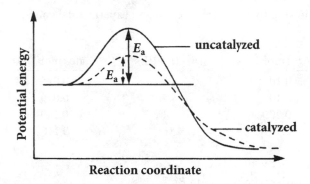

Figure 33.3

The energy barrier for the catalyzed reaction is much lower than the energy barrier for the uncatalyzed reaction. Note that the rates of both the forward and the reverse reactions are increased by the catalyst, since E_a of the forward and reverse reactions are lowered by the same amount. Therefore, the presence of a catalyst causes the reaction to proceed more quickly toward equilibrium.

REVIEW PROBLEMS

1. All of the following are true statements concerning reaction orders EXCEPT:

    (A) The rate of a zero-order reaction is constant.
    (B) After three half-lives, a sample will have one-ninth of its original activity.
    (C) The units for the rate constant for first-order reactions are s^{-1}.
    (D) Higher-order reactions are those with an order greater than two.

2. Consider the following hypothetical reaction and experimental data:

    $$A + B \rightarrow C + D \qquad\qquad T = 273 \text{ K}$$

	$[A]_o$ (mol/L)	$[B]_o$ (mol/L)	rate (mol/L·s)
Exp 1	0.10	1	0.035
Exp 2	0.10	4	0.070
Exp 3	0.20	1	0.140
Exp 4	0.10	16	0.140

    (A) What is the order with respect to A?
    (B) What is the order with respect to B?
    (C) What is the rate equation?
    (D) What is the overall order of the reaction?
    (E) Calculate the rate constant.

3. Consider the following chemical reaction and experimental data:

    $$A\ (aq) \rightarrow B\ (aq) + C\ (g)$$

Trial 1		**Trial 2**	
[A] mol/L	rate (M/s)	[A] mol/L	rate (M/s)
0.10	0.6	0.10	0.9
0.20	0.6	0.20	0.9
0.30	0.6	0.30	0.9
0.40	0.6	0.40	0.9

    (A) What is the rate expression for trial 1?
    (B) What is the rate constant for trial 1?
    (C) What is the most likely reason for the increased rate in trial 2?

4. Consider the following reaction and experimental data:

    $$SO_3 + H_2O \rightarrow H_2SO_4$$

	$[SO_3]$ (mol/L)	$[H_2O]$ (mol/L)	rate (mol/L·s)
Trial 1	0.1	0.01	0.013
Trial 2	0.2	0.01	0.052
Trial 3	X	0.02	0.234
Trial 4	0.1	0.03	0.039

(A) What is the value of *X*?

(B) What is the order of the reaction?

(C) What is the rate constant?

(D) What would be the rate if $[SO_3]$ in trial 4 were raised to 0.2 mol/L?

5. In the following diagram, which labeled arrow represents the activation energy for the reverse reaction?

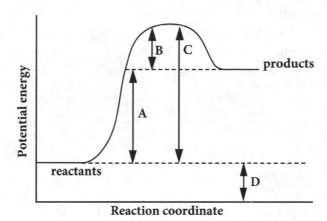

(A) A

(B) B

(C) C

(D) D

6. The activation energy for a reaction in the forward direction is 78 kJ. The activation energy for the same reaction in reverse is 300 kJ. If the energy of the products is 25 kJ, then:

(A) What is the energy of the reactants?

(B) Is the forward reaction endothermic or exothermic?

(C) Is the reverse reaction endothermic or exothermic?

(D) What is the enthalpy change for the forward reaction?

7. According to chemical kinetic theory, a reaction can occur

(A) if the reactants collide with the proper orientation.

(B) if the reactants possess sufficient energy of collision.

(C) if the reactants are able to form a correct transition state.

(D) for all of the above.

8. The number of undecayed nuclei in a sample of bromine-87 decreased by a factor of 4 over a period of 112 s. What is the decay constant for bromine-87?

(A) 6.19×10^{-3} s^{-1}

(B) 1.24×10^{-2} s^{-1}

(C) 6.93×10^{-1} s^{-1}

(D) 56 s

9. Which of the following is most likely to increase the rate of a reaction?

(A) Decreasing the temperature

(B) Increasing the volume of the reaction vessel

(C) Reducing the activation energy

(D) Decreasing the concentration of the reactant in the reaction vessel

10. All of the following are true statements concerning catalysts EXCEPT that a

(A) catalyst will speed the rate-determining step.

(B) catalyst will be used up in a reaction.

(C) catalyst may induce steric strain in a molecule.

(D) catalyst will lower the activation energy of a reaction.

SOLUTIONS TO REVIEW PROBLEMS

1. B Discussed in the section on reaction orders in this chapter.

2.   First, the general rate equation must be written out. It is:

rate $= k[A]^x[B]^y$

where:

$k =$ the rate constant

$x =$ the order with respect to reactant A

$y =$ the order with respect to reactant B

A $x = 2$

To solve for x, it is necessary to find two trials in which B is held constant; here, experiments 1 and 3. The data shows that if the concentration of A is doubled, the rate increases by a factor of 4. Thus, the rate varies as the square of the concentration of A. The order with respect to A, x, is therefore equal to 2.

B $y = 0.5$

To solve for y, follow the steps as in x. In experiments 1 and 2 (and 2 and 4) A is held constant, the concentration of B quadruples, and the rate doubles. The rate, therefore, varies as the square root of the concentration of B. The order, y, is therefore equal to 0.5.

C rate $= k[A]^2 [B]^{0.5}$

D order $= 2.5$

The overall order is equal to $x + y = 2.5$.

E **3.5**

Given the rate expression, the rate constant can be calculated by substituting the rate and concentrations for any of the four trials into the rate expression; the rate constant will work out to 3.5 in each case.

Trial 1: $0.035 = k[0.10]^2[1]^{0.5}$; $k = 3.5$ $M^{-1.5}$ s^{-1}

Trial 2: $0.070 = k[0.10]^2[4]^{0.5}$; $k = 3.5$ $M^{-1.5}$ s^{-1}

Trial 3: $0.140 = k[0.20]^2[1]^{0.5}$; $k = 3.5$ $M^{-1.5}$ s^{-1}

Trial 4: $0.140 = k[0.10]^2[16]^{0.5}$; $k = 3.5$ $M^{-1.5}$ s^{-1}

3. A rate $= k[A]^0 = k$

This reaction has only one reactant. It is evident from the data that the rate of the reaction is not affected by reactant concentration. This is a zero-order reaction, and the rate is equal to its rate constant, k.

B $k = 0.6$

C The most likely reason for the increased rate in trial 2 is a change in temperature. We know that in a zero-order reaction, changing the concentration of the reactant will not cause a change in rate; the factor most likely to affect the rate is temperature.

4. **A** $X = 0.3$

To calculate X, first write the rate expression for this reaction. From the data, the rate expression is calculated as:

$$\text{rate} = k[SO_3]^2 [H_2O]$$

The order with respect to SO_3 is 2, since the rate quadruples when the concentration of SO_3 doubles (with the concentration of H_2O remaining constant) between trials 1 and 2. The order with respect to H_2O is 1, as the rate triples as the concentration of H_2O triples (with the concentration of SO_3 remaining constant) between trials 1 and 4.

X can be calculated by plugging the values from trial 3 into the rate expression. First, however, calculate the rate constant, k, by plugging in the known values from trial 1, 2, or 4. For instance:

Trial 4: $0.039 = k[0.1]^2 [0.03]$; $k = 130$ $M^{-2}.$ s^{-1}

To calculate X, plug in the values of rate and $[H_2O]$ for trial 3, using $k = 130$ $M^{-2}.$ s^{-1}.

$0.234 = 130[X]^2 [0.02]$

$X = 0.3$ M

B **3**

The order of the reaction is the sum of the exponents in the rate expression: in this case, $(2 + 1) = 3$.

C **130 $M^{-2}.s^{-1}$**

For calculations see solution to part A.

D **0.156 units**

Substitute 0.2 M instead of 0.1 M for $[SO_3]$:

$\text{rate} = (130)(0.2)^2(0.03) = 0.156$ M/s

5. **B** The activation energy is the minimum amount of energy needed for a reaction to proceed. The activation energy for the reverse reaction is the change in potential energy between the products and the transition state indicated by arrow B.

6. **A** **247 kJ**

The best way to visualize the solution to this set of problems is to draw a diagram.

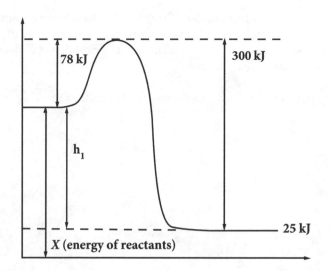

$$\Delta H = \text{Activation Energy}_{\text{forward}} - \text{Activation Energy}_{\text{reverse}}$$
$$= 78 \text{ kJ} - 300 \text{ kJ} = -222 \text{ kJ}$$

And because $\Delta H = \text{Energy}_{\text{products}} - \text{Energy}_{\text{reactants:}}$
$$-222 \text{ kJ} = 25 \text{ kJ} - X$$
$$X = 247 \text{ kJ} = \text{energy of reactants}$$

B The forward reaction is exothermic because ΔH is negative.

C The reverse reaction is endothermic.

D The enthalpy change, ΔH, of the reaction is -222 kJ.

7. **D** Discussed in the section on the efficiency of reactions in this chapter.

8. **B** If the number of nuclei decaying in a sample has decreased by a factor of 4, the sample has been through 2 half-lives, and the half-life will be

$$\frac{112 \text{ s}}{2} = 56 \text{ s} = t_{1/2}$$

The equation to determine the decay constant for the first-order reaction is

$$t_{1/2} = \frac{0.693}{k}$$

Thus, given that the half-life is 56 s, the decay constant will be

$$56 \text{ s} = \frac{0.693}{k}$$
$$k = 0.0124 \text{ s}^{-1}$$

9. **C** Various conditions can affect the rate of reaction: increased temperature, increased concentration of reactants, decreased volume or increased pressure (if any reactants are gases), or addition of a suitable catalyst. The effect of a catalyst is to decrease the activation energy; therefore, choice (C) is correct.

10. **B** Discussed in the section on factors affecting reaction rate in this chapter.

CHAPTER THIRTY-FOUR

Equilibrium

Often, reactions are discussed under the assumption that they are **irreversible** (i.e., only proceed in one direction) and that they proceed to completion. However, a **reversible** reaction often does not proceed to completion because (by definition) the products can react to reform the reactants. This is particularly true of reactions occurring in closed systems, where products are not allowed to escape. When there is no **net** change in the concentrations of the products and reactants during a reversible chemical reaction, equilibrium exists. This is not to say that a reaction in equilibrium is static; change continues to occur in both the forward and reverse directions. Equilibrium can be thought of as a balance between the two reaction directions.

Consider the following reaction:

$$A \rightleftharpoons B$$

At equilibrium, the concentrations of A and B are constant, yet the reactions A → B and B → A continue to occur at equal rates.

LAW OF MASS ACTION

Consider the following **one-step** reaction:

$$2A \rightleftharpoons B + C$$

Since the reaction occurs in one step, the rates of the forward (rate$_f$) and reverse (rate$_r$) reactions are given by:

$$\text{rate}_f = k_f[A]^2 \text{ and rate}_r = k_r[B][C]$$

When rate$_f$ = rate$_r$, equilibrium is achieved. Since the rates are equal, it can be stated that

$$k_f[A]^2 = k_r[B][C] \text{ or } \frac{k_f}{k_r} = \frac{[B][C]}{[A]^2}$$

Since k_f and k_r are both constants, this equation may be rewritten:

$$K_c = \frac{[B][C]}{[A]^2}$$

where K_c is called the **equilibrium constant**, and the subscript c indicates that it is in terms of concentration. When dealing with gases, the equilibrium constant is referred to as K_p, and the subscript p indicates that it is in terms of pressure. For dilute solutions, K_c and K_{eq} are used interchangeably; the symbol K is also often used, though it is not completely correct to do so.

While the forward and reverse reaction rates are equal at equilibrium, the **molar concentrations** of the reactants and products usually are not equal. This means that the forward and reverse rate constants, k_f and k_r, respectively, are also usually unequal. For the one-step reaction described above:

$$k_f [A]^2 = k_r [B][C]$$

$$k_f = k_r \left(\frac{[B][C]}{[A]^2} \right)$$

In a reaction of more than one step, the equilibrium constant for the overall reaction is found by multiplying together the equilibrium constants for each step of the reaction. When this is done, the equilibrium constant for the overall reaction is equal to the concentrations of products divided by reactants in the overall reaction, each raised to its stoichiometric coefficient. The forward and reverse rate constants for any step n are designated k_n and k_{-n} respectively. For example, if the reaction

$$aA + bB \rightleftharpoons cC + dD$$

occurs in three steps, then

$$K_{eq} = \frac{k_1 k_2 k_3}{k_{-1} k_{-2} k_{-3}} \text{ will equal } \frac{[C]^c[D]^d}{[A]^a[B]^b}$$

This expression is known as the **law of mass action**.

Example: What is the expression for the equilibrium constant for the following reaction?

$$3 H_2 (g) + N_2 (g) \rightleftharpoons 2 NH_3 (g)$$

Solution:

$$K_{eq} = \frac{[NH_3]^2}{[H_2]^3[N_2]}$$

The **reaction quotient**, Q, is a measure of the degree to which a reaction has gone to completion. Q_c is equal to:

$$Q_c = \frac{[C]^c[D]^d}{[A]^a[B]^b}$$

Q can be calculated based on the concentrations of reactants and products at any point in time during the course of a reaction, and the values can vary considerably depending on when during the reaction the calculation is made. Q_c is a constant only at equilibrium, when Q_c is equal to K_c.

PROPERTIES OF THE EQUILIBRIUM CONSTANT

The equilibrium constant, K_{eq}, has the following characteristics:

- Pure solids and liquids do not appear in the equilibrium constant expression.
- K_{eq} is characteristic of a given system at a given temperature.
- If the value of K_{eq} is much larger than 1, an equilibrium mixture of reactants and products will contain very little of the reactants compared to the products.
- If the value of K_{eq} is much smaller than 1 (i.e., less than 0.1), an equilibrium mixture of reactants and products will contain very little of the products compared to the reactants.
- If the value of K_{eq} is close to 1, an equilibrium mixture of products and reactants will contain approximately equal amounts of reactants and products.

LE CHÂTELIER'S PRINCIPLE

The French chemist Henry Louis Le Châtelier indicated that, if an external stress is applied to a system currently at equilibrium, the system will attempt to adjust itself to partially offset the stress. This rule, known as Le Châtelier's principle, is used to determine the direction in which a reaction at equilibrium will proceed when subjected to a stress, such as a change in concentration, pressure, temperature, or volume.

Changes in Concentration

Increasing the concentration of a species will tend to shift the equilibrium in the direction that will reestablish the equilibrium concentration of the species that is added, and decreasing its concentration will shift the equilibrium in the opposite direction. For example, in the reaction:

$$A + B \rightleftharpoons C + D$$

if the concentration of A and/or B is increased, the equilibrium will shift toward (or favor production of) C and D. Conversely, if the concentration of C and/or D is increased, the equilibrium will shift away from the production of C and D, favoring production of A and B. Similarly, decreasing the concentration of a species will tend to shift the equilibrium toward the production of that species. For example, if A and/or B is removed from the above reaction, the equilibrium will shift so as to favor increasing the concentrations of A and B.

This effect is often used in industry to increase the yield of a useful product or drive a reaction to completion. If D were constantly removed from the above reaction, the net reaction would produce more D and concurrently more C. Likewise, using an excess of the least expensive reactant helps to drive the reaction forward.

Change in Pressure or Volume

In a system at constant temperature, a change in pressure causes a change in volume, and vice versa. Since liquids and solids are practically incompressible, a change in the pressure or volume of systems involving only these phases has little or no effect on their equilibrium. Reactions involving gases, however, may be greatly affected by changes in pressure or volume; since gases are highly compressible, changing the volume of a container effectively changes the concentration of the gases it contains.

Pressure and volume are inversely related. An increase in the pressure of a system will shift the equilibrium so as to decrease the number of moles of gas present. This reduces the volume of the system and relieves the stress of the increased pressure. Consider the following reaction:

$$N_2 \, (g) + 3 \, H_2 \, (g) \rightleftharpoons 2 \, NH_3 \, (g)$$

The left side of the reaction has four moles of gaseous molecules, whereas the right side has only two moles. When the pressure of this system is increased, the equilibrium will shift so that the side of the reaction producing fewer moles is favored. Since there are fewer moles on the right, the equilibrium will shift toward the right. Conversely, if the volume of the same system is increased, its pressure immediately decreases, which, according to Le Châtelier's principle, leads to a shift in the equilibrium to the left.

Change in Temperature

Changes in temperature also affect equilibrium. To predict this effect, heat may be considered as a product in an exothermic $(\Delta H < 0)$ reaction and as a reactant in an endothermic reaction $(\Delta H > 0)$. Consider the following exothermic reaction:

$$A \rightleftharpoons B + \text{heat}$$

If this system were placed in an ice bath, its temperature would decrease, driving the reaction to the right to replace the heat lost. Conversely, if the system were placed in a boiling-water bath, the reaction equilibrium would shift to the left due to the increased "concentration" of heat.

Not only does a temperature change alter the position of the equilibrium, it also alters the numerical value of the equilibrium constant. In contrast, changes in the concentration of a species in the reaction, in the pressure, or in the volume alter the position of the reaction quotient without changing the numerical value of the equilibrium constant itself.

SOLUTION EQUILIBRIA

The process of solvation, like other reversible chemical and physical changes, tends toward equilibrium. Immediately after a solute has been introduced into a solvent, most of the change taking place is dissociation because no dissolved solute is initially present. However, according to Le Châtelier's principle, as solute dissociates, the reverse reaction (precipitation of the solute) also begins to occur. Eventually, equilibrium is reached and the rate of solute dissociation is equal to the rate of precipitation. At equilibrium, the net concentration of the dissociated solute remains unchanged regardless of the amount of solute added.

An ionic solid introduced into a polar solvent dissociates into its component ions. The dissociation of such a solute in solution may be represented by

$$A_m B_n \, (s) \rightleftharpoons m A \, (aq) + n B \, (aq)$$

For example: $\qquad\qquad CaCl_2 \, (s) \rightleftharpoons Ca^{2+} \, (aq) + 2 \, Cl^- \, (aq)$

The Solubility Product Constant

A slightly soluble ionic solid exists in equilibrium with its saturated solution. In the case of AgCl, for example, the solution equilibrium is as follows:

$$AgCl\ (s) \rightleftarrows Ag^+\ (aq) + Cl^-\ (aq)$$

The **ion product** (Q_{sp}) of a compound in solution is defined as follows:

$$Q_{sp} = [A]^m[B]^n$$

The same expression for a saturated solution at equilibrium defines the **solubility product constant** (K_{sp}).

$$K_{sp} = [A]^m[B]^n \text{ in a saturated solution}$$

However, Q_{sp} is defined with respect to initial concentrations and does not necessarily represent either an equilibrium or a saturated solution, while K_{sp} does.

Each salt has its own distinct K_{sp} at a given temperature. If at a given temperature a salt's Q_{sp} is equal to its K_{sp}, the solution is saturated, and the rate at which the salt dissolves equals the rate at which it precipitates out of solution. If a salt's Q_{sp} exceeds its K_{sp}, the solution is supersaturated (holding more salt than it should be able to at a given temperature) and unstable. If the supersaturated solution is disturbed by adding more salt, other solid particles, or jarring the solution by a sudden decrease in temperature, the solid salt will precipitate until Q_{sp} equals the K_{sp}. If Q_{sp} is less than K_{sp}, the solution is unsaturated and no precipitate will form.

Example: The solubility of $Fe(OH)_3$ in an aqueous solution was determined to be 4.5×10^{-10} mol/L. What is the value of the K_{sp} for $Fe(OH)_3$?

Solution: The molar solubility (the solubility of the compound in mol/L) is given as 4.5×10^{-10} M. The equilibrium concentration of each ion can be determined from the molar solubility and the balanced dissociation reaction of $Fe(OH)_3$. The dissociation reaction is:

$$Fe(OH)_3\ (s) \rightleftarrows Fe^{3+}\ (aq) + 3\ OH^-\ (aq)$$

Thus, for every mole of $Fe(OH)_3$ that dissociates, one mole of Fe^{3+} and three moles of OH^- are produced. Since the solubility is 4.5×10^{-10} M, the K_{sp} can be determined as follows:

$$K_{sp} = [Fe^{3+}][OH^-]^3$$

$$[OH^-] = 3[Fe^{3+}]; \quad [Fe^{3+}] = 4.5 \times 10^{-10} \text{ M}$$

$$K_{sp} = [Fe^{3+}](3[Fe^{3+}])^3 = 27[Fe^{3+}]^4$$

$$K_{sp} = 27(4.5 \times 10^{-10})^4 = 27(410 \times 10^{-40}) = 11,070 \times 10^{-40}$$

$$K_{sp} = 1.1 \times 10^{-36}$$

Example: What are the concentrations of each of the ions in a saturated solution of $PbBr_2$, given that the K_{sp} of $PbBr_2$ is 2.1×10^{-6}? If 5 g of $PbBr_2$ are dissolved in water to make 1 L of solution at 25°C, would the solution be saturated, unsaturated, or supersaturated?

Solution: The first step is to write out the dissociation reaction:

$$PbBr_2\ (s) \rightleftarrows Pb^{2+}\ (aq) + 2\ Br^-\ (aq)$$

$$K_{sp} = [Pb^{2+}][Br^-]^2$$

Let $x =$ the concentration of Pb^{2+}; then $2x =$ the concentration of Br^- in the saturated solution at equilibrium (since $[Br^-]$ is twice as large as $[Pb^{2+}]$).

$$K_{sp} = [x][2x]^2 = 4x^3$$

$$2.1 \times 10^{-6} = 4x^3$$

Solving for x, the concentration of Pb^{2+} in a saturated solution is 8.07×10^{-3} M, and the concentration of Br^- ($2x$) is 1.61×10^{-2} M.

To solve the second part of the question, convert 5 g of $PbBr_2$ into moles:

$$5\,g \times \frac{1\,mol\ PbBr_2}{367\,g} = 1.36 \times 10^{-2}\,mol$$

1.36×10^{-2} mol of $PbBr_2$ is dissolved in 1 L of solution, so the concentration of the solution is 1.36×10^{-2} M. Since this is higher than the concentration of a saturated solution of $PbBr_2$ (8.07×10^{-3} M), this solution would be supersaturated.

Factors Affecting Solubility

The quantity of a salt that can be dissolved is considerably reduced when it is dissolved in a solution that already contains one of its ions rather than in a pure solvent. This reduction in solubility, called the **common ion effect,** is another example of Le Châtelier's principle. The common ion effect will not change K_{sp}, but it will change the molar solubility (the concentrations of the individual ions, or x, in the solution).

Example: The K_{sp} of AgI in aqueous solution is 1×10^{-16} mol/L. If a 1×10^{-5} M solution of $AgNO_3$ is saturated with AgI, what will be the final concentration of the iodide ion?

Solution: The concentration of Ag^+ in the original $AgNO_3$ solution will be 1×10^{-5} mol/L. After AgI is added to saturation, the iodide concentration can be found with the K_{sp} equation:

$$AgI\ (s) \rightleftarrows Ag^+\ (aq) + I^-\ (aq)$$

$$K_{sp} = [Ag^+][I^-]$$

$$1 \times 10^{-16} = [Ag^+][I^-]$$

$$1 \times 10^{-16} = [1 \times 10^{-5}][I^-]$$

$$[I^-] = 1 \times 10^{-11}\ mol/L$$

If the AgI had been dissolved in pure water, the concentration of both Ag⁺ and I⁻ would have been 1×10^{-8} mol/L. The presence of the common ion, silver, at a concentration one thousand times higher than what it would be in a solution of just water and silver iodide has reduced the iodide concentration to one thousandth of what it would have been otherwise. An additional 1×10^{-11} mol/L of silver will dissolve in solution along with the iodide ion, but this will not significantly affect the final silver concentration, which is one million times greater.

REVIEW PROBLEMS

1. The equilibrium constant, K_{eq}, of a certain single-reactant reaction is 0.16. Suppose an appropriate catalyst is added in twice the concentration of the reactant.

   (A) What will be the equilibrium constant?

   (B) Will the activation energy increase or decrease?

2. At equilibrium

   (A) the forward reaction will continue.

   (B) a change in reaction conditions will shift the equilibrium.

   (C) the reverse reaction will not continue.

   (D) both A and B will occur.

3. What is the general equation for K_{eq} for the following reaction?

$$2 \, NO_2 \, (g) + 2 \, H_2 \, (g) \rightleftharpoons N_2 \, (g) + 2 \, H_2O \, (g)$$

4. If $K_{eq} > 1$,

   (A) the equilibrium mixture will contain more product than reactant.

   (B) the equilibrium mixture will contain more reactant than product.

   (C) the equilibrium amounts of reactants and products are equal.

   (D) the reaction is irreversible.

5. Answer the following questions using the reaction given below.

$$CH_3OH \, (l) + H_2 \, (g) \rightleftharpoons CH_4 \, (g) + H_2O \, (l) \qquad \Delta H = -30 \, kcal$$

   (A) In which direction would the reaction be shifted if the temperature were increased?

   (B) In which direction would the reaction be shifted if the volume were doubled?

   (C) In which direction would the reaction be shifted if methane (CH_4) were removed from the reaction vessel?

6. What is the concentration of the Ag^+ ion in a saturated solution of AgCl? (K_{sp} for AgCl = 1.7×10^{-10})

$$AgCl \, (s) \rightleftharpoons Ag^+ \, (aq) + Cl^- \, (aq)$$

   (A) $1.7 \times 10^{-10} \, M$

   (B) $3.4 \times 10^{-10} \, M$

   (C) $1.3 \times 10^{-5} \, M$

   (D) $2.6 \times 10^{-5} \, M$

7. Explain the common ion effect in terms of K_{sp}.

SOLUTIONS TO REVIEW PROBLEMS

1. **A** K_{eq} remains constant at 0.16. Catalysts do not affect equilibrium position.

   B Addition of a catalyst decreases the activation energy.

2. **D** At equilibrium, both the forward and reverse reactions are proceeding. Any change in the equilibrium conditions will shift the equilibrium to alleviate the stress on the reaction.

3. $$K_{eq} = \frac{[N_2][H_2O]^2}{[NO_2]^2[H_2]^2}$$

4. **A** Discussed in the section on the equilibrium constant in this chapter.

5. **A** The reaction shifts to the left. This is an exothermic reaction, as seen by the negative ΔH, and any increase in temperature will favor the reverse reaction.

   B The reaction will remain unchanged. Changing the volume constraints on a reaction that involves gases will affect the equilibrium only when one side of the reaction has a greater number of moles than the other.

   C The reaction would shift to the right. By removing methane gas from the reaction vessel, the reactant concentrations are effectively increased relative to the product concentrations, and the reaction will go to the right to correct for this.

6. **C** $K_{sp} = [Ag^+][Cl^-]$

   Let $x = [Ag^+]$

   Since $[Ag^+] = [Cl^-]$: $1.7 \times 10^{-10} = x^2$

   $x = 1.3 \times 10^{-5}\,M$

7. Consider as an example a dilute solution of AgCl. The K_{sp} of AgCl at 25°C is 1.7×10^{-10}. If the original concentration of AgCl is 1×10^{-6} M, then $Q_{sp} = (1 \times 10^{-6})^2 = 1 \times 10^{-12}$, which is less than the K_{sp}; thus, all the salt is dissolved.

   Now suppose NaCl is added to this solution until the NaCl concentration is 1×10^{-2}. $[Cl^-]$ will now be the sum of $[Cl^-]$ due to AgCl and $[Cl^-]$ due to NaCl; $[Cl^-] = 1 \times 10^{-2} + 1 \times 10^{-6} = 1.0001 \times 10^{-2}$, or approximately 1×10^{-2}.

   Thus, the Q_{sp} for AgCl is $(1 \times 10^{-6})(1 \times 10^{-2}) = 1 \times 10^{-8}$, which is greater than the K_{sp}. AgCl will therefore precipitate until Q_{sp} is reduced to the K_{sp}. Because of the high concentration of Cl^-, the final concentration of Ag^+ will be lower than it would have been otherwise.

CHAPTER THIRTY-FIVE

Phase Changes

Matter can exist in three different physical forms called **phases** or **states**: gas, liquid, and solid. The primary difference between the three phases is how tightly the constituent pieces are held together. When the attractive forces between gaseous molecules overcome the kinetic energy that keeps them apart, the molecules move closer together such that they can no longer move about freely, entering the **liquid** or **solid** phase. Because of their smaller volume relative to gases, liquids and solids are also referred to as **condensed phases**.

The table below contrasts the general properties of each phase.

Phase	Volume and Shape	Motion Principles	Density	Ability to be Compressed
Gas	Conforms to the volume and shape of the container it is in	Continual motion	Low	Easily compressed to smaller volume
Liquid	Conforms to the shape of the container; however, has definite volume	Sliding motion of particles past one another	Moderate	Small ability to be compressed (considered incompressible on the PCAT)
Solid	Defined volume and shape	Particles in a fixed position	High	Difficult to compress (considered incompressible on the PCAT)

Table 35.1

GASES

Gases display similar behavior and follow similar laws regardless of their identity. The atoms or molecules in a gaseous sample move rapidly and are far apart from each other. In addition, only very weak intermolecular forces exist between gas particles; this results in certain characteristic physical properties, such as the ability to expand to fill any volume, to take on the shape of a container, and to flow as fluids. Furthermore, gases are easily, though not infinitely, compressible. This chapter will mainly focus on principles of liquids and solids, but gases will be discussed more in Chapter 36, Gas Laws.

LIQUIDS

In a liquid, atoms or molecules are held close together with little space between them. As a result, liquids have definite volumes and cannot easily be expanded or compressed. However, the molecules can still move around and are in a state of relative disorder. Consequently, the liquid can change shape to fit its container, and its molecules are able to **diffuse** and **evaporate**.

One of the most important properties of liquids is their ability to mix, both with each other and with other phases, to form **solutions** (see Chapter 31, Solutions). The degree to which two liquids can mix is called their **miscibility**. Oil and water are almost completely **immiscible**; that is, their molecules tend to repel each other due to their polarity difference. Oil and water normally form separate layers when mixed, with oil on top because it is less dense. Under extreme conditions, such as violent shaking, two immiscible liquids can form a fairly homogeneous mixture called an **emulsion**. Although they look like solutions, emulsions are actually mixtures of discrete particles too small to be seen distinctly.

SOLIDS

In a solid, the attractive forces between atoms, ions, or molecules are strong enough to hold them rigidly together. Thus, the particles' only motion is vibration about fixed positions, and the kinetic energy of solids is predominantly **vibrational energy**. As a result, solids have definite shapes and volumes.

A solid may be **crystalline** or **amorphous**. A crystalline solid, such as NaCl, possesses an ordered structure; its atoms exist in a specific, three-dimensional geometric arrangement with repeating patterns of atoms, ions, or molecules. An amorphous solid, such as glass, has no ordered three-dimensional arrangement, although the molecules are also fixed in place.

Most solids are crystalline in structure. The two most common forms of crystals are **metallic** and **ionic** crystals.

Ionic solids are aggregates of positively and negatively charged ions; there are no discrete molecules. The physical properties of ionic solids include high melting points, high boiling points, and poor electrical conductivity in the solid phase. These properties are due to the compounds' strong electrostatic interactions, which also cause the ions to be relatively immobile. Ionic structures are given by empirical formulas that describe the ratio of atoms in the lowest possible whole numbers. For example, the empirical formula $BaCl_2$ gives the ratio of barium to chloride within the crystal.

Metallic solids consist of metal atoms packed together as closely as possible. Metallic solids have high melting and boiling points as a result of their strong covalent attractions. Pure metallic structures (consisting of a single element) are usually described as layers of spheres of roughly similar radii.

Crystals (both ionic and metallic) are defined by their **unit cells**, which represent the smallest repeating units that compose the larger crystalline structure. Although there are many types of unit cells, the cubic unit cells are the most important: **simple cubic**, **body-centered cubic**, and **face-centered cubic**.

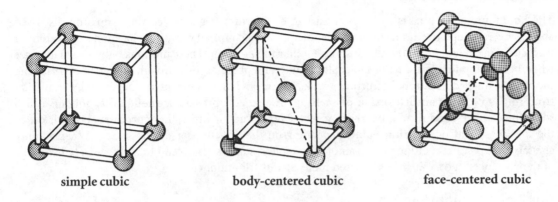

simple cubic   body-centered cubic   face-centered cubic

Figure 35.1

Each point in a unit cell diagram represents the exact same atom or ion. Additional atoms or ions of other elements may also be present, but these are not included in the unit cell diagram. For example, the ions of cesium chloride (CsCl) arrange in simple cubic units such that each of the eight corners of the cube are occupied by Cl^- ions. The center of the cube is occupied by one Cs^+ ion (creating a final structure similar to the body-centered cubic diagram), but the Cs^+ ion is not represented in the simple cubic diagram since Cs^+ is not the same ion as the corners, which are Cl^-.

PHASE EQUILIBRIA

In an isolated system, phase changes (solid to liquid to gas) are reversible, and an equilibrium exists between phases. For example, at 1 atm and 0°C in an isolated system, an ice cube floating in water is in equilibrium. Some of the ice may absorb heat and melt, but an equal amount of water will release heat and freeze. Thus, the relative amounts of ice and water remain constant.

Gas-Liquid Equilibrium

The temperature of a liquid is related to the average kinetic energy of the liquid molecules; however, the kinetic energy of the molecules will vary. A few molecules near the surface of the liquid may have enough energy to leave the liquid phase and escape into the gaseous phase. This process is known as **evaporation** or **vaporization**. Each time the liquid loses a high-energy particle, the temperature of the remaining liquid decreases; thus, evaporation is a cooling process. Nevertheless, given enough kinetic energy, the liquid will completely evaporate.

If a cover is placed on a beaker of liquid, the escaping molecules are trapped above the solution. These molecules exert a countering pressure, which forces some of the gas back into the liquid phase; this process is called **condensation**. Atmospheric pressure acts on a liquid in a similar fashion as a solid lid. As evaporation and condensation proceed, an equilibrium is reached in which the rates of the two processes become equal. Once this equilibrium is reached, the pressure that the gas exerts over the liquid is called the **vapor pressure** of the liquid. Vapor pressure increases as temperature increases, since more molecules have sufficient kinetic energy to escape into the gas phase. The temperature at which the vapor pressure of the liquid equals the external pressure is called the **boiling point**.

Liquid-Solid Equilibrium

The liquid and solid phases can also coexist in equilibrium (e.g., the ice water mixture discussed above). Even though the atoms or molecules of a solid are confined to definite locations, each atom or molecule can undergo motions about some equilibrium position. These motions (vibrations) increase when heat is applied. If atoms or molecules in the solid phase absorb enough energy in this fashion, the solid's three-dimensional structure breaks down, and the liquid phase begins. The transition from solid to liquid is called **fusion** or **melting**. The reverse process, from liquid to solid, is called **solidification**, **crystallization**, or **freezing**. The temperature at which these processes occur is called the **melting point** or **freezing point**, depending on the direction of the transition. Whereas pure crystals have distinct melting points, amorphous solids, such as glass, tend to melt over a larger range of temperatures due to their less-ordered molecular distribution.

Gas-Solid Equilibrium

A third type of phase equilibrium is that between a gas and a solid. When a solid goes directly into the gas phase, the process is called **sublimation**. Dry ice (solid CO_2) sublimes at room temperature, becoming CO_2 (g); the absence of the liquid phase makes it a convenient refrigerant. The reverse transition, from the gaseous to the solid phase, is called **deposition**.

The Gibbs Function

The thermodynamic criterion for each of the above equilibria is that the change in Gibbs free energy must equal zero, meaning no net energy is required for or released from the forward or reverse reaction. For an equilibrium between a gas and a solid:

$$\Delta G = G\,(g) - G\,(s)$$

$$\text{so } G\,(g) = G\,(s) \text{ at equilibrium}$$

The same is true of the Gibbs functions for the other two equilibria.

PHASE DIAGRAMS

Single Component

A standard **phase diagram** depicts the phases and phase equilibria of a substance at defined temperatures and pressures. In general, the gas phase is found at high temperature and low pressure; the solid phase is found at low temperature and high pressure; and the liquid phase is found at high temperature and high pressure. A typical phase diagram is shown below:

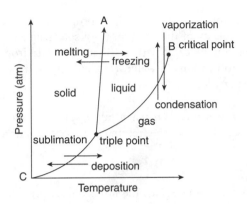

Figure 35.2

The three phases are demarcated by lines indicating the temperatures and pressures at which two phases are in equilibrium. Line A represents freezing/melting, line B vaporization/condensation, and line C sublimation/deposition. The intersection of the three lines is called the **triple point**. At this temperature and pressure, unique for a given substance, all three phases are in equilibrium. The point at B is known as the **critical point**, the temperature and pressure above which the liquid and gas phases are not possible and supercritical fluids exist instead.

Multiple Components

The phase diagram for a mixture of two or more components is complicated by the requirement that the composition of the mixture, as well as the temperature and pressure, must be specified. Consider a solution of two liquids, A and B. The vapor above the solution is a mixture of the vapors of A and B. The pressures exerted by vapor A and vapor B on the solution are the vapor pressures that each exerts above its individual liquid phase. **Raoult's law** (described below) enables one to determine the relationship between the vapor pressure of vapor A and the concentration of liquid A in the solution.

COLLIGATIVE PROPERTIES

Colligative properties are physical properties derived solely from the number of particles present, not the nature of those particles. These properties are usually associated with dilute solutions.

Freezing-Point Depression

Pure water (H_2O) freezes at 0°C; however, for every mole of solute particles dissolved in 1 L of water, the freezing point is lowered by 1.86°C. This is because the solute particles interfere with the process of crystal formation that occurs during freezing; the solute particles lower the temperature at which the molecules can align themselves into a crystalline structure.

The formula for calculating this freezing-point depression is:

$$\Delta T_f = iK_f m$$

where ΔT_f is the freezing-point depression, K_f is a proportionality constant characteristic of a particular solvent, m is the molality of the solution (mol solute/kg solvent), and i is the van't Hoff factor, which accounts for the number of particles that dissociate from the original molecule. For example, NaCl dissociates into two ions in water, Na^+ and Cl^-, so its $i = 2$ to represent that 1 mol NaCl becomes 2 mol solute particles.

One of the best examples of this principle is when salt is sprinkled on roads to make ice melt. This thawing occurs because the salt depresses the freezing point of the water.

Boiling-Point Elevation

A liquid boils when its vapor pressure equals the atmospheric pressure. If the vapor pressure of a solution is lower than that of the pure solvent, more energy (and consequently a higher temperature) will be required before its vapor pressure equals atmospheric pressure. The extent to which the boiling point of a solution is raised relative to that of the pure solvent is given by the following formula:

$$\Delta T_b = iK_b m$$

where ΔT_b is the boiling-point elevation, K_b is a proportionality constant characteristic of a particular solvent, m is the molality of the solution, and i is the van't Hoff factor.

One commonly misunderstood example of this principle is the addition of salt (NaCl) to a boiling pot of water on the stove, such as before cooking pasta, supposedly to speed cooking by raising the temperature of the water. Although adding Na^+ and Cl^- ions does increase the boiling point, the molality of salt normally added only results in an increase in boiling point of approximately 0.1°C (in fact, the main values of adding salt are to decrease sticking and add flavor).

Osmotic Pressure

Consider a container separated into two compartments by a semipermeable membrane (which, by definition, selectively permits the passage of only certain molecules). One compartment contains pure water, while the other contains water with dissolved solute. The membrane allows water but not solute to pass through. Because substances tend to flow, or **diffuse**, from higher to lower concentrations (which increases entropy), water will diffuse from the compartment containing pure water to the compartment containing the water-solute mixture. This net flow will cause the water level in the compartment containing the solution to rise above the level in the compartment containing pure water.

However, the pressure exerted by the water level in the solute-containing compartment due to gravity will eventually oppose the influx of water due to diffusion, and the water will stop flowing once this point is reached. This pressure is defined as the **osmotic pressure** (Π) of the solution and is given by the formula:

$$\Pi = iMRT$$

where M is the molarity of the solution, R is the ideal gas constant, T is the temperature on the Kelvin scale, and i is the van't Hoff factor. This equation shows that molarity and osmotic pressure are directly proportional (i.e., as the concentration of the solution increases, the osmotic pressure also increases). Thus, the osmotic pressure depends only on the amount of solute, not its identity.

Vapor-Pressure Lowering (Raoult's Law)

When solute B is added to pure solvent A, the vapor pressure of A above the solvent decreases. If the vapor pressure of A above pure solvent A is designated by P°_A and the vapor pressure of A above the solution containing B is P_A, the vapor pressure decreases as follows:

$$\Delta P = P^\circ_A - P_A$$

In the late 1800s, the French chemist François Marie Raoult determined that this vapor pressure decrease is also equivalent to:

$$\Delta P = X_B P^\circ_A$$

where X_B is the mole fraction of the solute B in solvent A (mol B/total moles). Because $X_B = 1 - X_A$ and $\Delta P = P^\circ_A - P_A$, substitution into the above equation leads to the common form of Raoult's law:

$$P_A = X_A P^\circ_A$$

Similarly, the expression for the vapor pressure of the solute in solution (assuming it is volatile) is given by:

$$P_B = X_B P^\circ_B$$

Raoult's law holds only when the attraction between molecules of the different components of the mixture is equal to the attraction between the molecules of any one component in its pure state. When this condition does not hold, the relationship between mole fraction and vapor pressure will deviate from Raoult's law. Solutions that obey Raoult's Law are called **ideal solutions**.

REVIEW PROBLEMS

1. Which of the following indicates the relative randomness of molecules in the three states of matter?

    (A) solid > liquid > gas

    (B) liquid < solid < gas

    (C) liquid > gas > solid

    (D) gas > liquid > solid

2. What factor determines whether or not two liquids are miscible?

    (A) Molecular size

    (B) Molecular polarity

    (C) Density

    (D) Both B and C

3. Discuss the physical properties of ionic crystals.

4. Alloys are mixtures of pure metals in either the liquid or solid phase. Which of the following is usually true of alloys?

    (A) The melting/freezing point of an alloy will be lower than that of either of the component metals because the new bonds are stronger.

    (B) The melting/freezing point of an alloy will be lower than that of either of the component metals because the new bonds are weaker.

    (C) The melting/freezing point of an alloy will be greater than that of either of the component metals because the new bonds are weaker.

    (D) The melting/freezing point of an alloy will be greater than that of either of the component metals because the new bonds are stronger.

Refer to the phase diagram below for questions 5–8.

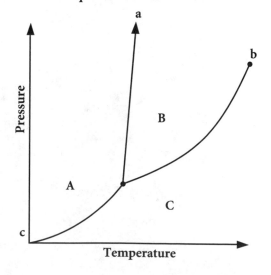

5. What is the typical form of a substance in state B?

    (A) Pure crystalline solid

    (B) Amorphous solid

    (C) Gas

    (D) Liquid

6. What is the typical form of a substance in state C?

    (A) Pure crystalline solid

    (B) Amorphous solid

    (C) Gas

    (D) Liquid

7. If line a was instead a band covering a range of temperatures, what would state A be?

    (A) Pure crystalline solid

    (B) Amorphous solid

    (C) Gas

    (D) Liquid

8. What is the triple point?

9. A semipermeable membrane separates a container of fresh water from one of salt water. If the volume of fresh water decreases significantly, what must be true of the semipermeable membrane? Assume that evaporation is negligible.

10. Once equilibrium is reached, if the temperature in Question 9 is suddenly increased, the osmotic pressure

    (A) will decrease.

    (B) will increase.

    (C) will remain the same.

    (D) cannot be determined.

11. What is the freezing point of a solution containing 0.5 mol of glucose dissolved in 200 g of H_2O? (The K_f for water is $1.86°C·m^{-1}$.)

12. The osmotic pressure at STP of a solution in which 1 L of solution contains 117 g of NaCl is

    (A) 44.8 atm.

    (B) 48.9 atm.

    (C) 89.5 atm.

    (D) 117 atm.

13. At 18°C and 1 atm, the vapor pressure of pure water is 0.02 atm, and the vapor pressure of pure ethyl alcohol (MW = 46 g/mol) is 0.50 atm. For a water-alcohol mixture with the alcohol present in a mole fraction of 0.2, find the vapor pressure due to the alcohol and the vapor pressure due to the water.

SOLUTIONS TO REVIEW PROBLEMS

1. **D** Because gas molecules have the greatest freedom to move around, gases have the greatest disorder. Liquids are denser than gases, and therefore the molecules are less free to move around. The arrangement of molecules in solids is the least random. Thus, melting and boiling are accompanied by an increase in entropy (i.e., $\Delta S > 0$).

2. **B** The miscibility of two liquids strongly depends on their polarities. In general, polar and nonpolar liquids are not miscible, while a polar liquid can usually be mixed with another polar liquid and a nonpolar liquid with another nonpolar liquid. Choice (A), molecular size, and choice (C), the density of a liquid, do not directly affect the miscibility. However, (C) should remind you that two immiscible liquids will form separate layers, with the denser liquid on the bottom. Thus, (B) is the only correct choice.

3. Ionic crystals contain repeating units of cations and anions. Because of the strong electrostatic attraction between the ions, these crystals have high melting points. Since the charges in these crystals are tightly fixed in the lattice, ionic solids are poor conductors of electricity. In the liquid or solution phase, the charged particles can move around, and thus liquid ionic compounds will conduct electricity, as will solutions of such salts.

4. **B** The bonds between different metal atoms in an alloy are much weaker than those between the atoms in pure metals. Therefore, breaking these bonds requires less energy than breaking the bonds in pure metals. Since melting and freezing points are inversely proportional to the stability of bonds, they tend to be lower for alloys than for pure metals. Alternately, an alloy can be looked at as a solid solution; impurities lower the melting point.

5. **D** Discussed in the section on phase diagrams in this chapter.

6. **C** Discussed in the section on phase diagrams in this chapter.

7. **B** Discussed in the section on phase diagrams in this chapter.

8. The unique combination of temperature and pressure at which the solid, liquid, and gas phases coexist at equilibrium.

9. The membrane must be permeable to water but not to salt. If it were permeable to salt, the salt would diffuse across the membrane into the fresh water container (down its concentration gradient) until the molarities of the two containers were the same. However, the volume of the salt water container increased, indicating that fresh water diffused across the membrane from a region of low solute concentration to one of high solute concentration. The water level rose until it exerted enough pressure to counterbalance the tendency to diffuse; this pressure is known as the osmotic pressure.

10. **B** Using the formula $\Pi = iMRT$, we see that osmotic pressure and temperature are directly proportional (i.e., if temperature increases, osmotic pressure will also increase). Thus, (B) is the correct answer.

11.   **−4.65°C**

This question applies the concept of freezing-point depression. If 0.5 mol of a nonelectrolyte solute such as glucose is dissolved in 200 g of H_2O, then the molality of the solution is

$$\frac{0.5\,\text{mol}}{0.200\,\text{kg H}_2\text{O}} = 2.5 \text{ mol solute/kg H}_2\text{O} = 2.5 \text{ m}$$

Using the equation $\Delta T_f = iK_f m$, the freezing point depression is $1 \times 2.5 \text{ m} \times 1.86°\text{C·m}^{-1} = 4.65°\text{C}$ ($i = 1$ for glucose because it does not dissociate in solution). The new freezing point is $0°\text{C} - 4.65°\text{C} = -4.65°\text{C}$. Note that ΔT_f is the change in freezing point and not the freezing point itself.

12.   **C**   The osmotic pressure (Π) of a solution is given by $\Pi = iMRT$. At STP, $T = 273$ K; R, the ideal gas constant, equals 8.2×10^{-2} L·atm/(K·mol). To determine the molarity, find the formula weight of NaCl from the periodic table; FW = 58.5 g/mol. The number of moles in the solution described is:

$$\frac{117\,\text{g/L}}{58.5\,\text{g/mol}} = 2 \text{ mol undissociated} = \text{NaCl/L}$$

But since NaCl is a strong electrolyte, it dissociates in aqueous solution into two particles, so i is 2, and there are actually 4 moles of particles per liter of solution (i.e., 2 moles of Na^+ and 2 moles of Cl^-). Thus:

$$\Pi = (2)(2 \text{ mol/L})(8.2 \times 10^{-2} \text{ L·atm})/(\text{K·mol}))(273 \text{ K})$$
$$= 89.54 \text{ atm}$$

Remember that colligative properties depend on the number of particles, not their identity.

13.   Use Raoult's law to answer this question, with A = H_2O and B = ethyl alcohol.
$$P_A = X_A P°_A$$
$$P_B = X_B P°_B$$
Because we are given that $X_B = 0.2$, then $X_A = 1 - X_B = 1 - 0.2 = 0.8$.
$$P°_A = 0.02 \text{ atm}$$
$$P°_B = 0.50 \text{ atm}$$
$$P_A = (0.8)(0.02 \text{ atm}) = 0.016 \text{ atm}$$
$$P_B = (0.2)(0.50 \text{ atm}) = 0.10 \text{ atm}$$
Thus, the vapor pressure due to water is 0.016 atm, and the vapor pressure due to alcohol is 0.10 atm.

CHAPTER THIRTY-SIX

Gas Laws

Gases, as defined in Chapter 35, Phase Changes, are unique in that their molecules have very weak intermolecular forces, allowing gases both to flow and to change volume to fill and take the shape of their containers. The state of a gaseous sample is generally defined by four variables: **pressure (P), volume (V), temperature (T),** and **number of moles (n)**. Pressure describes force per area, such as the force per area an enclosed gas exhibits on the walls of its container. The SI unit of pressure is the pascal (Pa), but pressure is also often expressed in units of atmospheres (atm) or millimeters of mercury (mmHg or torr), which are related as follows:

$$1 \text{ atm} = 10^5 \text{ Pa} = 760 \text{ mmHg} = 760 \text{ Torr}$$

Volume is generally expressed in liters (L) or milliliters (mL). The temperature of a gas is usually given in Kelvin (K, not °K). Gases are also often discussed in terms of **standard temperature and pressure (STP)**, which refers to conditions of 273.15 K (0°C) and 1 atm. It is important not to confuse STP with **standard conditions**—the two standards involve different temperatures and are used for different purposes. STP (0°C or 273 K) is generally used for gas law calculations; standard conditions (25°C or 298 K) are used when measuring standard enthalpy, entropy, Gibbs free energy, or voltage.

IDEAL GASES

When examining the behavior of gases under varying conditions of temperature and pressure, scientists speak of ideal gases. An ideal gas represents a hypothetical gas whose molecules have no intermolecular forces and occupy no volume. Although gases actually deviate from this idealized behavior, under conditions of relatively low pressure (i.e., atmospheric pressure) and high temperature, many gases behave in a nearly ideal fashion. Therefore, the assumptions used for ideal gases can be applied to real gases with reasonable accuracy.

Boyle's Law

Experimental studies performed by Robert Boyle in 1660 led to the formulation of Boyle's law. His work showed that, for a given gaseous sample held at a constant temperature (isothermal conditions), the product of pressure and volume is constant: $PV = k$. Another way to think about this mathematical relationship is that pressure and volume are inversely proportional.

It is important to note that the individual values of pressure and volume can vary greatly for a given sample of gas. However, as long as the temperature remains constant and the amount of gas does not change, the product of both P and V will equal the same constant (k). Subsequently, for a given sample of gas under two sets of conditions, the following equation can be derived:

$$P_1V_1 = k_1 = P_2V_2 \quad \text{or simply} \quad P_1V_1 = P_2V_2$$

where k is a proportionality constant and the subscripts 1 and 2 represent two different sets of conditions. A plot of pressure versus volume for a gas is shown below.

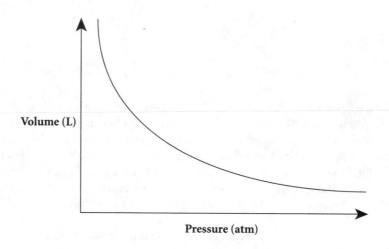

Figure 36.1

Example: Under isothermal conditions, what would be the volume of a 1 L sample of helium after its pressure is changed from 12 atm to 4 atm?

Solution:

$$P_1 = 12 \text{ atm} \qquad P_2 = 4 \text{ atm}$$
$$V_1 = 1 \text{ L} \qquad V_2 = ?$$

$$P_1V_1 = P_2V_2$$
$$12 \text{ atm (1 L)} = 4 \text{ atm}(V_2)$$
$$\frac{12 \text{ atm}}{4 \text{ atm}} \times 1 \text{ L} = V_2$$
$$V_2 = 3 \text{ L}$$

Charles's Law

The law of volumes, also known as Charles's law, was developed at the turn of the 19th century. The law states that, at constant pressure, the quotient of the volume and temperature of gas is constant. Or, put another way, the volume of a gas is directly proportional to its absolute temperature

$$\frac{V}{T} = k \quad \text{or} \quad \frac{V_1}{T_1} = \frac{V_2}{T_2}$$

where k is a constant and the subscripts 1 and 2 represent two different sets of conditions. The absolute temperature (T) is the temperature expressed in Kelvin, which can be calculated from the expression $T_K = T_{°C} + 273.15$. It is important to note that the temperature $-273.15°C$ is the theoretical lowest attainable temperature, known as **absolute zero**. Below is a summary to help understand this principle:

absolute zero	0 K	−273.15°C
water freezes	273.15 K	0°C
water boils	373.15 K	100°C

A plot of temperature versus volume is shown below.

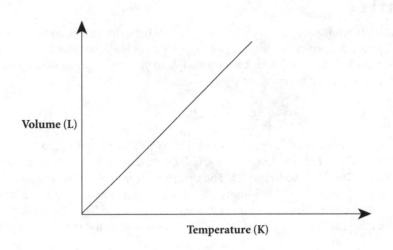

Figure 36.2

Example: If the absolute temperature of 2 L of gas at constant pressure is changed from 283.15 K to 566.30 K, what would be the final volume?

Solution:

$$T_1 = 283.15 \text{ K} \qquad V_1 = 2 \text{ L}$$
$$T_2 = 566.30 \text{ K} \qquad V_2 = \text{?}$$

$$\frac{V_1}{T_1} = \frac{V_2}{T_2}$$

$$\frac{2 \text{ L}}{283.15 \text{ K}} = \frac{V_2}{566.30 \text{K}}$$

$$V_2 = \frac{2 \text{ L } (566.30 \text{ K})}{283.15 \text{ K}}$$

$$V_2 = 4 \text{ L}$$

Avogadro's Principle

In 1811, Amedeo Avogadro proposed that, for all gases at a constant temperature and pressure, the volume of the gas will be directly proportional to the number of moles of gas present; therefore, all gases have the same number of moles in the same volume.

$$\frac{n}{V} = k \quad \text{or} \quad \frac{n_1}{V_1} = \frac{n_2}{V_2}$$

The subscripts 1 and 2 once again apply to two different sets of conditions with the same temperature and pressure.

Ideal Gas Law

A theoretical gas whose volume-pressure-temperature behavior can be completely understood by the ideal gas equation is known as an "ideal gas." The ideal gas law combines the relationships outlined in Boyle's law, Charles's law, and Avogadro's principle to yield an expression that can be used to predict the behavior of a gas and is represented by the equation

$$PV = nRT$$

The constant R is known as the **gas constant**. Under STP conditions (273.15 K and 1 atmosphere), one mole of ideal gas has a volume of 22.4 L. Substituting these values into the ideal gas equation gives $R = 8.21 \times 10^{-2}$ L · atm/(mol · K). The gas constant may also be expressed in many other units; another common value is 8.314 J/(K·mol), which is derived when the SI units of pascals (for pressure) and cubic meters (for volume) are substituted into the ideal gas law. When carrying out calculations based on the ideal gas law, it is important to choose a value of R that matches the units of the variables.

Example: What volume would 12 g of helium occupy at 20°C and a pressure of 380 mmHg?

Solution: The ideal gas law can be used, but first all the variables must be converted to yield units that correspond to the expression of the gas constant as 0.0821 L·atm/(mol·K):

$$P = 380 \text{ mmHg} \times \frac{1 \text{ atm}}{760 \text{ mmHg}} = 0.5 \text{ atm}$$

$$T = 20°C + 273.15 = 293.15 \text{ K}$$

$$n = 12 \text{ g He} \times \frac{1 \text{ mol He}}{4.0 \text{ g}} = 3 \text{ mol He}$$

Substituting into the ideal gas equation:

$PV = nRT$

$(0.5 \text{ atm})(V) = (3 \text{ mol})(0.0821 \text{ L} \cdot \text{atm/(mol} \cdot \text{K)})(293.15 \text{ K})$

$V = 144.4 \text{ L}$

Sometimes, it is advantageous to compare gases under different conditions. To do this quickly, divide the ideal gas law from one condition by another condition:

$$\frac{P_1 V_1}{P_2 V_2} = \frac{n_1 R T_1}{n_2 R T_2}$$

One great advantage of this approach is that the ideal gas constant (R) cancels out, leaving:

$$\frac{P_1 V_1}{P_2 V_2} = \frac{n_1 T_1}{n_2 T_2}$$

And from this point, some straightforward algebra can find pressure, volume, moles, or temperature under either condition. Removing R from the equation can certainly help with mental math on the PCAT, but not all ideal gas questions on the PCAT compare gases under two separate conditions. However, by remembering that 1 mole of gas at STP (1 atm and 273.15K) occupies 22.4 L, one can use the comparative ideal gas equation and still remove the ideal gas constant from the solution (as long as all the units align!):

$$\frac{PV}{P_{STP} V_{STP}} = \frac{nT}{n_{STP} T_{STP}}$$

Using the above simplification as a guide, let's go through the previous example again:

Example: What volume would 12 g of helium occupy at 20°C and a pressure of 380 mmHg?

Solution: Convert the given information on mass, temperature, and pressure to units that match the STP information (mol, atm, K, and L):

12 g of He is 3 mol

20°C is 293.15 K

380 mmHg is 0.5 atm

Then, rearrange the simplification to solve for V and plug in the values given:

$$\frac{PV}{P_{STP} V_{STP}} = \frac{nT}{n_{STP} T_{STP}}$$

$$V = \frac{V_{STP} P_{STP} nT}{P n_{STP} T_{STP}} = (22.4 \text{ L}) \left(\frac{1 \text{ atm}}{0.5 \text{ atm}} \right) \left(\frac{3 \text{ mol}}{1 \text{ mol}} \right) \left(\frac{293.15 \text{ K}}{273.15 \text{ K}} \right)$$

$$= (22.4 \text{ L}) \left(\frac{3}{0.5} \right) \left(\frac{293.15 \text{ K}}{273.15 \text{ K}} \right) \approx (22 \text{ L})(6)(1.1)$$

$$V = 145 \text{ L}$$

(actual volume = 144.4 L)

Density

In addition to standard calculations to determine the pressure, volume, or temperature of a gas, the ideal gas law may also be used to determine the **density** and **molar mass** of a gas. Density is defined as the mass per unit volume (m/V) of a substance and, for gases, is usually expressed in units of g/L. By rearrangement, the ideal gas equation can be used to calculate the density of a gas.

$$PV = nRT$$

where:

$$n = \frac{m}{MM} \frac{\text{(mass in g)}}{\text{(molar mass)}}$$

therefore:

$$PV = \frac{m}{MM} RT$$

and:

$$\frac{P(MM)}{RT} = \frac{m}{V} = d$$

Another way to find the density of a gas is to start with the volume of a mole of gas at STP, 22.4 L, calculate the effect of pressure and temperature on the volume, and finally calculate the density by dividing the mass by the new volume.

Example: What is the density of HCl gas at 2 atm and 45°C? (the molar mass of H is 1 g/mol and Cl is 35.5 g/mol)

Solution: At STP, a mole of gas occupies 22.4 liters. Since the increase in pressure to 2 atm decreases volume, 22.4 L must be multiplied by $\left(\frac{1\,\text{atm}}{2\,\text{atm}}\right)$. Since the increase in temperature increases volume, the temperature factor will be $\left(\frac{318\,\text{K}}{273\,\text{K}}\right)$. Given the molar mass information in the question, the mass of 1 mol of HCl is 36.5 g. Plugging that into the ideal gas law comparing different conditions gives the following:

$$V = \frac{V_{STP} P_{STP}\, nT}{Pn_{STP} T_{STP}} = (22.4\,\text{L})\left(\frac{1\,\text{atm}}{2\,\text{atm}}\right)\left(\frac{1\,\text{mol}}{1\,\text{mol}}\right)\left(\frac{318\,\text{K}}{273\,\text{K}}\right) = (22\,\text{L})\left(\frac{1}{2}\right)(1.2) = 13\,\text{L}$$

$$d = \left(\frac{36.5\,\text{g}}{13\,\text{L}}\right) = 2.8\,\text{g/L} \quad \text{(actual value is 2.77 g/L)}$$

Molar mass

Sometimes the identity of a gas is unknown, and the molar mass must be determined to identify it. Using the concept of density, the molar mass of a gas can be determined experimentally using the ideal gas law.

Example: What is the molar mass of an 8 g sample of gas that occupies 2 L at a temperature of 15°C and a pressure of 1.5 atm?

Solution: The mass of the gas (8 g) and therefore the moles of gas are constant regardless of the volume, temperature, or pressure. To find the molar mass (g/mol), calculate how many moles (mol) of gas are present in the 2 L sample at 15°C and 1.5 atm:

$$\frac{PV}{P_{STP}V_{STP}} = \frac{nT}{n_{STP}T_{STP}}$$

$$n = n_{STP}\frac{PVT_{STP}}{P_{STP}V_{STP}T} = (1 \text{ mol})\left(\frac{1.5 \text{ atm}}{1 \text{ atm}}\right)\left(\frac{2 \text{ L}}{22.4 \text{ L}}\right)\left(\frac{273.15 \text{ K}}{288.15 \text{ K}}\right)$$

$$= \left(\frac{3}{22.4}\right)\left(\frac{273.15 \text{ K}}{288.15 \text{ K}}\right) \approx \left(\frac{6}{45}\right)(0.95)$$

$$n = \frac{6}{45} = \frac{2}{15} \text{ mol}$$

Therefore, the molar mass of the unknown substance is:

$$MM = \left(\frac{m}{n}\right) = \left(\frac{8}{2/15}\right) = \frac{8 \times 15}{2} = 4 \times 15$$

$$MM = 60 \text{ g/mol}$$

(actual value = 63.1 g/mol)

REAL GASES

In general, the ideal gas law is a good approximation of the behavior of real gases, but all real gases deviate from ideal gas behavior to some extent, particularly when the gas atoms or molecules are forced into close proximity under high pressure and at low temperature so that molecular volume and intermolecular attractions become significant.

Deviations Due to Pressure

As the pressure of a gas increases, the particles are pushed closer and closer together. As the condensation pressure for a given temperature is approached, intermolecular attraction forces become more and more significant until the gas condenses into the liquid state (see Gas-Liquid Equilibrium in Chapter 35).

At moderately high pressure (a few hundred atm) the volume of a gas is less than would be predicted by the ideal gas law; this is due to intermolecular attraction. At extremely high pressure the size of the particles becomes relatively large compared to the distance between them, and this causes the gas to take up a larger volume than would be predicted by the ideal gas law.

Deviations Due to Temperature

As the temperature of a gas is decreased, the average velocity of the gas molecules decreases, and the attractive intermolecular forces become increasingly significant. As the condensation temperature (which is the same as the boiling point) is approached for a given pressure, intermolecular attractions eventually cause the gas to condense to a liquid state, and the increasing intermolecular attractions cause the gas to have a smaller volume than would be predicted by the ideal gas law. The closer the temperature of a gas is to its boiling point, the less ideal is its behavior.

DALTON'S LAW OF PARTIAL PRESSURES

When two or more gases are found in one vessel without chemical interaction, each gas will behave independently of the other(s). Therefore, the pressure exerted by each gas in the mixture will be equal to the pressure that gas would exert if it were the only one in the container. The pressure exerted by each individual gas is called the **partial pressure** of that gas. In 1801, John Dalton derived an expression, now known as Dalton's law of partial pressures, which states that the total pressure of a gaseous mixture is equal to the sum of the partial pressures of the individual components. The equation is:

$$P_T = P_A + P_B + P_C + \cdots$$

The partial pressure of a gas is related to its mole fraction and can be determined using the following equations:

$$P_A = P_T X_A$$

$$X_A = \frac{n_A \text{ (moles of A)}}{n_T \text{ (total moles)}}$$

Example: A vessel contains 0.75 mol of nitrogen, 0.20 mol of hydrogen, and 0.05 mol of fluorine at a total pressure of 2.5 atm. What is the partial pressure of each gas?

Solution: First, calculate the mole fraction of each gas.

$$X_{N_2} = \frac{0.75 \text{ mol}}{1.0 \text{ mol}} = 0.75 \qquad X_{H_2} = \frac{0.20 \text{ mol}}{1.0 \text{ mol}} = 0.20 \qquad X_{F_2} = \frac{0.05 \text{ mol}}{1.0 \text{ mol}} = 0.05$$

Then, calculate the partial pressures.

$$P_A = X_A P_T$$

$$P_{N_2} = (0.75)(2.5 \text{ atm}) \qquad P_{H_2} = (0.20)(2.5 \text{ atm}) \qquad P_{F_2} = (0.05)(2.5 \text{ atm})$$

$$= 1.875 \text{ atm} \qquad\qquad = 0.5 \text{ atm} \qquad\qquad = 0.125 \text{ atm}$$

KINETIC MOLECULAR THEORY OF GASES

As indicated by the gas laws, all gases show similar physical characteristics and behavior. A theoretical model to explain the behavior of gases was developed during the second half of the 19th century. The combined efforts of Boltzmann, Maxwell, and others led to a simple explanation of gaseous molecular behavior based on the motion of individual molecules. This model is called the kinetic molecular theory of gases. Like the gas laws, this theory was developed in reference to ideal gases, but it can be applied with reasonable accuracy to real gases as well.

Assumptions of the Kinetic Molecular Theory

- Gases are made up of particles whose volumes are negligible compared to the container volume.
- Gas atoms or molecules are inert and exhibit no intermolecular attractions or repulsions.

- Gas particles are in continuous, random motion, undergoing collisions with other particles and the container walls.

- Collisions between any two gas particles are elastic, meaning that there is no overall gain or loss of energy.

- The average kinetic energy of gas particles is proportional to the absolute temperature of the gas and is the same for all gases at a given temperature.

Applications of the Kinetic Molecular Theory of Gases

Average molecular speeds

According to the kinetic molecular theory of gases, the average kinetic energy (and therefore average velocity) of a gas particle is proportional to the absolute temperature of the gas:

$$KE = \frac{1}{2}mv^2 = \frac{3}{2}kT$$

where k is the Boltzmann constant. However, because of the large number of rapidly and randomly moving gas particles, the speed of an individual gas molecule is nearly impossible to define. Instead, it is the average speed of all the gas particles that can be related exactly to the temperature. Some particles will be moving at higher speeds and some at lower speeds.

A **Maxwell-Boltzmann distribution curve** shows the distribution of speeds of gas particles at a given temperature. The curve below shows a distribution curve of molecular speeds at two temperatures, T_1 and T_2, where $T_2 > T_1$. Notice that the bell-shaped curve flattens and shifts to the right as the temperature increases, indicating that, at higher temperatures, more molecules are moving at high speeds.

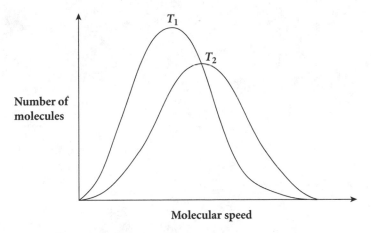

Figure 36.3

Graham's law of diffusion and effusion

Diffusion of gases can provide a demonstration of random motion when the molecules of these gases mix with one another by virtue of their individual kinetic properties. Diffusion occurs when gas molecules move through a mixture. Diffusion accounts for the fact that an open bottle of perfume can quickly be smelled across a room. The kinetic molecular theory of gases predicts that heavier gas molecules diffuse more slowly than lighter ones because of their differing average speeds. In 1832,

Thomas Graham showed mathematically that, under isothermal and isobaric conditions, the rates at which two gases diffuse are inversely proportional to the square root of their molar masses. Thus:

$$\frac{r_1}{r_2} = \left(\frac{MM_2}{MM_1}\right)^{\frac{1}{2}} = \sqrt{\frac{MM_2}{MM_1}}$$

where r_1 and MM_1 represent the diffusion rate and molar mass of gas 1, respectively, and r_2 and MM_2 represent the diffusion rate and molar mass of gas 2.

Effusion is the flow of gas particles under pressure from one compartment to another through a small opening. Graham used the kinetic molecular theory of gases to show that for two gases at the same temperature, the rates of effusion are proportional to the average speeds. He then expressed the rates of effusion in terms of molar mass and found that the relationship is the same as that for diffusion.

REVIEW PROBLEMS

1. Boyle's law can be used for which of the following?

    (A) Predicting the expected volumes of two party balloons

    (B) Predicting the relative pressures inside a hot air balloon

    (C) Predicting the change in volume of an inflatable toy from summer to winter

    (D) Predicting the change in volume of a party balloon inside a bell jar as a vacuum is being drawn

2. The word *kinetic* appears in the kinetic molecular theory of gases because

    (A) the properties of a gas are dependent primarily on the motion of its component particles.

    (B) gases only possess kinetic energy in closed systems.

    (C) gases possess more kinetic than potential energy.

    (D) collisions in real gases do not dissipate kinetic energy.

3. A sample of argon occupies 50 L at standard temperature. Assuming constant pressure, what volume will the gas occupy if the temperature is doubled?

    (A) 25 L

    (B) 50 L

    (C) 100 L

    (D) 200 L

4. What is the molecular weight of an unknown gas if 2.5 g of it occupies 2 L at 630 torr and a temperature of 600 K?

5. Explain the conditions that define an ideal gas.

6. If a 360 mL sample of helium contains 0.25 mol of the gas, how many molecules of chlorine gas would occupy the same volume at the same temperature and pressure?

    (A) 1.51×10^{23}

    (B) 3.01×10^{23}

    (C) 6.022×10^{23}

    (D) 1.2×10^{24}

7. In the kinetic molecular theory of gases, the speed of molecules is most often discussed in terms of the average speed. Which of the following statements concerning average speeds is true?

    (A) Most of the molecules are moving faster than the average speed, but a few outliers skew the average.

    (B) The average speed is independent of pressure and volume in a closed system.

    (C) When the temperature increases, more of the molecules will move at the new average speed.

    (D) When the temperature increases, fewer molecules will move at the new average speed.

8. What is the density of a gas at 76.0 torr and 37.0°C (MM = 25.0 g/mol)?

    (A) 0.098 g/L
    (B) 0.800 g/L
    (C) 22.4 g/L
    (D) 75.0 g/L

9. The following reaction represents the production of hydrogen chloride gas:

$$H_2 + Cl_2 \rightarrow 2\ HCl$$

    How many grams of chlorine gas are needed to produce 3 L of HCl gas at a pressure of 2 atm and a temperature of 19°C?

10. Dalton's law of partial pressures says that the total pressure of all the gases in a system

    (A) is less than the sum of the partial pressures of the gases.
    (B) is more than the sum of the partial pressures of the gases.
    (C) is equal to the sum of the partial pressures of the gases.
    (D) is not related to the partial pressures of the gases.

11. A student performing an experiment has a bulb containing 14 g of N_2, 64 g of O_2, 8 g of He, and 35 g of Cl_2 at a total pressure of 380 torr. What are the partial pressures of each gas?

12. A 1.74 g sample of gas is found to occupy 1 L at 10°C and 2 atm. What is the molar mass of the gas?

13. All of the following statements underlie the kinetic molecular theory of gases EXCEPT:

    (A) Gas molecules have no intermolecular forces.
    (B) Gas particles are in random motion.
    (C) The collisions between gas particles are elastic.
    (D) The average kinetic energy is directly proportional to the number of moles present of a gas.

14. What will be the final pressure of a gas that expands from 1 L at 10°C to 10 L at 100°C if the original pressure was 3 atm?

15. In the reaction $N_2 + 2\ O_2 \rightarrow 2\ NO_2$, what volume of NO_2 is produced from 7 g of nitrogen gas at 27°C and 0.9 atm?

SOLUTIONS TO REVIEW PROBLEMS

1. **D** Boyle's law states that, when a gas is held at constant temperature, its pressure and volume are inversely proportional. This means that, as the pressure increases, the volume decreases, and vice versa. Of the answer choices, the only one that involves both pressure and volume—in addition to a controlled variation of one of the variables—is (D). When a balloon is placed in a bell jar, the volume of the balloon will increase as a vacuum is being drawn in the jar. Boyle's law can be used to predict this behavior.

2. **A** In developing the kinetic molecular theory of gases, it was found that the properties of a gas sample, such as pressure, volume, and temperature, can be explained in terms of the motion of the individual gas molecules. Because *kinetic* is defined as "relating to motion," this theory of gases was called the kinetic molecular theory.

3. **C** This question is an application of Charles's law, which states that, at constant pressure, the volume and temperature of a gas will vary in direct proportion to each other. If a 50 L volume of gas is heated from standard temperature, which is 273 K, to two times standard temperature, 546 K, the volume will double as well. Therefore, the volume of the gas will increase from 50 L to 100 L. The answer can also be calculated using proportions.

$$\frac{V_1}{V_2} = \frac{T_1}{T_2}$$

$$\frac{50\,\text{L}}{x} = \frac{273\,\text{K}}{546\,\text{K}}$$

$$x = (2)(50\,\text{L})$$

$$x = 100\,\text{L}$$

4. **74.1 g/mol**
    The molecular weight of a gas is the number of grams that occupy 22.4 L at STP. At 630 torr and 600 K, the density of this gas is 2.5 g per 2 L. First, find the volume at STP:

$$V = (2\,\text{L})\left(\frac{630\,\text{torr}}{760\,\text{torr}}\right)\left(\frac{273\,\text{K}}{600\,\text{K}}\right) = 0.754\,\text{L}$$

Next, find the density at STP:

$$d = \frac{2.5\,\text{g}}{0.754\,\text{L}} = \frac{3.31\,\text{g}}{\text{L}}$$

Finally, find the gram molecular weight of 22.4 L of gas at STP:

$$MM = d\,(V \text{ for 1 mol gas at STP}) = (3.31\,\text{g/L})(22.4\,\text{L/mol}) = 74.1\,\text{g/mol}$$

5. The conditions that define an ideal gas are low pressure and high temperature. Under these conditions, the gas molecules are assumed to have no intermolecular forces and to occupy no volume. Therefore, it is possible to predict their behavior.

6. **A** This question is an application of Avogadro's principle, which states that, at a constant temperature and pressure, all gases will have the same number of moles in the same

volume. This is true regardless of the identity of the gas. Thus, to answer the question, the number of particles in 0.25 mol of helium must be calculated; that value will represent the number of molecules of chlorine gas in the same volume. The number of helium atoms is $(0.25 \text{ mol}) (6.022 \times 10^{23} \text{ atoms/mol}) = 1.51 \times 10^{23}$ atoms. Thus, (D) is correct.

7. **D** The average speed of a gas is defined as the mathematical average of all the speeds of the gas particles in a sample. To answer this question, you must understand the Maxwell-Boltzmann distribution curve, which shows the distribution of speeds of all the gas particles in a sample at a given temperature. The distribution curve is a bell-shaped curve that flattens and shifts to the right as the temperature increases. The flattening of the curve means that gas particles within the sample are traveling at a greater range of speeds. As a result, a smaller proportion of the molecules will move at exactly the new average speed.

8. **A** A gas weighing 25 g/mol will have a density of 25 g per 22.4 L at STP. The density at 76 torr and 37°C is found by calculating the change in volume of a mole of gas under these conditions:

$$\frac{P_1 V_1}{T_1} = \frac{P_2 V_2}{T_2}$$

$$V_2 = \frac{P_1 V_1 T_2}{T_1 P_2}$$

$$V_2 = \frac{(760 \text{ torr})(22.4 \text{ L})(310 \text{ K})}{(273 \text{ K})(76 \text{ torr})} = 254 \text{ L/mol}$$

$$d = \frac{25 \text{ g/mol}}{254 \text{ L/mol}} = 0.098 \text{ g/L}$$

9. **8.88 g**

First, let's find out how many moles of HCl would occupy 3 L at the pressure and temperature given.

$$n = \frac{(2 \text{ atm})(3 \text{ L})}{(0.0821 \text{ Latm/molK})(293 \text{ K})} = 0.25 \text{ mol}$$

Because 2 mol of HCl are produced from each mol of Cl_2, 0.25 mol HCl would be produced from 0.125 mol of Cl_2. The molecular weight of Cl_2 is 71 g/mol, so the answer is $(71 \text{ g } Cl_2/\text{mol}) (0.125 \text{ mol}) = 8.88 \text{ g } Cl_2$.

10. **C** Discussed in the section on Dalton's law of partial pressures in this chapter.

11. **N_2: 38 torr, O_2: 152 torr, He: 152 torr, Cl_2: 38 torr**

According to Dalton's law of partial pressures, the sum of the partial pressures of the gases in a mixture is equal to the total pressure of the mixture. Therefore, the partial pressures of nitrogen, oxygen, helium, and chlorine will add up to 380 torr. The partial pressure of a gas is calculated as follows:

$$P_p = X P_T$$

where X is the mole fraction of the gas. Thus, the mole fractions of each of the gases must be determined.

$$X = \frac{n}{n_T}$$

$$X_{N_2} = \frac{0.5 \text{ mol}}{5 \text{ mol}} = 0.1$$

$$X_{O_2} = \frac{2 \text{ mol}}{5 \text{ mol}} = 0.4$$

$$X_{He} = \frac{2 \text{ mol}}{5 \text{ mol}} = 0.4$$

$$X_{Cl_2} = \frac{0.5 \text{ mol}}{5 \text{ mol}} = 0.1$$

Now the partial pressures may be calculated.

$P_{N_2} = (380 \text{ torr})(0.1) = 38 \text{ torr}$

$P_{O_2} = (380 \text{ torr})(0.4) = 152 \text{ torr}$

$P_{He} = (380 \text{ torr})(0.4) = 152 \text{ torr}$

$P_{Cl_2} = (380 \text{ torr})(0.1) = 38 \text{ torr}$

12. **20.2 g/mol**

Convert the density given to the density at STP.

$$(1 \text{ L})\left(\frac{273 \text{ K}}{283 \text{ K}}\right)\left(\frac{2 \text{ atm}}{1 \text{ atm}}\right) = 1.93 \text{ L at STP}$$

$$\frac{1.74 \text{ g}}{1.93 \text{ L}} = 0.902 \text{ g/L at STP}$$

Now find the molar mass by multiplying by 22.4.

$MM = (0.902 \text{ g/L})(22.4 \text{ L/mol}) = 20.2 \text{ g/mol}$

13. **D** Kinetic energy is proportional to temperature, not number of moles. In an isolated system, increasing the number of moles of a gas while maintaining constant temperature and pressure will cause a decrease in temperature and therefore kinetic energy, indicating an inverse relationship.

14. **0.4 atm**

This question is different from the previous ones in that the new volume is given and you are looking for the final pressure. Rearranging the equation

$$\frac{P_1 V_1}{T_1} = \frac{P_2 V_2}{T_2}$$

gives

$$P_2 = \frac{P_1 V_1 T_2}{T_1 V_2}$$

$$P_2 = \frac{(3 \text{ atm})(1 \text{ L})(373 \text{ K})}{(283 \text{ K})(10 \text{ L})}$$

$$P_2 = 0.4 \text{ atm}$$

15.   **13.7 L**

$$\frac{7 \text{ g N}_2}{28 \text{ g N}_2/\text{mol}} = 0.25 \text{ mol N}_2$$

From the balanced reaction equation, 2 mol of NO_2 are produced from each mol of N_2, so 0.50 mol of NO_2 will be produced from 0.25 mol of N_2. Therefore, the volume at STP will be (0.5 mol NO_2) (22.4 L/mol at STP) = 11.2 L NO_2.

Now find the volume under the conditions given.

$$V = (11.2 \text{ L})\left(\frac{1 \text{ atm}}{0.9 \text{ atm}}\right)\left(\frac{300 \text{ K}}{273 \text{ K}}\right) = 13.7 \text{ L}$$

CHAPTER THIRTY-SEVEN

Acids and Bases

Many important reactions in chemical and biological systems involve **acids** and **bases** (defined below). Acids and bases cause color changes in certain compounds called **indicators**, which may be in solution or on paper. A particularly common indicator is **litmus paper**, which turns red in acidic solution and blue in basic solution. A more extensive discussion of the chemical properties of acids and bases is outlined below.

Acids	Bases
• Have a sour taste.	• Have a bitter taste.
• Aqueous solutions can conduct electricity.	• Aqueous solutions can conduct electricity.
• React with bases to form water and a salt.	• React with acids to form water and a salt.
• Nonoxidizing acids react with metals to produce hydrogen gas.	• Feel slippery to the touch.
• Cause color changes in plant dyes—turn litmus paper red.	• Cause color changes in plant dyes—turn litmus paper blue

Table 37.1

DEFINITIONS

Arrhenius Definition

The first definitions of acids and bases were formulated by Svante Arrhenius toward the end of the 19th century. Arrhenius defined an acid as a species that produces H^+ (a proton) in an aqueous solution and a base as a species that produces OH^- (a hydroxide ion) in an aqueous solution. These definitions, though useful, fail to describe acidic and basic behavior in nonaqueous media.

An example of an Arrhenius acid (HCl), base (NaOH), and acid-base reaction, respectively, are as follows:

$$HCl\ (aq) \rightarrow H^+(aq) + Cl^-(aq)$$

$$NaOH\ (aq) \rightarrow Na^+(aq) + OH^-(aq)$$

$$HCl\ (aq) + NaOH(aq) \rightarrow NaCl(aq) + H_2O(l)$$

Brønsted-Lowry Definition

A more general definition of acids and bases was proposed independently by Johannes Brønsted and Thomas Lowry in 1923. A Brønsted-Lowry acid is a species that donates protons, while a Brønsted-Lowry base is a species that accepts protons. For example, NH_3 (*g*) is a Brønsted-Lowry base because it can accept a proton. However, it cannot be called an Arrhenius base since it is not in an aqueous solution.

Brønsted-Lowry acids and bases always occur in pairs, called **conjugate acid-base pairs**. The two members of a conjugate pair are related by the transfer of a proton. For example, H_3O^+ is the conjugate acid of the base H_2O, and NO_2^- is the conjugate base of HNO_2:

$$H_3O^+ (aq) \rightarrow H_2O\ (aq) + H^+ (aq)$$
$$HNO_2 (aq) \rightarrow NO_2^- (aq) + H^+ (aq)$$

Lewis Definition

At approximately the same time as Brønsted and Lowry, Gilbert Lewis also proposed definitions of acids and bases. Lewis defined an acid as an electron-pair acceptor and a base as an electron-pair donor. Lewis's are the most inclusive definitions. Just as every Arrhenius acid is a Brønsted-Lowry acid, every Brønsted-Lowry acid is also a Lewis acid (and likewise for bases). However, the Lewis definition encompasses some species not included within the Brønsted-Lowry definition. For example, BCl_3 and $AlCl_3$ can each accept an electron pair and are therefore Lewis acids, despite their inability to donate protons.

NOMENCLATURE OF ARRHENIUS ACIDS

The name of an acid is related to the name of the parent anion (the anion that combines with H^+ to form the acid). Acids formed from anions whose names end in **-ide** have the prefix **hydro-** and the ending **-ic**.

F^-	Fluoride	HF	Hydrofluoric acid
Br^-	Bromide	HBr	Hydrobromic acid

Acids formed from oxyanions are called **oxyacids**. If the anion ends in **-ite** (less oxygen), then the acid will end with **-ous acid**. If the anion ends in **-ate** (more oxygen), then the acid will end with **-ic acid**. Prefixes in the names of the anions are retained. Some examples:

ClO^-	Hypochlorite	$HClO$	Hypochlorous acid
ClO_2^-	Chlorite	$HClO_2$	Chlorous acid
ClO_3^-	Chlorate	$HClO_3$	Chloric acid
ClO_4^-	Perchlorate	$HClO_4$	Perchloric acid
NO_2^-	Nitrite	HNO_2	Nitrous acid
NO_3^-	Nitrate	HNO_3	Nitric acid

PROPERTIES OF ACIDS AND BASES

Hydrogen Ion Equilibria (pH and pOH)

Hydrogen ion concentration, $[H^+]$, is generally measured as **pH**, where:

$$pH = -\log[H^+]$$

Likewise, hydroxide ion concentration, $[OH^-]$, is measured as **pOH** where:

$$pOH = -\log[OH^-]$$

In any aqueous solution, the H_2O solvent dissociates slightly in a process called autoionization:

$$H_2O\ (l) \leftrightarrows H^+\ (aq) + OH^-\ (aq)$$

This dissociation is an equilibrium reaction and is therefore described by a constant, K_w, the water dissociation constant:

$$K_w = [H^+][OH^-] = 10^{-14}$$

Rewriting this equation in logarithmic form gives:

$$pH + pOH = 14$$

In pure H_2O, $[H^+]$ is equal to $[OH^-]$ because, for every mole of H_2O that dissociates, one mole of H^+ and one mole of OH^- are formed. At STP, a solution with equal concentrations of H^+ and OH^- is neutral and has a pH of 7 ($-\log(10^{-7}) = 7$). A pH below 7 indicates a relative excess of H^+ ions and, therefore, an acidic solution; a pH above 7 indicates a relative excess of OH^- ions and, therefore, a basic solution.

Math note: estimating p-scale values

A useful skill for various problems involving acids and bases, as well as their corresponding buffer solutions, is the ability to quickly convert pH, pOH, pK_a, and pK_b into nonlogarithmic form and vice versa (pK_a and pK_b are acid and base dissociation constants, discussed below).

When the original value is a power of 10, the operation is relatively simple; changing the sign on the exponent gives the corresponding p-scale value directly. For example:

      If $[H^+] = 0.001$, or 10^{-3}, then $pH = 3$.

      If $K_b = 1.0 \times 10^{-7}$, then $pK_b = 7$.

More difficulty arises when the original value is not an exact power of 10; exact calculation would be excessively onerous without a calculator, but a simple method of approximation exists. If the nonlogarithmic value is written in proper scientific notation, it will look like $n \times 10^{-m}$, where n is a number between 1 and 10. The log of this product can be written as $\log(n \times 10^{-m}) = -m + \log n$, and the negative log is thus $m - \log n$. Now, since n is a number between 1 and 10, its logarithm is a fraction between 0 and 1; thus, $m - \log n$ is between $m - 1$ and m. Furthermore, the larger the n, the larger the log n, and therefore the closer the answer is to $m - 1$.

Example: If $K_a = 1.8 \times 10^{-5}$, then $pK_a = 5 - \log 1.8$. Because 1.8 is small, its log will be small, and the answer will be closer to 5 than to 4. (The actual answer is 4.74.)

Relative Strengths of Acids and Bases

The strength of an acid or base will depend largely upon its ability to ionize. The strength of an acid, for example, can be measured by the fraction of the molecules of that acid undergoing ionization. Subsequently, the acid strength can be expressed by the following equation:

$$\text{Percent ionization} = \frac{\text{ionized acid concentration at equilibrium}}{\text{inital concentration of acid}} \times 100\%$$

When an acid or base is strong (has more complete dissociation), its conjugate base or acid will be weak. The stronger the acid, the weaker the conjugate base. For incredibly strong acids (near complete dissociation), the conjugate base is so weak that it is practically inert. Within a series of weak acids, the stronger the acid, the weaker its conjugate base for all acids and bases included. For example, HF is a stronger acid than HCN; therefore, F^- is a weaker base than CN^-.

Strong Acids and Bases

Strong acids and bases are those that completely dissociate into their component ions in aqueous solution. For example, when NaOH is added to water, it dissociates completely:

$$NaOH(s) + \text{excess } H_2O(l) \rightarrow Na^+ (aq) + OH^- (aq)$$

Hence, in a 1 M solution of NaOH, complete dissociation gives 1 mole of OH^- ions per liter of solution.

$$pH = 14 - (-\log[OH^-]) = 14 + \log[1] = 14$$

Because NaOH is a strong base, virtually no undissociated NaOH remains. Note that the $[OH^-]$ contributed by the autoionization of H_2O is considered to be negligible in this case. In fact, the contribution of OH^- and H^+ ions from the dissociation of H_2O can always be neglected if the concentration of the acid or base is significantly greater than 10^{-7} M.

As a counterexample, consider the pH of a 1×10^{-8} M HCl solution. HCl is a strong acid and will dissociate completely, so the $[H^+] = 1 \times 10^{-8}$ M. At first glance, the pH of the solution might appear to be 8 because $-\log (1 \times 10^{-8}) = 8$. However, a pH of 8 is in the basic pH range, and an HCl solution should be acidic (pH < 7), not basic. The discrepancy arises from the fact that, at low HCl concentrations, H^+ from the dissociation of water contribute significantly to the total $[H^+]$.

The total concentration of H^+ can be calculated from:

$K_w = [H^+][OH^-]$

$1.0 \times 10^{-14} = [x + 1 \times 10^{-8}][x]$

(note the H^+ from water and HCl are added together in the left term due to the common ion effect).

Solving for x gives $x = 9.5 \times 10^{-8}$ M, so $[H^+]_{total} = [H^+ \text{ from HCl} + H^+ \text{ from water}] = (9.5 \times 10^{-8} + 1 \times 10^{-8})$ M $= 1.05 \times 10^{-7}$ M, and pH $= -\log (1.05 \times 10^{-7}) = 6.98$. The pH is slightly less than 7, as should be expected for a very dilute yet acidic solution.

Strong acids and bases commonly encountered on the PCAT include the following:

Acids	Bases
$HClO_4$ (perchloric acid)	NaOH (sodium hydroxide)
HNO_3 (nitric acid)	KOH (potassium hydroxide)
H_2SO_4 (sulfuric acid)	$Ca(OH)_2$ (calcium hydroxide)
HCl (hydrochloric acid)	other soluble hydroxides of Group IA and IIA metals

Table 37.2

Calculation of the pH and pOH of strong acids and bases assumes complete dissociation of the acid or base in solution: $[H^+]$ = normality of strong acid, and $[OH^-]$ = normality of strong base.

Weak Acids and Bases

Weak acids and bases are those that only partially dissociate in aqueous solution. A weak, monoprotic acid (HA) in aqueous solution will achieve the following equilibrium after dissociation (H_3O^+ is equivalent to H^+ in aqueous solution):

$$HA\ (aq) + H_2O\ (l) \rightleftharpoons H_3O^+\ (aq) + A^-\ (aq)$$

The **acid dissociation constant, K_a,** is a specific type of K_{eq} (see Chapter 34, Equilibrium) that measures the degree to which an acid dissociates by showing the ratio of concentrations of the products (the conjugate base and the H^+ donated) to that of the reactant (the original acid).

$$K_a = \frac{[H_3O^+][A^-]}{[HA]}$$

The weaker the acid, the smaller the K_a. Note that K_a does not contain an expression for the pure liquid, water, since pure liquids (and pure solids) are not included in any K_{eq} calculations.

A weak monovalent base (BOH) undergoes dissociation to give B^+ and OH^-. The **base dissociation constant, K_b,** is a measure of the degree to which a base dissociates. The weaker the base, the smaller its K_b. For a monovalent base, K_b is defined as follows:

$$K_b = \frac{[B^+][OH^-]}{[BOH]}$$

A **conjugate acid** is defined as the acid formed when a base gains a proton. Similarly, a **conjugate base** is formed when an acid loses a proton. For example, in the HCO_3^-/CO_3^{2-} conjugate acid/base pair, CO_3^{2-} is the conjugate base, and HCO_3^- is the conjugate acid:

$$HCO_3^-\ (aq) \rightleftharpoons H^+\ (aq) + CO_3^{2-}\ (aq)$$

To find the K_a of the conjugate acid HCO_3^-, the reaction with water must be considered:

$$HCO_3^- \ (aq) + H_2O \ (l) \leftrightharpoons H_3O^+ \ (aq) + CO_3^{2-} \ (aq)$$

Likewise, for the K_b of CO_3^{2-}:

$$CO_3^{2-} \ (aq) + H_2O \ (l) \leftrightharpoons HCO_3^- \ (aq) + OH^- \ (aq)$$

The equilibrium constants for these reactions are as follows:

$$K_a = \frac{[H^+][CO_3^{2-}]}{[HCO_3^-]} \quad \text{and} \quad K_b = \frac{[HCO_3^-][OH^-]}{[CO_3^{2-}]}$$

Adding the two reactions shows that the net reaction is simply the dissociation of water:

$$HCO_3^- \ (aq) + H_2O \ (l) \leftrightharpoons H_3O^+ \ (aq) + CO_3^{2-} \ (aq)$$
$$+ \quad CO_3^{2-} \ (aq) + H_2O \ (l) \leftrightharpoons HCO_3^- \ (aq) + OH^- \ (aq)$$
$$\overline{2 \ H_2O \ (l) \leftrightharpoons H_3O^+ \ (aq) + OH^- \ (aq)}$$

The equilibrium constant for this net reaction is $K_w = [H^+][OH^-]$, which is the product of K_a and K_b. Thus, if the **dissociation constant** either for an acid or for its conjugate base is known, then the dissociation constant for the other can be determined using the equation:

$$K_a \times K_b = K_w = 1 \times 10^{-14}$$

Thus, K_a and K_b are inversely related. In other words, the larger the K_a (the stronger the acid), the smaller the conjugate's K_b (the weaker the base), and vice versa. For strong acids and bases, the K_as and K_bs are significantly larger than 1. For example, the K_a of HCl is 1.3×10^6. Because the K_a is large, the K_b is expected to be small. Keeping in mind that $K_a \times K_b = 1 \times 10^{-14}$, $K_b = 8.3 \times 10^{-21}$. As expected, the conjugate base (Cl^-) is weak; in fact, 8.3×10^{-21} is such a very small number that Cl^- can, practically speaking, be considered inert.

Applications of K_a and K_b

To calculate the concentration of H^+ in a 2.0 M aqueous solution of acetic acid, CH_3COOH ($K_a = 1.8 \times 10^{-5}$), first write the equilibrium reaction:

$$CH_3COOH \ (aq) \leftrightharpoons H^+ \ (aq) + CH_3COO^- \ (aq)$$

Next, write the expression for the acid dissociation constant:

$$K_a = \frac{[H^+][CH_3COO^-]}{[CH_3COOH]} = 1.8 \times 10^{-5}$$

Because acetic acid is a weak acid, the concentration of CH_3COOH at equilibrium is equal to its initial concentration, 2.0 M, less the amount dissociated, x. Likewise $[H^+] = [CH_3COO^-] = x$, since each molecule of CH_3COOH dissociates into one H^+ ion and one CH_3COO^- ion. Thus, the equation can be rewritten as follows:

$$K_a = \frac{[x][x]}{[2.0 - x]} = 1.8 \times 10^{-5}$$

We can approximate that $2.0 - x \approx 2.0$ since acetic acid is a weak acid that only slightly dissociates in water, and x will be small. Multiplying or dividing by small numbers can have large effects, but adding or subtracting small numbers is not statistically significant. On the PCAT, the math can be made much simpler be ignoring x values that are added or subtracted from (comparably) large numbers:

$$K_a = \frac{[x][x]}{[2.0]}$$
$$1.8 \times 10^{-5} = \frac{x^2}{2}$$
$$3.6 \times 10^{-5} = x^2$$
$$x = 6 \times 10^{-3} M$$

The fact that x is so much less than the initial concentration of acetic acid (2.0 M) validates the approximation; otherwise, it would have been necessary to solve for x using the quadratic formula. (A rule of thumb is that the approximation is valid as long as x is less than 5 percent of the initial concentration.)

SALT FORMATION

Acids and bases may react with one another, forming a salt and (often, but not always) water in what is termed a **neutralization reaction**. For example:

$$HA + BOH \rightarrow BA + H_2O$$

The salt may precipitate out or remain ionized in solution depending on its solubility and the amount produced. Neutralization reactions generally go to completion. The reverse reaction, in which the salt ions react with water to give back the acid or base, is known as **hydrolysis**.

Four combinations of strong and weak acids and bases are possible:
1. strong acid + strong base: e.g., $HCl + NaOH \rightarrow NaCl + H_2O$
2. strong acid + weak base: e.g., $HCl + NH_3 \rightarrow NH_4Cl$
3. weak acid + strong base: e.g., $HClO + NaOH \rightarrow NaClO + H_2O$
4. weak acid + weak base: e.g., $HClO + NH_3 \leftrightarrows NH_4ClO$

The products of a reaction between equal concentrations of a strong acid and a strong base are a salt and water. The conjugate acids and bases (Na^+ and Cl^- from combination 1, above) are so very weak that they are practically inert and will not contribute to the pH of the solution. The only other remaining product is water, meaning the resulting solution is neutral (pH = 7).

The product of a reaction between a strong acid and a weak base is also a salt, but usually no water is formed since weak bases are usually not hydroxides. In this case, the cation of the salt is the conjugate acid of a weak base, which will not be inert and will contribute to the pH. Instead of a neutral salt and water (as in the strong acid and strong base reaction), an inert anion and a weak acid cation (Cl^- and NH4$^+$ from combination 2 above, respectively) are formed, meaning the solution will be slightly acidic (pH < 7).

Another way to consider this reaction is that the weak-acid cation will react with the water solvent, reforming the weak base. This reaction constitutes hydrolysis. Revisiting combination 2:

$$HCl\ (aq) + NH_3\ (aq) \leftrightarrows NH_4^+\ (aq) + Cl^-\ (aq) \qquad \text{Reaction I}$$
$$NH_4^+\ (aq) + H_2O\ (aq) \leftrightarrows NH_3\ (aq) + H_3O^+\ (aq) \qquad \text{Reaction II}$$

By increasing the amount of H_3O^+, the pH of the strong acid/weak base reaction product will be slightly acidic (pH < 7).

On the other hand, when a weak acid reacts with a strong base, the opposite occurs. The cation product is practically inert, and the anion product is a weak base (Na^+ and ClO^- from combination 3 above, respectively). The presence of the weak base anion will cause the water solvent to become slightly alkaline (pH > 7); the weak base anion (ClO^- in our example) will react with the H_2O solvent, which leaves OH^- to raise the pH.

The pH of a solution containing a weak acid and a weak base depends on the relative strengths of the reactants. For example, the acid HClO has a $K_a = 3.2 \times 10^{-8}$, and the base NH_3 has a $K_b = 1.8 \times 10^{-5}$. Thus, an aqueous solution of HClO and NH_3 is basic since the K_a for HClO is smaller than the K_b for NH_3, and therefore NH_3 is the stronger reactant.

POLYVALENCE AND NORMALITY

The relative acidity or basicity of an aqueous solution is determined by the relative concentrations of **acid** and **base equivalents**. An acid equivalent is equal to one mole of H^+ (or H_3O^+) ions; a base equivalent is equal to one mole of OH^- ions. Some acids and bases are polyvalent, that is, each mole of the acid or base liberates more than one acid or base equivalent. For example, the diprotic acid H_2SO_4 undergoes the following dissociation in water:

$$H_2SO_4\ (aq) \rightarrow H^+\ (aq) + HSO_4^-\ (aq)$$
$$HSO_4^-\ (aq) \leftrightarrows H^+\ (aq) + SO_4^{2-}\ (aq)$$

One mole of H_2SO_4 can thus produce two acid equivalents (two moles of H^+). The acidity or basicity of a solution depends upon the concentration of acidic or basic equivalents that can be liberated. The quantity of acidic or basic capacity is directly indicated by the solution's normality (N) where $N = \text{Molarity} \times \dfrac{\text{equivalents}}{\text{mol}}$ (see Chapter 31, Solutions). Because each mole of H_3PO_4 can liberate three moles (equivalents) of H^+, a 2 M H_3PO_4 solution would be 6 N (6 normal).

Another useful measurement is **equivalent weight**. The equivalent weight is calculated by taking the molecular weight and dividing by the number of equivalents per mole. For example, the gram molecular weight of H_2SO_4 is 98 g/mol. Because each mole liberates two acid equivalents, the gram equivalent weight of H_2SO_4 would be $\frac{98}{2} = 49$ g; that is, the dissociation of 49 g of H_2SO_4 would release one acid equivalent. Common polyvalent acids include H_2SO_4, H_3PO_4, and H_2CO_3.

AMPHOTERIC SPECIES

An amphoteric, or **amphiprotic,** species is one that can act either as an acid or a base, depending on its chemical environment. In the Brønsted–Lowry sense, an amphoteric species can either gain or lose a proton. Water is the most common example. When water reacts with a base, it behaves as an acid:

$$H_2O + B^- \leftrightarrows HB + OH^-$$

When water reacts with an acid, it behaves as a base:

$$HA + H_2O \leftrightarrows H_3O^+ + A^-$$

The partially dissociated conjugate base of a polyprotic acid is usually amphoteric (e.g., HSO_4^- can either gain an H^+ to form H_2SO_4 or lose an H^+ to form SO_4^{2-}). The hydroxides of certain metals (e.g., Al, Zn, Pb, and Cr) are also amphoteric. Furthermore, species that can act as either oxidizing or reducing agents (see Chapter 32, Reaction Types) are considered to be amphoteric as well, since by accepting or donating electron pairs, they act as Lewis acids or bases, respectively.

TITRATION AND BUFFERS

Titration is a procedure used to determine the molarity of an acid or base. This is accomplished by reacting a known volume of a solution of unknown concentration with a known volume of a solution of known concentration. When the number of acid equivalents equals the number of base equivalents added, or vice versa, the **equivalence point** is reached. It is important to emphasize that, while a strong acid/strong base titration will have an equivalence point at pH 7, the equivalence point need *not* always occur at pH 7. Also, when titrating polyprotic acids or bases, there are several equivalence points, as each acidic or basic species is titrated separately (see Polyprotic Acids and Bases later in this chapter).

The equivalence point in a titration is estimated in two common ways: either by plotting the pH (measured with a **pH meter**) of the solution as a function of added titrant on a graph or by watching for a color change of an added **indicator**. Indicators are weak organic acids or bases that have different colors in their undissociated and dissociated states. Indicators are used in low concentrations and therefore do not significantly alter the equivalence point. The point at which the indicator actually changes color is not the equivalence point but is called the **end point**; this point is not significant mathematically but rather is a practical way to ensure the reaction has gone to completion. If the titration is performed well, the volume difference (and therefore the error) between the end point and the equivalence point is small and may be corrected for or ignored.

Strong Acid and Strong Base

Consider the titration of 10 mL of a 0.1 N solution of HCl with a 0.1 N solution of NaOH. Plotting the pH of the reaction solution versus the quantity of NaOH added gives the curve shown in Figure 37.1. Because HCl is a strong acid and NaOH is a strong base, the equivalence point of the titration will be at pH 7, and the solution will be neutral.

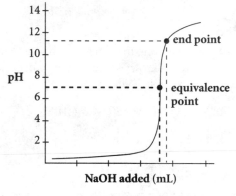

Figure 37.1

In the early part of the curve (when little base has been added), the acidic species predominates, so the addition of small amounts of base will not appreciably change either the [OH⁻] or the pH. Similarly, in the last part of the titration curve (when an excess of base has been added), the addition of small amounts of base will not change the [OH⁻] significantly, and the pH remains relatively constant. The addition of base most alters the concentrations of H^+ and OH^- near the equivalence point, and thus the pH changes most drastically in that region.

Weak Acid and Strong Base

Titration of a weak acid, HA, with a strong base produces the titration curve shown in Figure 37.2.

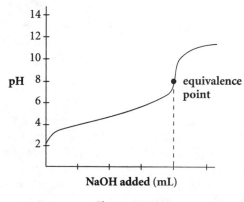

Figure 37.2

Comparing Figure 37.2 with Figure 37.1 shows that the initial pH of the weak acid solution is greater than the initial pH of the strong acid solution. The pH changes most significantly early on in the titration, and the equivalence point is in the basic range. Although the original weak acid and strong base are completely neutralized at the equivalence point (forming water with pH = 7), the side product of weak conjugate base from the original weak acid will be able to react with water in solution, consuming H⁺, thereby lowering [H⁺] and raising pH.

Buffers

A **buffer solution** consists of a mixture of a weak acid and its salt (which consists of its conjugate base and a cation) or a mixture of a weak base and its salt (which consists of its conjugate acid and an anion). Two examples of buffers are a solution of acetic acid (CH_3COOH) and its salt, sodium acetate (CH_3COONa), and a solution of ammonia (NH_3) and its salt, ammonium chloride (NH_4Cl). Buffer solutions have the useful property of resisting changes in pH when small amounts of acid or base are added.

Consider a buffer solution of acetic acid and sodium acetate:

$$CH_3COOH \leftrightarrows H^+ + CH_3COO^-$$

$$CH_3COONa \leftrightarrows Na^+ + CH_3COO^-$$

When a small amount of NaOH is added to the buffer, the OH⁻ ions from the NaOH react with the acetic acid in the buffer solution such that:

$$CH_3COOH + NaOH \leftrightarrows H_2O + CH_3COO^- + Na^+$$

Subsequently, the solution contains less acetic acid and more acetate ion. Instead of a strong base (OH⁻) in solution, there is now a weak base (CH_3COO^-). Though the strong base may have considerably changed the pH, the substitution by a weak base does not appreciably change pH. Likewise, when a small amount of HCl is added to the buffer, the acid will react with the acetate ion (CH_3COO^-):

$$CH_3COONa + HCl \leftrightarrows NaCl + CH_3COOH$$

Instead of the addition of a strong acid (HCl), there is now a weak acid present (CH_3COOH). Just as with the strong base, the pH shift will be quite small.

The **Henderson-Hasselbalch equation** is used to estimate the pH of a solution in the buffer region where the concentrations of the species and its conjugate are present in approximately equal concentrations. For a weak acid buffer solution:

$$pH = pK_a + \log \frac{[\text{conjugate base}]}{[\text{weak acid}]}$$

Note that when [conjugate base] = [weak acid] (in a titration, halfway to the equivalent point), the pH = pK_a because log 1 = 0. Likewise, for a weak base buffer solution:

$$pOH = pK_b + \log \frac{[\text{conjugate acid}]}{[\text{weak base}]}$$

pOH = pK_b when [conjugate acid] = [weak base].

Polyprotic Acids and Bases

The titration curve for a polyprotic acid or base looks different from that for a monoprotic acid or base. Figure 37.3 shows the titration of Na_2CO_3 with HCl in which the polyprotic acid H_2CO_3 is the ultimate product.

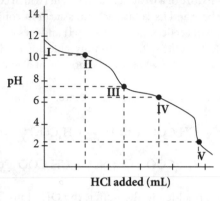

Figure 37.3

In the region between I and II, little acid has been added, and the predominant species is CO_3^{2-}. Point II represents the half-equivalence point where $[CO_3^{2-}]$ and $[HCO_3^-]$ are equal. Around this point the pH remains relatively constant at pH = 10.3; this is the first buffer region, and the pH corresponds to the pK_a of HCO_3^-.

In the region between II and III, HCO_3^- begins to predominate until point III, the first equivalence point, where all of the original CO_3^- has been consumed, leaving only HCO_3^-.

The same pattern occurs again as HCO_3^- reacts to form H_2CO_3. Point IV represents the second half-equivalence point (with a pH of 6.4 to correspond with the pK_a of H_2CO_3), and point V represents the second equivalence point where no original HCO_3^- remains, leaving only H_2CO_3.

REVIEW PROBLEMS

1. A certain aqueous solution has $[OH^-] = 6.2 \times 10^{-5}$ M.

    (A) Calculate $[H^+]$.
    (B) Calculate the pH of the solution.
    (C) Is the solution acidic or basic?

2. What is the ratio of $[H^+]$ of a solution of pH $= 4$ to the $[H^+]$ of a solution of pH $= 7$?

3. Write equations expressing what happens to each of the following bases in aqueous solutions:

    (A) LiOH
    (B) $Ba(OH)_2$
    (C) NH_3
    (D) NO_2^-

4. What volume of a 3 M solution of NaOH is required to titrate 0.05 L of a 4 M solution of HCl to the equivalence point?

5. If 10 mL of 1 M NaOH is titrated with 1 M HCl to a pH of 2, what volume of HCl was added?

6. Identify the conjugate acids and bases in the following equation:

    $$NH_3 + H_2O \leftrightharpoons NH_4^+ + OH^-$$

7. Identify each of the following as an Arrhenius acid or base, Brønsted-Lowry acid or base, or Lewis acid or base.

    (A) NaOH, in $NaOH \rightarrow Na^+ + OH^-$
    (B) HCl, in $HCl \rightarrow H^+ + Cl^-$
    (C) NH_3, in $NH_3 + H^+ \rightarrow NH_4^+$
    (D) NH_4^+, in $NH_4^+ \rightarrow NH_3 + H^+$
    (E) $(CH_3)_3N:$, in $(CH_3)_3N: + BF_3 \rightarrow (CH_3)_3N:BF_3$
    (F) BF_3 in the above equation

8. At equilibrium, a certain acid, HA, in solution yields $[HA] = 0.94$ M and $[A^-] = 0.060$ M.

    (A) Calculate K_a.
    (B) Is this acid stronger or weaker than sulfurous acid ($K_a = 1.7 \times 10^{-2}$)?
    (C) Calculate K_b.
    (D) Calculate pH.
    (E) Calculate the pK_a.

9. For each of the following pairs, choose that which describes the weaker acid:

    (A) $K_a = x$, $K_a = 3x$
    (B) $[H^+] = x$, $[H^+] = 3x$
    (C) $pK_a = x$, $pK_a = 3x$
    (D) pH $= x$, pH $= 3x$

10. For a certain acid HA, $K_b(A^-) = 2.22 \times 10^{-11}$. Calculate the pH of a 0.5 M solution of HA.

11. Which of the following sets of materials would make the best buffer solution?

(A) H_2O, 1 M NaOH, 1 M H_2SO_4

(B) H_2O, 1 M $HC_2H_3O_2$, 1 M $NaC_2H_3O_2$

(C) H_2O, 1 M $HC_2H_3O_2$, 6 M $NaC_2H_3O_2$

(D) H_2O, 1 M $HC_2H_3O_2$, 1 M NaOH

12. A certain buffer solution is 3 M in HF and 2 M in NaF. Calculate the pH of this buffer given that the K_a of HF = 7.0×10^{-4}.

13. Which of the following combinations would produce a buffer solution of pH = 4? (K_a HNO_2 = 4.5×10^{-4})

(A) 0.30 M HNO_2, 0.22 M $NaNO_2$

(B) 0.22 M HNO_2, 0.30 M $NaNO_2$

(C) 0.11 M HNO_2, 0.50 M $NaNO_2$

(D) 0.50 M HNO_2, 0.11 M $NaNO_2$

14. Write chemical equations describing the buffer activity that prevents drastic pH changes when (**A**) a strong acid and (**B**) a strong base is added.

SOLUTIONS TO REVIEW PROBLEMS

1. **A 1.6×10^{-10} M**

   Water is composed of hydronium and hydroxide ions, and the dissociation constant of water, K_w, is defined as $[H^+][OH^-] = 1.0 \times 10^{-14}$ M. If $[OH^-] = 6.2 \times 10^{-5}$, then:

   $$[H^+] = \frac{K_w}{[OH^-]} = \frac{1.0 \times 10^{-14}}{6.2 \times 10^{-5}} = 1.6 \times 10^{-10} \text{ M}.$$

   B 9.79

   The pH of a solution is a logarithmic measurement of $[H^+]$, which expresses the degree of acidity.

   pH is defined as $-\log[H^+]$. In this case, pH $= -\log(1.6 \times 10^{-10}) = 9.79$.

   C Basic

   A pH of 9.79 indicates a basic solution, as does any $[OH^-] > 1.0 \times 10^{-7}$ M.

2. **1,000:1**

   This problem can be solved by calculating the $[H^+]$ of the pH $= 4$ solution and the $[H^+]$ of the pH $= 7$ solution. Then divide the former by the latter: because pH $= -\log[H^+]$, $[H^+] =$ antilog $(-\text{pH})$. For pH $= 4$, antilog $(-4) = 1.0 \times 10^{-4}$. For pH $= 7$, antilog $(-7) = 1.0 \times 10^{-7}$. $1 \times 10^{-4}: 1 \times 10^{-7} = 1,000:1$. Alternately, we could subtract the pHs first, and then find the antilog: $7 - 4 = 3$ implies 10^3, or 1,000:1.

3. **A** $LiOH \rightarrow Li^+ + OH^-$
   B $Ba(OH)_2 \rightarrow Ba^{2+} + 2OH^-$
   C $NH_3 + H_2O \rightarrow NH_4^+ + OH^-$
   D $NO_2^- + H_2O \rightarrow HNO_2 + OH^-$

4. **0.067 L**

   At the equivalence point,

   $(\text{Normality})_{acid}(\text{Volume})_{acid} = (\text{Normality})_{base}(\text{Volume})_{base}$

   4 M HCl = 4 N HCl

   3 M NaOH = 3 N NaOH

   Plugging into the formula,

   $(4)(0.05) = (3)(V_B)$

   $V_B = 0.067$ L

5. **10.2 mL**

   First, add enough HCl to neutralize the solution. Because both the acid and the base are 1 M, 10 mL of HCl will neutralize 10 mL of NaOH, from $N_A V_A = N_B V_B$. This produces 20 mL of 0.5 M NaCl solution.

   Next calculate how much more HCl must be added to produce a $[H^+]$ of 1×10^{-2}. Let x be the amount of HCl to be added. The total volume of the solution will be $(20 + x)$ mL. Since this is now a dilution problem, the amount of HCl to be added can be found by using the formula:

$$M_1V_1 = M_2V_2$$

$$(1 \text{ M})(x \text{ mL}) = (0.01 \text{ M})[(20 + x)\text{mL}]$$

When this equation is solved, x is found to have an approximate value of 0.2 mL, so a total of 10.2 mL of HCl was added to the original NaOH solution.

6. NH_4^+ is the conjugate acid of the weak base, NH_3; OH^- is the conjugate base of the weak acid, H_2O.

The reaction in question is:

$$NH_3 + H_2O \rightleftharpoons NH_4^+ + OH^-$$

According to the Brønsted-Lowry theory of acids and bases, an acid releases a proton, whereas a base accepts a proton. In the case of weak acids and bases, an equilibrium is established whereby a weak acid, in this case H_2O, dissociates partially, donating a proton to a weak base, which is NH_3. The weak acid, H_2O, loses a proton and becomes a relatively stronger conjugate base, OH^-. This is one conjugate acid-base pair (H_2O, OH^-). Meanwhile, the weak base, NH_3, picks up a proton to become a relatively stronger conjugate acid, NH_4^+. This is the second conjugate acid-base pair (NH_4^+, NH_3).

7. **A** NaOH is an Arrhenius base.

   B HCl is an Arrhenius acid and a Brønsted-Lowry acid.

   C NH_3 is a Brønsted-Lowry base and a Lewis base.

   D NH_4^+ is an Arrhenius acid and a Brønsted-Lowry acid.

   E $(CH_3)_3N$: acts only as a Lewis base.

   F BF_3 acts only as a Lewis acid.

8. **A** 3.8×10^{-3}

   K_a is the equilibrium constant for an acid, also called the dissociation constant for the particular equilibrium state that is achieved by the dissociation of an acid. We are told that at equilibrium [HA] is 0.94 M, whereas [A$^-$] is 0.060 M. The dissociation of HA can be written as follows:

   $$HA \rightarrow H^+ + A^-$$

   The molar ratio of A$^-$ to H$^+$ is 1:1, so [H$^+$] must also be 0.060 M at equilibrium. It follows, then, that:

   $$K_a = \frac{[A^-][H^+]}{[HA]} = \frac{(0.060)(0.060)}{0.94} = 3.8 \times 10^{-3}$$

   B Weaker

   K_a is a measure of the strength of an acid. An acid with a high K_a is a strong acid because its equilibrium position lies farther to the right (more product increases the numerator of the equilibrium expression and makes K_a larger), meaning that dissociation is more complete. Greater dissociation means a stronger acid. The K_a of sulfurous acid is 1.7×10^{-2} and the K_a of HA is 3.8×10^{-3}. The K_a of HA is less than that of sulfurous acid; therefore, HA is a weaker acid.

   C 2.6×10^{-12}

   Just as K_a is the dissociation constant for an acid, K_b is the dissociation constant of a base. Whereas K_a measures the degree to which H$^+$ is liberated, K_b measures the degree to which

OH^- is liberated. Because H^+ and OH^- are related by $K_w = 1.0 \times 10^{-14}$, K_b can be easily calculated. In this case,

$$K_b = \frac{1.0 \times 10^{-14}}{3.8 \times 10^{-3}} = 2.6 \times 10^{-12}$$

D 1.22

$$pH = -\log [H^+] = -\log (0.060) = 1.22$$

E 2.42

$$pK_a = -\log K_a = -\log (3.8 \times 10^{-3}) = 2.42$$

9. A $K_a = x$

K_a is a measure of the dissociation of an acid and, therefore, the strength of an acid. A higher K_a indicates a stronger acid; a lower K_a indicates a weaker acid. x is one-third the value of $3x$ and, therefore, a weaker acid.

B $[H^+] = x$

$[H^+]$ is a direct measure of the strength of an acid. The greater the concentration of H^+ in solution, the stronger the acid. An acid that liberates x moles of H^+ per liter is weaker, therefore, than an acid that liberates $3x$ moles of H^+ per liter.

C $pK_a = 3x$

$pK_a = -\log K_a$; therefore, a pK_a of $3x$ corresponds to a K_a lower in value than that of a pK_a of x. A lower K_a means a weaker acid, and a lower pK_a means a stronger acid. $3x$ is greater than x, so the acid whose pK_a is $3x$ is weaker than the acid whose pK_a is x.

D $pH = 3x$

The acid with a pH of $3x$ is the weaker acid, using the same reasoning as for part (C).

10. 1.82

If $K_b = 2.22 \times 10^{-11}$, then

$$K_a = \frac{K_w}{K_b} = \frac{1.0 \times 10^{-14}}{2.22 \times 10^{-11}}$$

$$K_a = 4.5 \times 10^{-4}$$

If HA dissociates according to the following expression,

$HA \rightleftharpoons H^+ + A^-$,

then the equilibrium expression for this dissociation is:

$$K_a = \frac{[H^+][A^-]}{[HA]}$$

We can let $[H^+] = x$ at equilibrium and, since $[H^+]:[A^-] = 1:1$, $[A^-] = x$.

If the original $[HA]$ was 0.5 M, and x mol/L are dissociated, then at equilibrium, $[HA] = 0.5 - x$.

Thus the equilibrium expression becomes:

$$4.5 \times 10^{-4} = \frac{[x][x]}{(0.5 - x)}$$

We can approximate that $0.5 - x \approx 0.5$ since HA has a small K_a, which indicates it is a weak acid.

$$4.5 \times 10^{-4} \approx \frac{x^2}{0.5}$$

$$x^2 = 2.25 \times 10^{-4}$$

$$x = 0.015 = [H^+]$$

$$pH = -\log [H^+] = -\log [0.015] = 1.82$$

11. **B** A buffer solution is prepared from a weak acid and its conjugate base, preferably in near-equal quantities. Choices (A) and (D) are incorrect because they do not show conjugate acid/base pairs. (C) is incorrect because it shows a weak acid and its conjugate base, where the concentrations of the acid and the base are quite different. Thus, the best buffer solution would be that prepared from (B), which shows a conjugate acid/base pair, both present in 1 M concentrations.

12. **2.98**

$$K_a = \frac{[H^+][F^-]}{[HF]}$$

$$7 \times 10^{-4} = \frac{[H^+](2)}{3}$$

$$[H^+] = 1.05 \times 10^{-3}$$

$$pH = -\log[H^+] = 2.98$$

Another way to solve this problem is by using the Henderson-Hasselbalch equation:

$$pH = pK_a + \log\frac{[\text{conjugate base}]}{[\text{weak acid}]}$$

Using the Henderson-Hasselbalch equation for this problem:

$$pH = -\log K_a + \log\frac{[F^-]}{[HF]}$$

$$pH = -\log(7.0 \times 10^{-4}) + \log\frac{2}{3}$$

$$pH = 3.155 - 0.176 = 2.98$$

13. **C** The Henderson-Hasselbalch equation may again be used here:

$$pH = pK_a + \log\frac{[A^-]}{[HA]}$$

$$4 = 3.35 + \log\frac{[A^-]}{[HA]}$$

$$0.65 = \log\frac{[A^-]}{[HA]}$$

$$\frac{[A^-]}{[HA]} = 4.5$$

Only choice (C) fulfills this criterion, as $\frac{0.50}{0.11} = 4.5$.

14. **A** Strong acid:

Salt in buffer dissociates completely:

$NaX \leftrightharpoons Na^+ + X^-$

Added strong acid dissociates completely:

$HCl \leftrightharpoons H^+ + Cl^-$

Protons from the acid are absorbed by the strong conjugate base of the salt:

$H^+ + X^- \leftrightharpoons HX$

B Strong base:

Weak acid in buffer hardly dissociates:

$HX \leftrightharpoons HX$

Added strong base dissociates completely:

$NaOH \leftrightharpoons Na^+ + OH^-$

OH^- is a strong base, which attracts protons from the weak acid:

$OH^- + HX \leftrightharpoons H_2O + X^-$

CHAPTER THIRTY-EIGHT

Nuclear Chemistry

Nuclear phenomena describe interactions with and changes to nuclei, which is distinctly different from many other topics in general chemistry focused on the behavior of electrons outside the nucleus. Therefore, to begin, it's important to understand the standard terminology used in nuclear chemistry and physics. Briefly, an amount of energy, called the **binding energy**, is required to break up a given nucleus into its constituent protons and neutrons. That energy is converted to mass via Einstein's $E = mc^2$ equation, resulting in a larger mass for the constituent protons and neutrons than that of the original nucleus; this difference is called the **mass defect**. The remainder of the chapter is concerned with a brief discussion of nuclear reactions (**fission** and **fusion**) and an extended treatment of radioactive decay, which itself is presented in two distinct parts. The first deals with the four different types of **radioactive decay** and a discussion of the reaction equations that describe them. The second covers the general problem of determining the number of nuclei that have not decayed as a function of time along with the associated concept of the half-life of a decay process.

NUCLEI

At the center of an atom lies its nucleus, consisting of one or more **nucleons** (protons or neutrons) held together with considerably more energy than the energy needed to hold electrons in orbit around the nucleus. The radius of the nucleus is about 100,000 times smaller than the radius of the atom. As described in Chapter 24, Atomic and Molecular Structure, the atomic number (Z) of an element describes the number of protons, whereas the mass number (A) describes the number of protons + neutrons. Z is used as a presubscript and A is used as a presuperscript to the chemical symbol in **isotopic notation**. The number of protons determines the identity (name) of an element, and varying numbers of neutrons determine different isotopes of that same element. The term **radionucleotide** is another generic name used to refer to any radioactive isotope, especially those used in nuclear medicine.

Nuclear versus Chemical Reactions

All nuclei of atoms, with the exception of hydrogen, contain protons and neutrons. When the nucleus of an atom is unstable, it may spontaneously emit particles or electromagnetic radiation (otherwise known as **radioactivity**). Nuclei may also change composition when nuclear transmutation occurs. This process involves the bombardment of the nucleus by electrons, neutrons, or other nuclei. These are all specific types of nuclear reactions, which involve changes to nuclei rather than solely electrons. Below is a summary of the major differences between nuclear and chemical reactions.

Nuclear reactions	Chemical reactions
• Elements or isotopes are changed from one to another.	• Atoms can be rearranged by the formation or breaking of chemical bonds.
• Reactions result in the release or absorption of large amounts of energy.	• Reactions generally result in the release or absorption of small amounts of energy.
• Reaction rates are generally not affected by catalysts, temperature, or pressure.	• Reaction rates are generally affected by catalysts, temperature, or pressure.
• Protons, neutrons, or electrons can be involved.	• Only electrons in the affected orbital of the atom are involved in the formation and breaking of bonds.

Table 38.1

Nuclear Binding Energy and Mass Defect

Every nucleus (other than ^1_1H) has a smaller mass than the combined mass of its constituent protons and neutrons. This difference is called the **mass defect**. Scientists had difficulty explaining why this mass defect occurred until Einstein discovered the equivalence of matter and energy, embodied by the equation $E = mc^2$. The mass defect is a result of matter that has been converted to energy. This energy, called **binding energy**, holds the nucleons together in the nucleus.

Note: The binding energy per nucleon peaks at iron, which implies that iron is the most stable atom. In general, intermediate-sized nuclei are more stable than large and small nuclei.

The mass defect and binding energy of ^4He are calculated in the following example.

Example: Measurements of the atomic mass of a neutron and a proton yield these results:

proton = 1.00728 amu

neutron = 1.00867 amu

A measurement of the atomic mass of a ^4He nucleus yields:

^4He = 4.00260 amu

^4He consists of two protons and two neutrons, which should theoretically give a ^4He mass of:

$$Z(m_p) + N(m_n) = 2(1.00728) + 2(1.00867)$$
$$= 4.03190 \text{ amu}$$

What is the mass defect and binding energy of this nucleus?

Solution: The difference $4.03190 - 4.00260 = 0.02930$ amu is the mass defect for ^4He and is interpreted as the conversion of mass into the binding energy of the nucleus. The rest energy (the energy equivalent of a given mass times the speed of light squared) of

1 amu is 932 MeV, so using $E = mc^2$, we find that $c^2 = 932$ MeV/amu. Therefore, the binding energy (BE) of ^{4}He is:

$$BE = \Delta mc^2$$
$$= (0.02930 \text{ amu})(932 \text{ MeV/amu})$$
$$= 27.3 \text{ MeV}$$

NUCLEAR REACTIONS AND DECAY

Nuclear reactions such as fusion, fission, and radioactive decay involve either combining or splitting the nuclei of atoms. Since the binding energy per nucleon is greatest for intermediate-sized atoms, when small atoms combine or large atoms split, a great amount of energy is released.

Fusion

Fusion occurs when small nuclei combine into a larger nucleus. As an example, many stars, including the sun, power themselves by fusing four hydrogen nuclei to make one helium nucleus. By this method, the sun produces 4×10^{26} J every second. Here on Earth, researchers are trying to find ways to use fusion as an alternative energy source. Because these fusion reactions can only take place at extremely high temperatures, they are generally referred to as **thermonuclear reactions**.

Fission

Fission is a process in which a large, heavy (mass number >200) atom splits to form smaller, more stable nuclei (especially noble gases) and one or more neutrons. It is important to note that, because the original large nucleus is more unstable than its products, there is the release of a large amount of energy. Spontaneous fission rarely occurs. However, by the absorption of a low-energy neutron, fission can be induced in certain nuclei. Of special interest are those fission reactions that release more neutrons since those other neutrons will cause other atoms to undergo fission. This in turn releases more neutrons, creating a **chain reaction**. By bombarding large, unstable, nuclei with neutrons, scientists can use fission reactions to power commercial nuclear electric-generating plants.

Example: A fission reaction occurs when uranium-235 (U-235) absorbs a low-energy neutron, briefly forming an excited state of U-236, which then splits into xenon-140, strontium-94, and x more neutrons. In isotopic notation form the reactions are:

$$^{235}_{92}\text{U} + ^{1}_{0}\text{n} \rightarrow ^{236}_{92}\text{U} \rightarrow ^{140}_{54}\text{Xe} + ^{94}_{38}\text{Sr} + x^{1}_{0}\text{n}$$

How many neutrons are produced in the last reaction?

Solution: The question is asking "What is x?" By treating each arrow as an equal sign, the problem is simply asking you to balance the last "equation." The mass numbers (A) on either side of each arrow must be equal. This is an application of **nucleon** or **baryon number conservation,** which says that the total number of neutrons plus protons remains the same, even if neutrons are converted to protons and vice versa, as they are in some decays. Because $235 + 1 = 236$, the first arrow is indeed balanced. To find the number of neutrons, solve for x in the last equation (arrow):

$$236 = 140 + 94 + x$$
$$x = 236 - 140 - 94$$
$$x = 2$$

So two neutrons are produced in this reaction. These neutrons are free to go on and be absorbed by more ^{235}U and cause more fission, and the process continues in a chain reaction. Note that it really was not necessary to know that the intermediate state $^{236}_{92}U$ was formed.

Some radioactive nuclei may be induced to fission via more than one **decay channel** or **decay mode**. For example, a different fission reaction may occur when uranium-235 absorbs a slow neutron and then immediately splits into barium-139, krypton-94, and three more neutrons with no intermediate state:

$$^{235}_{92}U + {}^1_0n \rightarrow {}^{139}_{56}Ba + {}^{94}_{36}Kr + 3{}^1_0n$$

Radioactive Decay

Radioactive decay is a naturally occurring spontaneous decay of certain nuclei accompanied by the emission of specific particles. It could be classified as a certain type of fission. Radioactive decay problems are of three general types:

1. The integer arithmetic of particle and isotope species
2. Radioactive half-life problems
3. The use of exponential decay curves and decay constants

Isotope decay arithmetic and nucleon conservation

Let the letters X and Y represent nuclear isotopes such that the **parent isotope** $^A_Z X$ decays into a **daughter isotope** $^{A'}_{Z'}Y$ as in:

$$^A_Z X \rightarrow {}^{A'}_{Z'}Y + \text{emitted decay particle}$$

Alpha decay

Alpha decay is the emission of an α-particle, which is a ^4_2He nucleus that consists of two protons and two neutrons. The alpha particle is very massive (compared to a beta particle) and doubly charged (since it contains 2 protons and has a $+2$ charge). Alpha particles interact with matter very easily; hence, they do not penetrate shielding (such as lead sheets) very far.

The emission of an α-particle means that the daughter's atomic number (Z') will be 2 less than the parent's atomic number, and the daughter's mass number (A') will be 4 less than the parent's mass number. This can be expressed in two equations:

$$Z_{daughter} = Z_{parent} - 2$$
$$A_{daughter} = A_{parent} - 4$$

The generic alpha decay reaction is then:

$$^A_Z X \rightarrow {}^{A-4}_{Z-2}Y + {}^4_2\alpha$$

Note that alpha decay and fission are the only radioactive decay processes on the exam during which the mass number (A') changes.

Example: Suppose a parent X alpha decays into a daughter Y such that:

$$^{238}_{92}X \rightarrow {}^{A'}_{Z'}Y + \alpha$$

What are the mass number (A') and atomic number (Z') of the daughter isotope Y?

Solution: Since $\alpha = {}^4_2He$, balancing the mass numbers and atomic numbers is all that needs to be done:

$238 = A' + 4$

$A' = 234$

$92 = Z' + 2$

$Z' = 90$

So $A' = 234$ and $Z' = 90$. Note that it was not necessary to know the chemical species of the isotopes to do this problem. However, the periodic table does show that $Z = 92$ means X is uranium-238 $\left({}^{238}_{92}U\right)$ and that $Z = 90$ means Y is thorium-234 $\left({}^{234}_{90}Th\right)$.

Beta decay

Beta decay is the emission of a β-particle, which could be either β^- (electron) or β^+ (positron), from the nucleus. A **positron** (e^+) is similar to an electron (so has minimal mass) but has a positive charge. Electrons and positrons do not normally reside in the nucleus but are emitted when a proton or neutron in the nucleus decays. This is because protons and neutrons are composed of elementary particles called quarks, which can recombine to form different particles. Specifically, in β^- decay, a neutron decays into a proton and a β^- particle (and an antineutrino), whereas, in β^+ decay, a proton decays into a neutron and a β^+ particle (and a neutrino). Note that neither of these reactions is concerned with electrons in orbitals outside the nucleus, which are generally ignored during radioactive decay.

β^- decay means that a neutron is consumed and a proton takes its place. Hence, the parent's mass number is unchanged, and the parent's atomic number is increased by 1. In other words, the daughter's A is the same as the parent's, and the daughter's Z is one more than the parent's.

$$Z_{daughter} = Z_{parent} + 1$$
$$A_{daughter} = A_{parent}$$

In β^+ decay, a proton is consumed and a neutron takes its place. Therefore, β^+ decay means that the parent's mass number is unchanged, and the parent's atomic number is decreased by 1. In other words, the daughter's A is the same as the parent's, and the daughter's Z is one less than the parent's.

$$Z_{daughter} = Z_{parent} - 1$$
$$A_{daughter} = A_{parent}$$

The generic negative beta-minus decay reaction is:

$$^A_ZX \rightarrow {}^A_{Z+1}Y + \beta^-$$

Note that β^- decay is the only radioactive decay on the test where the atomic number (Z') increases. The generic beta-plus decay reaction is:

$$_Z^A X \rightarrow {}_{Z-1}^A Y + \beta^+$$

Since β particles are singly charged and about 1,836 times lighter than protons, the beta radiation from radioactive decay is more penetrating than alpha radiation.

Example: Suppose a cobalt-60 nucleus undergoes beta-minus decay such that:

$$_{27}^{60} Co \rightarrow {}_{Z+1}^A Y + \beta^-$$

What are the A' and Z' of the daughter isotope?

Solution: Balance mass numbers:

$60 = A' + 0$

$A' = 60$

Now balance the atomic numbers, taking into account that cobalt has 27 protons (the Z value, or presubscript, given in the question) and that there is one more proton on the right-hand side:

$Z' = Z + 1$

$Z' = 27 + 1$

$Z' = 28$

The answer is an element with 28 protons and 60 nucleons. Although the question does not ask for the identity of the daughter, the periodic table shows that it is:

$Y = {}_{28}^{60} Ni$

Gamma decay

Gamma decay is the emission of γ-particles, which are high-energy photons. Gamma decay usually follows another type of nuclear decay and is a way for the nucleus to shed excess energy (similar to how an electron in an excited state emits a photon to shed energy). Gamma particles carry no charge and simply lower the energy of the emitting (parent) nucleus without changing the mass number or the atomic number. In other words, the daughter's A is the same as the parent's, and the daughter's Z is the same as the parent's.

$$Z_{parent} = Z_{daughter}$$
$$A_{parent} = A_{daughter}$$

The generic gamma decay reaction is thus:

$$_Z^A X^* \rightarrow {}_Z^A X + \gamma$$

Example: Suppose a parent isotope $_Z^A X$ emits a β^+ and turns into an excited state of the isotope $_{Z'}^{A'} Y^*$, which then γ-decays to $_{Z''}^{A''} Y$, which in turn α-decays to $_{Z'''}^{A'''} W$. If W is ^{60}Fe (Z = 26), what is $_Z^A X$?

Solution: Since the final daughter in this chain of decay is given, it will be necessary to work backward through the reactions. First, work backward from the α-decay, then use that answer to work backward from the β^+-decay. Note that the γ-decay simply releases energy from the nucleus but does not alter the atomic number or the mass number of the parent and so can be disregarded for these calculations.

First, the α-decay:

$$_{Z''}^{A''} Y \rightarrow {}_{26}^{60}Fe + {}_2^4He^{2+}$$

By balancing the atomic numbers you find:

$Z'' = 26 + 2 = 28$

A balancing of the mass numbers implies:

$A'' = 60 + 4 = 64$

So the γ-decay was:

$$_{28}^{64} Y^* \rightarrow {}_{28}^{64} Y + \gamma$$

The first reaction was a β^+-decay that must have looked like:

$$_Z^A X \rightarrow {}_{28}^{64} Y^* + \beta^+$$

Again, balance the atomic numbers:

$Z = 28 + 1 = 29$

Since A remains unchanged during β^+-decay, $A' = A = 64$.

While the question did not ask for it, it is possible again to look at the periodic table to find that the total chain of decays can be written as:

$$_{29}^{64}Cu \rightarrow {}_{28}^{64}Ni^* + \beta^+$$
$$_{28}^{64}Ni^* \rightarrow {}_{28}^{64}Ni + \gamma$$
$$_{28}^{64}Ni \rightarrow {}_{26}^{60}Fe + \alpha$$

Electron capture

Certain unstable radionuclides are capable of capturing an inner electron that combines with a proton to form a neutron. The atomic number is now one less than the original, but the mass number remains the same. Electron capture is a rare process best thought of as an inverse β^- decay, following the exact same process as beta-minus decay but in reverse.

$$_Z^A X + e^- \rightarrow {}_{Z-1}^A Y$$

Radioactive decay half-life

In a collection of a great many identical radioactive isotopes, the **half-life** ($T_{1/2}$) of the sample is the time it takes for half of the sample to decay by any of the above processes. After n half-lives, $\left(\frac{1}{2}\right)^n$ of the original sample will remain, whereas $1 - \left(\frac{1}{2}\right)^n$ will have decayed.

Example: If the half-life of a certain isotope is 4 years, what fraction of a sample of that isotope will remain after 12 years?

Solution: If 4 years is one half-life, then 12 years is three half-lives and $n = 3$. During the first half-life—the first 4 years—half of the sample will have decayed. During the second half-life (years 4 to 8), half of the remaining half will decay, leaving one-fourth of the original. During the third and final period (years 8 to 12), half of the remaining fourth will decay, leaving one-eighth of the original sample. Thus the fraction remaining after 3 half-lives is $\left(\frac{1}{2}\right)^3$ or $\frac{1}{8}$.

Exponential decay

Let N be the number of radioactive nuclei that have not yet decayed in a sample. It turns out that the **rate** at which the nuclei decay $\left(\frac{\Delta N}{\Delta t}\right)$ is proportional to the number that remain (N). This suggests the equation:

$$\frac{\Delta N}{\Delta t} = -\lambda N$$

where λ is known as the **decay constant.** The solution of this equation tells us how the number of radioactive nuclei changes with time, which is known as **exponential decay:**

$$N = N_0 e^{-\lambda t}$$

where N_0 is the number of undecayed nuclei at time $t = 0$. (The decay constant is related to the half-life by $\lambda = \dfrac{\ln(2)}{T_{1/2}} = \dfrac{0.693}{T_{1/2}}$.)

Example: If at time $t = 0$ there is a two-mole sample of radioactive isotopes of decay constant 2 (hour)$^{-1}$, how many nuclei remain after 45 minutes?

Solution: Because 45 minutes is 3/4 of an hour, the exponent ($-\lambda t$) is

$$-\lambda t = -2\left(\frac{3}{4}\right) = -\frac{6}{4} = -\frac{3}{2}$$

The exponential factor will be a number smaller than 1:

$$e^{-\lambda t} = e^{-3/2} = 0.22$$

So only 0.22 or 22% of the original two-mole sample will remain. To find N_0, multiply the number of moles by the number of particles per mole (Avogadro's number):

$$N_0 = 2(6.02 \times 10^{23}) = 1.2 \times 10^{24}$$

From the equation that describes exponential decay, you can calculate the number of nuclei that remain after 45 minutes:

$$\begin{aligned}
N &= N_0 e^{-\lambda t} \\
&= (1.2 \times 10^{24})(0.22) \\
&= 2.6 \times 10^{23} \text{ particles}
\end{aligned}$$

REVIEW PROBLEMS

1. Element $^{102}_{20}\varsigma$ is formed as a result of 3 α and 2 β^- decays. Which of the following is the parent element?

   (A) $^{90}_{16}\Gamma$

   (B) $^{114}_{24}\Phi$

   (C) $^{114}_{28}\Theta$

   (D) $^{12}_{8}\Delta + ^{90}_{12}\vartheta$

2. Element X is radioactive and decays via α-decay with a half-life of 4 days. If 12.5% of an original sample of element X remains after t days, then determine t.

3. A patient undergoing treatment for thyroid cancer receives a dose of radioactive iodine (^{131}I), which has a half-life of 8.05 days. If the original dose contained 12 mg of ^{131}I, what mass of ^{131}I remains after 16.1 days?

4. In an exponential decay, if the natural logarithm of the ratio of intact nuclei (N) at time t to the intact nuclei at time $t = 0$ (N_0) is plotted against time, what does the slope of the graph correspond to?

5. The half-life of radioactive sodium is 15.0 hours. How many hours would it take for a 64 g sample to decay to one-eighth of its original activity?
   (A) 3
   (B) 15
   (C) 30
   (D) 45

SOLUTIONS TO REVIEW PROBLEMS

1. **B** Emission of three alpha particles by the (as yet unknown) parent results in the following changes:

   Mass number: decreases by 3×4 or 12 units

   Atomic number: decreases by 3×2 or 6 units

   Emission of two negative betas results in the following changes:

   Mass number: no change

   Atomic number: increases by 2×1 or 2 units

   So the net change is: mass number decreases by 12 units; atomic number decreases by 4 units. Therefore, the mass number of the parent is 12 greater than 102, or 114; the atomic number of the parent is 4 greater than 20, or 24. The only choice given with these numbers is (B).

2. $t = 12$ **days**

   Because the half-life of element X is 4 days, 50% of an original sample remains after 4 days, 25% of an original sample remains after 8 days, and 12.5% of an original sample remains after 12 days. Thus, $t = 12$ days. A different approach is to set $\left(\dfrac{1}{2}\right)^n = 0.125$, where n is the number of half-lives that have elapsed. Solving for n gives $n = 3$. Thus, 3 half-lives have elapsed, and given the half-life is 4 days, $t = 12$ days.

3. **3 mg**

   Given that the half-life of ^{131}I is 8.05 days, we know that two half-lives have elapsed after 16.1 days, which means that 25% of the original amount of ^{131}I is still present. Thus, only 25% of the original number of ^{131}I nuclei remain, which also means that only 25% of the original mass of ^{131}I remain. Because the original dose contained 12 mg of ^{131}I, only 3 mg remain after 16.1 days.

4. $-\lambda$

   The expression $N = N_0 e^{-\lambda t}$ is equivalent to $\dfrac{N}{N_0} = e^{-\lambda t}$. Taking the natural logarithm of both sides of the latter expression you find: $\ln\!\left(\dfrac{N}{N_0}\right) = -\lambda t$.

   This expression shows that plotting $\ln\!\left(\dfrac{N}{N_0}\right)$ versus t will give a straight line of slope $-\lambda$.

5. **D** For a 64 g sample to decay to one-eighth of its original activity, or 8 g, the sample would have to go through three half-lives. Therefore, the amount of time needed for the decay is 3 half-lives $\times$ 15 hours per half-life = 45 hours.

Section VI:

ORGANIC CHEMISTRY

CHAPTER THIRTY-NINE

Structural Formulas

Nomenclature, the set of accepted conventions for naming compounds, is crucial to a discussion of organic chemistry. Nomenclature represents the basic language of organic chemistry; if you don't know it, you may feel like you're taking a test in a foreign language! Note that the rules of nomenclature presented in this chapter are for general cases only. More specific examples will be discussed in the chapters dealing with particular types of compounds.

ALKANES

Alkanes are the simplest organic molecules, consisting only of carbon and hydrogen atoms held together by single bonds.

Straight-Chain Alkanes

The names of the four simplest alkanes are:

CH_4 CH_3CH_3 $CH_3CH_2CH_3$ $CH_3CH_2CH_2CH_3$
methane   **eth**ane   **prop**ane   **but**ane

The names of the longer-chain alkanes consist of prefixes derived from the Greek root for the number of carbon atoms with the ending **-ane.**

C_5H_{12} = **pent**ane C_9H_{20} = **non**ane

C_6H_{14} = **hex**ane $C_{10}H_{22}$ = **dec**ane

C_7H_{16} = **hept**ane $C_{11}H_{24}$ = **undec**ane

C_8H_{18} = **oct**ane $C_{12}H_{26}$ = **dodec**ane

These prefixes are applicable to more complex organic molecules, too, and should be memorized.

Branched-Chain Alkanes

The International Union of Pure and Applied Chemistry (IUPAC) proposed a set of simple rules for naming complex molecules. This basic system can be used to name all classes of organic compounds. Throughout these notes, the IUPAC names will be listed as the primary name, and common names will appear in parentheses.

1. Find the longest chain in the compound.

The longest continuous carbon chain within the compound is taken as the backbone. If two or more chains are of equal length, the most highly substituted chain (the one with the greatest number of other groups attached) takes precedence. The longest chain may not be as obvious from the structural formula as when it is drawn. For example, the backbone shown below is an octane (it contains eight carbon atoms).

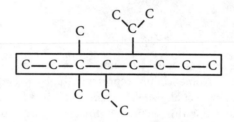

Figure 39.1

2. Number the chain.

Number the chain from one end in such a way that the lowest set of numbers is obtained for the substituents (which in alkanes are carbon groups not part of the main carbon chain).

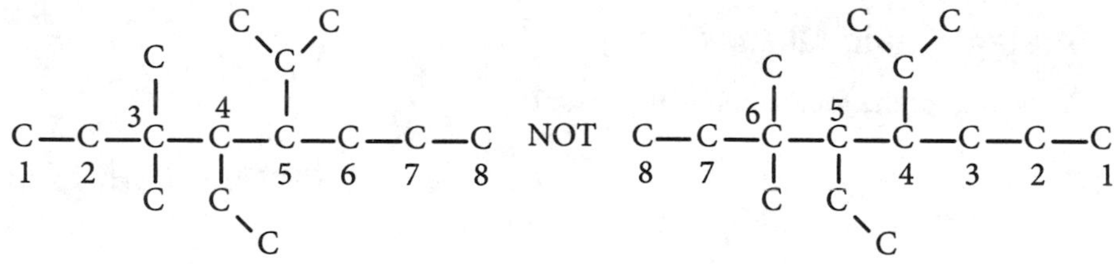

Figure 39.2

3. Name the substituents.

Substituents are named according to their appropriate prefix with the ending **-yl.** For example:

$$CH_3- \qquad CH_3CH_2- \qquad CH_3CH_2CH_2-$$
$$\text{methyl} \qquad \text{ethyl} \qquad \textit{n}\text{-propyl}$$

The prefix *n-* in the above example indicates an unbranched ("normal") compound. There are special names for some common branched alkanes (see Figure 39.3), and these are usually used in the naming of substituents.

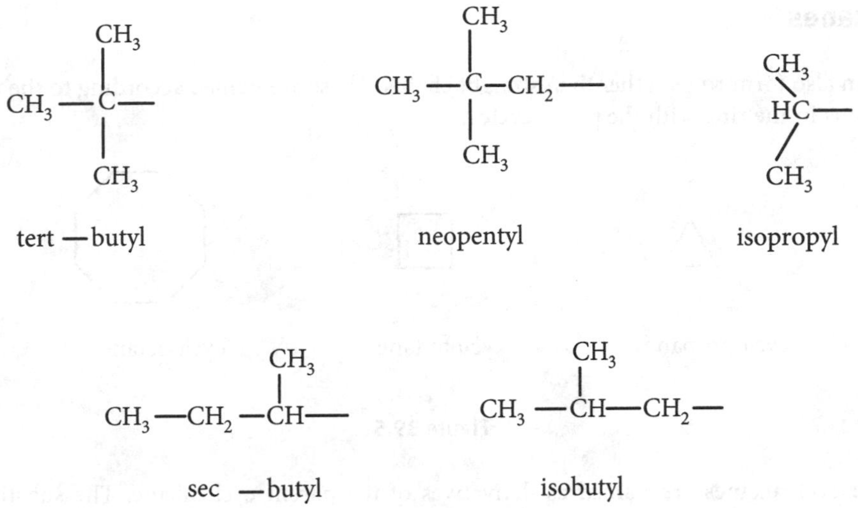

tert —butyl   neopentyl   isopropyl

sec —butyl   isobutyl

Figure 39.3

If two or more equivalent groups are present, the prefixes **di-, tri-, tetra-,** etc. are used.

4. Assign a number to each substituent.

Each substituent is assigned a number to identify its point of attachment to the principal chain. If the prefixes **di-, tri-, tetra-,** etc., are used, a number is still necessary for each individual group.

5. Complete the name.

List the substituents in alphabetical order with their corresponding numbers. Prefixes such as di-, tri-, etc., as well as the hyphenated prefixes (*tert-* [or *t-*], *sec-, n-*), are ignored in alphabetizing. In contrast, **cyclo-, iso-,** and **neo-** are considered part of the group name and are alphabetized. Commas should be placed between numbers, and hyphens should be placed between numbers and words. For example:

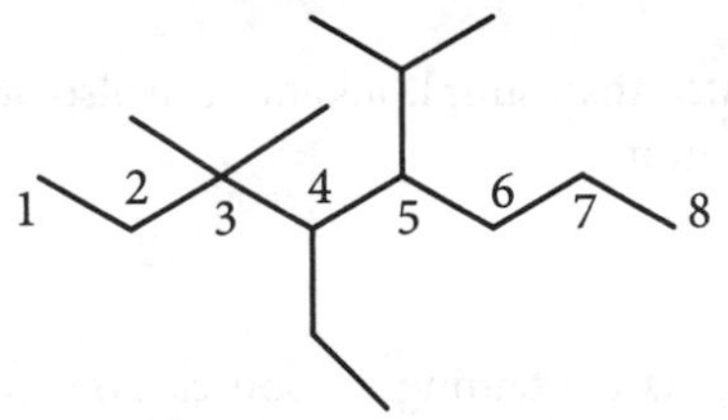

4-ethyl-5-isopropyl-3,3-dimethyl octane

Figure 39.4

You may also need to indicate the isomer you are describing—e.g., *cis* or *trans*, *R* or *S*, etc. Isomers are discussed in detail in Chapter 40.

Cycloalkanes

Alkanes can also form rings rather than straight chains. These are named according to the number of carbon atoms in the ring with the prefix **cyclo-**.

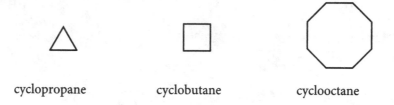

cyclopropane   cyclobutane   cyclooctane

Figure 39.5

Substituted cycloalkanes are named as derivatives of the parent cycloalkane. The substituents are named, and the carbon atoms are numbered around the ring *starting from the point of greatest substitution*. Again, the goal is to provide the lowest series of numbers as in rule number 2 above.

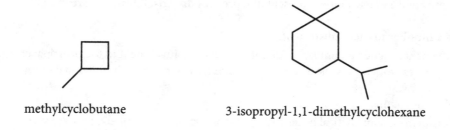

methylcyclobutane   3-isopropyl-1,1-dimethylcyclohexane

Figure 39.6

MULTIPLE BONDS

Organic molecules more complicated than simple alkanes can also be named using the 5-step process but with a few additional considerations.

Alkenes

Alkenes (or **olefins**) are compounds containing carbon-carbon double bonds. The nomenclature rules are essentially the same as for alkanes except that the ending **-ene** is used rather than **-ane**. Note the exceptions of the common names *ethylene* and *propylene,* which are used preferentially over the IUPAC names *ethene* and *propene.*

When identifying the carbon backbone, select the longest chain that contains the double bond (or the greatest number of double bonds if more than one is present).

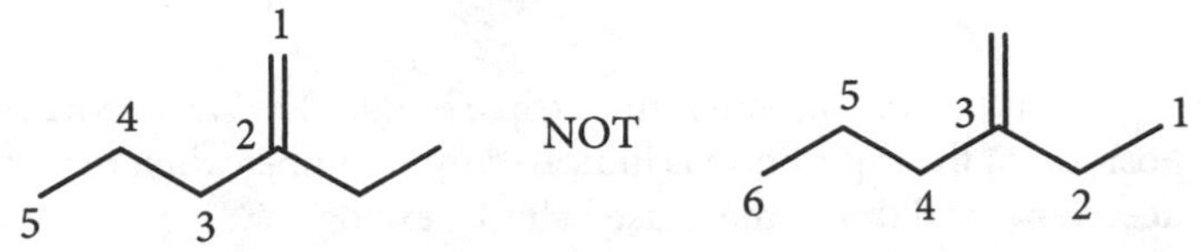

Figure 39.7

Number the backbone so the double bond receives the lowest number possible. Remember that multiple double bonds must be named using the prefixes di-, tri-, etc. and that each must receive a number. Also, you may need to name the configurational isomer (*cis/trans, Z/E*). This topic will be discussed further in Chapter 40.

Substituents are named as they are for alkanes, and their positions are specified by the number of the backbone carbon atom to which they are attached.

Frequently, an alkene group must be named as a substituent. In these cases, the systematic names may be used, but common names are more popular. **Vinyl-** derivatives are monosubstituted ethylenes (**ethenyl-**), and **allyl-** derivatives are propylenes substituted at the C–3 position (**2-propenyl-**). **Methylene** refers to the –CH$_2$ group.

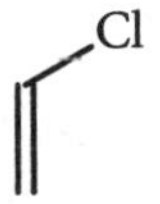

chloroethene
(vinyl chloride)

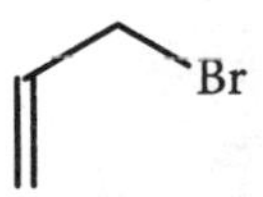

3-bromo-1-propene
(allyl bromide)

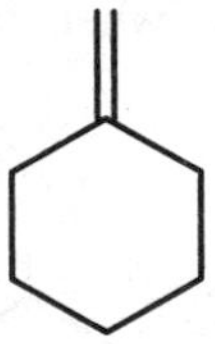

methylene cyclohexane

Figure 39.8

Cycloalkenes

Cycloalkenes are named like cycloalkanes but with the suffix -**ene** rather than -**ane**. If the molecule has only one double bond and no other substituents, a number is not necessary.

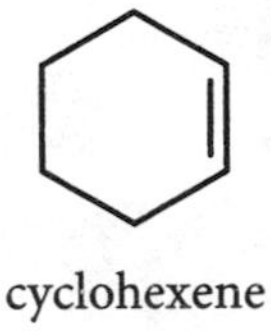

cyclohexene

Figure 39.9

Alkynes

Alkynes are compounds that possess carbon-carbon triple bonds. The suffix **-yne** replaces *-ane* in the parent alkane. The position of the triple bond is indicated by a number when necessary. The common name for ethyne is **acetylene,** and this name is used almost exclusively.

HC≡CH
ethyne
(acetylene)

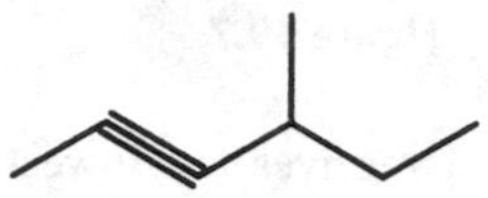

4-methyl-2-hexyne

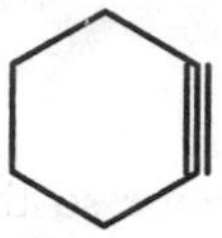

cyclohexyne

Figure 39.10

SUBSTITUTED ALKANES

Haloalkanes

Compounds containing a halogen substituent are named following similar rules as those above while including the halogen as a substituent. If the halogen is the highest priority substituent, ensure it has the lower number when deciding from which end of the carbon chain to start counting. For example:

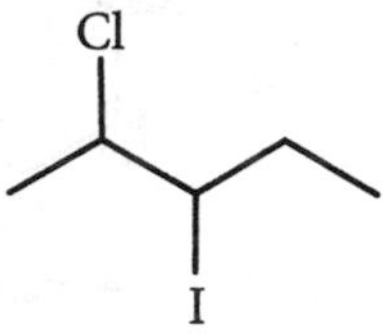

2-chloro-3-iodopentane

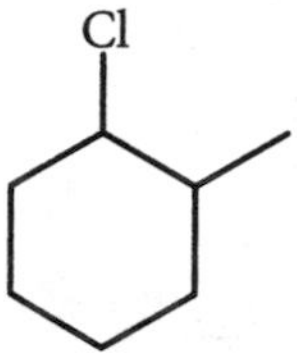

1-chloro-2-methylcyclohexane

Figure 39.11

Alternatively, the haloalkane may be named as an **alkyl halide.** In this system, chloroethane is called **ethyl chloride**. Other examples are:

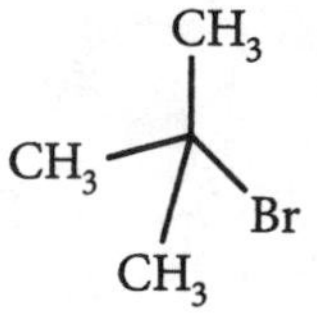

2-bromo-2-methylpropane
(*t*-butyl bromide)

2-iodopropane
(isopropyl iodide)

Figure 39.12

Alcohols

In the IUPAC system, **alcohols** are named by replacing the *-e* of the corresponding alkane with **-ol**. The chain is numbered such that the carbon attached to the hydroxyl group (–OH) receives the lowest number possible.

In compounds that possess a multiple bond and a hydroxyl group, numerical priority is given to the carbon attached to the –OH.

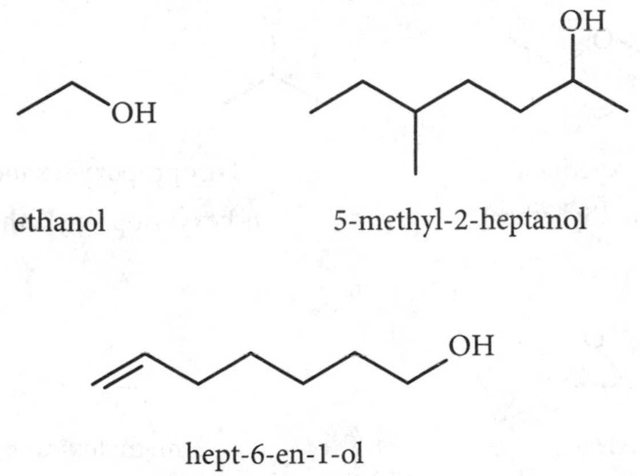

ethanol

5-methyl-2-heptanol

hept-6-en-1-ol

Figure 39.13

A common system of nomenclature exists for alcohols in which the name of the alkyl group is combined with the word *alcohol*. These common names are used for simple alcohols. For example, methanol may be named "methyl alcohol," while 2-propanol may also be named "isopropyl alcohol."

Molecules with two hydroxyl groups are called **diols** (or **glycols**) and are named with the suffix **-diol**. Two numbers are necessary to locate the two functional groups. Diols with hydroxyl groups on adjacent carbons are referred to as **vicinal**, and diols with hydroxyl groups on the same carbon are **geminal**. These terms apply for any two functional groups. Geminal diols (also called **carbonyl hydrates**) are not commonly observed because they spontaneously lose water (**dehydrate**) to produce carbonyl compounds (containing C=O; see Chapter 44).

Ethers

In the IUPAC system, **ethers** are named as derivatives of alkanes, and the larger alkyl group is chosen as the backbone. The ether functionality is specified as an **alkoxy-** prefix, indicating the presence of an ether (*oxy-*), and the corresponding smaller alkyl group (*alk-*). The chain is numbered to give the ether the lowest position. Common names for ethers are frequently used. They are derived by naming the two alkyl groups in alphabetical order and adding the word *ether*. The generic term "ether" refers to diethyl ether, a commonly used solvent.

For **cyclic ethers**, numbering of the ring begins at the oxygen and proceeds to provide the lowest numbers for the substituents. Three-membered rings are termed **oxiranes** by IUPAC. The simplest of these are commonly called **epoxides**.

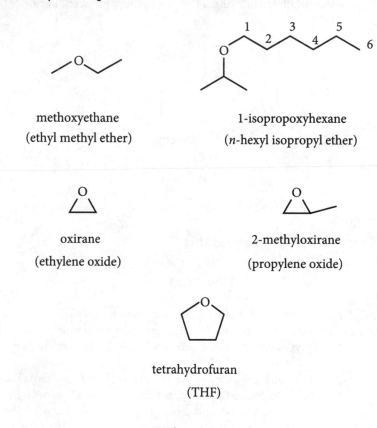

methoxyethane
(ethyl methyl ether)

1-isopropoxyhexane
(*n*-hexyl isopropyl ether)

oxirane
(ethylene oxide)

2-methyloxirane
(propylene oxide)

tetrahydrofuran
(THF)

Figure 39.14

Aldehydes and Ketones

Aldehydes are named according to the longest chain containing the aldehyde functional group. The suffix **-al** replaces the *-e* of the corresponding alkane. The carbonyl carbon receives the lowest number, although numbers are not always necessary since by definition an aldehyde is terminal and receives the number (1).

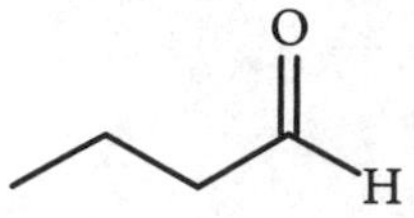

n-butanal

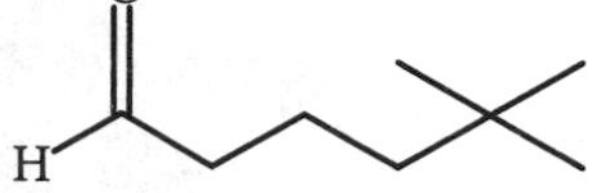

5,5-dimethylhexanal

Figure 39.15

The common names *formaldehyde*, *acetaldehyde*, and *propionaldehyde* are used almost exclusively instead of the IUPAC names *methanal*, *ethanal*, and *propanal*, respectively.

methanal
(formaldehyde)

ethanal
(acetaldehyde)

propanal
(propionaldehyde)

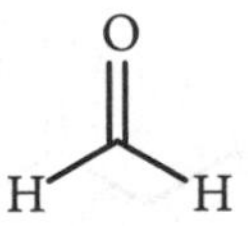

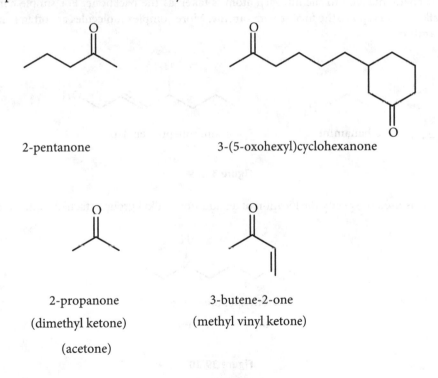

Figure 39.16

Ketones are named analogously with aldehydes but with **-one** as a suffix. If highest priority, the carbonyl group must be assigned the lowest possible number. In complex molecules, the carbonyl group can be named as a prefix with the term **oxo-**. Alternatively, the individual alkyl groups may be listed in alphabetical order and followed by the word **ketone**.

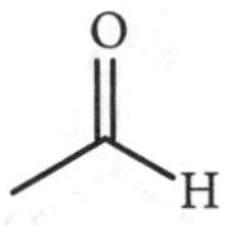

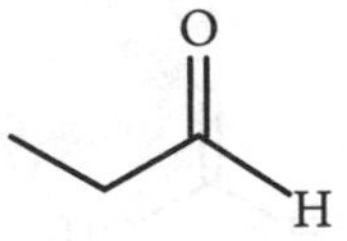

2-pentanone

3-(5-oxohexyl)cyclohexanone

2-propanone
(dimethyl ketone)
(acetone)

3-butene-2-one
(methyl vinyl ketone)

Figure 39.17

A commonly used alternative to the numerical designation of substituents is to term the carbon atom adjacent to the carbonyl carbon as α and the carbon atoms successively along the chain as β, γ, δ, etc. This system is encountered with dicarbonyl compounds and halocarbonyl compounds.

Carboxylic Acids

Carboxylic acids are named with the ending **-oic acid** replacing the *-e* ending of the corresponding alkane. Carboxylic acids are terminal functional groups and, like aldehydes, are numbered one (1).

The common names *formic acid* (methanoic acid), *acetic acid* (ethanoic acid), and *propionic acid* (propanoic acid) are used almost exclusively.

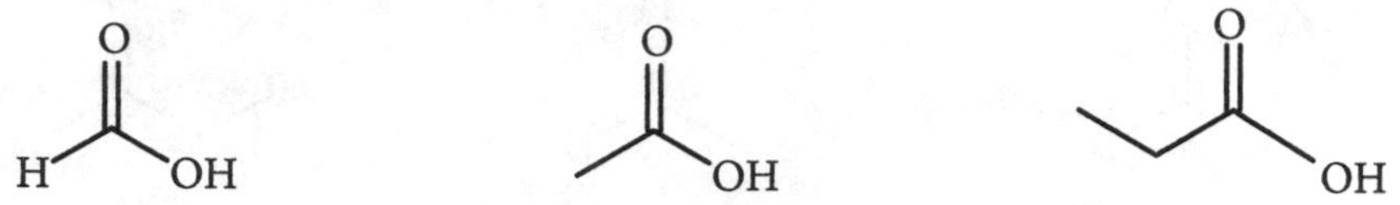

methanoic acid

(formic acid)

ethanoic acid

(acetic acid)

propanoic acid

(propionic acid)

Figure 39.18

Amines

The longest chain attached to the nitrogen atom is taken as the backbone. For simple compounds, name the alkane and replace the final *-e* with **-amine**. More complex molecules are often named using the prefix **amino-**.

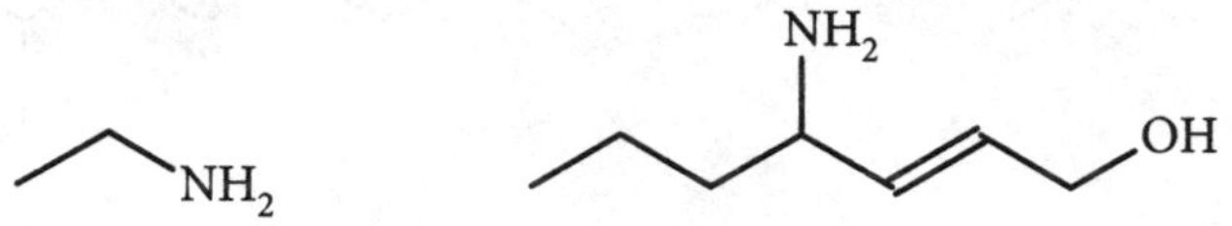

ethanamine

4-aminohept-2-en-1-ol

Figure 39.19

The prefix N- is used to specify the location of an additional alkyl group attached to the nitrogen:

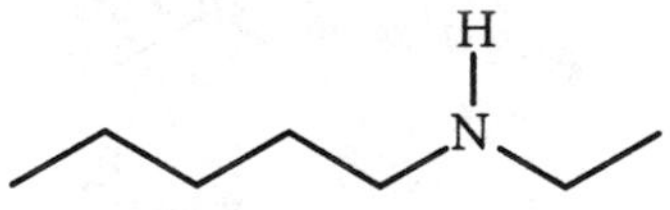

N-ethylpentanamine

(ethylpentylamine)

Figure 39.20

SUMMARY OF FUNCTIONAL GROUPS

Table 39.1 lists the major functional groups you need to know.

Functional Group	Structure	IUPAC Prefix	IUPAC Suffix
Carboxylic acid		carboxy-	-oic acid
Ester		alkoxycarbonyl-	-oate
Acyl halide		halocarbonyl-	-oyl halide
Amide		amido-	-amide
Nitrile	$RC\equiv N$	cyano-	-nitrile
Aldehyde		oxo-	-al
Ketone		oxo-	-one
Alcohol	ROH	hydroxy-	-ol
Thiol	RSH	sulfhydryl-	-thiol
Amine	RNH_2	amino-	-amine
Imine	$R_2C=NR'$	imino-	-imine
Ether	ROR	alkoxy-	-ether
Sulfide	R_2S	alkylthio-	
Halide	-I, -Br, -Cl, -F	halo-	
Nitro	RNO_2	nitro-	
Azide	RN_3	azido-	
Diazo	RN_2^+	diazo-	

Table 39.1

REVIEW PROBLEMS

1. What is the IUPAC name of the following compound?

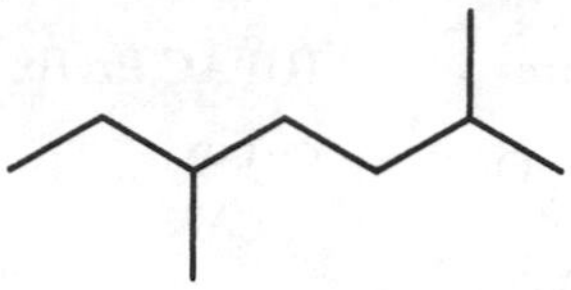

    (A) 2,5-dimethylheptane
    (B) 2-ethyl-5-methylhexane
    (C) 3,6-dimethylheptane
    (D) 5-ethyl-2-methylhexane

2. What is the structure of 5-ethyl-2,2-dimethyloctane?

3. What is the name of the following compound?

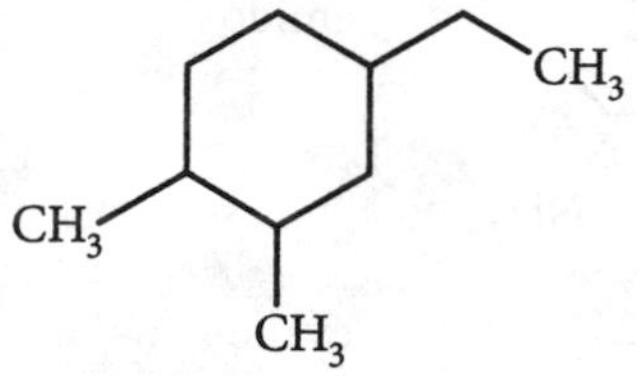

    (A) 1-ethyl-3,4-dimethylcycloheptane
    (B) 2-ethyl-4,5-dimethylcyclohexane
    (C) 1-ethyl-3,4-dimethylcyclohexane
    (D) 4-ethyl-1,2-dimethylcyclohexane

4. What is the name of the following compound?

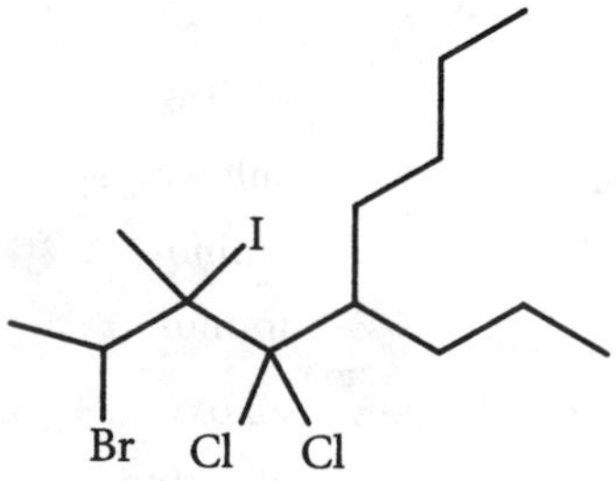

    (A) 2-bromo-5-butyl-4,4-dichloro-3-iodo-3-methyloctane
    (B) 7-bromo-4-butyl-5,5-dichloro-6-iodo-6-methyloctane
    (C) 2-bromo-4,4-dichloro-3-iodo-3-methyl-5-propylnonane
    (D) 2-bromo-5-butyl-4,4-dichloro-3-iodo-3-methylnonane

5. What is the name of the following compound?

$$\underset{H_3C}{\overset{H}{}}C=C\underset{H}{\overset{\underset{\displaystyle CHCH_2CH_3}{\overset{\displaystyle \overset{OH}{|}}{\underset{\displaystyle |}{CHCH_3}}}}{}}$$

(A) *trans*-3-ethyl-4-hexen-2-ol
(B) *trans*-4-ethyl-2-hexen-5-ol
(C) *trans*-3-ethanol-2-hexene
(D) *trans*-4-ethanol-2-hexene

6. Indicate the α, β, γ, and δ carbons in the following compound.

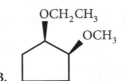

7. An alkane can be synthesized from its corresponding alkene by a reaction with hydrogen in the presence of a platinum catalyst. If 5-methenyl-3-methyloctane (shown below) were treated with hydrogen in the presence of a platinum catalyst, what would be the name and structure of the alkane that would be produced?

8. What is the correct structure for *cis*-1-ethoxy-2-methoxycyclopentane?

A.

B.

C.

D.

9. Do the following structures show the same compound or different compounds? Give a name for each structure.

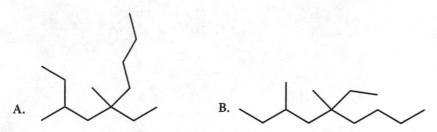

A.　　　　　　　　　　　　B.

10. Match each name with the correct structure below.

    (A) *t*-butyl
    (B) diene
    (C) β-keto acid
    (D) cyclohexanol
    (E) *sec*-butyl

1. R⎓⎓⎓R

2. ⬡—OH

3. CH_3—CH—
          |
          C_2H_5

4. $(CH_3)_3C$—

5. R
    O O
    ‖   ‖
    R   OH

11. Which of the following are considered terminal functional groups?

    (A) Aldehydes
    (B) Ketones
    (C) Carboxylic acids
    (D) Both A and C

SOLUTIONS TO REVIEW PROBLEMS

1. **A** The first task in naming alkanes is identifying the longest chain. In this case, the longest chain has seven carbons, so the parent alkane is heptane. Choices (B) and (D) can be eliminated. The next step is to identify the substituents on the alkane chain. This compound has two methyl groups at carbons 2 and 5, so the correct IUPAC name is 2,5-dimethylheptane. Choice (C) is incorrect because the position numbers of the substituents are not minimized.

2. The structure of 5-ethyl-2,2-dimethyloctane is shown below.

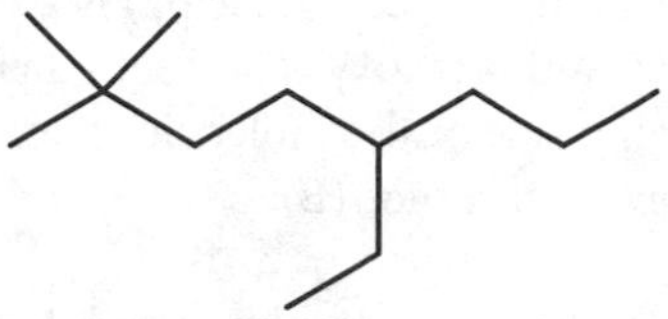

3. **D** Substituted cycloalkanes are named as derivatives of their parent cycloalkane, which in this case is cyclohexane. Thus, choice (A) can be ruled out immediately. Then, the substituents are listed in alphabetical order, and the carbons are numbered so as to give the lowest sum of substituent numbers. This cyclohexane has an ethyl and two methyl substituents; it is therefore an ethyl dimethyl cyclohexane. All the remaining answer choices recognize this; they only differ in the numbers assigned. In order to give the lowest sum of substituent numbers, the two methyl substituents must be numbered 1 and 2, and the ethyl substituent must be numbered 4. The correct name for this compound is thus 4-ethyl-1,2-dimethylcyclohexane.

4. **C** This question requires the application of the same set of rules laid out in Question 1. The longest backbone has nine carbons, so the compound is a nonane. Thus, choices (A) and (B) can be ruled out immediately. The substituent groups are, in alphabetical order: bromo, chloro, iodo, methyl, and propyl; these substituents must be given the lowest possible number on the hydrocarbon backbone. The resulting name is 2-bromo-4,4-dichloro-3-iodo-3-methyl-5-propylnonane.

5. **A** The first step is to locate the longest carbon chain containing the functional groups (C=C and OH). The backbone has six carbons (hex-). Since the alcohol group has higher priority than the double bond, it dictates the ending (-ol) and is given the lower position (2). The alkene is named according to the position of the double bond followed by -ene (4-hexene). Thus, the chain is called 4-hexene-2-ol. The substituents on the backbone are an ethyl group and an alkene group on C–3 and C–4, respectively. Since these constituents lie on opposite sides of the double bond, the molecule is *trans*. Therefore, this compound is called *trans*-3-ethyl-4-hexen-2-ol.

6. Numbering the carbons on the backbone from left to right, C–2 and C–4 are α carbons, C–1 and C–5 are β carbons, C–6 is a γ carbon, and C–7 is a δ carbon. This nomenclature is used to specify how far a given carbon in the backbone is from a reactive center, usually a carbonyl carbon.

7.   Treating this alkene with hydrogen in the presence of a platinum catalyst will cause hydrogen atoms to be added across the double bond. The product will be 3,5-dimethyloctane, shown below.

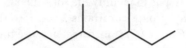

8. **B** A cyclopentane is a cyclic alkane with five carbons. A *cis* cyclic compound has both of its substituents on the same side of the ring. Only choices (B) and (C) have two substituents, so (A) and (D) can be ruled out. In fact, choice (C) is a *trans* compound, so the correct answer must be (B). Ethoxy and methoxy represent ether substituents, and they must be on adjacent carbons on the same side of the molecule. Thus, the structure of *cis*-1-ethoxy-2-methoxycyclopentane is given in choice (B).

9.   These structures both represent the same compound, 5-ethyl-3,5-dimethylnonane. The best way to see this is to name each one; this forces you to determine both the backbone and the substituents.

10.   A. 4

      B. 1

      C. 5

      D. 2

      E. 3

11. **D** Both aldehyde and carboxylic acid functional groups are located on the terminal ends of carbon backbones. As a result, the carbon to which they are attached is named C–1, and choice (D) is correct. Ketones are always internal to the carbon chain.

CHAPTER FORTY

Isomers

Isomers are chemical compounds that have the same molecular formula but differ in structure—that is, in their atomic connectivity or the spatial orientation of their atoms. Isomers may be similar, sharing most or all of their physical and chemical properties, or they may be very different.

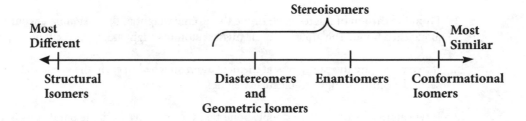

Figure 40.1

STRUCTURAL ISOMERISM

Structural isomers, also known as constitutional isomers, are compounds that share only a molecular formula. Structural isomers differ in where and how atoms are connected to each other and thus often have very different chemical and physical properties (such as melting point, boiling point, and solubility). For example, five different structures exist for compounds with the formula C_6H_{14}.

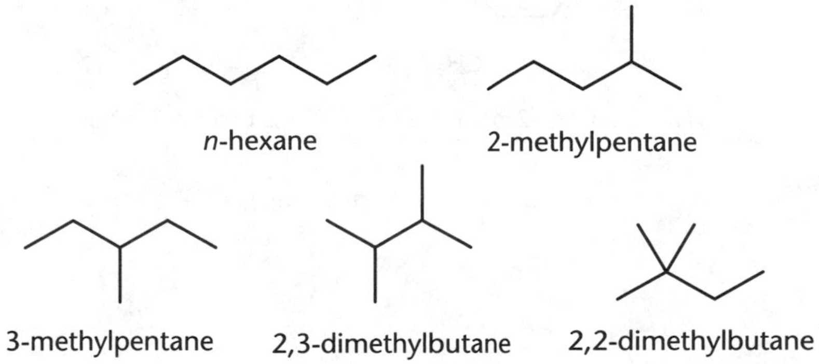

n-hexane   2-methylpentane

3-methylpentane   2,3-dimethylbutane   2,2-dimethylbutane

Figure 40.2

All have the same formula, but they differ in their carbon framework and in the number and type of atoms bonded to one another.

STEREOISOMERISM

Stereoisomers are compounds that have the same connectivity between their atoms and differ from each other only in the way that their atoms are oriented in space. *Cis-trans* isomers, enantiomers, diastereomers, *meso* compounds, and conformational isomers are all types of stereoisomers.

Cis-Trans Isomers

Cis-trans isomers, formerly known as **geometric isomers**, are compounds that differ in the position of substituents attached to the two carbons that form a double bond. Because a double bond cannot rotate, the substituents are fixed relative to one another and to the bond. If the substituents on the carbons are both above the double bond, they are on the same side, and the double bond is called *cis*. If one is above and one below, they are on opposite sides, and it is called a *trans* double bond.

For compounds with more than one substituent on either carbon of the double bond, an alternative method of naming applies. The highest priority substituent attached to each double bonded carbon has to be determined:

1. From the carbon of interest, determine the atomic weight of the first *atom* encountered along each bond. The group with the highest atomic weight atom has the highest priority.

2. If two atoms are the same, look at the next atom attached to each; the group that has the second atom with higher molecular weight is higher priority.

3. If two atoms are the same, a double bond takes priority over a single bond. This is a tie-breaker only; higher atomic weight will always take priory over a double bond.

The alkene is called (*Z*) (from German *zusammen*, meaning together) if the two highest priority substituents on each carbon are both above or both below the double bond or (*E*) (from German *entgegen*, meaning opposite) if they are on opposite sides. A simple mnemonic is that (*Z*) isomers are on "ze zame zide" of the double bond, while (*E*) isomers are "epposite."

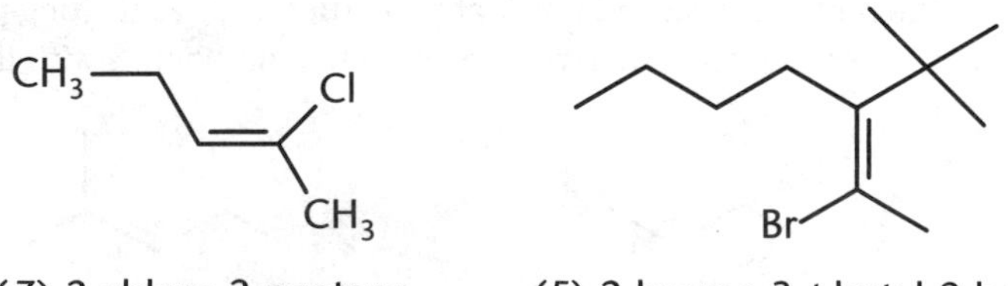

(*Z*)-2-chloro-2-pentene   (*E*)-2-bromo-3-*t*-butyl-2-heptene

Figure 40.3

Enantiomers and Chirality

A molecule that is not superimposable upon its mirror image is called **chiral**. Your right and left hands are illustrations of chirality. Although essentially identical, your hands differ in their ability to fit into a right-handed glove. They are mirror images of each other yet cannot be superimposed. **Achiral** molecules are mirror images that can be superimposed; for example, the letter A is identical to its mirror image and therefore is achiral.

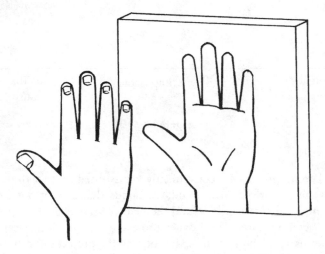

Figure 40.4

Carbon atoms are chiral only if they have four different substituents. Such a carbon atom is called **asymmetric** because it lacks a plane or point of symmetry. For example, the C−1 carbon atom in 1-bromo-1-chloroethane has four different substituents. The molecule is chiral because it is not superimposable on its mirror image. Pairs of chiral molecules that are nonsuperimposable mirror images are called **enantiomers** and are a specific type of stereoisomer discussed later in this chapter.

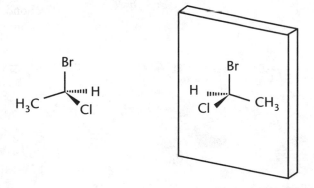

Figure 40.5

A carbon atom with only three different substituents, such as 1,1-dibromoethane, has a plane of symmetry and is therefore achiral. A simple 180° rotation along the *y*-axis allows the compound to be superimposed upon its mirror image.

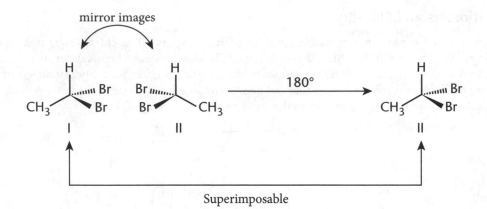

Figure 40.6

Fischer projections

A three-dimensional molecule can be conveniently represented in two dimensions in a **Fischer projection**. In this system, horizontal lines indicate bonds that project out from the plane of the page, while vertical lines indicate bonds behind the plane of the page. The point of intersection of the lines represents a carbon atom. The Fischer projection of a molecule can be manipulated by interchanging any two pairs of substituents or by rotating the projection in the plane of the page by 180°, and it will keep the same absolute configuration. If only one pair of substituents is interchanged or if the molecule is rotated by 90°, the mirror image and thus the opposite enantiomer of the original compound is obtained.

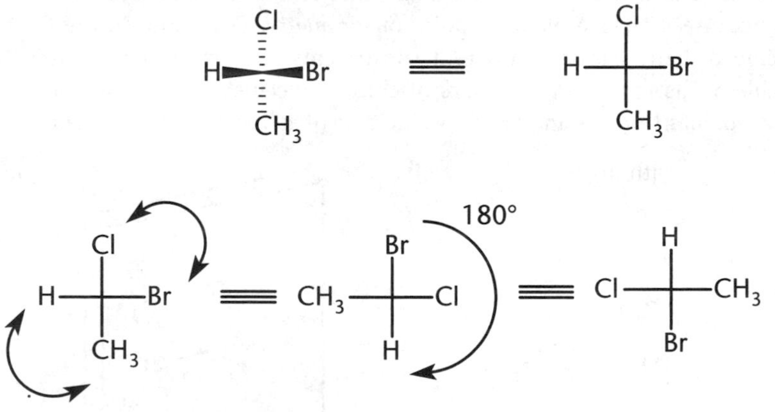

Figure 40.7

Fischer projections allow straightforward determination of the configuration at a chiral center, discussed next.

Relative and absolute configuration

A **configuration** describes the spatial arrangement of the atoms or functional groups of a stereoisomer. The **relative configuration** of a chiral molecule is its configuration in relation to another chiral molecule.

The **absolute configuration** of a chiral molecule describes the spatial arrangement of these atoms or groups within the molecule relative to each other. Absolute configuration is determined using the *R/S* naming convention, and relative configuration is compared between the *R* and the *S* enantiomers.

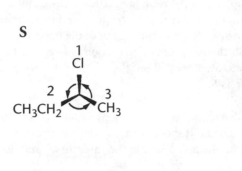 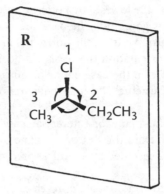

Figure 40.8

The set sequence to determine the absolute configuration of a molecule at a single chiral center is as follows:

Step 1:

Assign priority to the four substituents using the same rules as for *E/Z* isomers:

1. From the carbon of interest, determine the atomic weight of the first *atom* encountered along each bond. The group with the highest atomic weight atom has the highest priority.

2. If two atoms are the same, look at the next atom attached to each; the group that has the second atom with higher molecular weight is higher priority.

3. If two atoms are the same, a double bond takes priority over a single bond. This is a tie-breaker only; higher atomic weight will always take priority over a double bond.

For example:

Figure 40.9

Step 2:

Proceeding from highest priority (1st) to second lowest (3rd), determine the order of substituents around the wheel as either clockwise or counterclockwise by drawing a loop that connects 1st to 2nd to 3rd priority, ignoring the 4th group. If the order is clockwise, the chiral center temporarily is called

R (from Latin *rectus*, meaning right). If it is counterclockwise, it is temporarily called *S* (from Latin *sinister*, meaning left).

Step 3:

Finally, look at the lowest (4th) priority group. If group 4 is on the vertical line in a Fischer projection or otherwise is going into the page, the molecule is oriented correctly, and the designation remains the same. If group 4 is on the horizontal line or otherwise coming out of the page, the molecule is in the opposite orientation that it should be, so the temporary designation is swapped to the opposite designation (i.e., if the designation obtained in Step 2 was *R* but the 4th priority group is coming out of the page, the actual absolute configuration is *S*).

To provide a full name for a stereoisomer with a chiral center, the terms *R* and *S* are put in parentheses and separated from the rest of the name by a dash. If more than one asymmetric carbon is present, the location is specified by a number preceding the *R* or *S* within the parentheses and without a dash.

Note that in the traditional approach to determining chirality, the molecule initially must be rotated to place the lowest priority group pointing toward the back. However, this can be problematic as it is easy to lose track of the relative positions of the substituents during this step. The simpler Kaplan strategy, as described above, recognizes that if the lowest priority group is coming out of the page, it will appear the opposite of its true configuration, which avoids the difficult work of mentally rearranging the molecule.

Optical activity

Pairs of enantiomers (with opposite *R* and *S* designations) have identical chemical and physical properties with one exception: **optical activity**. A compound is optically active if it has the ability to rotate plane-polarized light. Ordinary light is unpolarized. It consists of waves vibrating in all possible planes perpendicular to its direction of motion. A polarizing filter allows light waves oscillating only in a particular direction to pass, producing plane-polarized light.

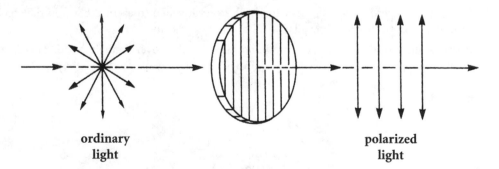

ordinary   **polarized**
light   **light**

Figure 40.10

If plane-polarized light is passed through a solution of an optically active compound, the molecule rotates the orientation of the polarized light by an angle α. The enantiomer of this compound will rotate light by the same amount, but in the opposite direction. A compound that rotates the plane-polarized light to the right, or clockwise (from the point of view of an observer seeing the light approach), is **dextrorotatory** and is indicated by (+). A compound that rotates light toward the left, or counterclockwise, is **levorotatory** and is labeled (−). The direction of rotation cannot be determined from the structure of a molecule and is not related to its *R* or *S* designation. Instead, it must be determined experimentally.

The amount of rotation depends on the number of molecules that a light wave encounters. This depends on two factors: the concentration of the optically active compound and the length of the tube through which the light passes. Chemists have set standard conditions of 1 g/mL for concentration and 1 dm for length in order to compare the optical activities of different compounds. Rotations measured at different concentrations and tube lengths can be converted to a standardized **specific rotation** (α) using the following equation:

$$\frac{\text{observed rotation}(\alpha)}{\text{concentration}(\text{g/ml}) \times \text{length}(\text{dm})}$$

A racemic mixture, or racemate, is a mixture of equal concentrations of both the $(+)$ and $(-)$ enantiomers. The rotations cancel each other, and no optical activity is observed.

Diastereomers

Many compounds have more than one chiral center, and thus multiple forms of stereoisomers exist for them. For any molecule with n chiral centers, there are 2^n possible stereoisomers. Thus, if a compound has two chiral carbon atoms, it has four possible stereoisomers (see Figure 40.11).

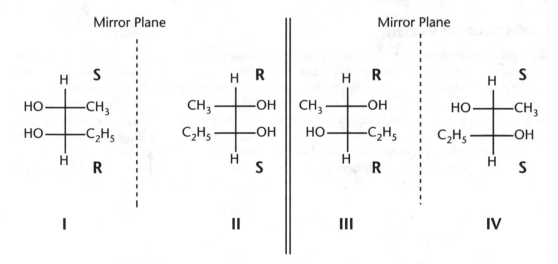

Figure 40.11

Compounds I and II are mirror images of each other and are therefore enantiomers. Similarly, compounds III and IV are enantiomers. However, compounds I and III are not. They are stereoisomers that are not mirror images, and so they are called diastereomers. Notice that other combinations of non–mirror image stereoisomers are also possible, and form diastereomer pairs. Hence compounds I and IV, compounds II and III, compounds I and III, and compounds II and IV are all pairs of diastereomers.

Diastereomers that differ at only one carbon make up special pairs called epimers, which are particularly important in the chemistry of carbohydrates.

Meso Compounds

Meso compounds are molecules with multiple chiral centers that also have an internal plane of symmetry. One half of the molecule has an *S* enantiomer, and the other half has its matching *R* enantiomer. If such a plane of symmetry exists, the molecule is not optically active, because the rotation of light by one chiral center is matched by the opposite rotation by the other chiral center. For example:

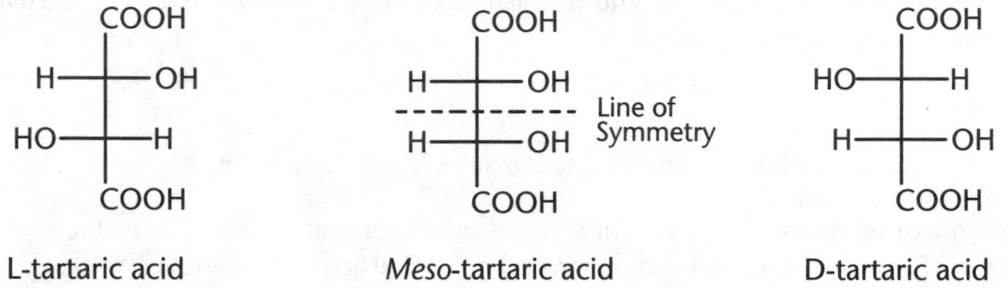

L-tartaric acid   *Meso*-tartaric acid   D-tartaric acid

Figure 40.12

D- and L-tartaric acid are both optically active, but *meso*-tartaric acid has a plane of symmetry and is not optically active. Although *meso*-tartaric acid has two chiral carbon atoms, the lack of optical activity is a function of the molecule as a whole.

Conformational Isomers

Conformational isomers are compounds that differ only by rotation about one or more single bonds. These isomers represent the same compound in a slightly different position—analogous to a person who may be either standing up or sitting down. These different conformations can be seen when the molecule is depicted in a **Newman projection**, in which the line of sight extends along a carbon-carbon bond axis. Because the view of the second carbon atom is blocked by the first, the second carbon is depicted as a large circle at the back, and the first carbon is depicted as the intersection of its three other bonds in front. The different conformations are encountered as the molecule is rotated about the axis between the two carbons. The classic example for demonstrating conformational isomerism in a straight chain molecule is *n*-butane. In a Newman projection, the line of sight extends through the C−2−C−3 bond axis.

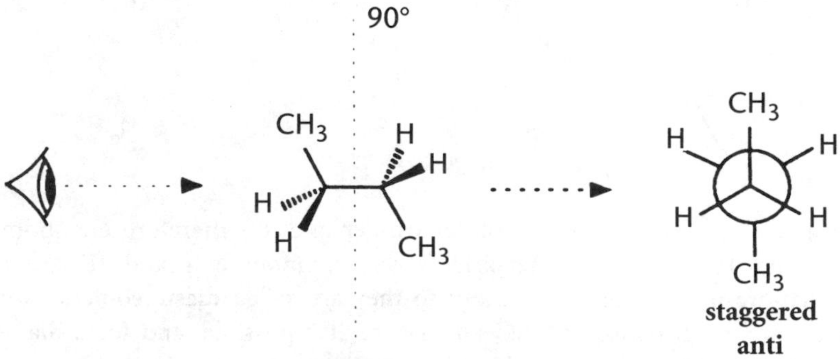

Figure 40.13

Straight-chain conformations

The most stable conformation of *n*-butane is found when the two methyl groups (C–1 and C–4) are oriented 180° from each other. There is no overlap of atoms along the line of sight (besides C–2 and C–3), so the molecule is said to be in a **staggered** conformation. Specifically, it is called the *anti* conformation, because the two methyl groups are antiperiplanar to each other. This particular orientation is very stable and thus represents an energy minimum because all atoms are far apart, minimizing repulsive steric interactions.

The other type of staggered conformation, called *gauche*, occurs when the two methyl groups are 60° apart. In order to convert from the *anti* to the *gauche* conformation, the molecule must pass through an eclipsed conformation, in which the two methyl groups are 120° apart and overlap with the H atoms on the adjacent carbon. When the two methyl groups overlap with each other, the molecule is said to be totally eclipsed and is in its highest energy state.

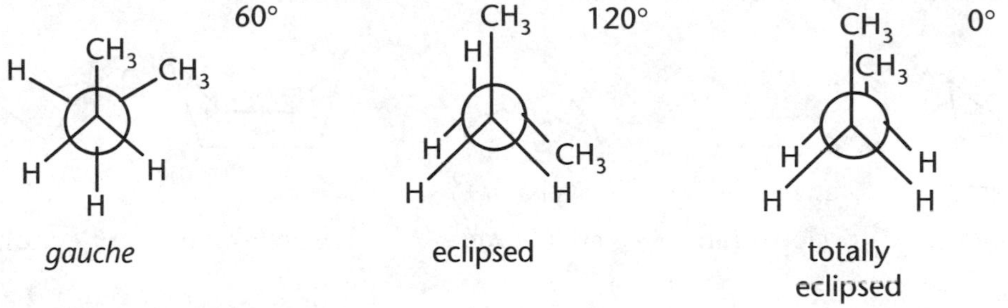

Figure 40.14

A plot of potential energy versus the degree of rotation about the C–2-C–3 bond shows the relative minima and maxima the molecule encounters throughout its various conformations.

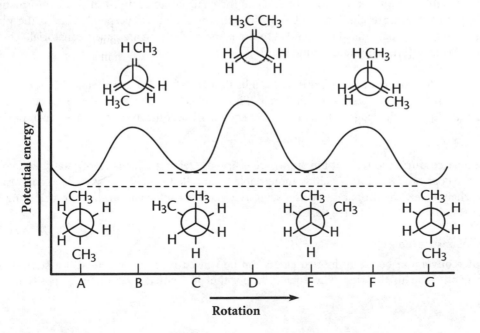

Figure 40.15

It is important to note that these barriers are rather small (3–4 kcal/mol) and are easily overcome at room temperature, when the molecule is rotating freely. Very low temperatures will slow conformational interconversion. If the molecules do not possess sufficient energy to cross the energy barrier, they may not rotate at all.

Cyclic conformations

In cycloalkanes, ring strain arises from three factors: angle strain, torsional strain, and nonbonded strain. Angle strain results when bond angles deviate from their ideal values (109.5° for sp³ hybridized carbons); torsional strain results when cyclic molecules must assume conformations that have eclipsed interactions; and nonbonded strain (van der Waals repulsion) results when atoms or groups compete for the same space. In order to alleviate these three types of strain, cycloalkanes attempt to adopt nonplanar conformations. Cyclobutane puckers into a slight V shape, cyclopentane adopts what is called the **envelope** conformation, and cyclohexane exists mainly in three conformations called the **chair,** the **boat,** and the **twist** or **skew-boat.**

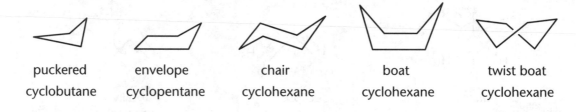

puckered cyclobutane envelope cyclopentane chair cyclohexane boat cyclohexane twist boat cyclohexane

Figure 40.16

Cyclohexane

i. Unsubstituted

The most stable conformation of cyclohexane is the chair conformation. In this conformation, all three types of strain are eliminated. The hydrogen atoms that are perpendicular to the plane of the ring are called axial, and those parallel to the plane of the ring are called equatorial. The axial-equatorial orientations alternate around the ring.

The chair conformation has two forms that can be thought of as "left facing" and "right facing." The boat conformation is adopted when the chair "flips" and converts to the other chair conformation. When this happens, hydrogen atoms that were equatorial become axial, and vice versa, in the new chair.

In the boat conformation, all of the atoms are eclipsed, creating a high-energy state. To avoid this strain, the boat can twist into a slightly more stable form called the twist or skew-boat conformation. In the chair form, the atoms are in the staggered gauche conformation, thus contributing to the greater stability compared to the boat form.

ii. Monosubstituted

The interconversion between the two chairs can be slowed or even prevented if a sterically bulky group is attached to the ring. The equatorial position is favored over the axial position because of steric repulsion with other axial substituents. Hence, a large group such as *t*-butyl can lock the molecule in one conformation.

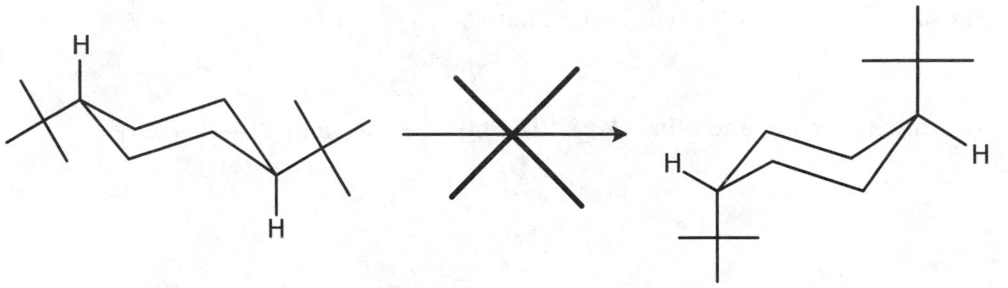

Bulky groups prefer equatorial positions

Figure 40.17

iii. Disubstituted

Different isomers can exist for disubstituted cycloalkanes. If both substituents are located on the same side of the ring, the molecule is called *cis*; if the two groups are on opposite sides of the ring, it is called *trans*.

cis-1,2-dimethylcyclohexane   trans-1,2-dimethylcyclohexane

Figure 40.18

Note that the chair form shows that equatorial constituents can be either above or below the plane of the ring, shown by the "slant" of the bond connecting them to their ring carbons. For example, in *trans*-1,4-dimethylcyclohexane, both of the methyl groups are equatorial in one chair conformation and axial in the other, but in either case they point in opposite directions relative to the plane of the ring.

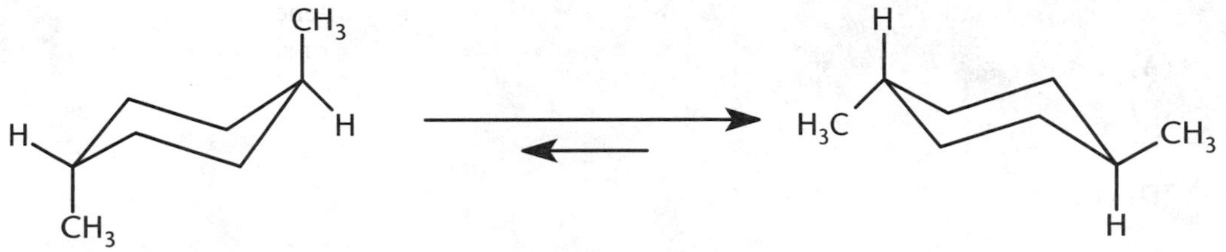

trans-1,4-dimethylcyclohexane

Figure 40.19

REVIEW PROBLEMS

1. Categorize the following pairs as enantiomers, diastereomers, structural isomers, molecules of the same compound, or different compounds.

   (A) dimethyl ether and ethanol

   (B) 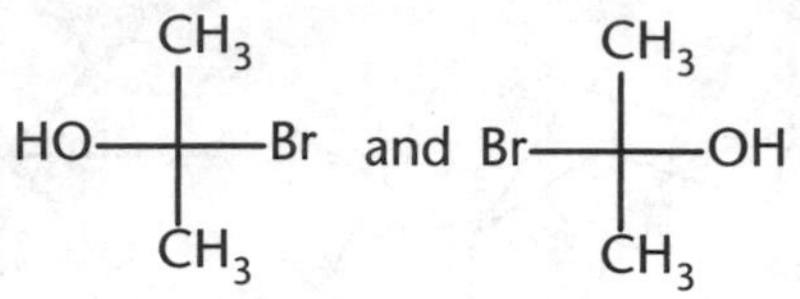 $HO-\overset{\overset{\displaystyle CH_3}{|}}{\underset{\underset{\displaystyle CH_3}{|}}{C}}-Br$ and $Br-\overset{\overset{\displaystyle CH_3}{|}}{\underset{\underset{\displaystyle CH_3}{|}}{C}}-OH$

   (C) $H-\overset{\overset{\displaystyle CH_3}{|}}{\underset{\underset{\displaystyle Cl}{|}}{C}}-Br$ and $H-\overset{\overset{\displaystyle CH_3}{|}}{\underset{\underset{\displaystyle Br}{|}}{C}}-Cl$

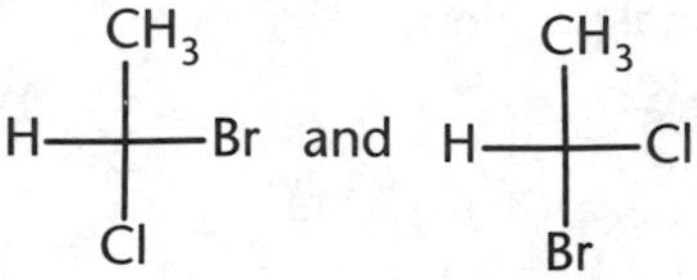

   (D) 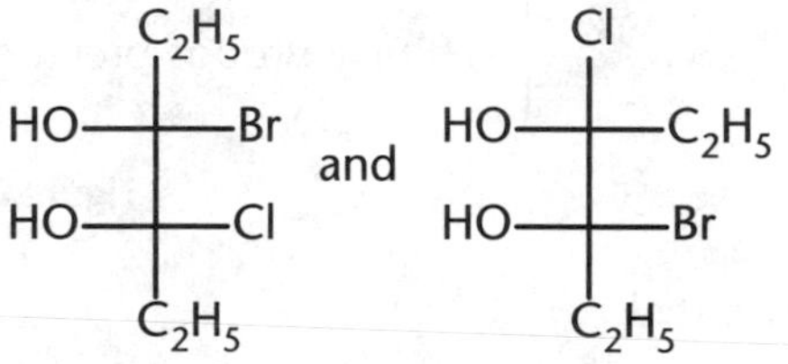 $HO-\overset{\overset{\displaystyle C_2H_5}{|}}{C}-Br$ $HO-\underset{\underset{\displaystyle C_2H_5}{|}}{C}-Cl$ and $HO-\overset{\overset{\displaystyle Cl}{|}}{C}-C_2H_5$ $HO-\underset{\underset{\displaystyle C_2H_5}{|}}{C}-Br$

2. Which of the following will NOT show optical activity?

   (A) (R)-2-butanol
   (B) (S)-2-butanol
   (C) A solution containing 1 M (R)-2-butanol and 2 M (S)-2-butanol
   (D) A solution containing 2 M (R)-2-butanol and 2 M (S)-2-butanol

3. How many stereoisomers exist for the following aldehyde?

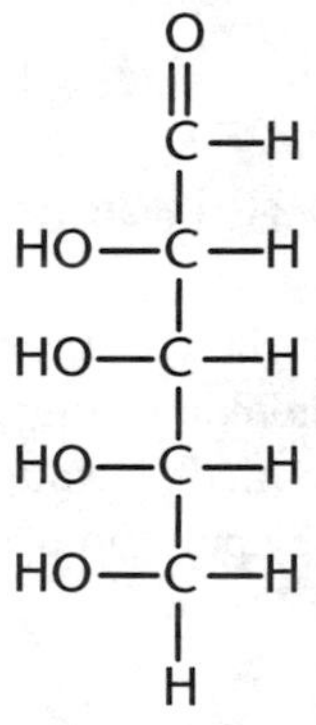

   $$\begin{array}{c} O \\ \| \\ C-H \\ | \\ HO-C-H \\ | \\ HO-C-H \\ | \\ HO-C-H \\ | \\ HO-C-H \\ | \\ H \end{array}$$

   (A) 2
   (B) 4
   (C) 8
   (D) 16

4. Which of the following compounds is optically inactive?

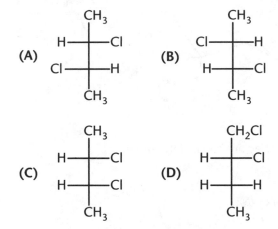

5. Which isomer of 2-pentene is more stable, the *cis* isomer or the *trans* isomer?

6. Assign (*R*) and (*S*) designations to the following compounds:

(A)

(B)

7. Cholesterol, shown below, contains how many chiral centers?

(A) 5
(B) 7
(C) 8
(D) 9

8. Which isomer of the following compound is the most stable?

(A)

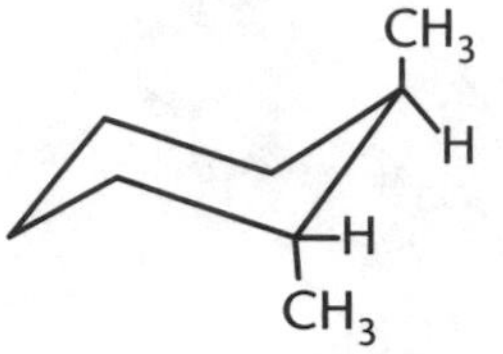

(B)

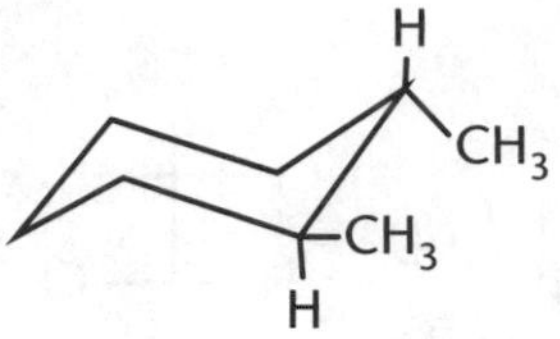

(C)

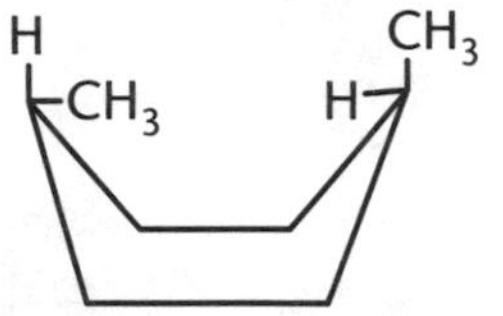

(D) They are all equally stable.

9. Designate the following compounds as (R) or (S):

(A) 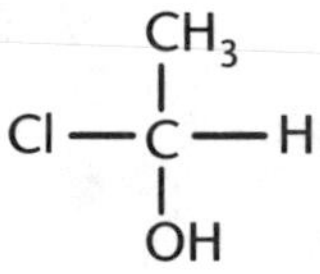 $Cl-\underset{\underset{OH}{|}}{\overset{\overset{CH_3}{|}}{C}}-H$

(B) $HO_2C-\underset{\underset{CH_3}{|}}{\overset{\overset{H}{|}}{C}}-CH_2CH_3$

(C) $HO-\underset{\underset{F}{|}}{\overset{\overset{Br}{|}}{C}}-Cl$

(D) $H-\underset{\underset{C(CH_3)_3}{|}}{\overset{\overset{HC=CH_2}{|}}{C}}-CH_2CH_3$

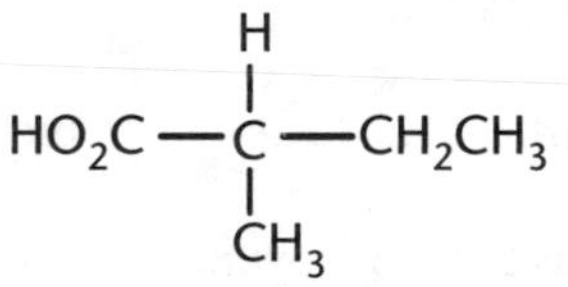

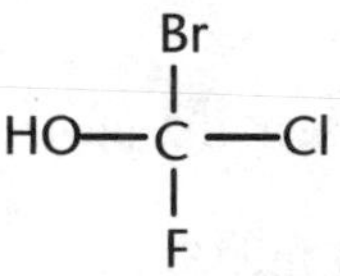

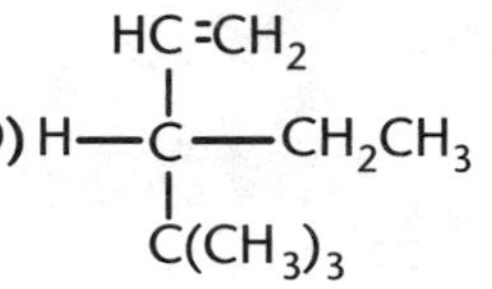

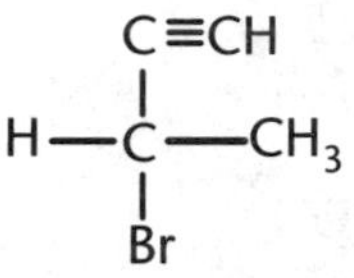

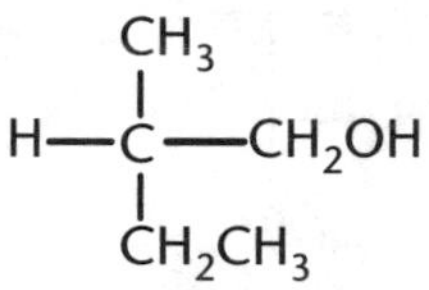

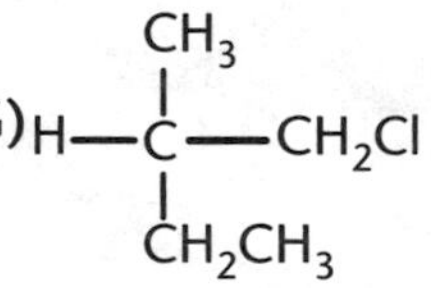

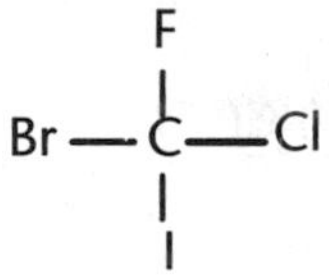

(E) $H-\underset{\underset{Br}{|}}{\overset{\overset{C\equiv CH}{|}}{C}}-CH_3$

(F) $H-\underset{\underset{CH_2CH_3}{|}}{\overset{\overset{CH_3}{|}}{C}}-CH_2OH$

(G) $H-\underset{\underset{CH_2CH_3}{|}}{\overset{\overset{CH_3}{|}}{C}}-CH_2Cl$

(H) $Br-\underset{\underset{I}{|}}{\overset{\overset{F}{|}}{C}}-Cl$

(I) $H_3C-\underset{\underset{OH}{|}}{\overset{\overset{NH_2}{|}}{C}}-Br$

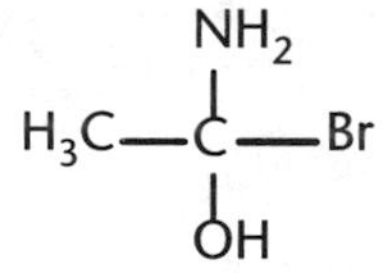

10. The following reaction results in:

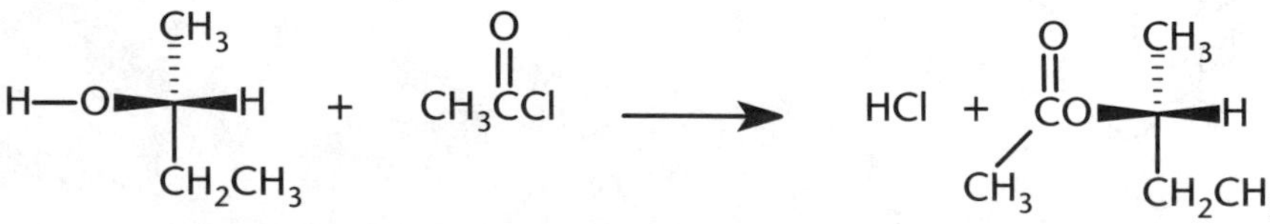

$$H-O{-}\overset{\overset{CH_3}{\vdots}}{\underset{\underset{CH_2CH_3}{|}}{C}}{-}H \ + \ CH_3\overset{\overset{O}{||}}{C}Cl \longrightarrow HCl \ + \ \overset{\overset{O}{||}}{C}O{-}\overset{\overset{CH_3}{\vdots}}{\underset{\underset{CH_2CH_3}{|}}{C}}{-}H$$

(A) retention of relative configuration and a change in the absolute configuration.

(B) a change in the relative and absolute configurations.

(C) retention of the relative and absolute configurations.

(D) retention of the absolute configuration and a change in the relative configuration.

11. The following structures are:

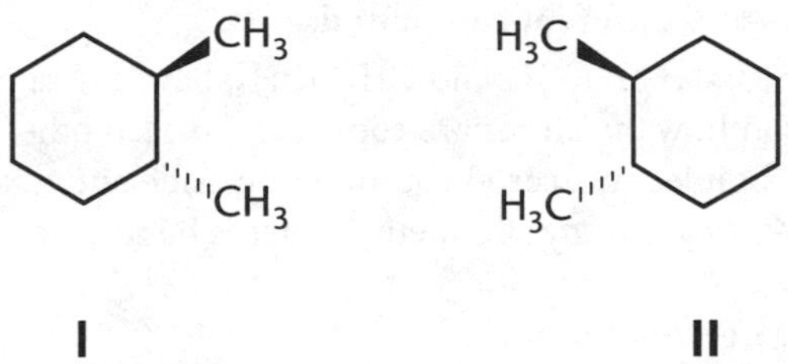

I   II

(A) enantiomers.
(B) diastereomers.
(C) *meso* compounds.
(D) structural isomers.

12. MSG ([S]-monosodium glutamate) is a compound widely used as a flavor enhancer. MSG has the following structure:

Na^+ $^-O_2CH_2CH_2C$ with H, NH_2, COH (=O)

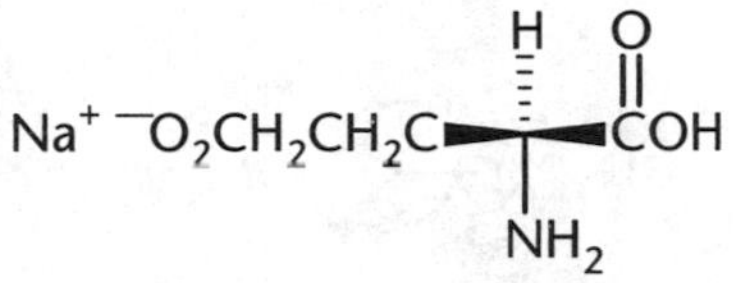

(S)-MSG

This enantiomer of MSG has a specific rotation of +24°. In a racemic mixture of MSG, what would be the specific rotation? What is the specific rotation of (R)-monosodium glutamate?

SOLUTIONS TO REVIEW PROBLEMS

1. **A   Structural isomers and different compounds**

    The two compounds, CH_3CH_2OH and CH_3OCH_3, have the same molecular formula, C_2H_6O, but differ in how the atoms are connected to each other. For instance, the oxygen atom of ethanol is bonded to a carbon atom on one side and to a hydrogen atom on the other, whereas the oxygen atom of dimethyl ether is bonded to carbon atoms on both sides.

    B   Molecules of the same compound

    The two structures are achiral. Rotating one gives the other.

    Also note that, in order for a compound to be chiral, at least one of its carbons must be bonded to four different substituents. In both of these compounds, all the carbons are attached to two identical groups, so the compounds are achiral.

    C.   Enantiomers

    These two compounds look alike, but the Cl and the Br have been interchanged. You may remember that one exchange of two substituents produces the mirror image of the original compound. Thus, these two molecules are enantiomers.

    Another way to solve this problem is to remember that, according to the rules governing Fischer projections, interchanging two pairs of substituents in a compound will give the original compound. Interchanging two pairs of substituents in the compound on the right in pair (C), as shown below, allows you to see that the two compounds of pair (C) are mirror images of each other; hence, they are enantiomers.

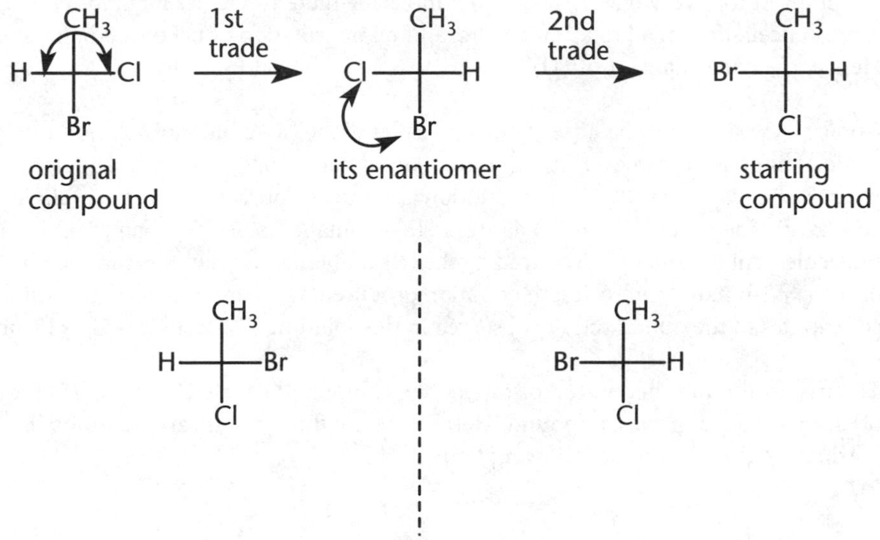

D. Diastereomers

Rotate the second compound in the plane of the paper by 180°. The two compounds now are:

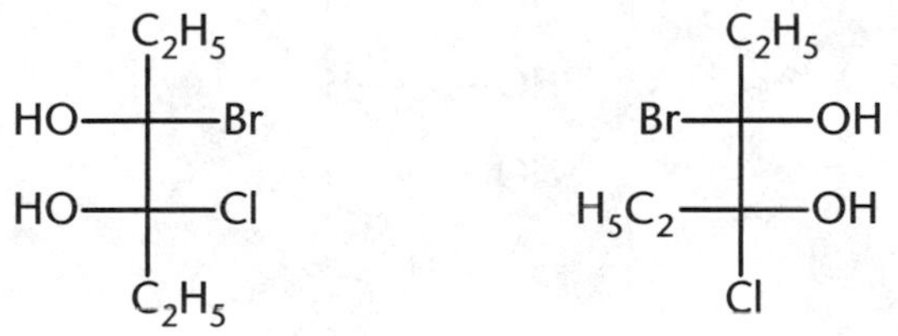

Assign (*R*) and (*S*) designations to the compounds:

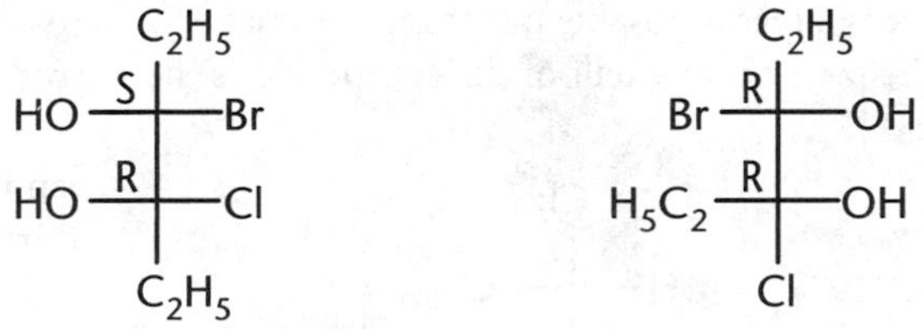

The above figure shows that one compound is an *S*, *R* stereoisomer and the other is an *R*, *R* stereoisomer; hence, they are diastereomers.

2. **D** A racemic mixture of 2-butanol consists of equimolar amounts of (R)-2-butanol and (S)-2-butanol. The (R)-2-butanol molecule rotates the plane of polarized light in one direction, and the (S)-2-butanol molecule rotates it by the same angle but in the opposite direction. If for every one (R)-2-butanol molecule there is one (S)-2 butanol molecule, exact cancellation of all rotation occurs, and no net rotation of polarized light is observed. Hence, the correct answer is (D).

Choice (A) is incorrect because all the molecules of the (R)-2-butanol solution rotate the plane of light in the same direction, so rotations do not cancel, and optical activity is observed. In the same way, the (S)-2-butanol solution also shows optical activity. Thus, choices (A) and (B) are incorrect. Choice (C) has more (S)-2-butanol molecules than (R)-2-butanol molecules. All the rotation produced by the (R)-2-butanol molecules is canceled by half of the (S)-2-butanol molecules; the rotation produced by the other half of (S)-2-molecules contributes to the optical activity observed in this solution. Thus, choice (C) is incorrect.

3. **C** The maximum number of stereoisomers of a compound equals 2^n, where n is the number of chiral carbons in the compound. Here, there are three chiral carbon atoms ($n = 3$) marked by asterisks in the following figure:

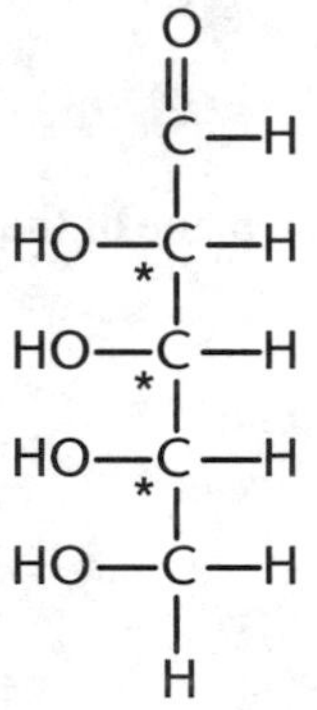

$$
\begin{array}{c}
\text{O} \\
\parallel \\
\text{C—H} \\
| \\
\text{HO—}\overset{*}{\text{C}}\text{—H} \\
| \\
\text{HO—}\overset{*}{\text{C}}\text{—H} \\
| \\
\text{HO—}\overset{*}{\text{C}}\text{—H} \\
| \\
\text{HO—C—H} \\
| \\
\text{H}
\end{array}
$$

So the number of stereoisomers it can form is $2^n = 2^3 = 8$. Hence, the correct choice is (C).

4. **C** The correct answer choice is an example of a *meso* compound: a compound that contains chiral centers but is superimposable on its mirror image. A *meso* compound can also be recognized by the fact that one half of the compound is the mirror image of the other half:

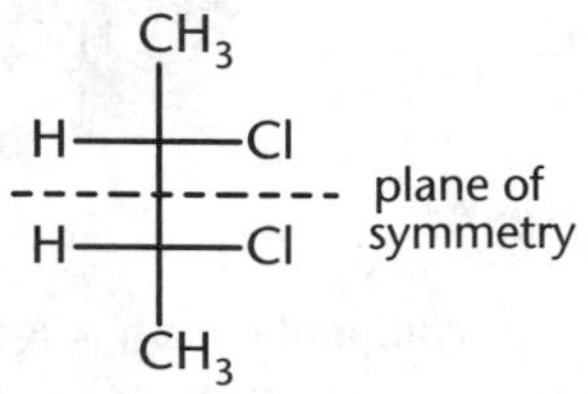

$$
\begin{array}{c}
\text{CH}_3 \\
| \\
\text{H—}\!\!\!\!-\!\!\!\!-\text{Cl} \\
\text{- - - - - - -} \quad \text{plane of} \\
\text{H—}\!\!\!\!-\!\!\!\!-\text{Cl} \quad \text{symmetry} \\
| \\
\text{CH}_3
\end{array}
$$

As a result of this internal plane of symmetry, the molecule is achiral and hence optically inactive. Choices (A) and (B) are enantiomers of each other and will certainly show optical activity on their own. Choice (D), since it contains a chiral carbon, is optically active as well.

5. The *trans* isomer of 2-pentene is the most stable. When you draw out this isomer, you can see that one side of the double bond has a methyl group and a hydrogen, and the other side has an ethyl group and a hydrogen. In this configuration, the van der Waals repulsion (nonbonding interaction) between the methyl and the ethyl groups is minimized. If these groups were oriented *cis* to each other (on the same side of the double bond), the van der Waals repulsion would be maximized.

trans   cis

6. A **(*R*)-2-bromo-1,1-dichloropropane**

In the above compound, C–1 is not chiral because it has two C–l atoms bound to it. Only C–2 is chiral, so the molecule is designated as (*R*) or (*S*) with respect to only C–2. Assign priority numbers to the atoms connected directly to C–2. The atom with the highest atomic number is given priority 1, followed by the atom with next highest atomic number, which is given the priority number 2, and so on. In this compound, Br has the highest atomic number and so is assigned priority 1. Next come two carbon atoms connected to the chiral carbon. Since these have the same atomic number, you must consider their substituents. C–1 has two Cl atoms and one hydrogen, whereas C–3 has three hydrogen. Since chlorine has a higher atomic number than hydrogen, C–1 is the higher priority. Thus, C–1 is 2 and C–3 is 3. The hydrogen is the lowest priority, 4.

Draw a curved arrow from $1 \rightarrow 2 \rightarrow 3$. The direction of the arrow is counterclockwise, so the molecule is temporarily designated (*S*). Finally, check the orientation of group 4, which in this case is coming out of the page, which is the opposite way it should be; thus the (*S*) should be swapped to the (*R*) designation.

B   **(*R*)-2,3-dihydroxypropanal**

For the purposes of prioritization, double- or triple-bonded atoms are considered to be linked by multiple single bonds. For instance, in $-C=O$, C would be considered to have two single bonds with O, and O would be considered to have two single bonds with carbon. In this question, $-OH$ is assigned the highest priority, 1; $-C=O$ (here considered to be two $-C-O$) is assigned the next priority, 2; $-CH_2OH$ is assigned priority 3; and hydrogen, with the lowest atomic number, is assigned the lowest priority, 4. The direction of the curved arrow from $1 \rightarrow 2 \rightarrow 3$ is clockwise, and the molecule is designated (*R*).

7.   C   To be a chiral center, a carbon must have four different substituents. There are eight stereocenters in this molecule, marked below with asterisks.

CHOLESTEROL

The other carbons are not chiral, for various reasons. Many are bonded to two hydrogen; others participate in double bonds, which count as two bonds to the same thing (another C atom).

8. **B** This is a chair conformation in which the two equatorial methyl groups are *trans* to each other. Since the methyl hydrogens do not compete for the same space as the (unshown) hydrogens attached to the ring, this conformation ensures the least amount of steric strain. Choice (A) would be more unstable than choice (B) since the diaxial methyl group hydrogens are closer to the hydrogens on the ring, causing greater steric strain. Choice (C) is incorrect because it is in the more unstable boat conformation. Choice (D) is incorrect because these are all different structures with different stabilities.

9.

10. **C** The relative configuration is retained because the bonds between the chiral carbon and its substituents are not broken. The bond that is cleaved is one between a substituent of the chiral carbon (the O atom) and another atom attached to the substituent (the H attached to the O). The absolute configuration is also retained because the (R)/(S) designation is the same for the reactant and the product.

11. **A** Compared side by side, the two structures are mirror images of each other. Rotating one of the structures by 180° (structure III) shows that structures I and III are nonsuperimposable.

Choice (B) is incorrect because diastereomers are stereoisomers that are not mirror images of each other. Choice (C) is incorrect because, in order for a compound to be designated as a *meso* compound, it must have a plane of symmetry, which neither of these structures contains. Choice (D) is incorrect because structural isomers are compounds with the same molecular formula but different connectivity. These compounds do have the same connectivity. The only difference is that they do not have the same spatial arrangement of atoms. As a result, they are stereoisomers, not structural isomers.

12. The specific rotation of a racemic mixture of MSG, or any other racemic mixture, is zero. A racemic mixture by definition is a mixture that contains equal amounts of the (+) and (−) enantiomers, which cancel each other's optical rotations. The specific rotation of (*R*)-monosodium glutamate is −24°. An enantiomer of a chiral compound rotates plane-polarized light by the same amount but in the opposite direction.

CHAPTER FORTY-ONE

Bonding

As discussed in general chemistry, there are two types of chemical bonds: **ionic**, in which an electron is transferred from one atom to another, and **covalent**, in which pairs of electrons are shared between two atoms. In organic chemistry, it is important to understand the details of covalent bonding, as these play a crucial role in determining the properties and reactions of organic compounds.

ATOMIC ORBITALS

The first three quantum numbers, n, l, and m, describe the size, shape, and number of the atomic orbitals an element possesses. The quantum number n corresponds to the energy levels in an atom and is essentially a measure of size. Within each electron shell, there can be several types of orbitals (s, p, d, and f, corresponding to the quantum numbers $l = 0$, 1, 2, 3, and 4). Each type of atomic orbital has a specific shape. An s orbital is spherical and symmetrical, centered around the nucleus. A p orbital is composed of two lobes located symmetrically about the nucleus and contains a **node** (an area where the probability of finding an electron is zero). A d orbital is composed of four symmetrical lobes and contains two nodes. Both d and f orbitals are complex in shape and are rarely encountered in organic chemistry.

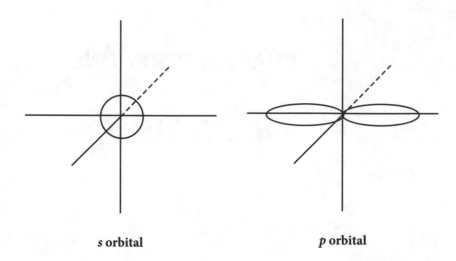

s orbital   *p* orbital

Figure 41.1

MOLECULAR ORBITALS

Single Bonds

Two atomic orbitals can be combined to form a **molecular orbital**. Molecular orbitals are obtained mathematically by adding the wave functions of the atomic orbitals. If the signs of the wave functions are the same, a lower-energy **bonding orbital** is produced. If the signs are different, a higher-energy **antibonding orbital** is produced. Figure 41.2 below shows examples of combining two s orbitals in both bonding and antibonding orbitals as well as the bonding orbitals formed from an s orbital and p orbital and from two p orbitals.

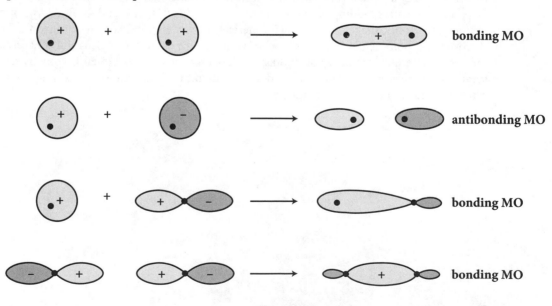

Figure 41.2

When a molecular orbital is formed by head-to-head overlap, the resulting bond is called a **sigma (σ) bond**. All single bonds are sigma bonds and contain two electrons. Shorter single bonds are stronger than longer single bonds.

Double and Triple Bonds

When two p orbitals overlap in a parallel fashion, a bonding MO is formed, called a **pi (π) bond**. When both a sigma and a pi bond exist between two atoms, a **double bond** is formed. When a sigma bond and two pi bonds exist, a **triple bond** is formed. As can be seen in Figure 41.3, the overlap of the p orbitals involved in a pi bond prevents rotation about double and triple bonds. Pi bonds contain two electrons each.

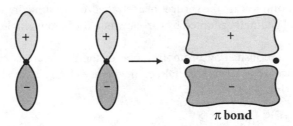

π bond

Figure 41.3

A pi bond cannot exist independently of a sigma bond. The formation of the sigma bond between two atoms orients their p orbitals to overlap from side to side, allowing the pi bond to form. In general, pi bonds are weaker than sigma bonds. It is possible to break the pi bond of a double bond but leave the sigma bond intact; however, the sigma bond cannot be broken unless the pi bond is broken first.

HYBRIDIZATION

Carbon has the electronic configuration $1s^2 2s^2 2p^2$ with 4 valence electrons; it therefore needs four additional electrons to complete its octet. A typical carbon-containing molecule is methane, CH_4. Experimentation shows that the four sigma bonds in methane are equal. This is inconsistent with the asymmetrical distribution of valence electrons: two electrons in the 2s orbital, one in the p_x orbital, one in the p_y orbital, and none in the p_z orbital. The theory of **orbital hybridization** was developed to account for this discrepancy.

sp^3

Hybrid orbitals are formed by mixing different types of atomic orbitals. If one s orbital and three p orbitals are mathematically combined, the result is four identical sp^3 hybrid orbitals that have a new shape.

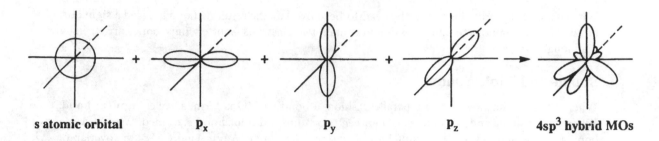

| s atomic orbital | P_x | P_y | P_z | 4sp³ hybrid MOs |

Figure 41.4

These four orbitals will point toward the vertices of a tetrahedron, minimizing repulsion. This explains the preferred tetrahedral geometry adopted by carbon when it has four single bonds to other atoms.

The hybridization is accomplished by promoting one of the 2s electrons into the $2p_z$ orbital (see Figure 41.5). This produces four valence orbitals, each with one electron, which can be mathematically mixed to create the hybrids.

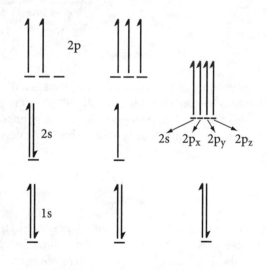

unhybridized ground state | unhybridized excited state | hybridized ground state

Figure 41.5

sp²

Although carbon is often found bonded to four other atoms with sp³ hybridization, there are other possibilities. If one s orbital and two p orbitals are mixed, three identical sp² hybrid orbitals are obtained.

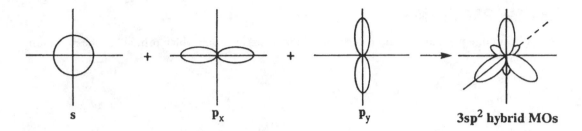

Figure 41.6

For example, this occurs in ethylene. The third p orbital of each carbon atom is left unhybridized and participates in the pi bond. The three sp² orbitals are 120° apart, allowing maximum separation. These orbitals participate in the formation of the C=C and C−H sigma bonds.

sp

If two p orbitals are used to form the pi bonds of a triple bond and the remaining p orbital is mixed with an s orbital, two identical sp hybrid orbitals are obtained. The remaining two p orbitals of each carbon atom are left unhybridized and participate in creating two pi bonds, resulting in a triple bond. The two sp hybrid orbitals are oriented 180° apart, explaining the linear structure of molecules such as acetylene.

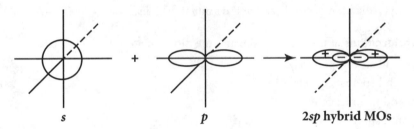

Figure 41.7

BONDING SUMMARY

The following table summarizes the major features of bonding orbitals in organic molecules.

Bond Order	Component Bonds	Hybridization	Angles	Examples
single	sigma	sp³	109.5°	C−C; C−H
double	sigma pi	sp²	120°	C=C; C=O
triple	sigma pi pi	sp	180°	C≡C; C≡N

Table 41.1

REVIEW PROBLEMS

1. Within one principal quantum level of a many-electron atom, which orbital has the minimum energy?

    (A) s
    (B) p
    (C) d
    (D) f

2. Which of the following compounds possesses at least one σ bond?

    (A) CH_4
    (B) C_2H_2
    (C) C_2H_4
    (D) All of the above

3. In a double-bonded carbon atom

    (A) hybridization between the s orbital and one p orbital occurs.
    (B) hybridization between the s orbital and two p orbitals occurs.
    (C) hybridization between the s orbital and three p orbitals occurs.
    (D) no hybridization occurs between the s and p orbitals.

4. The hybridizations of the carbon atom and the nitrogen atom in the ion CN^- are

    (A) sp^3 and sp^3, respectively.
    (B) sp^3 and sp, respectively.
    (C) sp and sp^3, respectively.
    (D) sp and sp, respectively.

5. Which of the following hybridizations does the Be atom in BeH_2 assume?

    (A) sp
    (B) sp^2
    (C) sp^3
    (D) None of the above

6. Two atomic orbitals combine to form:

        I. a bonding molecular orbital.
        II. an antibonding molecular orbital.
        III. new atomic orbitals.

    (A) I only
    (B) I, II, and III
    (C) III only
    (D) I and II only

7. Molecular orbitals can contain a maximum of

   (A) 1 electron.

   (B) 2 electrons.

   (C) 4 electrons.

   (D) $2n^2$ electrons, where n is the principal quantum number of the combining atomic orbitals.

8. π bonds are formed by which of the following orbitals?

   (A) Two s orbitals

   (B) Two p orbitals

   (C) One s and one p orbital

   (D) All of the above

9. How many σ bonds and π bonds are present in the following compound?

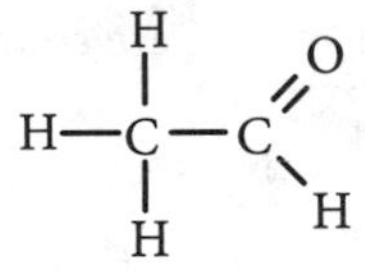

   (A) 6 σ bonds and 1 π bond

   (B) 6 σ bonds and 2 π bonds

   (C) 7 σ bonds and 1 π bond

   (D) 7 σ bonds and 2 π bonds

10. The four C–H bonds of CH_4 point toward the vertices of a tetrahedron. This indicates that the hybridization of a carbon atom is

   (A) sp.

   (B) sp^2.

   (C) sp^3.

   (D) none of the above.

SOLUTIONS TO REVIEW PROBLEMS

1. **A**   In a many-electron atom, the energy of the orbitals within the principal quantum numbers is as follows: 2s < 2p; 3s < 3p < 3d; 4s < 4p < 4d < 4f. For any given principal quantum level, the s orbital is always the lowest in energy, thus the correct choice is (A).

2. **D**   σ bonds are formed when orbitals overlap end-to-end. All single bonds are σ bonds; double and triple bonds contain one σ bond each. The compounds CH_4, C_2H_2, and C_2H_4 (choices (A), (B), and (C), respectively) all contain at least one single bond, so the correct choice is (D).

3. **B**   In a double-bonded carbon, sp^2 hybridization occurs, i.e., one s orbital hybridizes with two p orbitals to form three sp^2 hybrid orbitals. Therefore, the correct choice is (B). Note that the sp^2 orbitals take part in σ bond formation, making choice (D) incorrect. The third p orbital of the carbon atom remains unhybridized and takes part in the formation of the pi bond of the double bond.

4. **D**   The carbon atom and the nitrogen atoms are connected by a triple bond in CN^-.

    $$:N \equiv C:^-$$

    A triple-bonded atom is sp hybridized; one s orbital hybridizes with one p orbital to form two sp hybridized orbitals. The two remaining unhybridized p orbitals take part in the formation of two π bonds. The correct choice, therefore, is (D).

5. **A** BeH_2 is a linear molecule, which means that the angle between the two Be–H bonds is 180°. Since the sp orbitals are oriented at an angle of 180°, the Be atom is sp hybridized. Therefore, the correct choice is (A). Note that sp^2 orbitals are oriented at an angle of 120°, and sp^3 orbitals are oriented at an angle of 109.5°.

6. **D**   When atomic orbitals combine to form molecular orbitals, the number of molecular orbitals obtained equals the number of atomic orbitals that take part in the process. Half of the molecular orbitals formed are bonding molecular orbitals and the other half are antibonding molecular orbitals. In this case, therefore, two atomic orbitals combine to form one low-energy bonding molecular orbital and one high-energy antibonding molecular orbital. New atomic orbitals do not form, so answer choices (B) and (C) can be eliminated. Finally, (A) is incorrect since the bonding molecular orbital will have a corresponding antibonding molecular orbital. The correct choice is (D).

7. **B**   Each molecular orbital, like an atomic orbital, can contain a maximum of two electrons with opposite spins.

8. **B**   Pi bonds are formed by the parallel overlap of unhybridized p orbitals. The electron density is concentrated above and below the bonding axis. A sigma bond can be formed by the head-to-head overlap of two s orbitals, two p orbitals, or one s and one p orbital. In a σ bond, the density of the electrons is concentrated between the two nuclei of the bonding atoms.

9. **A** Each single bond has 1 σ bond, and each double bond has one σ and one π bond. In this question, there are five single bonds (5 σ bonds) and one double bond (one σ bond and one π bond), which gives a total of six σ bonds and one π bond. Thus, the correct choice is (A).

10. **C** The four bonds point to the vertices of a tetrahedron, which means that the angle between two bonds is 109.5°. sp^3 orbitals have an angle of 109.5° between them. Hence, the carbon atom of CH_4 is sp^3 hybridized. The correct choice, therefore, is (C).

CHAPTER FORTY-TWO

Alkanes

Alkanes are hydrocarbons that have the maximum possible number of hydrogen atoms attached to each carbon, and thus are said to be saturated. These compounds consist only of hydrogen and carbon atoms joined by single bonds and their general formula is C_nH_{2n+2}. However, alkanes can be modified with additional functional groups as well, such as alcohols, halogens, or amines.

A brief overview of nomenclature and properties of alkanes will be followed by a discussion of substitution reactions and then additional types of reactions.

NOMENCLATURE

Alkanes are named for their longest, straight carbon chain. The names of the four simplest alkanes are:

$$CH_4 \qquad CH_3CH_3 \qquad CH_3CH_2CH_3 \qquad CH_3CH_2CH_2CH_3$$

methane   **eth**ane   **prop**ane   **but**ane

The names of the longer-chain alkanes consist of prefixes derived from the Greek root for the number of carbon atoms with the ending -**ane**.

$C_5H_{12} =$ **pent**ane $C_9H_{20} =$ **non**ane

$C_6H_{14} =$ **hex**ane $C_{10}H_{22} =$ **dec**ane

$C_7H_{16} =$ **hept**ane $C_{11}H_{24} =$ **undec**ane

$C_8H_{18} =$ **oct**ane $C_{12}H_{26} =$ **dodec**ane

For detailed information on naming branched chain alkanes and alkanes with substituent groups, refer to Chapter 39.

Carbon atoms can be characterized by the number of other carbon atoms to which they are directly bonded. A **primary** carbon atom (written as **1°**) is bonded to only one other carbon atom. A **secondary (2°)** carbon is bonded to two; a **tertiary (3°)** to three, and a **quaternary (4°)** to four other carbon atoms. In addition, hydrogen atoms or other functional groups attached to 1°, 2°, or 3° carbon atoms are referred to as 1°, 2°, or 3°, respectively.

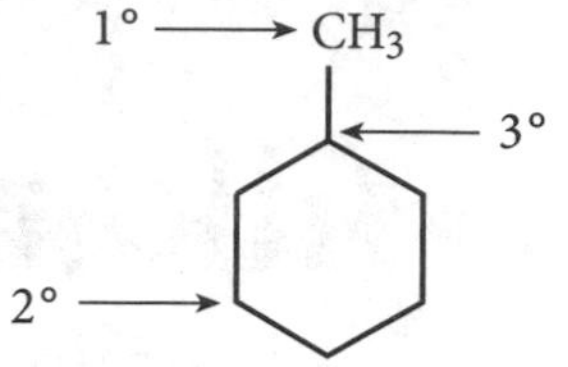

Figure 42.1

PHYSICAL PROPERTIES

Most of the physical properties of alkanes vary in a predictable manner. In general, as the molecular weight of a straight chain alkane increases, the melting point, boiling point, and density also increase. At room temperature, the straight-chain compounds C_1H_4 through C_4H_{10} are gases, C_5H_{12} through $C_{16}H_{34}$ are liquids, and the longer-chain compounds are waxes and harder solids.

Branched molecules have slightly lower boiling and melting points than their straight-chain isomers. Greater branching reduces the surface area of a molecule, decreasing the weak intermolecular attractive forces (London dispersion forces). The molecules are held together less tightly, thus lowering the boiling point. In addition, branched molecules are more difficult to pack into a tight, three-dimensional structure, which is reflected in the lower melting points of branched alkanes.

SUBSTITUTION REACTIONS OF ALKANES

Alkyl halides and other substituted carbon molecules can take part in reactions known as *nucleophilic substitutions*. Substitution reactions involve removing an atom or a functional group from a molecule and replacing it with another. Substitution reactions can occur in many different types of molecules; however, this chapter will specifically discuss substitution reactions of alkanes. In all substitution reactions, identifying the nucleophile and the leaving group are critical to an understanding of the mechanism.

Nucleophiles

Nucleophiles are molecules that are attracted to positive charge, as seen by their name: nucleophile means "nucleus lover." Nucleophiles are electron-rich species that are often but not always negatively charged. Nucleophiles are attracted to atoms with partial or full positive charges.

Basicity

If a group of nucleophiles are based on the same atom (for example, oxygen) then nucleophilicity is roughly correlated to basicity. In other words, the stronger the base, the stronger the nucleophile. This is because bases act as electron donors, and stronger nucleophiles are also better electron donors. For example, nucleophilic strength decreases in the order:

$$RO^- > HO^- > RCO_2^- > ROH > H_2O$$

Size and polarizability

If a series of nucleophiles is based on different atoms, nucleophilic ability doesn't necessarily correlate to basicity. In a protic solvent (a solvent that is able to form hydrogen bonds), large atoms or ions tend to be better nucleophiles. Larger ions more easily shed their solvent molecules and are more polarizable. Hence, nucleophilic strength decreases in the order:

$$CN^- > I^- > RO^- > HO^- > Br^- > Cl^- > F^- > H_2O$$

In contrast, in an aprotic solvent (a solvent that cannot form hydrogen bonds) the nucleophiles are "naked"; they are not solvated. In this case, nucleophilic strength is directly related to basicity. For example, in DMSO (an aprotic solvent), the order of nucleophilic strength is the same as base strength:

$$F^- > Cl^- > Br^- > I^-$$

Leaving Groups

The ease with which nucleophilic substitution takes place is dependent on the nature of the leaving group. The best leaving groups are those that are weak bases, as these can accept a negative charge and dissociate to form a stable ion in solution. In the case of the halogens, therefore, this is the opposite of base strength:

$$I^- > Br^- > Cl^- > F^-$$

Other leaving groups besides halogens can be used for substitution reactions. For example, an $-OH$ group that is a poor leaving group can be protonated to form $-H_2O^+$, which leaves as a water molecule.

S$_N$1 Reactions

S$_N$1 designates a **unimolecular nucleophilic substitution** reaction. It is unimolecular because the rate of the reaction is dependent upon only one molecule in the reaction; in other words, the rate expression is first order. The rate-determining step of an S$_N$1 reaction is the dissociation of the substrate (the starting molecule) to form a stable, positively charged ion called a **carbocation.** The formation and stabilization of the carbocation determine all other aspects of S$_N$1 reactions.

Mechanism

S$_N$1 reactions involve two steps: the dissociation of a substrate molecule into a carbocation and a leaving group, followed by the combination of the carbocation with a nucleophile to form the substituted product.

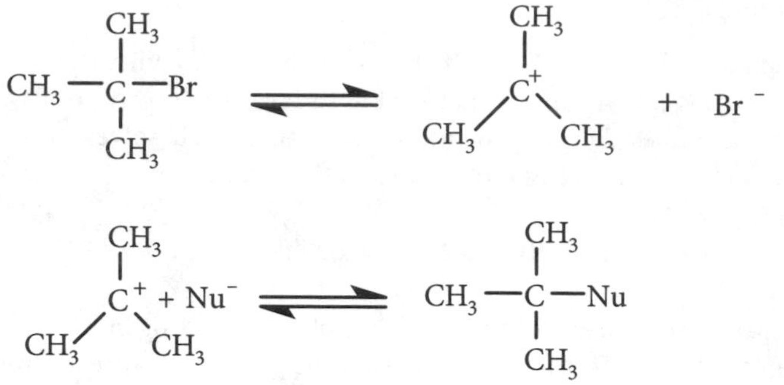

Figure 42.2

In the first step, a carbocation intermediate is formed. Carbocations are stabilized by polar solvents that have lone electron pairs available to donate (e.g., water or ethyl alcohol). Carbocations are also stabilized by charge delocalization throughout the molecule. More highly substituted carbocations are more stable, because hydrocarbon substituent groups donate electron density toward the positive charge. The order of stability for carbocations is:

$$\text{tertiary} > \text{secondary} > \text{primary} > \text{methyl}$$

To drive the reaction forward, the original leaving group should be a weaker nucleophile than the replacement nucleophile. The second step, in which the nucleophile combines with the carbocation, occurs very rapidly compared to the first step, and is essentially irreversible.

Rate

The rate at which a reaction occurs can never be greater than the rate of its slowest step. Such a step is termed the **rate-limiting** or **rate-determining step** of the reaction (see Chapter 33 for a more detailed discussion of rate expressions). In an S_N1 reaction, the slowest step is the dissociation of the molecule to form a carbocation intermediate, a step that is energetically unfavorable. The formation of a carbocation is therefore the rate-limiting step of an S_N1 reaction. The only reactant in this step is the original substrate molecule, and so the rate of the entire reaction depends only on the concentration of the substrate (a so-called *first-order reaction*): rate $= k$[substrate]. The rate is *not* dependent on the concentration or the nature of the nucleophile, because it plays no part in the rate-limiting step.

The rate of an S_N1 reaction can be increased by anything that promotes the formation and stability of the carbocation. The most important factors are as follows:

a. Structural factors: Highly substituted alkanes allow for distribution of the positive charge over a greater number of carbon and hydrogen atoms, and thus form the most stable carbocations. The order of reactivity of substrates for S_N1 reactions is tertiary > secondary > primary > methyl; in general, primary and methyl substrates do not react by the S_N1 mechanism.

b. Solvent effects: Highly polar solvents are better at surrounding and isolating ions than are less polar solvents. Polar protic solvents such as water or alcohols work best for two reasons. Protic solvents can form hydrogen bonds with the leaving group, solvating it and preventing it from returning to the carbocation. Also, lone electron pairs on oxygen or nitrogen atoms in the solvent molecule can stabilize the carbocation intermediate.

c. Nature of the leaving group: Weak bases dissociate more easily from the alkyl chain and thus make better leaving groups, increasing the rate of carbocation formation.

d. Nature of the nucleophile: S_N1 reactions do not require a strong nucleophile. S_N1 reactions run equally well with either strong (fully charged) or weak (electron-rich but uncharged) nucleophiles.

Stereochemistry

S_N1 reactions involve carbocation intermediates, which are sp^2 hybridized and have trigonal planar geometry. The attacking nucleophile can approach the carbocation from either above or below with equal probability, and thus create either the (*R*) or (*S*) enantiomer with equal probability.

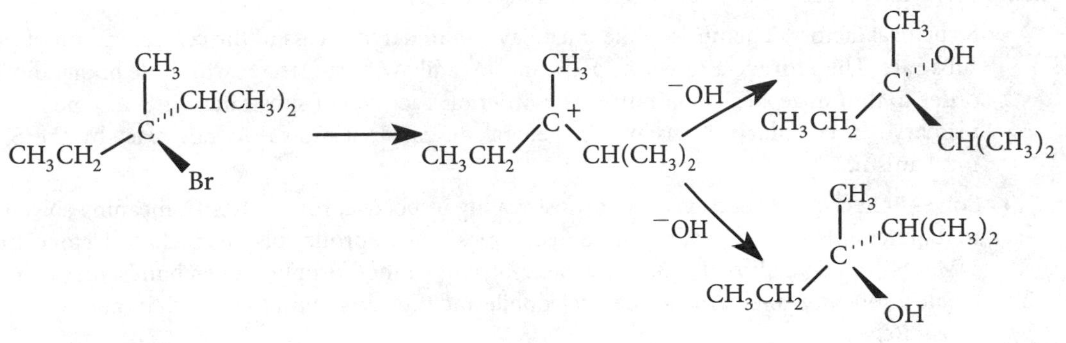

Figure 42.3

If the original compound is optically active because of the presence of a chiral center, then a racemic mixture will be produced. In some cases, the nucleophile may react so rapidly that it approaches the carbocation from the opposite side of the leaving group with greater frequency; in this case, the product will be characterized as a partial racemate.

S_N2 Reactions

S_N2 designates a **bimolecular nucleophilic substitution** reaction. S_N2 reactions involve a nucleophile pushing its way into a compound while simultaneously displacing the leaving group. Its rate-determining and only step involves two molecules: the substrate and the nucleophile.

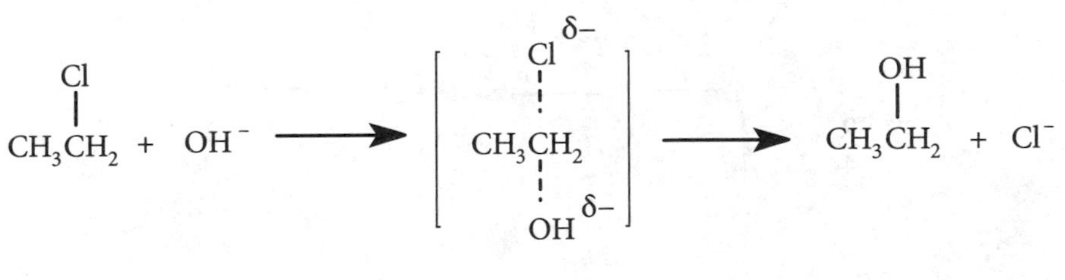

Figure 42.4

Mechanism

S_N2 reactions are **concerted** reactions, meaning that the entire mechanism occurs in single coordinated process. The nucleophile attacks the reactant from the backside of the leaving group, forming a trigonal bipyramidal **transition state**. As the reaction progresses, the bond to the nucleophile strengthens while the bond to the leaving group weakens. The leaving group is displaced as the bond to the nucleophile becomes complete.

Rate

The single step of an S_N2 reaction involves *two* reacting species: the substrate and the nucleophile. The concentrations of both therefore play a role in determining the rate of an S_N2 reaction; the two species must "meet" in solution, and raising the concentration of either will make such a meeting more likely. Since the rate of the S_N2 reaction depends on the concentration of two reactants, it follows **second-order kinetics**. The rate expression for an S_N2 reaction is: rate = k[substrate][nucleophile].

Other factors that can affect the rate of S_N2 reactions include:

- Structural factors: The nucleophile must have unhindered access to the central carbon of the substrate. Therefore S_N2 reactions occur most readily with substrates with little branching in order to minimize steric hindrance. The order of reactivity of substrates for S_N2 is methyl > primary > secondary > tertiary; in general, tertiary substrates do not react by the S_N2 mechanism.

- Solvent effects: S_N2 reactions occur most readily in polar aprotic solvents, meaning solvents that are unable to form hydrogen bonds. Typical polar aprotic solvents include acetone and DMSO (dimethylsulfoxide). Because these solvents cannot form hydrogen bonds, they do not create a solvation shell around the nucleophile and thus do not interfere with its attack on the substrate.

- Nature of the leaving group: Weak bases dissociate more easily from the alkyl chain and thus make better leaving groups, increasing the ease of displacement by the nucleophile.

- Nature of the nucleophile: Because the nucleophile must attack a neutral molecule and displace the leaving group, it must be strongly nucleophilic. This typically means that the nucleophile is a negatively charged ionic species, and can be either a strong or weak base.

Stereochemistry

The single step of an S_N2 reaction involves a chiral transition state. Since the nucleophile attacks from one side of the central carbon and the leaving group departs from the opposite side, the reaction "flips" the bonds attached to the carbon.

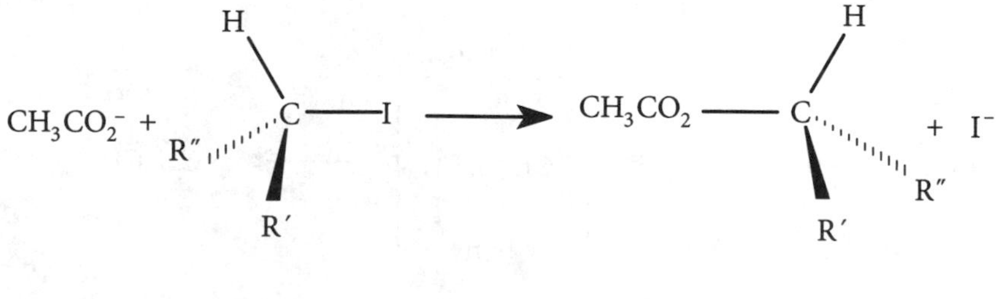

Figure 42.5

If the reactant is chiral, optical activity will be retained, but will invert between (*R*) and (*S*) as long as the nucleophile and leaving group have the same priority relative to the other groups in the substrate.

If the nucleophile and leaving group have different priorities compared to the rest of the molecule, however, the absolute configuration must be determined for the substituted product.

S_N1 vs. S_N2

Certain reaction conditions favor one substitution mechanism over the other, and provide distinctive "fingerprints" that allow the determination of whether S_N1 or S_N2 will proceed. Sterics, nucleophilic strength, leaving group ability, reaction conditions, and solvent effects are all important in determining which reaction will occur.

	S_N1	S_N2
Substrate reactivity	$3° > 2° > 1° > CH_3$	$CH_3 > 1° > 2° > 3°$
Leaving group	Cl^-, Br^-, I^-, weak bases $-OH$ if protonated to form OH_2^+	Cl^-, Br^-, I^-, weak bases
Nucleophile	Any nucleophile	Strong (charged) nucleophile
Solvent	Polar protic	Polar aprotic
Reaction mechanism	2-step: carbocation, then nucleophilic attack	Concerted 1-step
Rate law	1st order: rate $= k$[substrate]	2nd order: rate $= k$[substrate][nucleophile]
Stereochemistry	Chiral → racemic mix	Inversion of R/S

Table 42.1

Free Radical Substitution Reactions

Alkanes can react by a **free radical substitution mechanism** in which one or more hydrogen atoms are replaced by Cl, Br, or I atoms. These reactions involve three steps:

1. **Initiation:** Diatomic halogens are cleaved by either UV light (shown as UV or hv) or peroxide (H-O O-H or R-O-O-H), resulting in the formation of free radicals (heat can also be used, but is not specific for radical formation). Free radicals are uncharged species with unpaired electrons (such as Cl• or $R_3C•$). They are extremely reactive and readily attack alkanes.

$$\text{Initiation: } X_2 \xrightarrow{\text{hv}} 2X•$$

2. **Propagation**—A propagation step is one in which a radical produces another radical that can continue the reaction. A free radical reacts with an alkane, removing a hydrogen atom to form HX, and creating an alkyl radical. The alkyl radical can then react with X_2 to form an alkyl halide (the substituted product) and generate another X•, thus propagating the radical.

$$\text{Propagation: } \quad X• + RH \longrightarrow HX + R•$$
$$R• + X_2 \longrightarrow RX + X•$$

3. Termination—Two free radicals combine with one another to form a stable molecule.

$$\text{Termination:} \quad X\bullet + X\bullet \longrightarrow X_2$$
$$X\bullet + R\bullet \longrightarrow RX$$
$$R\bullet + R\bullet \longrightarrow R_2$$

A single free radical can initiate many reactions before the reaction chain is terminated.

Larger alkanes have many hydrogens that the free radical can attack. Bromine radicals react fairly slowly, and primarily attack the hydrogens on the carbon atom that can form the most stable free radical, i.e., the most substituted carbon atom.

$$\bullet CR_3 > \bullet CR_2H > \bullet CRH_2 > \bullet CH_3$$
$$3° > 2° > 1° > \text{methyl}$$

Thus, a tertiary radical is the most likely to be formed in a free-radical bromination reaction. As a result, the substitution product will have the bromine on the most highly substituted carbon. Note the same pattern of stability and the same resulting product compared to a carbocation-based mechanism.

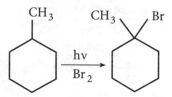

Figure 42.6

Free-radical chlorination is a more rapid process and depends on both the stability of the intermediate and on the number of hydrogens present. Free-radical chlorination reactions are likely to replace primary hydrogens that are found abundantly in most molecules, despite the relative instability of primary radicals. Unfortunately, free-radical chlorination reactions produce mixtures of products, and are useful only when a single type of hydrogen is present.

ADDITIONAL REACTIONS OF ALKANES

Combustion

The reaction of alkanes with molecular oxygen to form carbon dioxide, water, and heat is a process of great practical importance. It is an unusual reaction because heat, not a chemical species, is generally the desired product. The reaction mechanism is very complex and is believed to proceed through a radical process. The equation for the complete **combustion** of propane is:

$$C_3H_8 + 5\,O_2 \longrightarrow 3\,CO_2 + 4\,H_2O + \text{heat}$$

All combustion reactions take this basic form, with different hydrocarbons used as the starting molecule, and each reaction must be balanced appropriately for the number of carbons, hydrogens, and oxygens present. Combustion is often incomplete, producing significant quantities of carbon monoxide instead of carbon dioxide. This frequently occurs, for example, in the burning of gasoline in an internal combustion engine.

Pyrolysis

Pyrolysis occurs when a molecule is broken down by heat in the absence of oxygen. Pyrolysis, also called **cracking,** is most commonly used to reduce the average molecular weight of heavy oils and to increase the production of more desirable volatile compounds. In the pyrolysis of alkanes, the C—C bonds are cleaved, producing smaller-chain alkyl radicals. These radicals can recombine to form a variety of alkanes:

$$CH_3CH_2CH_3 \xrightarrow{\Delta} CH_3\bullet + \bullet CH_2CH_3$$

$$2\ CH_3\bullet \longrightarrow CH_3CH_3$$

$$2\ \bullet CH_2CH_3 \longrightarrow CH_3CH_2CH_2CH_3$$

Figure 42.7

Alternatively, in a process called **disproportionation,** a radical transfers a hydrogen atom to another radical, producing an alkane and an alkene:

$$\bullet CH_3 + \bullet CH_2CH_3 \longrightarrow CH_4 + H_2C=CH_2$$

Figure 42.8

REVIEW PROBLEMS

1. Under the following conditions,

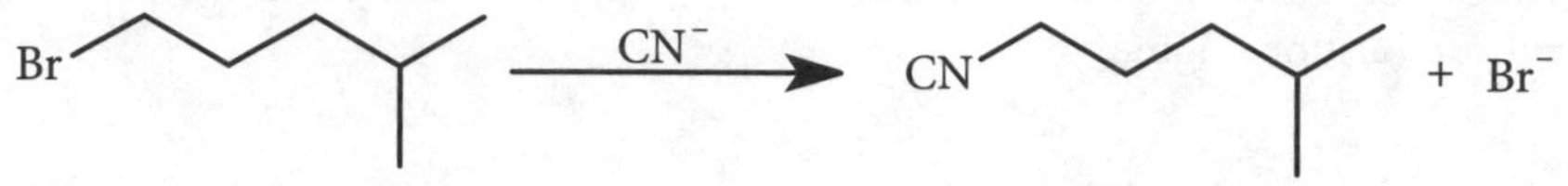

    1-bromo-4-methylpentane will most probably react via

    (A) S_N1.
    (B) S_N2.
    (C) both S_N1 and S_N2.
    (D) neither S_N1 nor S_N2.

2. The following molecule can be classified as having

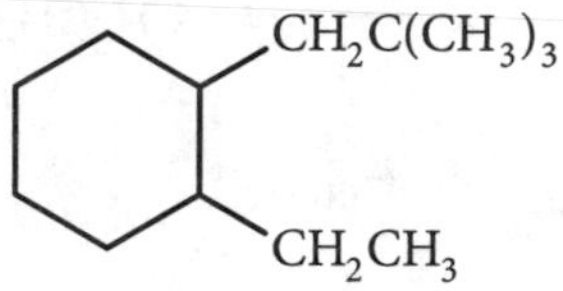

    (A) 4 primary, 2 secondary, 4 tertiary, and 3 quaternary carbon atoms.
    (B) 3 methyl groups, 2 ethyl groups, and 4 secondary carbon atoms.
    (C) 4 primary, 6 secondary, 2 tertiary, and 1 quaternary carbon atoms.
    (D) 3 primary, 3 secondary, 4 tertiary, and 3 quaternary carbon atoms.

3. The following reactions are part of a free-radical halogenation sequence:

		ΔH (kcal/mol)
(A)	$Cl_2 \longrightarrow 2\ Cl\bullet$	$+58$
(B)	$Cl\bullet + CH_4 \longrightarrow \bullet CH_3 + HCl$	$+1$
(C)	$\bullet CH_3 + Cl_2 \longrightarrow CH_3Cl + Cl\bullet$	-26
(D)	$\bullet CH_3 + Cl\bullet \longrightarrow CH_3Cl$	-84

    Identify the initiation, propagation, and termination steps.

4. S_N1 reactions show first-order kinetics because

    (A) the rate-limiting step is the first step to occur in the reaction.
    (B) the rate-limiting step involves only one molecule.
    (C) there is only one rate-limiting step.
    (D) the reaction involves only one molecule.

5. The following reaction sequence is typical of S_N1 reactions. Which is the rate-limiting step(s)?

Step 1 $(CH_3)_3C—Cl \longrightarrow (CH_3)_3C^+ + Cl^-$

Step 2 $(CH_3)_3C^+ \xrightarrow{CH_3CH_2OH} (CH_3)_3C—\overset{+}{\underset{H}{O}}—CH_2CH_3$

Step 3 $(CH_3)_3C—\overset{+}{\underset{H}{O}}—CH_2CH_3 \longrightarrow (CH_3)_3C—O—CH_2CH_3 + H^+$

(A) Step 1
(B) Step 2
(C) Step 3
(D) Steps 1 and 2

6. Which of the following would be the best solvent for an S_N2 reaction?

(A) H_2O
(B) CH_3CH_2OH
(C) CH_3SOCH_3
(D) $CH_3CH_2CH_2CH_2CH_2CH_3$

7. What choices for X and Y would most favor the following reaction?

$$R_3C–X \xrightarrow{-X^-} R_3C^+ \xrightarrow{+Y^-} R_3C–Y$$

(A) $X = I^-, Y = Cl^-$
(B) $X = EtO^-, Y =$ tosylate $(CH_3C_6H_4SO_2)$
(C) $X =$ tosylate, $Y = CN^-$
(D) $X = OH^-, Y = H_2O$

8. What would be the major product of the following reaction?

$$CH_3CH_2CH_3 + Br_2 \xrightarrow{h\nu}$$

(A) $CH_3CH_2CH_2Br$
(B) $CH_3CH_2CH_2CH_2CH_2CH_3$
(C) $H_3CCHBrCH_3$
(D) CH_3CH_2Br

9. Treatment of (S)-2-bromobutane with sodium hydroxide results in the production of a compound with an (R) configuration. The reaction has most likely taken place through

(A) an S_N1 mechanism.
(B) an S_N2 mechanism.

(C) both an S_N1 and S_N2 reaction.

(D) a reaction that cannot be determined.

10. What is the correct decreasing order of the boiling points of the following compounds?

   I. *n*-hexane

  II. 2-methylpentane

 III. 2,2-dimethylbutane

 IV. *n*-heptane

(A) I > IV > II > III

(B) IV > III > II > I

(C) IV > I > II > III

(D) I > II > III > IV

11. The reaction of isobutane with an unknown halogen is catalyzed by light. The two major products obtained are:

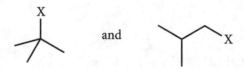

What is the unknown halogen?

(A) Cl_2

(B) Br_2

(C) I_2

(D) F_2

12. Place the following species in order of increasing stability.

(A) (i) $CH_3CH_2CH_2{}^{\bullet}$ (ii) $(CH_3)_2\underset{\underset{\displaystyle H}{|}}{C}{}^{\bullet}$ (iii) $CH_3{}^{\bullet}$ (iv) $(CH_3)_3C^{\bullet}$

(B) (i) $\underset{\underset{\displaystyle H}{|}}{R_2C^{+}}$ (ii) R_3C^{+} (iii) H_3C^{+} (iv) $\underset{\underset{\displaystyle R}{|}}{H_2C^{+}}$

SOLUTIONS TO REVIEW PROBLEMS

1. **B** In this question, a primary alkyl halide is treated with cyanide, which is a good nucleophile. Primary alkyl halides are not sterically hindered and are readily displaced in S_N2 reactions. Cyanide will displace the bromide to produce 5-methylheptanenitrile in good yield. The correct answer is therefore choice (B). An S_N1 reaction will probably not occur because formation of a primary carbocation, which would result from the loss of bromide, is highly unfavorable.

2. **C** The molecule shown in question 2 is 2-ethyl-1-neopentylcyclohexane. A primary carbon atom is one that is bonded to only one other carbon atom, a secondary carbon atom is bonded to two, a tertiary to three, and a quaternary to four. Thus, this molecule has four primary, six secondary, two tertiary, and one quaternary carbon atoms, so choice (C) is correct. Choice (A) is incorrect because there are six, not two, secondary carbon atoms. These include four on the ring and one on each substituent. Choice (B) is incorrect because there are six, not four, secondary carbon atoms, and choice (D) is incorrect because there are four primary carbon atoms, not three, from the four different methyl groups.

3.   Step **(A)** is an initiation step because a nonradical species forms two radicals. Both steps **(B)** and **(C)** are propagation steps in which one radical species reacts to form another radical species. Step **(D)** is a termination step in which two radicals form a nonradical species.

4. **B** An S_N1 reaction is a first-order nucleophilic substitution reaction. It is called first order because the rate-limiting step involves only one molecule; thus the correct answer is choice (B). Choice (A) is incorrect because the rate-limiting step is not necessarily the first step to occur in a reaction. It is simply the slowest step. Choice (C) is a true statement, but is incorrect because it is irrelevant to the term "first-order." Finally, choice (D) is incorrect because it is the rate-limiting step, not the reaction, that involves only one molecule.

5. **A** The formation of a carbocation is the rate-limiting step. This step is the slowest to occur and its rate determines the rate of the reaction. Step 2 is a nucleophilic attack on the carbocation by ethanol. In step 3 a proton is lost from the protonated ether. Both steps 2 and 3 occur very rapidly in solution and are not rate-limiting steps. Answer choice (D) is incorrect because there can be only one rate-limiting step.

6. **C** The correct answer is choice (C), dimethyl sulfoxide. S_N2 reactions give the best results if a polar aprotic solvent is used. S_N2 reactions occur via a one-step mechanism in which a nucleophile attacks a substrate. Polar aprotic solvents accelerate this reaction by allowing the nucleophile to be "naked," i.e., not surrounded by hydrogen-bonded solvation spheres. The nucleophile therefore has easy access to the substrate. In addition, the solvent should be polar to dissolve the reactants. Choice (A), water, and choice (B), ethanol, are both incorrect because although these are polar, they are also protic and would diminish the power of the nucleophile. Choice (D) is hexane and is incorrect because it is a nonpolar solvent.

7. **C** This reaction is S_N1 and in order to occur, there must be a good leaving group and a strong incoming nucleophile. In choice (C), X is a tosylate ion, an excellent leaving group and Y is a cyanide ion, an excellent nucleophile. Therefore, choice (C) is the correct answer. Choice (A) is incorrect; even though iodide is a good leaving group (favoring the forward reaction), it is also a good nucleophile (favoring the reverse reaction) because the solvent

will be polar protic and it is an S_N1 reaction. Choice (B) is incorrect because ethoxide is a poor leaving group and tosylate is a weak nucleophile. Finally, choice (D) is incorrect because hydroxide is a poor leaving group and water is a poor nucleophile.

8. **C**   This question concerns the free-radical bromination of an alkane. The bromination reaction occurs in such a way as to produce the most stable alkyl radical. This is because bromine radicals are very selective, as opposed to chlorine radicals, which react indiscriminately. In this question, the most stable radical is a secondary radical, which further reacts to form 2-bromopropane, choice (C), the correct answer. Choice (A) is incorrect because 1-bromopropane results from reaction of a primary radical, and although this may occur to an extent, the major product will be 2-bromopropane. Choice (B) would result from the combination of two primary radicals and is expected to be a very minor product. Finally, choice (D) is incorrect because a carbon atom is lost in the reaction, and this does not occur in free-radical bromination.

9. **B**   Inversion of configuration is a trademark of the S_N2 reaction, whereas racemization is typical of S_N1 reactions. When (S)-2-bromobutane is treated with hydroxide, a compound with an *R* configuration is obtained. The most likely occurrence is a substitution reaction, and the fact that the absolute configuration has changed suggests an S_N2 reaction. If the reaction proceeded by S_N1, the products would have both *R* and *S* configurations because the hydroxide ion could attack the planar carbocation from either side and would form a racemic mix. There is only one configuration in this case, and therefore the correct answer is S_N2.

10. **C**   The correct answer is choice (C), IV > I > II > III, corresponding to: *n*-heptane > *n*-hexane > 2-methylpentane > 2,2-dimethylbutane. As the chain length of a straight-chain alkane is increased, the boiling point also increases, approximately 25−30°C for each additional carbon atom. Therefore, *n*-heptane is expected to boil at a higher temperature than *n*-hexane. Isomeric alkanes follow a typical trend: as branching increases, boiling point decreases. Compounds I, II, and III are isomeric hexanes, listed in increasing order of branching. Therefore, *n*-hexane boils at a higher temperature than 2-methylpentane, which boils at a higher temperature than 2,2-dimethylbutane.

11. **A**   Free-radical halogenation reactions are practical only for bromine and chlorine; iodine and fluorine do not react efficiently and can therefore be eliminated. Bromine radicals react slowly in comparison to chlorine radicals, and are therefore more likely to react in a manner that forms the most stable alkyl radical, i.e., the most substituted radical. This leads to the production of one major bromination product. Chlorine radicals, on the other hand, react so quickly that they become rather indiscriminate and generally produce several different products. In this particular reaction, two different products are isolated in comparable yields.

12. **A**   III < I < II < IV

    The order of stability of free radicals follows this sequence: $CH_3 < 1° < 2° < 3°$. Stability is enhanced by an increase in the number of alkyl substituents bonded directly to the radical carbon atom. These substituents allow the extra electron density to be spread out or delocalized throughout the molecule.

    B   III < IV < I < II

    The stability of carbocations is increased when the positive charge can be distributed over more than one carbon atom. This means that tertiary carbocations are more stable than secondary, and so on.

CHAPTER FORTY-THREE

Alkenes and Alkynes

Alkenes and alkynes are hydrocarbons that contain double and triple bonds between carbons. They are called unsaturated, because they contain fewer than the maximum possible number of hydrogens. Double and triple bonds are considered functional groups, and alkenes and alkynes are more reactive than the corresponding alkanes. The double and triple bonds of alkenes and alkynes are made from first forming a single sigma bond, and then by forming one or two additional pi bonds (for a review of bonding, please see Chapter 41, Bonding).

For both alkenes and alkynes, a brief overview of nomenclature and properties will be followed by a discussion of their synthesis and then of their reactions.

ALKENES

Alkenes are hydrocarbons that contain carbon-carbon double bonds. The general formula for a straight-chain alkene with one double bond is C_nH_{2n}. The degree of unsaturation (the number N of double bonds or rings) of a compound of molecular formula C_nH_m can be determined according to the equation:

$$N = \frac{1}{2}(2n + 2 - m)$$

The carbons at either end of a double bond are sp^2 hybridized and both form planar bonds with bond angles of 120°. Alkenes are not able to rotate around their double bond and thus are constrained to unique configurations.

NOMENCLATURE OF ALKENES

Alkenes, also called olefins, may be described by the terms *cis, trans, E,* and *Z* to distinguish the configuration of functional groups around the double bond. The common names *ethylene, propylene,* and *isobutylene* are often used over the IUPAC names ethene, propene, and 2-methyl-1-propene, respectively. For a review of *cis-trans* isomers, see Chapter 40, Isomers; to review nomenclature, see Chapter 39, Structural Formulas.

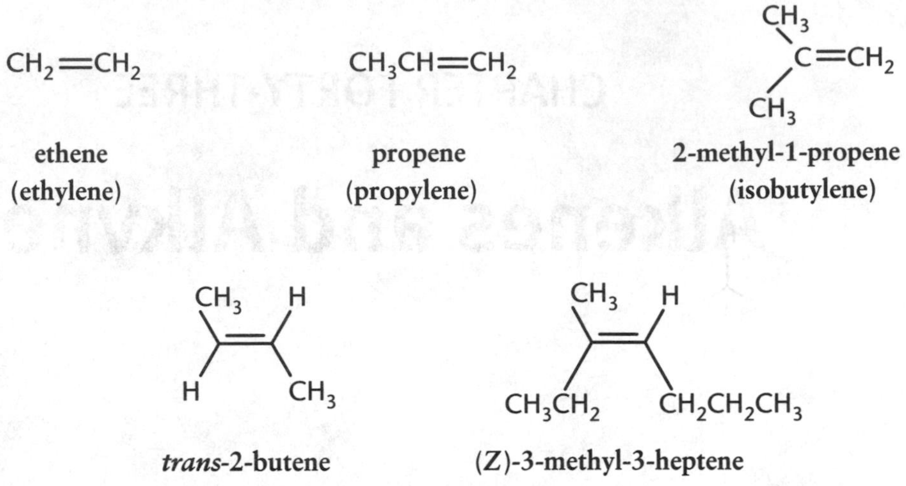

$$CH_2{=}CH_2$$

**ethene
(ethylene)**

$$CH_3CH{=}CH_2$$

**propene
(propylene)**

**2-methyl-1-propene
(isobutylene)**

trans-2-butene

(Z)-3-methyl-3-heptene

Figure 43.1

PHYSICAL PROPERTIES OF ALKENES

The physical properties of alkenes are similar to those of alkanes. For example, their melting and boiling points increase with increasing molecular weight and are similar in value to those of the corresponding alkanes. Terminal alkenes (or 1-alkenes) usually boil at a lower temperature than internal alkenes. *Trans*-alkenes generally have higher melting points than *cis*-alkenes because their higher symmetry allows better packing in the solid state. They also tend to have lower boiling points than *cis*-alkenes because they are less polar.

Polarity is a property that results from the asymmetrical distribution of electrons in a particular molecule. In alkenes, this distribution creates dipole moments that are oriented from the electropositive alkyl groups toward the electronegative alkene. In *trans*-2-butene, the two dipole moments are oriented in opposite directions and cancel each other. The compound possesses no net dipole moment and is not polar. On the other hand, *cis*-2-butene has a net dipole moment, resulting from addition of the two smaller dipoles. The compound is polar, and the additional intermolecular forces raise the boiling point.

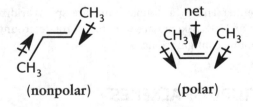

(nonpolar)   **(polar)**

Figure 43.2

SYNTHESIS OF ALKENES

Alkenes can be synthesized in a number of different ways. The most common method involves elimination reactions of either alcohols or alkyl halides. In these reactions the molecule loses either HX (where X is a halide) or a molecule of water from two adjacent carbons to form a double bond:

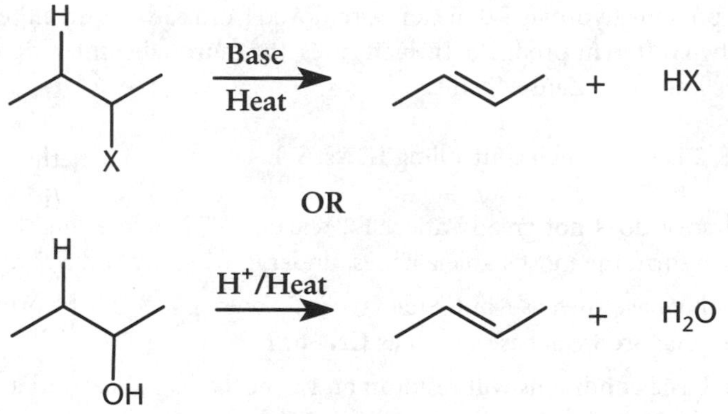

Figure 43.3

Elimination occurs by two distinct mechanisms, unimolecular and bimolecular, which are referred to as E1 and E2, respectively.

Unimolecular Elimination

Unimolecular elimination, abbreviated **E1**, is a two-step process proceeding through a carbocation intermediate. The rate of reaction is dependent on the concentration of only the substrate. The elimination of a leaving group and a proton results in the production of a double bond. In the first step, the leaving group departs, producing a carbocation. In the second step, a proton is removed by a base and the double bond forms.

Because both involve the formation of a carbocation intermediate, E1 is favored by the same factors that favor S_N1: protic solvents, highly branched carbon chains, good leaving groups, and weak nucleophiles in low concentration. After the identical first step, the reaction can proceed by either the E1 or S_N1 pathway. E1 and S_N1 are therefore competitive, and occur simultaneously under the same conditions. In fact, E1 and S_N1 have exactly the same rate law, given by rate $= k$[substrate], including having the same value of k. Directing a reaction toward either E1 or S_N1 alone is difficult, although high temperatures tend to favor E1; this means that a mixture of both E1 and S_N1 products will always be present.

Bimolecular Elimination

Bimolecular elimination, termed **E2**, occurs in one step. Its rate is dependent on the concentration of two species, the substrate and the base. A strong base such as the ethoxide ion ($C_2H_5O^-$) removes a proton, while simultaneously a halide ion *anti* to the proton leaves, resulting in the formation of a double bond.

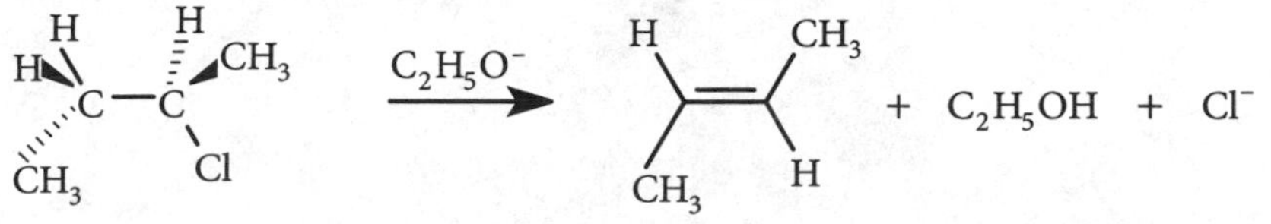

Figure 43.4

Often there are two possible hydrogens that can be removed from carbons on either side of the leaving group, resulting in two different products. In such cases, the more substituted double bond is formed preferentially; this is known as Zaitsev's rule.

Controlling E2 vs. S_N2 is easier than controlling E1 vs. S_N1:

1. Steric hindrance does not greatly affect E2 reactions. Therefore, highly substituted carbon chains, which form the most stable alkenes, undergo E2 easily and S_N2 rarely.

2. A strong, bulky base such as *t*-butoxide favors E2 over S_N2. S_N2 is favored over E2 by strong nucleophiles that are weak bases, such as CN^- or I^-.

In general, heat and basic conditions will result in an E2 mechanism; heat and acidic conditions will result in E1 combined with S_N1.

REACTIONS OF ALKENES

Alkenes undergo several types of reactions, including:

- reduction by hydrogen
- addition by electrophiles and free radicals
- hydroboration
- a variety of oxidations
- polymerization

Reduction

Catalytic hydrogenation is the reductive process of adding molecular hydrogen (H_2) to a double bond with the aid of a metal catalyst. Typical catalysts are platinum, palladium, and nickel (usually Raney nickel, a special powdered form), but on rare occasions rhodium, iridium, or ruthenium are used.

The reaction takes place on the surface of the metal. One face of the double bond is coordinated to the metal surface, and thus the two hydrogen atoms are added to the same face of the double bond. This type of addition is called *syn* addition and results in a *meso* compound if the starting molecule was symmetrical (see Chapter 40, Isomers, for a review of *meso* compounds).

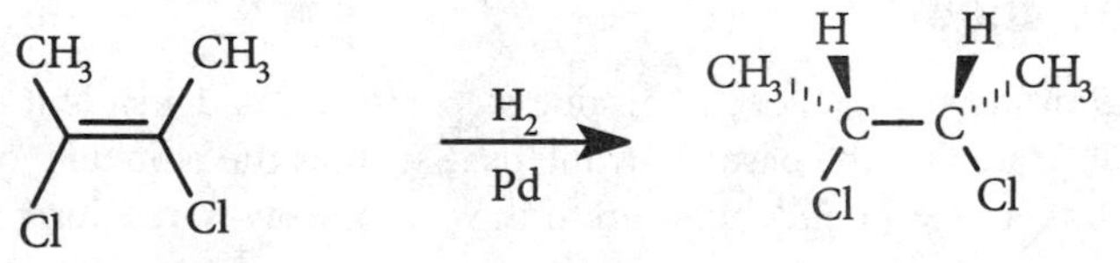

Figure 43.5

Electrophilic Additions

The π bond is somewhat weaker than the σ bond, and can therefore be broken without breaking the σ bond. As a result, compounds can *add* to double bonds while leaving the carbon skeleton intact. Although many different addition reactions exist, most operate via the same essential mechanism.

The electrons of the π bond are particularly exposed and are thus easily attacked by molecules that seek to accept an electron pair (Lewis acids). Because these groups are electron-seeking, they are known as electrophiles (literally, "lovers of electrons").

Addition of HX

The electrons of the double bond act as a Lewis base and react with electrophilic HX (hydrogen halide) molecules. The first step yields a carbocation intermediate after the double bond reacts with a proton. In the second step, the halide ion combines with the carbocation to give an alkyl halide. In cases where the alkene is asymmetrical, the initial protonation creates the *most stable carbocation*. The proton will add to the less substituted carbon atom (the carbon atom with the most hydrogens), and the positive charge of the carbocation will reside on the more substituted carbon. The halogen will then add to the carbocation, and thus create the product with the halide on the most substituted carbon. This phenomenon is called Markovnikov's rule. An example is:

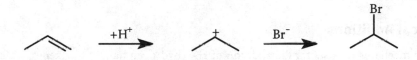

Figure 43.6

Addition of X₂

The addition of halogens to a double bond is a rapid process. The addition of bromine and resulting change in color of the solution is frequently used as a diagnostic tool to test for the presence of double bonds. In the example shown, the double bond acts as a nucleophile and attacks a Br₂ molecule, displacing Br⁻. The Br⁺ attaches to the double bond and a cyclic bronomium ion is formed. This is attacked by Br⁻, giving the dibromo compound. Note that this addition is *anti* because the Br⁻ attacks the cyclic bronomium ion in a standard S_N2 displacement from the opposite side.

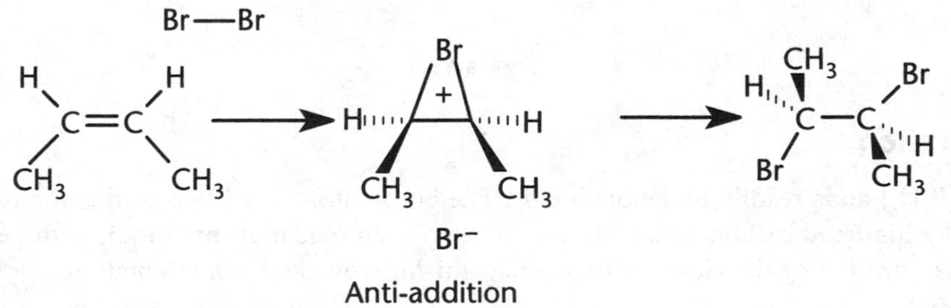

Anti-addition

Figure 43.7

If the reaction is carried out in a nucleophilic solvent, the solvent molecules can compete in the displacement step, producing, for example, a bromo alcohol rather than the dibromo compound.

Addition of H₂O

Water can be added to alkenes under acidic conditions. The double bond is protonated according to Markovnikov's rule, forming the most stable carbocation. This carbocation reacts with water, forming a protonated alcohol, which then loses a proton to yield the alcohol. The reaction is performed at low temperature because the reverse reaction is an acid-catalyzed dehydration favored by high temperatures.

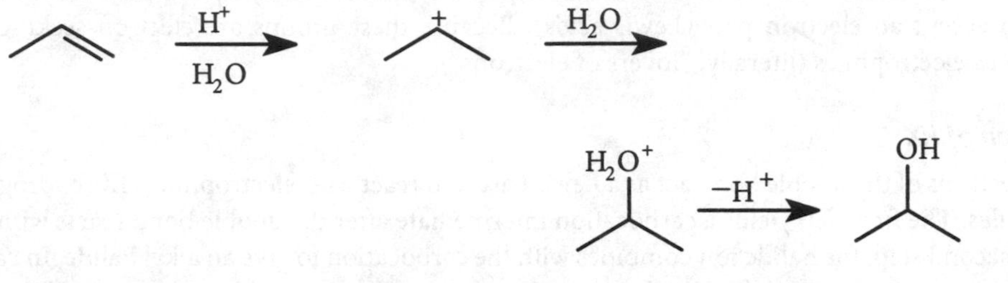

Figure 43.8

Direct addition of water is generally not useful in the laboratory because yields vary greatly with reaction conditions; therefore, this reaction is generally carried out indirectly using mercuric acetate, $Hg(CH_3COO)_2$.

Free Radical Additions

An alternate mechanism exists for the addition of HX (hydrogen halide) to alkenes, which proceeds through free-radical intermediates, and occurs when peroxides, oxygen, or other impurities are present. Free-radical additions are called anti-Markovnikov because X• adds first to the double bond, producing the most stable free radical on the most substituted carbon. The hydrogen then adds to the free radical, resulting in the less substituted product. The reaction is useful for HBr but is not practical for HCl or HI because the energies are unfavorable.

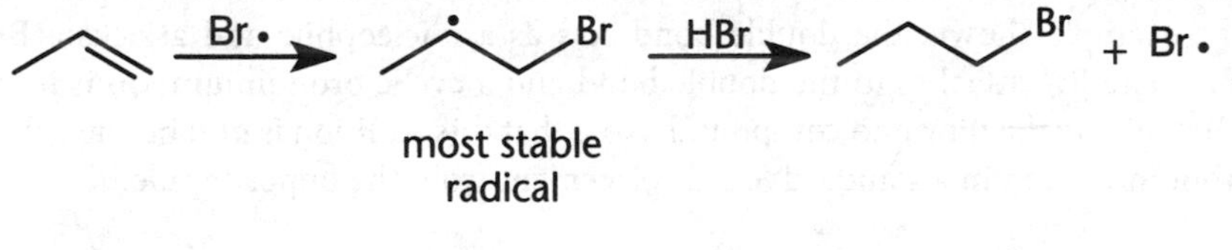

most stable
radical

Figure 43.9

Hydroboration

Diborane (B_2H_6) adds readily to double bonds. The boron atom is a Lewis acid and attaches to the less sterically hindered carbon atom. The second step is an oxidation-hydrolysis with peroxide and aqueous base, producing the alcohol with overall anti-Markovnikov, *syn* orientation.

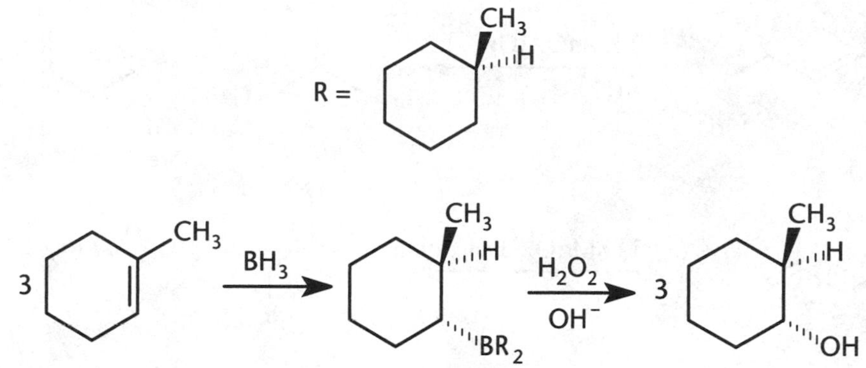

Figure 43.10

Oxidation

Potassium permanganate

Alkenes can be oxidized with $KMnO_4$ to provide different types of products, depending upon the reaction conditions. Cold, dilute, aqueous $KMnO_4$ reacts to produce 1,2 diols (vicinal diols), which are also called glycols, with *syn* orientation:

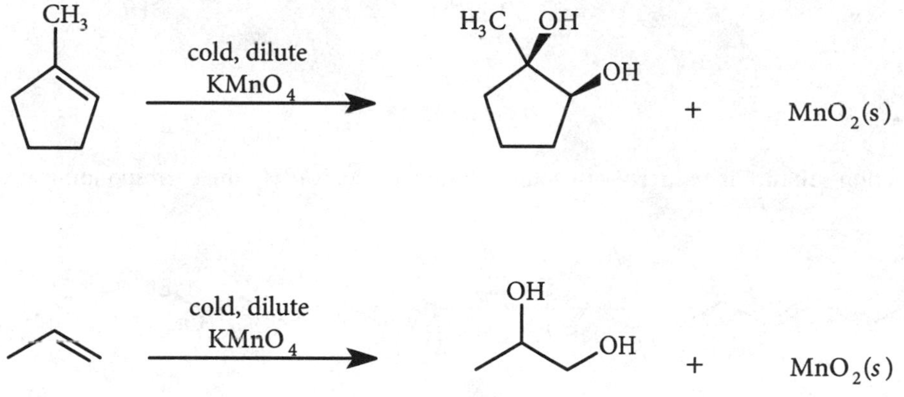

Figure 43.11

Under acidic conditions, manganate ions (MnO_4^{2-}) are reduced to manganese ions (Mn^{2+}), and this reaction can be coupled to the complete cleavage of a double bond. If a hot, basic solution of potassium permanganate is added to the alkene and then acidified, the product will be determined by the nature of the alkene substrate. Nonterminal alkenes are cleaved to form 2 molar equivalents of carboxylic acid, and terminal alkenes are cleaved to form a carboxylic acid and carbon dioxide. If the nonterminal double bonded carbon is disubstituted, however, a ketone will be formed:

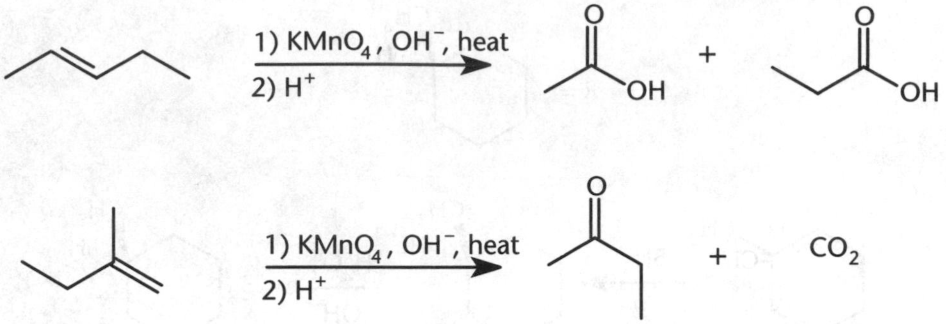

1) KMnO$_4$, OH$^-$, heat
2) H$^+$

1) KMnO$_4$, OH$^-$, heat
2) H$^+$

$+$ CO$_2$

Figure 43.12

Ozonolysis

Treatment of alkenes with ozone followed by reduction with zinc and water is a milder reaction. This treatment results in cleavage of the double bond to produce two aldehyde molecules as shown (or ketones if the double bond is substituted with alkyl groups):

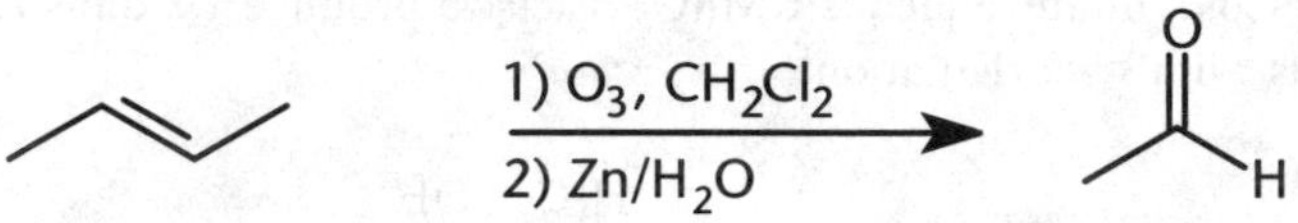

1) O$_3$, CH$_2$Cl$_2$
2) Zn/H$_2$O

Figure 43.13

If the reaction mixture is reduced with sodium borohydride, NaBH$_4$, the corresponding alcohols are produced:

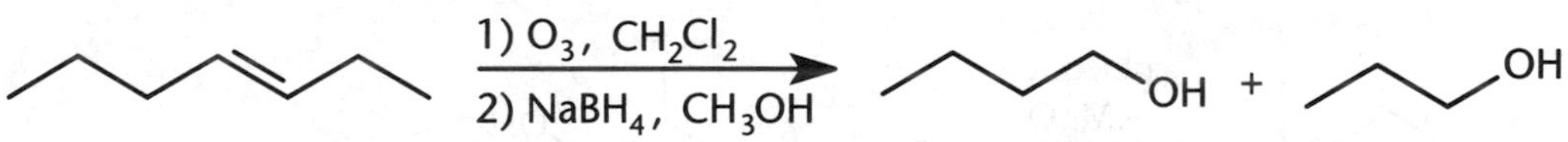

1) O$_3$, CH$_2$Cl$_2$
2) NaBH$_4$, CH$_3$OH

Figure 43.14

Peroxycarboxylic acids

Alkenes can be oxidized with peroxycarboxylic acids. Peroxyacetic acid (CH$_3$CO$_3$H) and *m*-chloroperoxybenzoic acid (mCPBA) are commonly used. The products formed are oxiranes (also called epoxides) and are highly reactive. This makes them ideal for further nucleophilic reactions such as substitutions and the formation of alcohols, glycols, and amines:

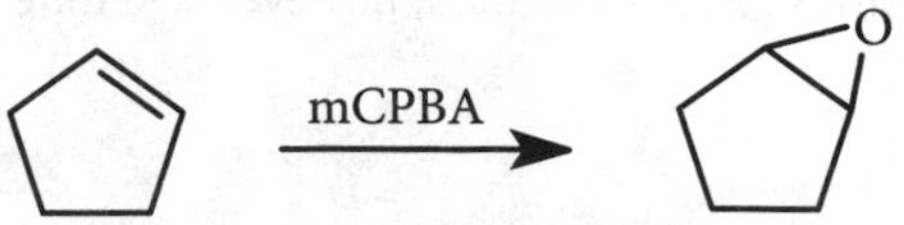

mCPBA

Figure 43.15

Polymerization

Polymerization is the creation of long, high molecular weight chains (polymers), composed of repeating subunits (called monomers). Polymerization usually occurs through a radical mechanism, although anionic and even cationic polymerizations are commonly observed. A typical example is the formation of polyethylene from ethylene (ethene) that requires high temperatures and pressures:

$$CH_2 = CH_2 \xrightarrow[\text{high pressure}]{R\bullet,\ \text{heat}} RCH_2CH_2(CH_2CH_2)_n CH_2CH_2R$$

Figure 43.16

ALKYNES

Alkynes are hydrocarbon compounds that possess one or more carbon-carbon triple bonds. The general formula for a straight-chain alkyne with one triple bond is C_nH_{2n-2}. Triple bonds are sp hybridized and are therefore linear, imparting unique characteristics to molecules that contain them.

NOMENCLATURE OF ALKYNES

The suffix **-yne** is used to designate an alkyne, and the position of the triple bond is specified when necessary. A common exception to the IUPAC rules is ethyne, which is called *acetylene*. Frequently, compounds are named as derivatives of acetylene.

$$CH_3CH_2CH_2\underset{\underset{Cl}{|}}{CH}C \equiv CCH_3 \qquad CH \equiv CH \qquad CH_3C \equiv CH$$

4-chloro-2-heptyne ethyne propyne

(acetylene) (methylacetylene)

Figure 43.17

PHYSICAL PROPERTIES OF ALKYNES

The physical properties of the alkynes are similar to those of their analogous alkenes and alkanes. In general, the shorter-chain compounds are gases, boiling at somewhat higher temperatures than the corresponding alkenes. Internal alkynes, like alkenes, boil at higher temperatures than terminal alkynes.

Asymmetrical distribution of electron density causes alkynes to have dipole moments that are larger than those of alkenes, but still small in magnitude. Thus, solutions of alkynes can be slightly polar.

Terminal alkynes are relatively acidic, having pK_a values of approximately 25. This property is exploited in some of the reactions of alkynes, which will be discussed later.

SYNTHESIS OF ALKYNES

Triple bonds can be made by the elimination of two molecules of HX from a geminal or vicinal dihalide:

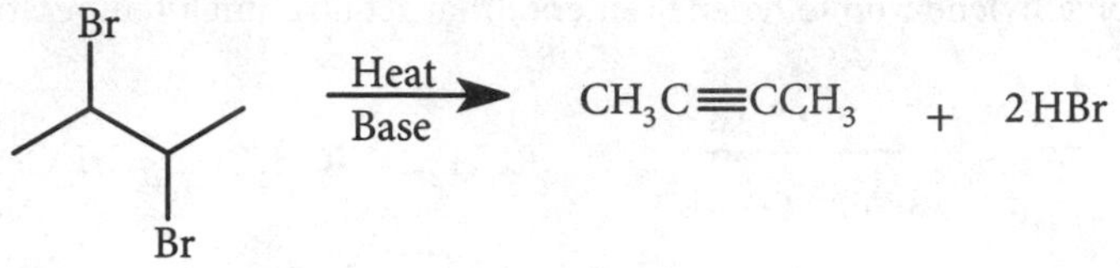

Figure 43.18

This reaction is not always practical and requires high temperatures and a strong base. A more useful method adds an already existing triple bond onto a particular carbon skeleton. A terminal triple bond is converted to a nucleophile by removing the acidic proton with strong base, producing an acetylide ion. This ion will perform nucleophilic displacements on alkyl halides at room temperature using an S_N2 mechanism:

Figure 43.19

REACTIONS OF ALKYNES

Alkynes undergo several types of reactions, most of which are closely related to the reactions of alkenes:

- a variety of reduction mechanisms by hydrogen and catalysts
- addition by electrophiles and free radicals
- hydroboration
- oxidation

Reduction

Alkynes, just like alkenes, can be hydrogenated with a metal catalyst to produce alkanes in a reaction that goes to completion:

$$CH_3\text{-}C{=}C\text{-}CH_3 \rightarrow CH_3CH_2CH_2CH_3 \text{ in the presence of Pt, Pd, or Ni}$$

A more useful reaction stops the reduction after addition of just one equivalent of H_2, producing alkenes. This partial hydrogenation can take place in two different ways. The first uses Lindlar's catalyst, which is palladium on barium sulfate $(BaSO_4)$ with quinoline, a poison that stops the reaction at the alkene stage. Because the reaction occurs on a metal surface, the product alkene is the *cis* isomer. The other method uses sodium in liquid ammonia below $-33°C$ (the boiling point of ammonia), and produces the *trans* isomer of the alkene via a free radical mechanism:

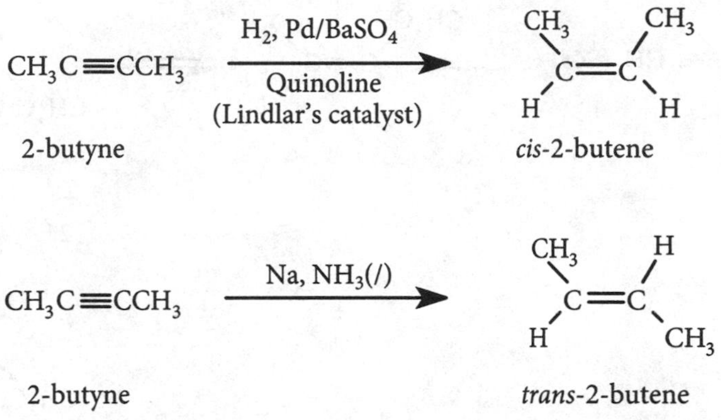

Figure 43.20

Addition

Electrophilic

Electrophilic addition to alkynes occurs in the same manner as it does to alkenes, with the reaction following Markovnikov's rule. The addition can generally be stopped at the intermediate alkene stage, or carried further:

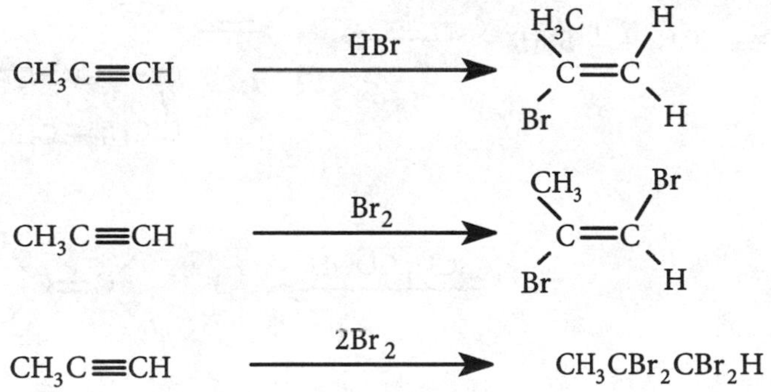

Figure 43.21

Free radical

Radicals add to triple bonds as they do to double bonds—with anti-Markovnikov placement of the halogen. The reaction product is usually the *trans* isomer, because the intermediate vinyl radical can isomerize to its more stable form as shown:

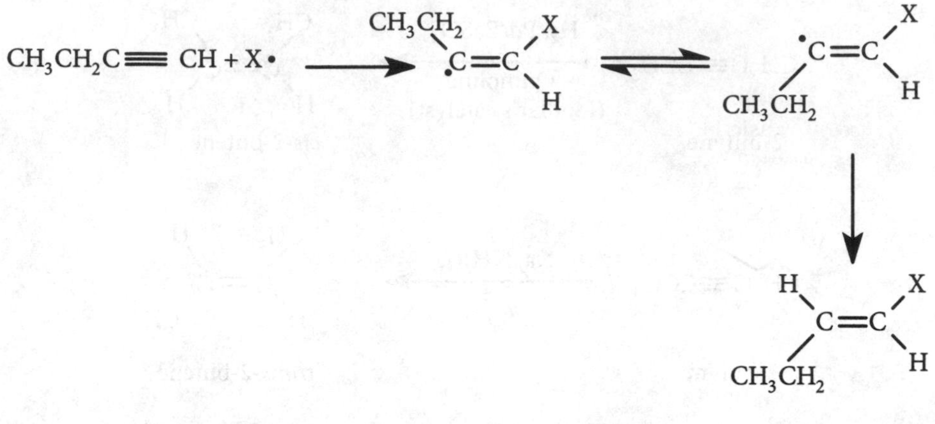

Figure 43.22

Hydroboration

Addition of boron to triple bonds occurs by the same method as addition of boron to double bonds. Addition is *syn,* and the boron atom adds first. The boron atom can be replaced with a proton from acetic acid, to produce a *cis* alkene:

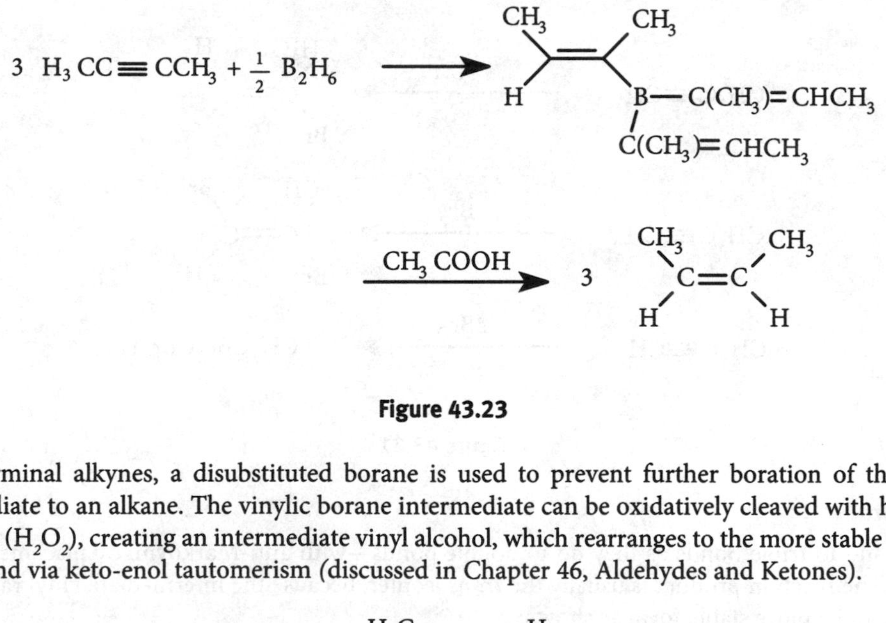

Figure 43.23

With terminal alkynes, a disubstituted borane is used to prevent further boration of the vinylic intermediate to an alkane. The vinylic borane intermediate can be oxidatively cleaved with hydrogen peroxide (H_2O_2), creating an intermediate vinyl alcohol, which rearranges to the more stable carbonyl compound via keto-enol tautomerism (discussed in Chapter 46, Aldehydes and Ketones).

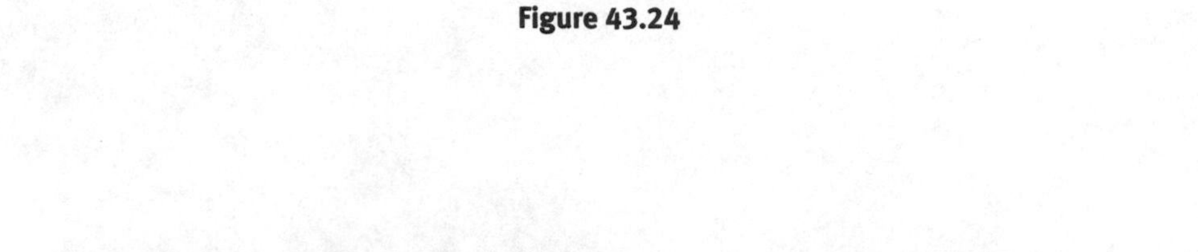

Figure 43.24

Oxidation

Alkynes can be oxidatively cleaved with either basic potassium permanganate (followed by acidification) or ozone. In both instances shown, carboxylic acids are produced, but treatment of a terminal alkyne with basic permanganate will produce carbon dioxide.

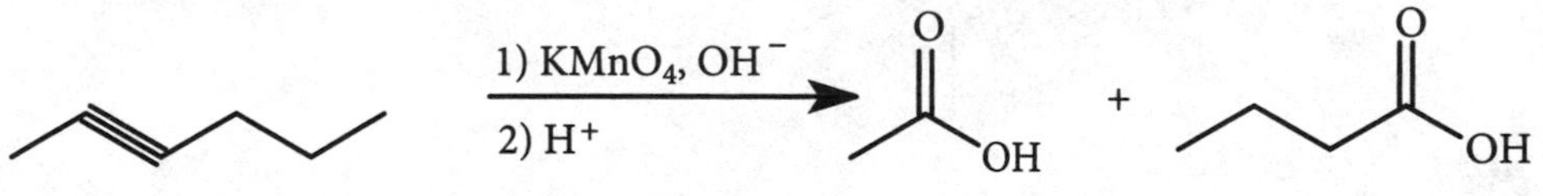

Figure 43.25

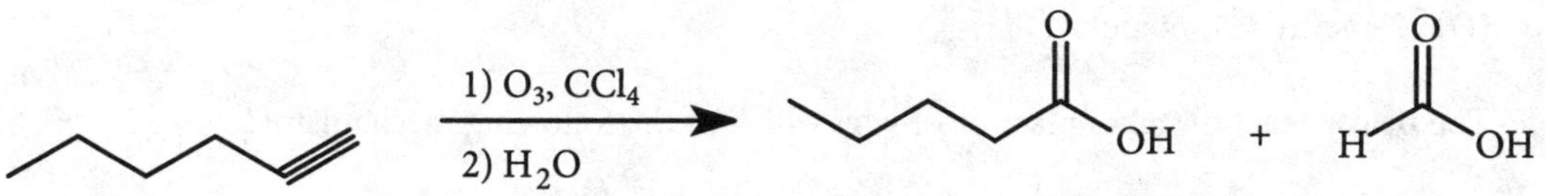

Figure 43.26

REVIEW PROBLEMS

1. The major product of the reaction below is

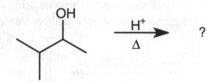

(A) 3-methyl-1-butene.

(B) 2-methyl-3-butene.

(C) 3-methyl-2-butene.

(D) 2-methyl-2-butene.

2. The below reaction takes place mostly by which of the following mechanisms?

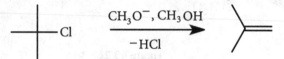

(A) S_N1

(B) S_N2

(C) E1

(D) E2

3. Which of the following products will be formed if 2-methyl-2-butene is reacted with hot basic $KMnO_4$?

(A) 1 mole of acetic acid and 1 mole of propanoic acid

(B) 2 moles of pentanoic acid

(C) 1 mole of acetic acid and 1 mole of acetone

(D) 2 moles of acetic acid and 1 mole of CO_2

4. Which of the following is true about E2 reactions?

(A) They are greatly affected by steric hindrance.

(B) They need a strong base to abstract the proton.

(C) They are favored over S_N2 by weak Lewis bases.

(D) They are favored over S_N1 and E1 by polar solvents.

5. What is the product of the following reaction?

$$\xrightarrow[\text{2. Zn, H}_2\text{O}]{\text{1. O}_3/\text{CH}_2\text{Cl}_2} \quad ?$$

(A) 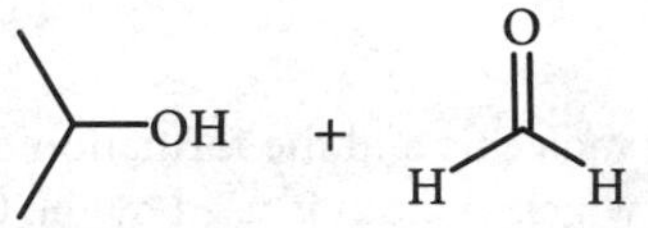 +   **(B)** 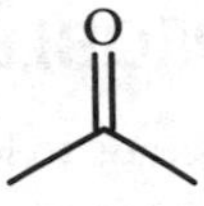 + CH_3OH

(C) 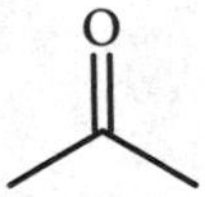 + CO_2 **(D)** 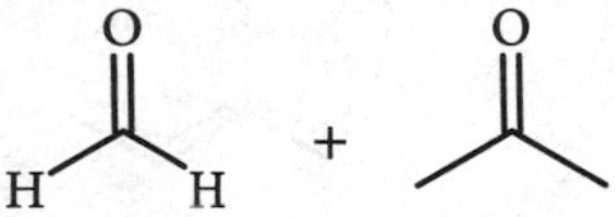 +

6. What is the product of the following reaction?

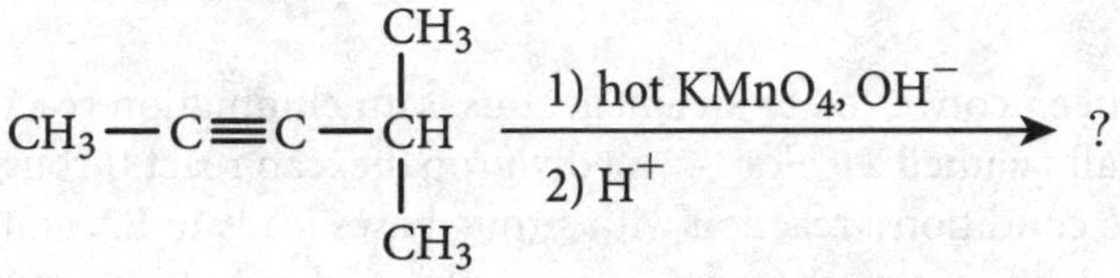

(A) 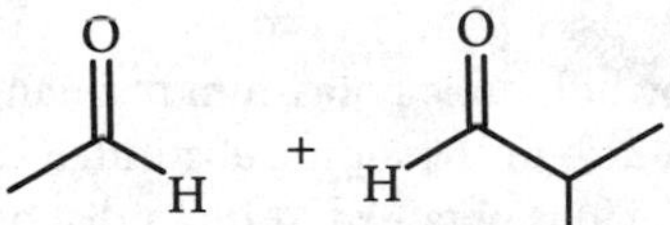   **(B)**

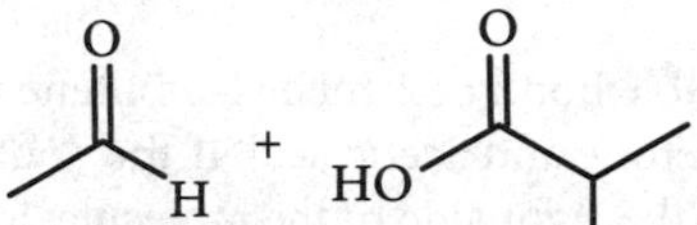

(C) 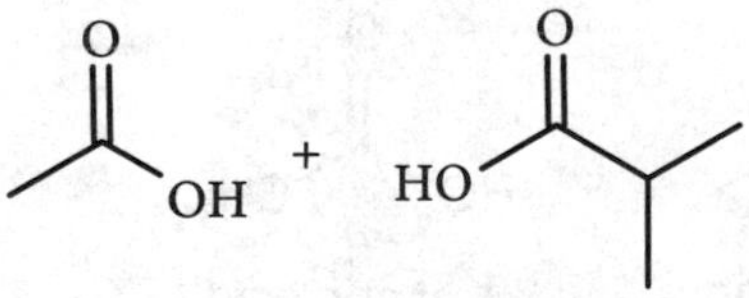   **(D)**

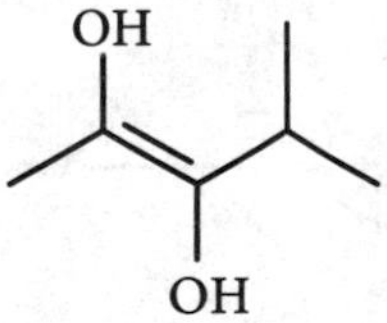

7. What is the product of the following reaction?

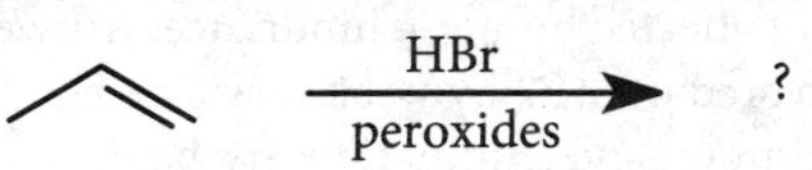

(A) 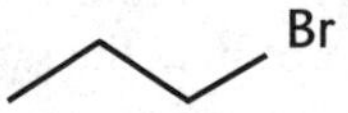   **(B)**

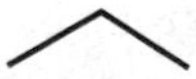

(C) 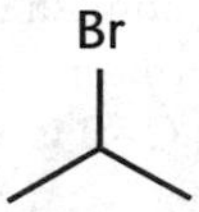   **(D)**

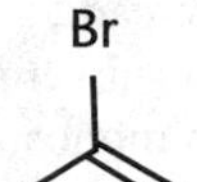

SOLUTIONS TO REVIEW PROBLEMS

1. **D** Heating an alcohol generally leads to loss of a water molecule and the formation of a double bond. Two products can be obtained depending on which H atom is used by the OH group to form water; either

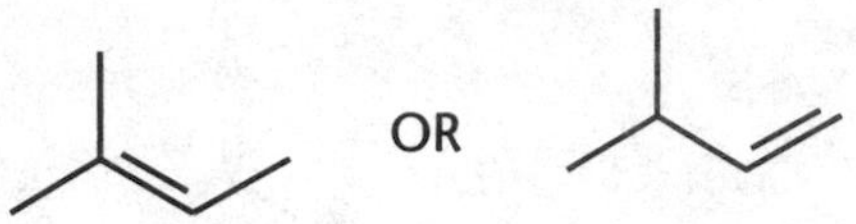

OR

The most stable alkene, which is the most substituted one, is formed. Of the two alkenes, 2-methyl-2-butene is more stable, and the correct choice is (D).

2. **D** Since tertiary butyl chloride has been converted to an alkene, this is an elimination reaction. This particular compound, formally named 2-chloro-2-methylpropane, can react through either E1 or E2 depending on the conditions: reaction with strong bases leads to E2, and reaction with weak bases leads to E1. Since methoxide is a strong base, elimination occurs by the E2 mechanism. Choice (D) is the correct response.

3. **C** The double bond of 2-methyl-2-butene is cleaved by hot, basic potassium permanganate to form acetone and acetic acid. If the double-bonded carbon is a monosubstituted carbon as seen on the right side of the molecule, a carboxylic acid is obtained; if it is a disubstituted carbon as seen on the left side, a ketone is obtained. Thus, the correct choice is (C).

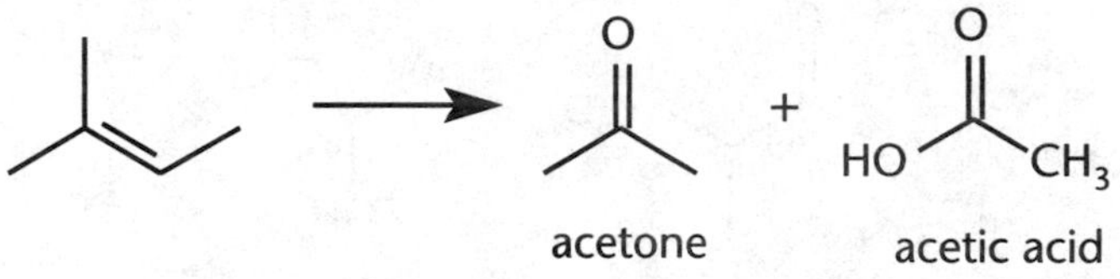

acetone   acetic acid

4. **B** Answer choice (A) is incorrect; E2 reactions are not affected by steric hindrance. Answer choice (C) is also incorrect, as S_N2 reactions are favored over E2 by weak Lewis bases. Answer choice (D) is a distortion, as all four substitution and elimination mechanisms require polar solvents to keep the polar reactants and products in solution. The correct answer choice is (B), as E2 requires a strong base to remove a proton at the same time that the leaving group departs on the opposite side of the molecule.

5. **D** Ozonolysis of an alkene and subsequent treatment with zinc and water produces carbonyl compounds. The double bond is broken and a disubstituted double-bonded carbon is converted to a ketone, whereas a monosubstituted double-bonded carbon is converted to an aldehyde. In this reaction, C−1 is a monosubstituted carbon and C−2 is a disubstituted carbon, and thus the products obtained are a ketone and an aldehyde.

6. **C** Treating alkynes with hot basic $KMnO_4$ leads to the cleavage of the triple bond and the formation of carboxylic acids.

7.   **A**   In the presence of peroxides, the addition of HBr to the double bond takes place in an anti-Markovnikov manner in a series of free-radical reactions initiated by peroxides.

   1.   ROOR → 2RO•
   2.   HBr + RO• → ROH + Br•
   3. $CH_3CH=CH_2$ + Br• → CH_3-CH_2Br
   4. CH_3-CH_2Br + HBr → $CH_3-CH_2-CH_2Br$ + Br •

In step 3, CH_3-CH_2Br is formed instead of CH_3-CHBr^-, since the more substituted free-radical is more stable than the less substituted one. Thus, the correct choice is (A). Note that in the absence of peroxides, HBr adds to the double bond in a Markovnikov manner.

CHAPTER FORTY-FOUR

Aromatic Compounds

The terms **aromatic** and **aliphatic,** meaning "fragrant" and "fatty," respectively, were used originally to distinguish types of organic compounds. The terms are still used by organic chemists but with new definitions. "Aromatic" now describes an unusually stable ring system with several unique characteristics. Aromatic compounds are cyclic, conjugated molecules that possess $4n + 2$ pi electrons and adopt planar conformations to allow maximum overlap of the conjugated pi orbitals. Aliphatic describes all compounds that are not aromatic.

All aromatic compounds are conjugated, but not all conjugated molecules are aromatic. A conjugated system consists of alternating single and double bonds, creating a delocalized pi electron network. This allows one or more resonance structures to exist; resonance indicates stability, which is a key characteristic of aromatics. Because every other bond is a double bond, every carbon in the conjugated system is sp^2 hybridized, and thus is trigonal planar in shape. When confined to a ring system, all of the sp^2 hybridized carbons must lie flat relative to each other, giving another characteristic of aromatics: they are cyclic and planar.

The criterion of possessing $4n + 2$ pi electrons is known as **Hückel's rule**, and is an important indicator of aromaticity. If a cyclic conjugated molecule follows Hückel's rule, then it is an aromatic compound. The integer n can be any nonnegative whole number, including 0, and thus $4n + 2$ can be 2, 6, 10, 14, 18, etc. It is often easier to remember and recognize these allowable values for Hückel's rule than to calculate them. To determine the number of pi electrons, determine the number of pi bonds and multiply by two. Unbonded p orbitals that contain lone pairs of electrons sometimes take part in the conjugation of an aromatic compound. Resonance forms are possible that include these electrons and usually have formal charges; when this is possible, the lone pairs are counted toward Hückel's rule.

Neutral compounds, anions, and cations may all be aromatic, and many compounds must be in their ionic form in order to be aromatic. Some typical aromatic compounds and ions are:

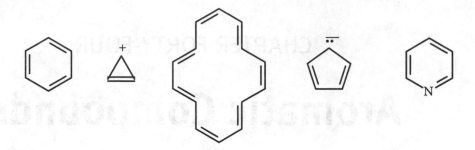

Figure 44.1

A cyclic, conjugated molecule that possesses 4*n* pi electrons is said to be **anti-aromatic** (a cyclic, conjugated molecule that is unstable and highly reactive). Some typical anti-aromatic compounds are:

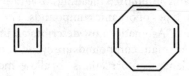

Figure 44.2

NOMENCLATURE

Aromatic compounds are referred to as **aryl** compounds, or **arenes**, and are represented by the symbol **Ar**. Aliphatic compounds are called **alkyl** and are represented by the symbol **R**. Common names exist for many mono- and disubstituted aromatic compounds.

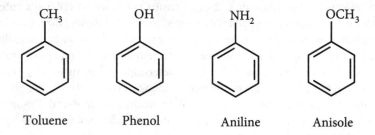

Toluene   Phenol   Aniline   Anisole

Figure 44.3

The benzene group is called a **phenyl** group (**Ph**) when named as a substituent. The term **benzyl** refers to a toluene molecule substituted at the methyl position.

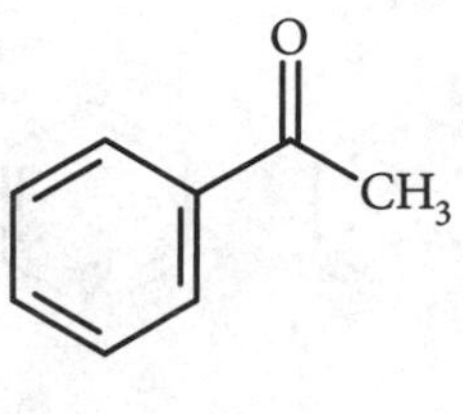

methyl phenyl ketone 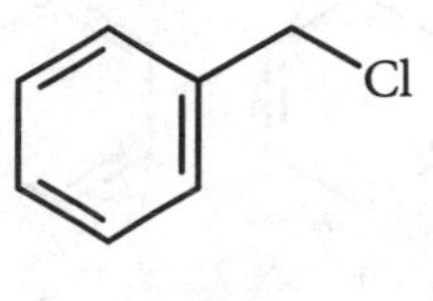   benzyl chloride

Figure 44.4

Substituted benzene rings are named as alkyl benzenes, with the substituents numbered to produce the lowest sequence. A 1,2-disubstituted compound is called *ortho*- or *o*-; a 1,3-disubstituted compound is called *meta*- or *m*-; and a 1,4-disubstituted compound is called *para*- or *p*-.

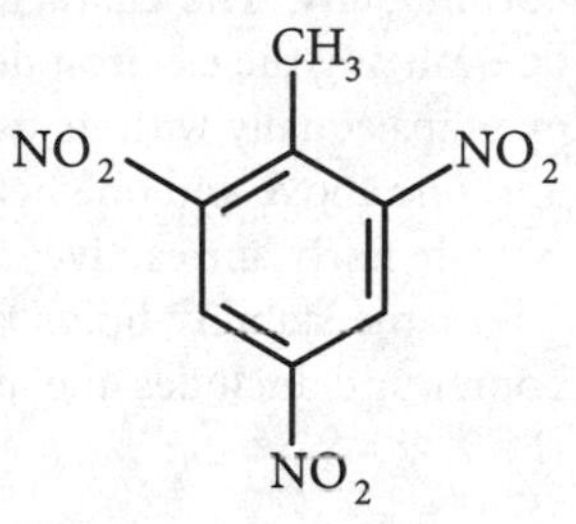

2,4,6-trinitrotoluene   *o*-nitrotoluene 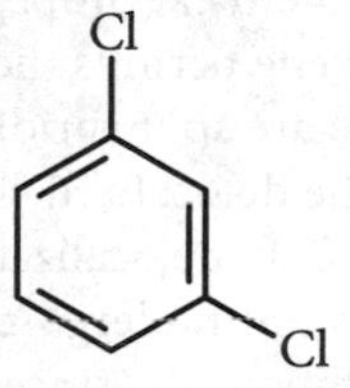   *m*-dichlorobenzene
(TNT)

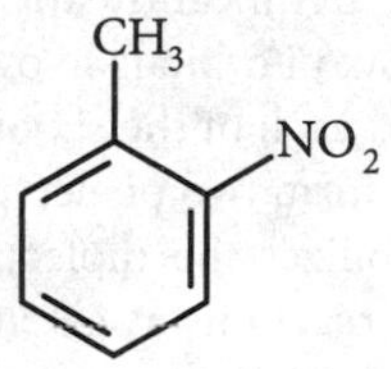

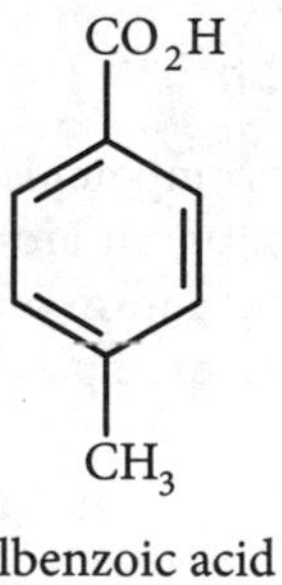

p-methylbenzoic acid

Figure 44.5

There are many polycyclic and heterocyclic aromatic compounds, many of which have common names:

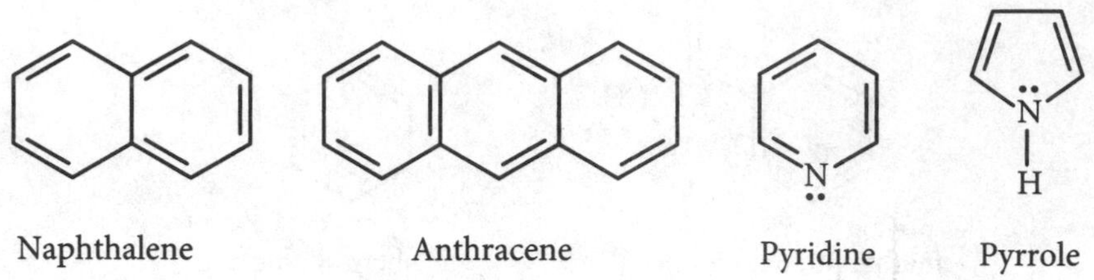

Naphthalene   Anthracene   Pyridine   Pyrrole

Figure 44.6

PROPERTIES

The physical properties of aromatic compounds are generally similar to those of other hydrocarbons. In contrast, chemical properties are significantly affected by aromaticity. The characteristic planar shape of benzene permits the ring's six pi orbitals to overlap, delocalizing the electron density. All six carbon atoms are sp^2 hybridized, and each of the six orbitals overlaps equally with its two neighbors. As a result, the delocalized electrons form two pi electron clouds, one above and one below the plane of the ring. This delocalization stabilizes the molecule, making it fairly unreactive: in particular, benzene does not undergo addition reactions as alkenes do. The same stability holds true for other aromatic compounds, since the definition of an aromatic compound includes the presence of a delocalized pi electron system.

REACTIONS

Electrophilic Aromatic Substitution

The most important reaction of aromatic compounds is electrophilic aromatic substitution. In this reaction an electrophile replaces a proton on an aromatic ring, producing a substituted aromatic compound. Because benzene is nonreactive, a form of acidic catalyst is required for the substitution reaction to proceed. The most common examples of substitution reactions are halogenation, sulfonation, nitration, and acylation.

Halogenation

Aromatic rings react with bromine or chlorine in the presence of a Lewis acid, such as $FeCl_3$, $FeBr_3$, or $AlCl_3$, to produce monosubstituted products in good yield. Reaction of fluorine and iodine with aromatic rings is less useful, as fluorine tends to produce multisubstituted products, and iodine's lack of reactivity requires special conditions for the reaction to proceed.

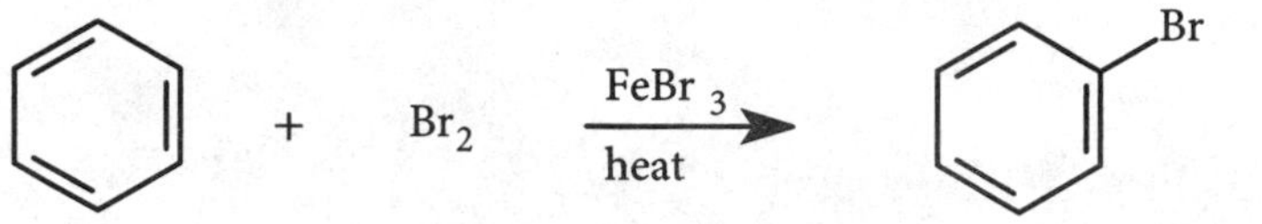

Figure 44.7

Sulfonation

Aromatic rings react with fuming sulfuric acid (a mixture of sulfuric acid and sulfur trioxide) to form sulfonic acids.

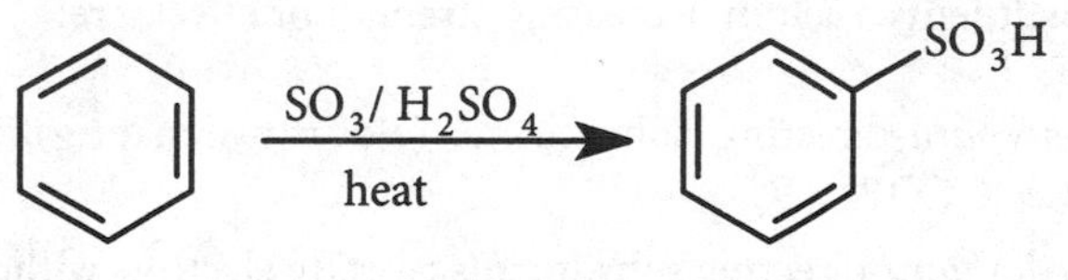

Figure 44.8

Nitration

The nitration of aromatic rings is another synthetically useful reaction. A mixture of nitric and sulfuric acids is used to create the nitronium ion, NO_2^+, a strong electrophile. This reacts with aromatic rings to produce nitro compounds.

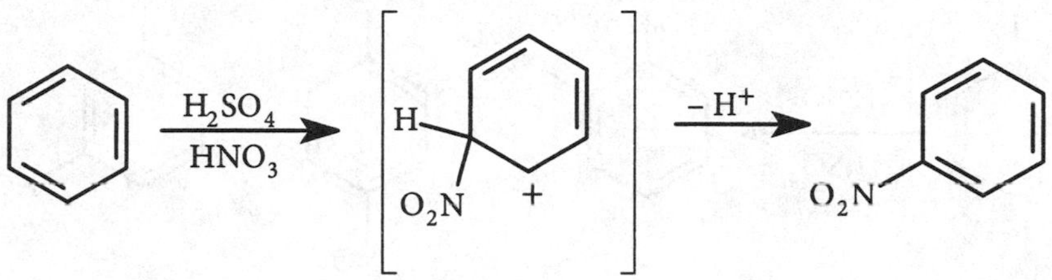

Figure 44.9

Acylation (Friedel-Crafts reactions)

In a Friedel-Crafts acylation reaction, a carbocation electrophile, usually an acyl group, is incorporated into the aromatic ring. These reactions are usually catalyzed by Lewis acids such as $AlCl_3$. This reaction can also be used to add alkyl groups, but the reaction is difficult to control and can lead to multiple products.

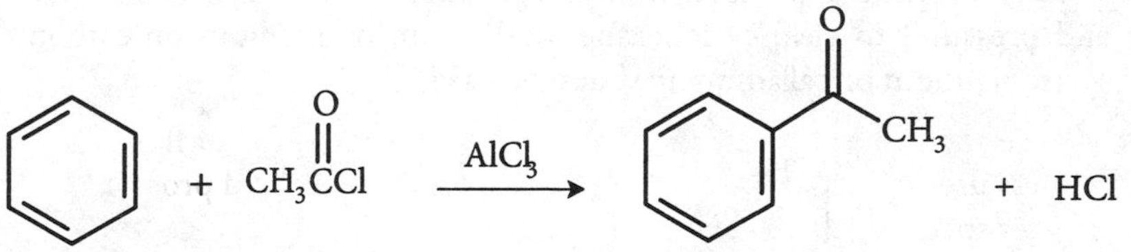

Figure 44.10

Substituent effects

The first substituent on an aromatic ring strongly influences the susceptibility of the ring to further electrophilic aromatic substitution, and also strongly affects what position on the ring another electrophile is most likely to attack. Substituents can be grouped into three different classes according to whether they are activating or deactivating, and where on the ring the next reaction is likely to take place. Activators cause the next reaction to occur more quickly and more easily; deactivators cause the next reaction to occur more slowly and with greater difficulty. These effects depend on whether the group tends to donate or withdraw electron density.

The three classes of substituents, each in decreasing strength of effect, are:

a. Activating, *ortho/para*-directing substituents (electron-donating): $NH_2 > NR_2 > OH > NHCOR > OR > OCOR > R$

b. Deactivating, *ortho/para*-directing substituents (weakly electron-withdrawing): $F > Cl > Br > I$

c. Deactivating, *meta*-directing substituents (electron-withdrawing): $NO_2 > SO_3H >$ carbonyl compounds, including COOH, COOR, COR, and CHO

Example: When toluene undergoes electrophilic aromatic substitution, the methyl group directs substitution to occur primarily at the *ortho* and *para* positions:

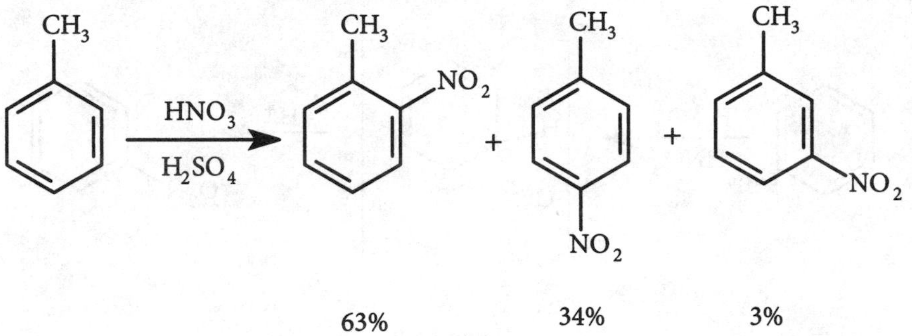

63%   34%   3%

Figure 44.11

Reduction

Catalytic Reduction

Benzene rings can be reduced by catalytic hydrogenation under vigorous conditions (elevated temperature and pressure) to yield cyclohexane. Ruthenium or rhodium on carbon are the most common catalysts; platinum or palladium may also be used.

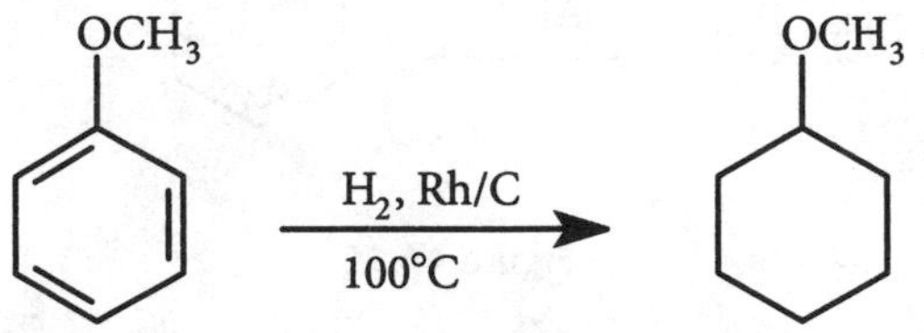

Figure 44.12

REVIEW PROBLEMS

1. Predict aromatic, anti-aromatic, or nonaromatic behavior for each of the following compounds.

(A)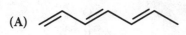

(B)

(C)

(D)

(E)

2. Which of the following represents the correct structure for *para*-nitrotoluene?

(A) CH_2NH_2

(B) NO_2
CH_3

(C) NO_2
H_3C

(D) NH_2
H_3C

3. What would be the major product of the following reaction?

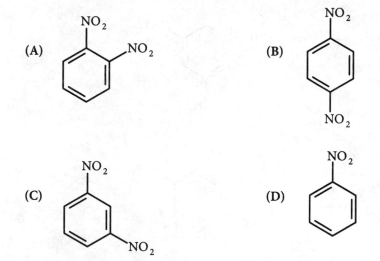

4. Nitration of benzene at 30°C leads to a 95 percent yield of nitrobenzene. When the temperature is increased to 100°C, dinitrobenzene is produced. Which of the following is the predominant product?

5. What is the major product of the nitration reaction below?

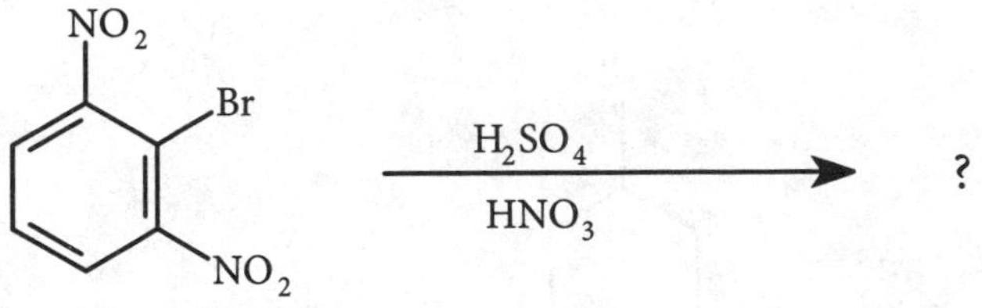

$$\xrightarrow[\text{HNO}_3]{\text{H}_2\text{SO}_4}$$?

(A)

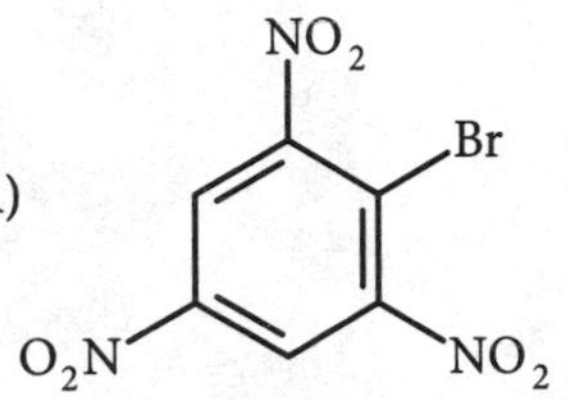

(C)

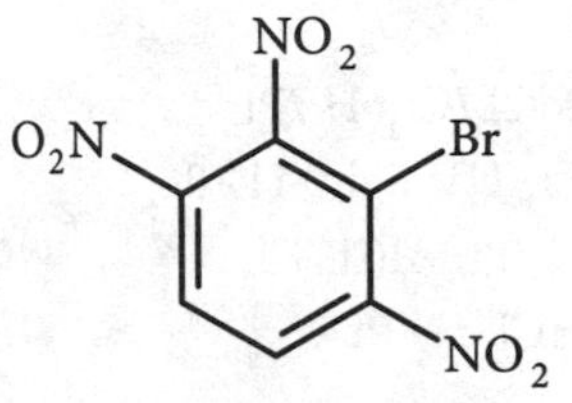

(B)

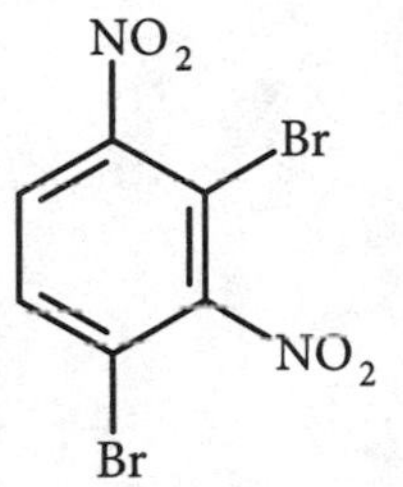

(D)

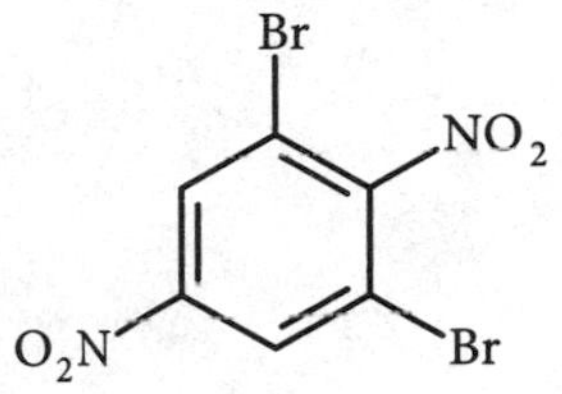

6. Which represents the predominant product(s) of the reaction below?

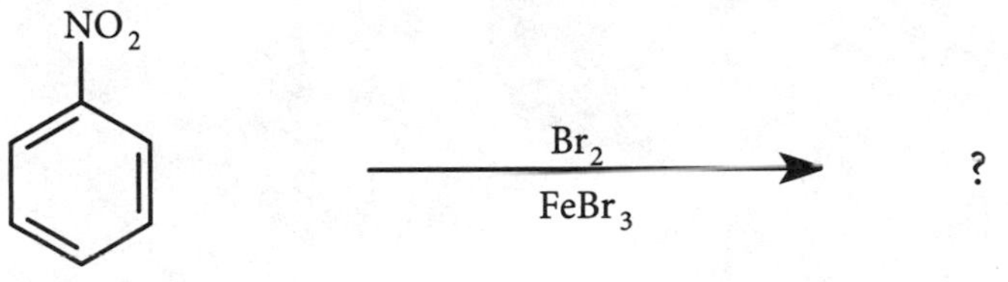

$$\xrightarrow[\text{FeBr}_3]{\text{Br}_2}$$?

(A)

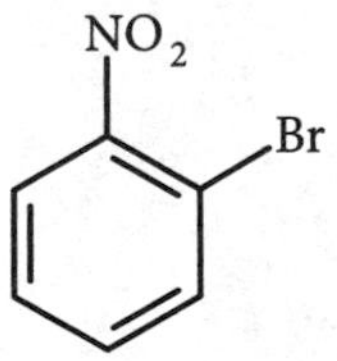

(B)

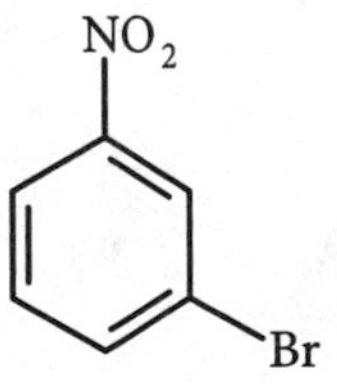

(C)

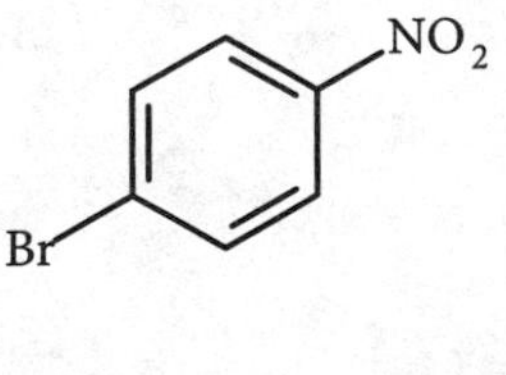

(D)

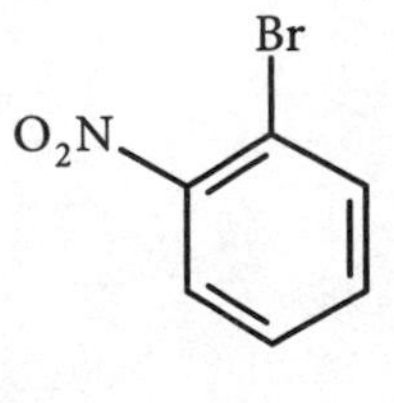

7. Which sequence of reaction conditions should be used to produce the compound below from benzene?

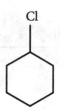

(A) $AlCl_3/Cl_2$; H_2/Pt
(B) Cl_2/UV light; H_2/Pt
(C) H_2/Pt; $AlCl_3/Cl_2$
(D) HCl; H_2/Pt

SOLUTIONS TO REVIEW PROBLEMS

1. **A** Nonaromatic. This compound has $4n + 2 = 6$ pi electrons ($n = 1$), and is a conjugated system; however, it is not cyclic.

   B Nonaromatic. This compound has $4n + 2 = 6$ pi electrons ($n = 1$) and is cyclic. However, there is no conjugation of the double bonds.

   C Aromatic. This compound (naphthalene) is cyclic, has $4n + 2 = 8$ pi electrons ($n = 2$), and has a conjugated system of double bonds.

   D Anti-aromatic. This compound is cyclic and conjugated. However, it has only $4n = 4$ pi electrons ($n = 1$).

   E Aromatic. This class of compounds (alkyl anilinium ions) has $4n + 2 = 6$ pi electrons ($n = 1$), is cyclic, and has conjugated double bond systems.

2. **C** Toluene is the common name for methylbenzene: a methyl group attached to a benzene ring. In *para*-nitrotoluene, the nitro group (NO_2) is attached to the ring directly across from the methyl group. Choice (C) is the correct response. Choice (B) is incorrect because the nitro group is *meta*, not *para* substituted. Choices (A) and (D) can be eliminated since nitro groups are not present in these compounds.

3. **B** The reaction shown, a Friedel-Crafts acylation of toluene, will yield a product containing a $-CH_3$ substituent and a $-C=O$ substituent. Chlorination of the ring also uses $AlCl_3$ as a reagent, but the second reagent would have to be Cl_2, not C_2H_5COCl; thus, choices (C) and (D) (both chlorotoluenes) can be eliminated. Since CH_3 is an activating, *ortho/para*-directing group, the *meta* isomer, choice (A), would be a minor product at best. Choice (B), the *para* isomer, would be favored by the substituent effect of the methyl group, and along with the *ortho* isomer (which is not among these choices) would be the major product.

4. **C** *meta*-dinitrobenzene is the predominant product since $-NO_2$ is a *meta*-directing group.

5. **A** All three substituents of 2-bromo-1,3-dinitrobenzene direct reaction to C−5, which is *meta* to both nitro groups and *para* to the bromine atom, so choice (A) will be the major product. Since all three groups are deactivating, the reaction will be slow and require elevated temperatures to proceed.

6. **B** This reaction shows the bromination of nitrobenzene. Choices (A) and (D) are actually different views of the same compound. Since aromatic rings are planar, rings that are mirror images are identical (although alkyl substituents of benzene rings may still have chiral centers, and molecules containing such groups may be chiral). Choice (B) shows *meta*-bromonitrobenzene, which is the favored product of this reaction since the nitro substituent is *meta*-directing. Choices (A) and (D) show the *para* isomer, while (C) shows the *ortho* isomer, both of which are less favored in this reaction.

7. **A** In order to produce chlorocyclohexane, two different procedures must be carried out: the benzene ring must be chlorinated and then hydrogenated. A suitable way to chlorinate the ring is to use Cl_2 and the Lewis acid $AlCl_3$, which is choice (A). Using chlorine in

the presence of UV light will not be effective, so choice (B) is incorrect. Choice (D) is incorrect because HCl will not chlorinate the ring. Now for the second step: hydrogenation. Hydrogenation of the benzene ring can be accomplished by using hydrogen in the presence of a platinum catalyst, so choice (A) is the correct answer. If the procedure were carried out according to choice (C), reduction would occur, forming cyclohexane, but chlorination would not, since cyclohexane is unreactive towards chlorine and the Lewis acid catalyst.

CHAPTER FORTY-FIVE

Alcohols and Ethers

Alcohols are compounds with the general formula **ROH**. The functional group –**OH** is called the **hydroxyl** group. An alcohol can be thought of as a substituted water molecule, with an alkyl group R replacing one **H** atom.

An ether is a compound with two alkyl or aryl groups bonded to a single oxygen atom. The general formula for an ether is R-O-R, and ethers can be thought of as disubstituted water molecules.

The nomenclature, properties, synthesis, and reactions of alcohols will be discussed in the following sections; subsequently the same topics will be reviewed for ethers.

NOMENCLATURE OF ALCOHOLS

Alcohols are named in the IUPAC system by replacing the **-e** ending of the root alkane with the ending **-ol**. The −OH group has high priority for naming; the carbon atom attached to the hydroxyl group usually must be included in the longest chain and receive the lowest possible number. Some examples are:

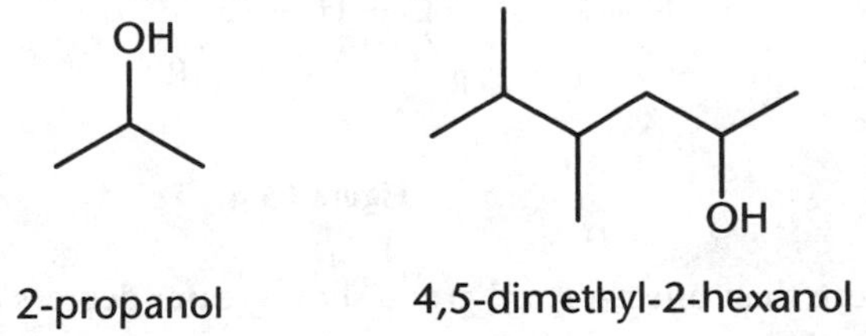

2-propanol   4,5-dimethyl-2-hexanol

Figure 45.1

The common names for alcohols are given by naming the alkyl group as a derivative, followed by the word *alcohol*.

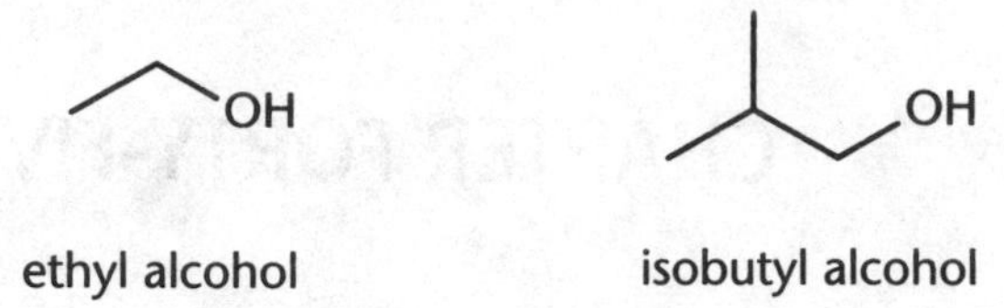

ethyl alcohol   isobutyl alcohol

Figure 45.2

Compounds of the general formula ArOH, with a hydroxyl group attached to an aromatic ring, are called **phenols**.

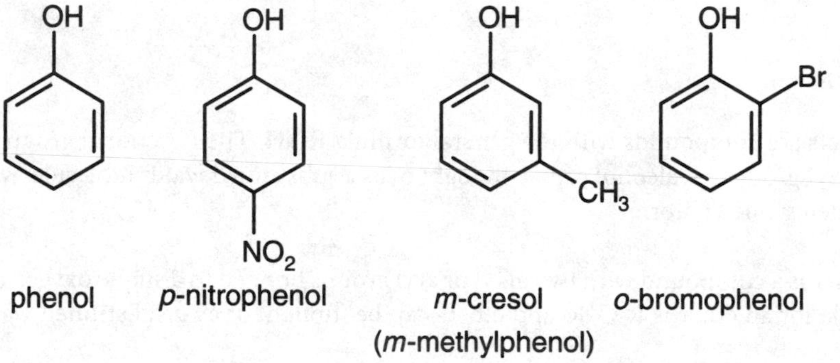

phenol   *p*-nitrophenol   *m*-cresol   *o*-bromophenol
                                         (*m*-methylphenol)

Figure 45.3

PHYSICAL PROPERTIES OF ALCOHOLS

Alcohols have a hydrogen attached directly to an oxygen, and thus are able to form **hydrogen bonds**. As a result of these strong intermolecular attractions, the boiling points of alcohols are significantly higher than those of their analogous hydrocarbons.

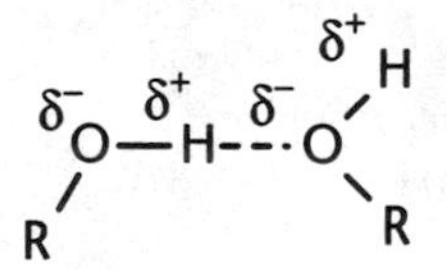

Figure 45.4

Molecules with more than one hydroxyl group show greater degrees of hydrogen bonding, as shown by the following boiling points:

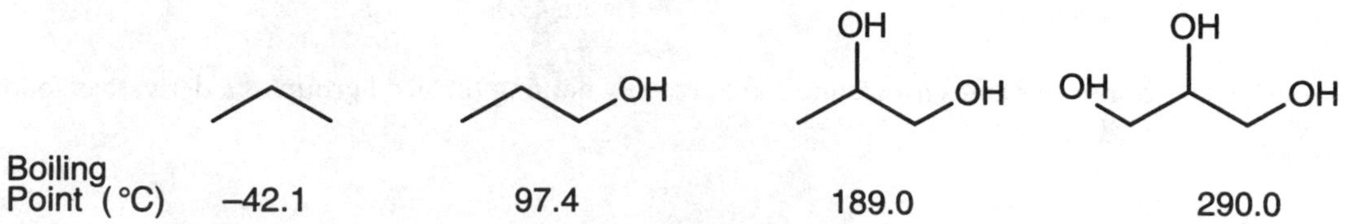

| Boiling Point (°C) | –42.1 | 97.4 | 189.0 | 290.0 |

Figure 45.5

The hydrogen atom of the hydroxyl group is weakly acidic, and alcohols can dissociate into protons and alkoxy ions just as water dissociates into protons and hydroxide ions. pK_a values of several compounds are listed below. The presence of electron withdrawing groups such as fluorine stabilize the negatively charged conjugate base of the alcohol, thus decreasing the pK_a. Conversely, alkyl groups destabilize the anionic form because of their electron donating properties, thereby increasing the pK_a. Note that as pK_a decreases, acidity increases; acids and pK_a values are discussed in Chapter 37, Acids and Bases.

	Dissociation		pK_a
H_2O	$\rightleftharpoons$	$HO^- + H^+$	15.7
CH_3OH	$\rightleftharpoons$	$CH_3O^- + H^+$	15.5
C_2H_5OH	$\rightleftharpoons$	$C_2H_5O^- + H^+$	15.9
i-PrOH	$\rightleftharpoons$	i-PrO$^- + H^+$	17.1
t-BuOH	$\rightleftharpoons$	t-BuO$^- + H^+$	18.0
CF_3CH_2OH	$\rightleftharpoons$	$CF_3CH_2O^- + H^+$	12.4
PhOH	$\rightleftharpoons$	$PhO^- + H+$	$\approx$10.0

Table 45.1

Phenols are more acidic than aliphatic alcohols, due to resonance structures that distribute the negative charge of the conjugate base throughout the ring, thus stabilizing the anion. This acidity allows phenols to readily form salts with inorganic bases such as NaOH. Phenols readily form intermolecular hydrogen bonds and have relatively high melting and boiling points. However, phenol and many of its derivatives are only slightly soluble in water due to the conflicting effects of the hydrophobicity of the phenyl ring and the ability of the $-OH$ group to hydrogen bond. The presence of other substituents on the ring has significant effects on the acidity, boiling point, and melting point of phenols. As with other aromatic compounds, electron-withdrawing substituents increase acidity by stabilizing the negatively charged conjugate base, and electron-donating groups decrease acidity.

OVERVIEW OF ALCOHOLS

Key Reaction Mechanisms for Alcohols

Several basic reaction mechanisms occur over and over in the chemistry of alcohols (and ethers in many cases as well). These reactions provide a framework for understanding and learning how the alcohols behave, and specific examples will be shown in the sections on both synthesis and reactions of alcohols that follow.

1. S_N1 and S_N2 nucleophilic substitution to create alcohols. Conversely, protonation of an alcohol allows it act as a leaving group in these reactions. See Chapter 42 for a review of S_N1 and S_N2 reaction mechanisms.

2. Electrophilic addition of water to a double bond to create an alcohol. Conversely, elimination reactions (E1, E2) remove hydroxyls to create a double bond. Addition and elimination reactions are discussed in Chapter 43.

3. Nucleophilic addition to a carbonyl to create an alcohol. This reaction type is discussed further in Chapters 44–46.

4. Oxidation and reduction: Alcohols are at the most reduced end of the oxidation/reduction continuum (shown in Table 45.2 below), as they have only single bonds to oxygen. Carbonyl-containing compounds are more oxidized, as demonstrated by the larger number of bonds to oxygen from a single carbon. Additional discussion of alcohols relative to aldehydes, ketones, and carboxylic acids is found in chapters 46 and 47.

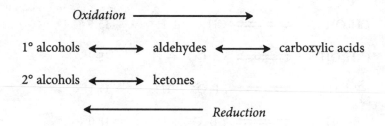

Oxidation ⟶

1° alcohols ⟷ aldehydes ⟷ carboxylic acids

2° alcohols ⟷ ketones

⟵ *Reduction*

Table 45.2

SYNTHESIS OF ALCOHOLS

Alcohols can be prepared from a variety of different types of compounds. Methanol, also called wood alcohol, is obtained from the destructive distillation of wood. It is toxic and can cause blindness if ingested. Ethanol, or grain alcohol, is produced from the fermentation of sugars and can be metabolized by the body; however, in large enough quantities, it too is toxic.

Addition Reactions

Alcohols can be prepared via several reactions that involve addition of water to double bonds (discussed in Chapter 41).

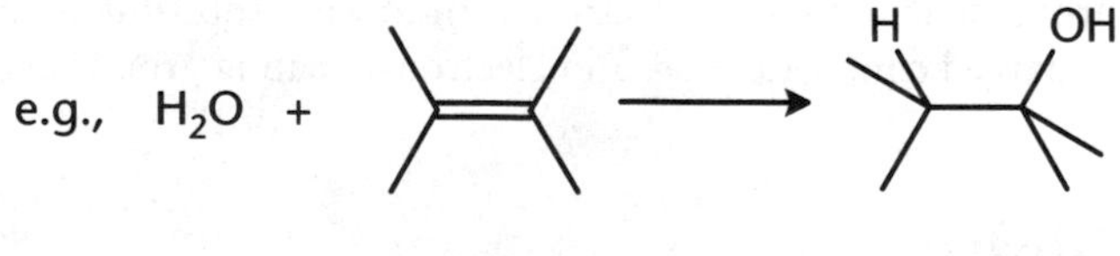

e.g., H_2O +

Figure 45.6

Alcohols can also be prepared from the addition of organometallic compounds to carbonyl groups (discussed in Chapter 46).

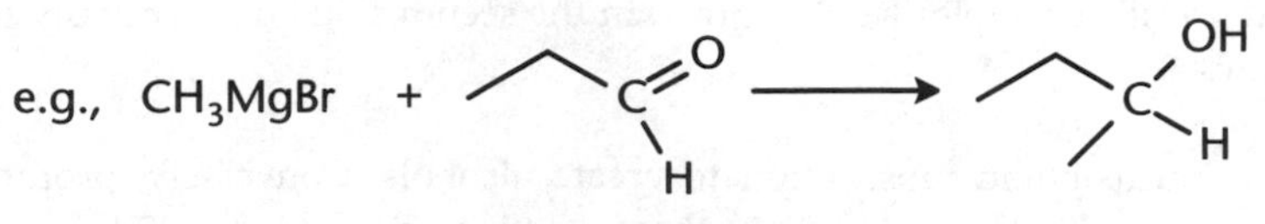

e.g., CH_3MgBr +

Figure 45.7

Substitution Reactions

Both S_N1 and S_N2 reactions can be used to produce alcohols under the appropriate reaction conditions (discussed in Chapter 42). For example:

$$CH_3Br + OH^- \rightarrow CH_3OH + Br^-$$

Reduction Reactions

Alcohols can be prepared from the reduction of aldehydes, ketones, carboxylic acids, or esters. Lithium aluminum hydride ($LiAlH_4$, or LAH) and sodium borohydride ($NaBH_4$) are the two most frequently used reducing reagents. LAH is stronger and less specific, whereas $NaBH_4$ is milder and more selective. For example, LAH will reduce carboxylic acids and esters to alcohols, while $NaBH_4$ will not. Both LAH and $NaBH_4$, however, will reduce aldehydes and ketones to alcohols.

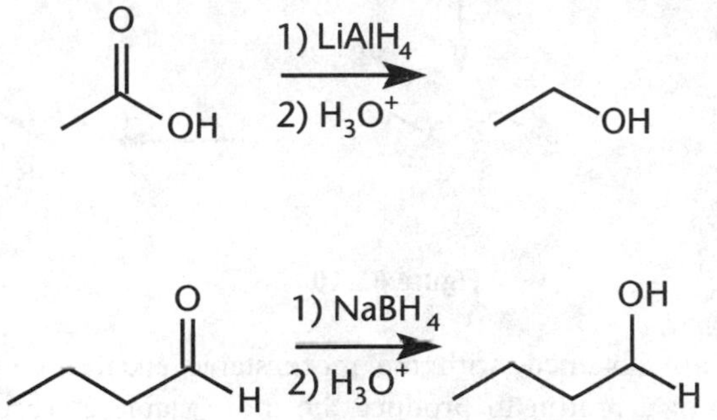

Figure 45.8

Phenol Synthesis

Phenols may be synthesized from arylsulfonic acids with heat and NaOH. However, this reaction is useful only for phenol or its alkylated derivatives, as most functional groups are destroyed by the harsh reaction conditions.

A more versatile method of synthesizing phenols proceeds using hydrolysis of diazonium salts.

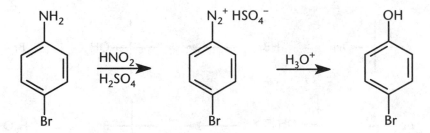

Figure 45.9

REACTIONS OF ALCOHOLS

Elimination Reactions

Alcohols can be **dehydrated** in strongly acidic solution (usually H_2SO_4) to produce alkenes. The mechanism of this dehydration reaction is E1, and proceeds by first protonating the alcohol and then removing a water molecule to form the double bond.

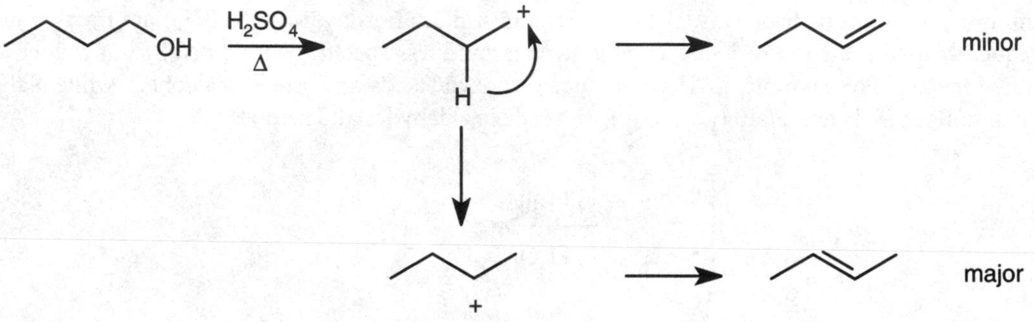

Figure 45.10

Notice that two products are obtained, with the more stable alkene being the major product. This occurs via movement of a proton to produce the more stable 2° carbocation. This type of rearrangement is commonly encountered with carbocations.

Substitution Reactions

The direct displacement of hydroxyl groups in substitution reactions is rare because the hydroxide ion is a poor leaving group. However, the hydroxyl group can be converted to a good leaving group using two different approaches. Protonating the alcohol makes water the leaving group, which works well for S_N1 reactions. Alternatively, the alcohol can be converted into a tosylate (*p*-toluenesulfonate) group, which is an excellent leaving group for S_N2 reactions (see Figures 45.11a and 45.11b).

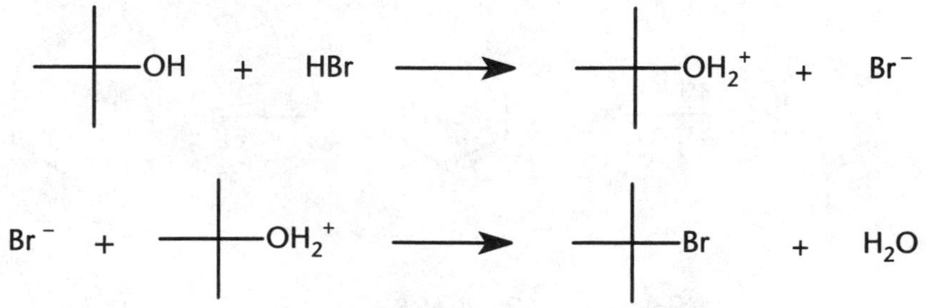

Figure 45.11a

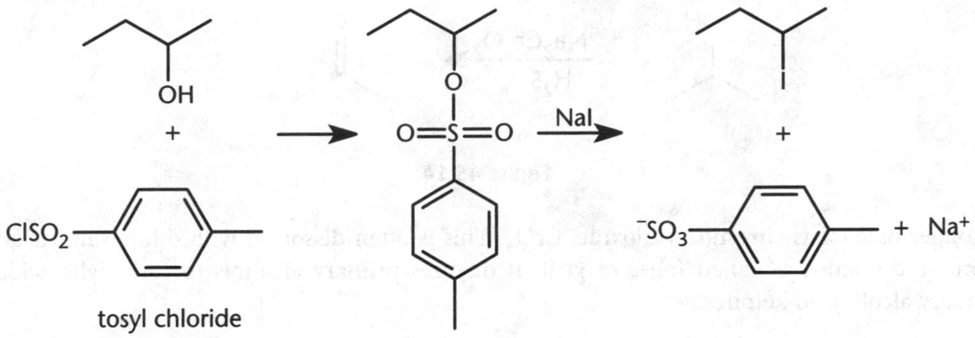

Figure 45.11b

Another substitution reaction that serves as a common method of converting alcohols into alkyl halides is through the formation of inorganic esters, which then readily undergo S_N2 reactions. Alcohols react with thionyl chloride to produce a chlorosulfite intermediate and HCl. The chloride ion of HCl then displaces SO_2 and regenerates Cl^-, forming the desired alkyl chloride.

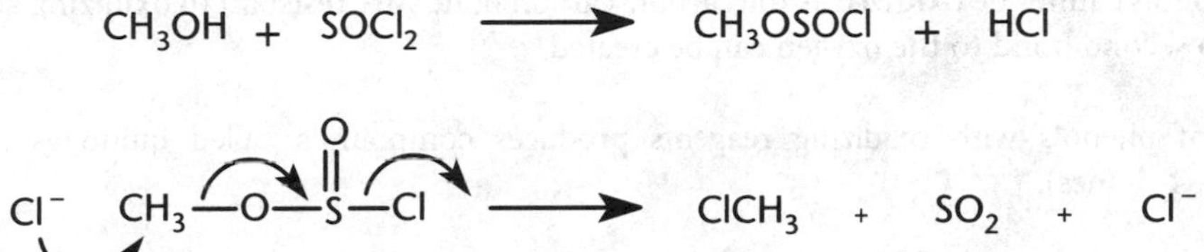

Figure 45.12

An analogous reaction in which the alcohol is treated with PBr_3 instead of thionyl chloride produces alkyl bromides.

Phenols readily undergo electrophilic aromatic substitution reactions. Because the $-OH$ group of phenol has lone pairs that can be donated to the ring, the $-OH$ is a strongly activating, *ortho/ para*-directing ring substituent (see Chapter 44).

Oxidation Reactions

The oxidation of alcohols generally involves a metal oxidizing agent such as chromium or manganese. For example, some form of chromium (VI) is reduced to chromium (III) during the reaction. PCC (pyridinium chlorochromate, $C_5H_6NCrO_3Cl$) is commonly used as a mild oxidant. It converts primary alcohols to aldehydes but does not continue the oxidation to the carboxylic acid. PCC can also be used to convert a secondary alcohol to a ketone.

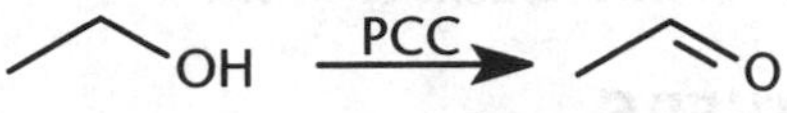

Figure 45.13

Potassium permanganate ($KMnO_4$) is a very strong oxidizing agent that will react with a primary alcohol to create a carboxylic acid or with a secondary alcohol to create a ketone. Another reagent used to oxidize primary or secondary alcohols is alkali (either sodium or potassium) dichromate salt.

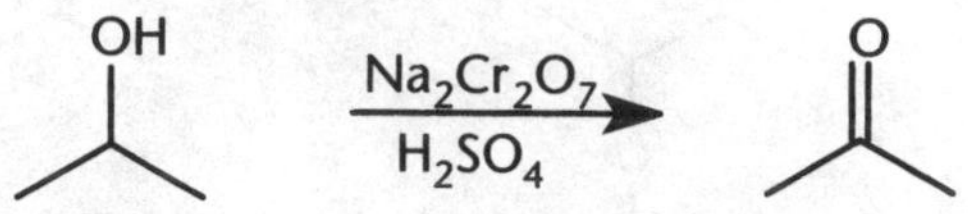

Figure 45.14

A stronger oxidant is chromium trioxide, CrO_3. This is often dissolved with dilute sulfuric acid in acetone; the mixture is called Jones reagent. It oxidizes primary alcohols to carboxylic acids and secondary alcohols to ketones.

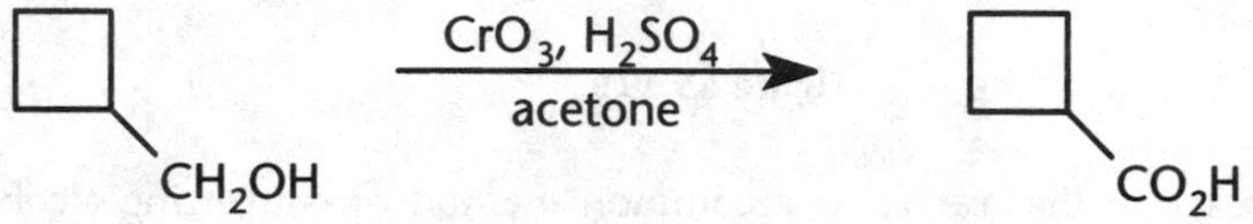

Figure 45.15

Tertiary alcohols cannot be oxidized as the carbon-carbon bonds are resistant to oxidizing agents, and therefore no second bond to the oxygen can be created.

Treatment of phenols with oxidizing reagents produces compounds called quinones (2,5-cyclo-hexadiene-1, 4-diones).

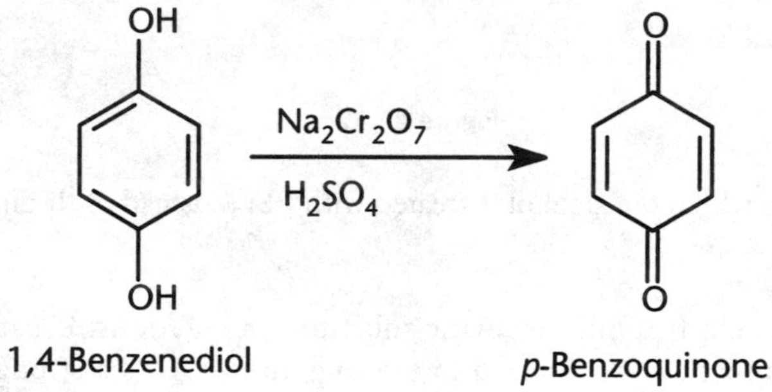

1,4-Benzenediol   *p*-Benzoquinone

Figure 45.16

ETHERS

An ether is a compound with two alkyl (or aryl) groups bonded to an oxygen atom. The general formula for an ether is **ROR**. Ethers can be thought of as disubstituted water molecules. The most familiar ether is diethyl ether, once used as a medical anesthetic. The following sections describe the nomenclature, properties, synthesis, and reactions of ethers.

NOMENCLATURE OF ETHERS

Ethers are named according to IUPAC rules as **alkoxyalkanes,** with the smaller chain as the prefix and the larger chain as the suffix. There is a common system of nomenclature in which ethers are named as alkyl alkyl ethers. In this system, methoxyethane would be named ethyl methyl ether. The alkyl substituents are alphabetized.

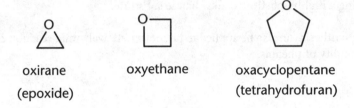

methoxyethane

(ethyl methyl ether)

ethoxybenzene

(ethyl phenyl ether)

Figure 45.17

Exceptions to these rules occur for cyclic ethers, also known as oxiranes, for which many common names also exist.

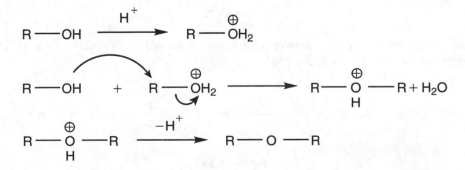

oxirane

(epoxide)

oxyethane

oxacyclopentane

(tetrahydrofuran)

Figure 45.18

PHYSICAL PROPERTIES

Ethers do not undergo hydrogen bonding because they have no hydrogen atoms bonded to the ether oxygen atoms. Ethers therefore boil at relatively low temperatures compared to alcohols; in fact, they boil at approximately the same temperatures as alkanes of comparable molecular weight.

Ethers are only slightly polar and therefore only slightly soluble in water. They are relatively inert to most organic reagents and are frequently used as solvents. However, ethers can form highly reactive peroxides (see Reactions of Ethers), requiring careful storage and handling.

SYNTHESIS OF ETHERS

Ethers are readily synthesized by the condensation of two molecules of an alcohol in the presence of acid, producing a symmetrical ether and water in a substitution reaction:

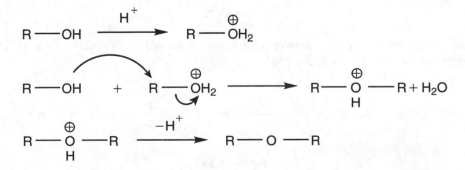

Figure 45.19

The Williamson ether synthesis produces asymmetrical ethers from the reaction of metal alkoxide ions with primary alkyl halides or tosylates. The alkoxides behave as nucleophiles and displace the halide or tosylate in an S_N2 reaction, producing an ether.

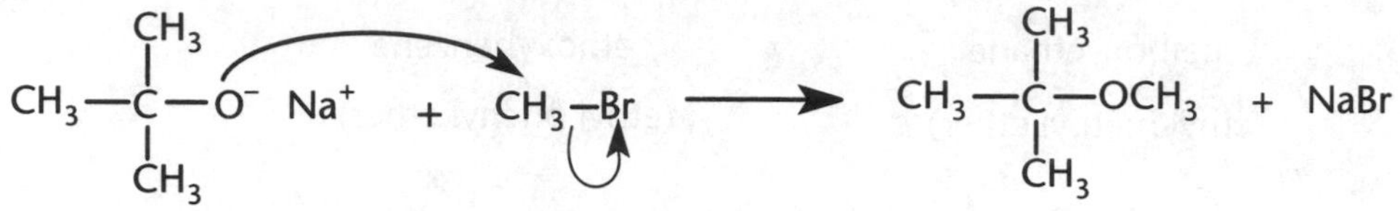

Figure 45.20

Because this is an S_N2 mechanism, alkoxides will attack only nonhindered halides. Thus, to synthesize a methyl ether, an alkoxide must attack a methyl halide; the reaction cannot be accomplished with the methoxide ion attacking a highly substituted alkyl halide substrate.

The Williamson ether synthesis can also be applied to phenols. Relatively mild reaction conditions are sufficient, due to the acidity of phenols.

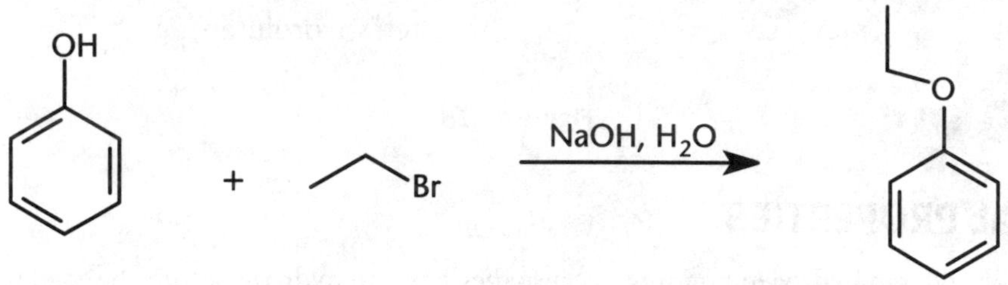

Figure 45.21

Cyclic ethers, also known as oxiranes, are prepared in a number of ways. Oxiranes can be synthesized by means of an internal S_N2 displacement. Since the nucleophile and substrate are part of the same molecule, they are in close proximity, facilitating the reaction.

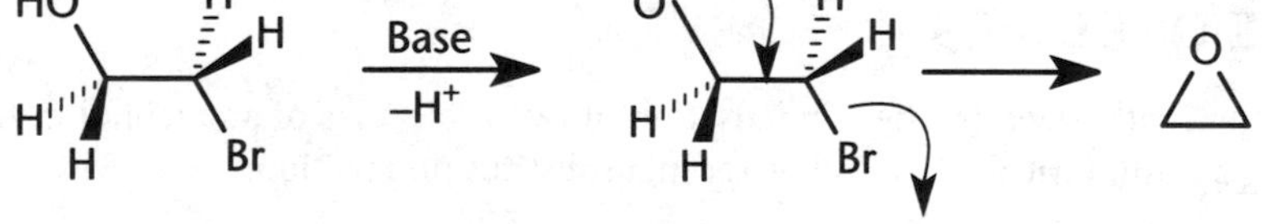

Figure 45.22

Oxidation of an alkene with a **peroxy acid** (general formula RCOOOH) such as mCPBA (*m*-chloroperoxybenzoic acid) will also produce an oxirane.

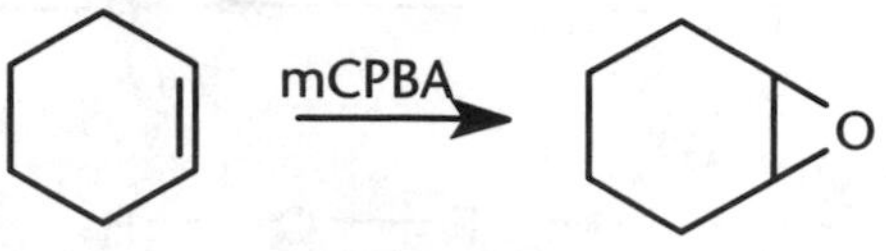

Figure 45.23

REACTIONS

Peroxide Formation

Ethers react with the oxygen in air to form highly explosive compounds called **peroxides** (general formula ROOR). For this reason, ethers are typically stored at low temperature and away from light.

Cleavage

Cleavage of straight-chain ethers will take place only under vigorous conditions: usually at high temperatures in the presence of HBr or HI. Cleavage is initiated by protonation of the ether oxygen. The reaction then proceeds by an S_N1 or S_N2 mechanism, depending on the conditions and the structure of the ether (note the difference in substitution of the substrates in Figure 45.24). Although not shown below, the alcohol products usually react with a second molecule of hydrogen halide to produce a second alkyl halide.

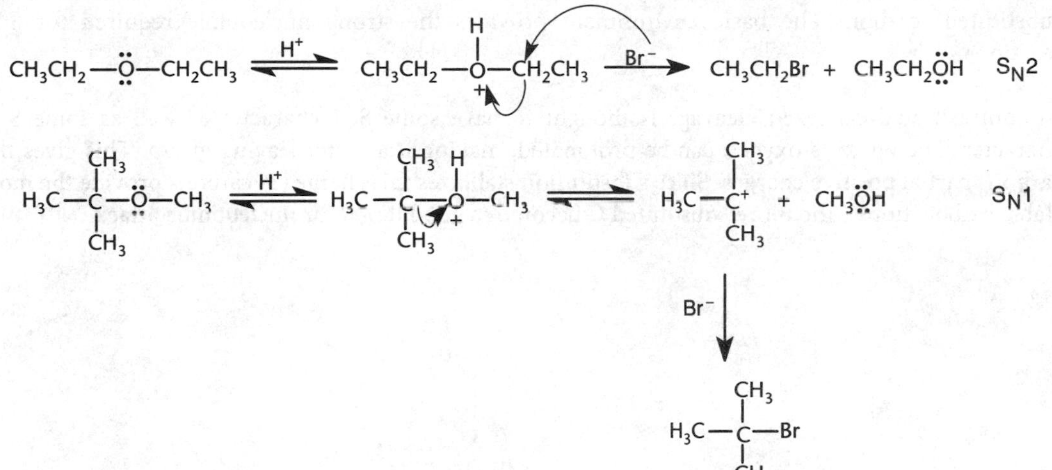

Figure 45.24

The same basic principles and reaction mechanisms of substitution reactions apply to epoxides. Since epoxides are highly strained cyclic ethers, they are susceptible to S_N2 reactions. Unlike straight-chain ethers, these reactions can be catalyzed by acids or bases. In symmetrical epoxides, either carbon can be attacked by a nucleophile; however, in asymmetrical epoxides, the most substituted carbon is attacked by the nucleophile in the presence of acid, and the least substituted carbon is attacked in the presence of base:

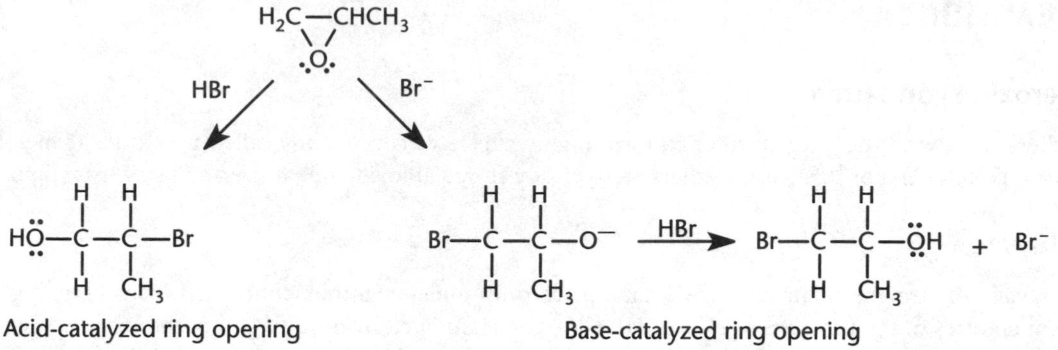

Figure 45.25

Reactions of epoxides provide additional insight into S_N1 and S_N2 reaction mechanisms. Base-catalyzed cleavage of epoxides has the most S_N2 character, so it occurs at the least hindered (least substituted) carbon. The basic environment provides the strong nucleophile required for S_N2 reactions.

In contrast, acid-catalyzed cleavage is thought to have some S_N1 character as well as some S_N2 character. The epoxide oxygen can be protonated, making it a better leaving group. This gives the carbons partial positive charges. Since substitution stabilizes this charge (3° carbons provide the most stable carbocations), the more substituted C becomes a good target for nucleophilic attack.

REVIEW PROBLEMS

1. Provide IUPAC names for the following alcohols and classify them as primary, secondary, or tertiary.

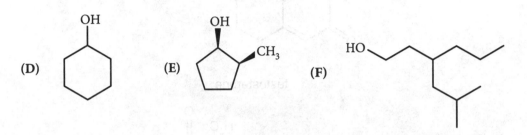

(A)   (B)   (C)

(D)   (E)   (F)

2. Alcohols have higher boiling points than their analogous ethers and hydrocarbons because

   (A) the oxygen atoms in alcohols have shorter bond lengths.
   (B) hydrogen bonding is present in alcohols.
   (C) alcohols are more acidic than their analogous ethers or hydrocarbons.
   (D) alcohols are lighter than their analogous ethers or hydrocarbons.

3. Why are alcohols of lower molecular weight more soluble in water than those of higher molecular weight?

4. Tertiary alcohols are oxidized with difficulty because

   (A) there is no hydrogen attached to the carbon with the hydroxyl group.
   (B) there is no hydrogen attached to the α-carbon.
   (C) they contain hydroxyl groups with no polarization.
   (D) they are relatively inert.

5. Which of the following reagents should be used to convert $CH_3(CH_2)_3CH_2OH$ into $CH_3(CH_2)_3CHO$?

   (A) $KMnO_4$
   (B) Jones reagent
   (C) PCC
   (D) $LiAlH_4$

6. The reaction of 1 mole of diethyl ether with excess hydrobromic acid results in the production of

   (A) 2 moles of ethyl bromide.
   (B) 2 moles of ethanol.
   (C) 1 mole of ethylbromide and 1 mole of ethanol.
   (D) 1 mole of methylbromide and 1 mole of propanol.

7. Which of the following reagents should be used to oxidize the steroid hormone testosterone to 4-androsterone-3,17-dione?

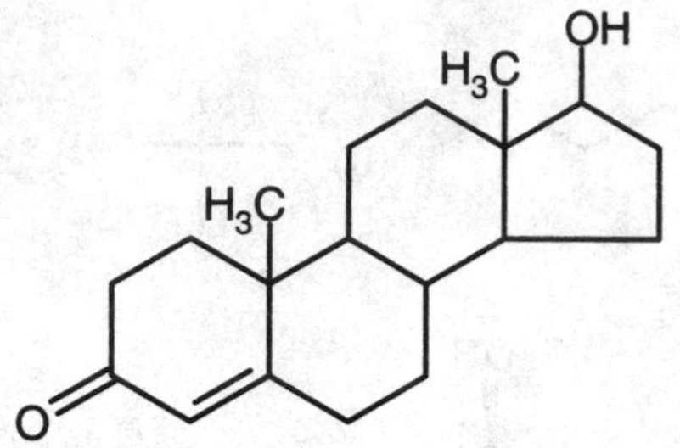

testosterone

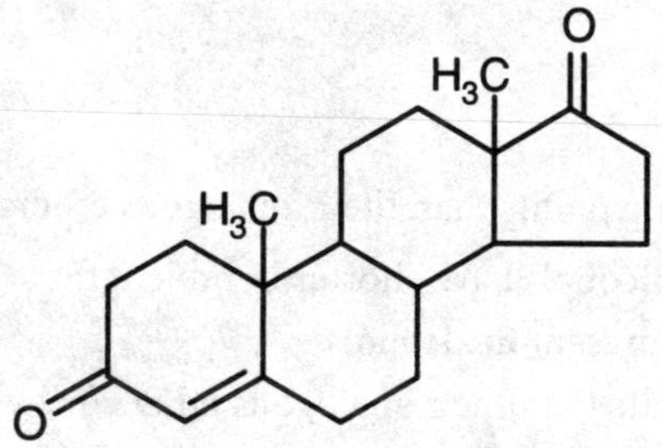

4-androsterone-3,17-dione

(A) Dilute $KMnO_4$

(B) O_3/CH_2Cl_2; Zn/H_2O

(C) PCC

(D) $LiAlH_4$

SOLUTIONS TO REVIEW PROBLEMS

1. **A 3-methyl-1-heptanol**

    A primary alcohol

    B 2-methyl-2-propanol, commonly called *t*-butyl alcohol or *t*-butanol

    A tertiary alcohol

    C 2-methyl-1-propanol, commonly called isobutyl alcohol

    A primary alcohol

    D cyclohexanol

    A secondary alcohol

    E *cis*-2-methylcyclopentanol

    A secondary alcohol

    F 5-methyl-3-propyl-1-hexanol

    A primary alcohol

2. **B** Alcohols have higher boiling points than their analogous ethers and hydrocarbons because alcohols have a polarized O—H bond in which the oxygen is partially negative and the hydrogen is partially positive. This enables the oxygen atoms of other alcohol molecules to be attracted to the hydrogen to form a hydrogen bond. These hydrogen bonds make it difficult for the alcohol to vaporize, thereby increasing the boiling point. The analogous hydrocarbons and ethers do not form hydrogen bonds and therefore vaporize at lower temperatures. Choice (A) is a nonsense choice. The bond length of the oxygen is not a factor in determining the boiling point of a substance. Choice (C) is incorrect because, although alcohols are more acidic than their analogous ethers or hydrocarbons, this property does not affect the boiling point of a substance. Choices (D) is not not always true and even if so would promote lower boiling points rather than higher since it would result in the alcohols having relatively weaker intermolecular forces.

3. Alcohols of lower molecular weight are more soluble in water than larger alcohols because the hydrophilic hydroxyl group can form hydrogen bonds with water. The nonpolar hydrocarbon chain is not solvated by the water because the alkyl group is hydrophobic. As the molecular weight of an alcohol increases, so does the length of the hydrocarbon chain, making the alcohol more hydrophobic. As the molecule becomes more hydrophobic, the alcohol becomes less soluble in water.

4. **A** Tertiary alcohols can be oxidized only under extreme conditions because they do not have a hydrogen attached to the carbon with the hydroxyl group. Alcohol oxidation involves the removal of such a hydrogen; if none is present, a carbon-carbon bond must be cleaved instead. This requires a great deal of energy and will therefore occur only under extreme conditions. Choice (B) is incorrect because the number of hydrogens attached to the α-carbon is irrelevant to the mechanism of alcohol oxidation. Choice (C) is incorrect because the hydroxyl group of a tertiary carbon *is* polarized.

5. **C** The best way to prepare aldehydes from primary alcohols is to use PCC (pyridinium chlorochromate, $C_5H_6NCrO_3Cl$), which is choice (C). $KMnO_4$, choice (A), is a strong oxidizing agent and converts a primary alcohol to a carboxylic acid. Jones reagent, choice (B), also converts a primary alcohol into a carboxylic acid. $LiAlH_4$, choice (D), is a reducing agent; it cannot reduce an alcohol further.

6. A When 1 mole of an ether reacts with excess HBr, the initial products are 1 mole alcohol and 1 mole alkyl bromide, choice (C). However, under these acidic conditions, Br displaces H_2O, resulting ultimately in 1 mole each of two alkyl bromides. In this case, since the ether is symmetric, the product is 2 moles ethyl bromide, choice (A). Choice (B) is incorrect because under these conditions, the alcohol is protonated, and H_2O (a good leaving group) is replaced by Br to form ethyl bromide. Choice (D) is incorrect because the ether molecule is split at the oxygen atom; it does not rearrange, as would be required to produce a 3-carbon and a 1-carbon fragment.

7. C The best way to oxidize this 2° alcohol to a ketone is with PCC, choice (C). $KMnO_4$, choice (A), would oxidize the double bond to a diol, while $LiAlH_4$, choice (D), is a reducing agent, not an oxidizing agent. Choice (B) is incorrect because ozone would cleave the double bond in testosterone.

CHAPTER FORTY-SIX

Aldehydes and Ketones

Aldehydes and **ketones** are compounds that contain the **carbonyl group,** C=O, a double bond between a carbon atom and an oxygen atom. A ketone has two alkyl or aryl groups bonded to the carbonyl, placing the carbon-oxygen group in the middle of the molecule. An aldehyde has one alkyl group and one hydrogen (or, in the case of formaldehyde, two hydrogens) bonded to the carbonyl; thus, an aldehyde is always a terminal group found at the end of a molecule.

The carbonyl group is one of the most important functional groups in organic chemistry and should always be visualized with a dipole moment: The carbon carries a partial positive charge, and the oxygen carries a partial negative charge. In addition to its presence in aldehydes and ketones, it is also found in carboxylic acids, esters, amides, and more complicated compounds. These additional carbonyl compounds are discussed in Chapters 47 and 48.

NOMENCLATURE

Because of their high degree of oxidation, aldehydes and ketones are usually the priority group in naming compounds. Note that the shorthand for an aldehyde group is always written –CHO; this should not be confused with the shorthand for an alcohol, which is C–OH.

In the IUPAC system, **aldehydes** are named with the suffix -**al**. The position of the aldehyde group does not need to be specified: it must occupy the terminal (C–1) position and usually is the highest priority group in the molecule. Common names exist for the first five aldehydes: formaldehyde, acetaldehyde, propionaldehyde, butyraldehyde, and valeraldehyde.

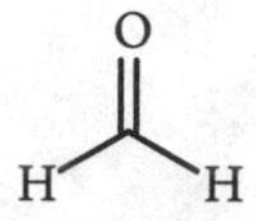

methanal
(formaldehyde)

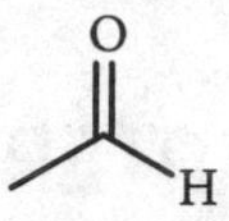

ethanal
(acetaldehyde)

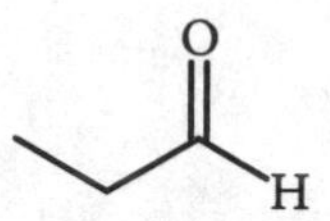

propanal
(propionaldehyde)

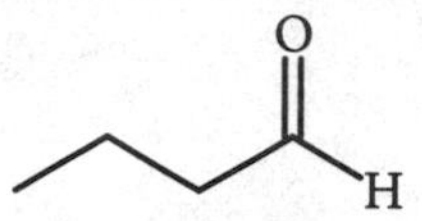

butanal
(butyraldehyde)

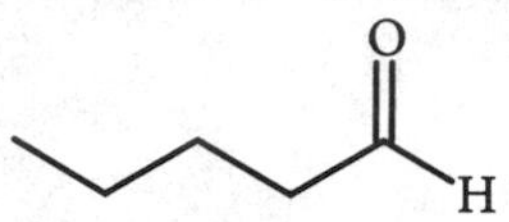

pentanal
(valeraldehyde)

Figure 46.1

In more complicated molecules, the suffix -**carbaldehyde** can be used. In addition, the aldehyde can be named as a functional group with the prefix **formyl-** when combined in a molecule with an even higher priority carboxylic acid group.

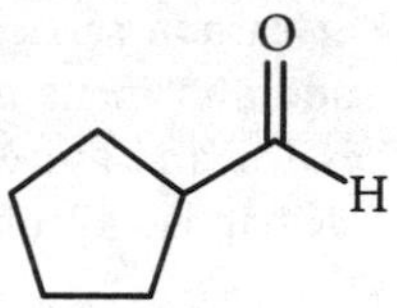

cyclopentanecarbaldehyde

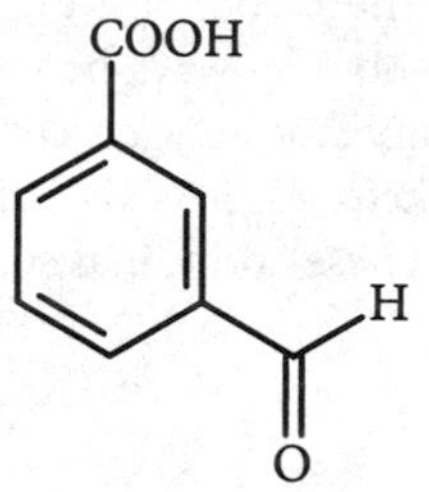

m-formylbenzoic acid

Figure 46.2

Ketones are named with the suffix -**one**. The location of the carbonyl group must be specified with a number, except in cyclic ketones, where it is assumed to occupy the number 1 position. The common system of naming ketones lists the two alkyl groups followed by the word *ketone*. When it is necessary to name the carbonyl as a substituent, the prefix **oxo-** is used.

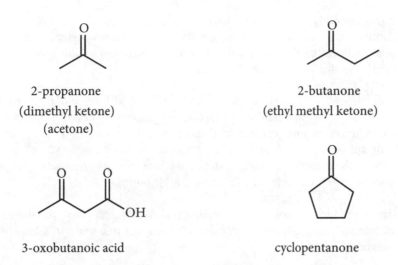

2-propanone
(dimethyl ketone)
(acetone)

2-butanone
(ethyl methyl ketone)

3-oxobutanoic acid

cyclopentanone

Figure 46.3

PHYSICAL PROPERTIES

The physical properties of aldehydes and ketones are governed by the presence of the carbonyl group and its strong dipole moment. Due to differences in electronegativity, the carbon carries a strong partial positive charge, and the oxygen carries a strong partial negative charge. The dipole moments associated with the polar carbonyl groups of nearby molecules align, causing an elevation in boiling point of aldehydes and ketones relative to similar alkanes. However, aldehydes and ketones show lower boiling points than comparable alcohols because –OH groups can form hydrogen bonds, but carbonyls cannot.

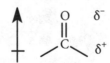

Figure 46.4

OVERVIEW OF ALDEHYDES AND KETONES

Aldehydes and ketones are midway along the oxidation/reduction continuum (shown below). The carbonyl carbon has two bonds to oxygen, placing it between the single C–O bond of alcohols and the three carbon-oxygen bonds of the carboxyl group.

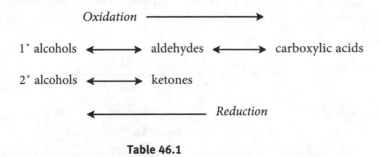

Table 46.1

There are numerous methods of preparing aldehydes and ketones, but three are of particular interest: oxidation of alcohols, oxidative cleavage of alkenes, and Friedel-Crafts acylation of benzenes. These three mechanisms are important to study both as synthetic pathways of aldehydes and ketones and also as reaction pathways for other compounds.

The reactions of aldehydes and ketones are likewise interrelated with those of other compounds and are often driven by the dipole moment of the carbon-oxygen double bond. Aldehydes and ketones can be oxidized or reduced to form carboxylic acids or alcohols, respectively. They can act as either the nucleophile or substrate in S_N1 and S_N2-type reactions. They can serve as the substrate for nucleophilic attack on the carbonyl to produce alcohols, ethers, amides, and related compounds. They can condense to form larger molecules and to create double bonds.

Although the variety of aldehyde and ketone reaction pathways can appear overwhelming, studying them in the context of other organic molecules allows a greater understanding of the overall mechanisms involved.

SYNTHESIS OF ALDEHYDES AND KETONES

Oxidation of Alcohols

An aldehyde can be obtained from the oxidation of a primary alcohol; a ketone can be obtained from a secondary alcohol. These reactions are usually performed with PCC (one of the only options to create an aldehyde), potassium permanganate, sodium or potassium dichromate, or chromium trioxide (Jones reagent). These reactions are discussed in Chapter 45, Alcohols and Ethers.

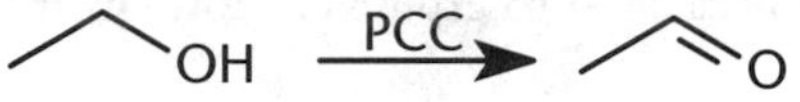

Figure 46.5

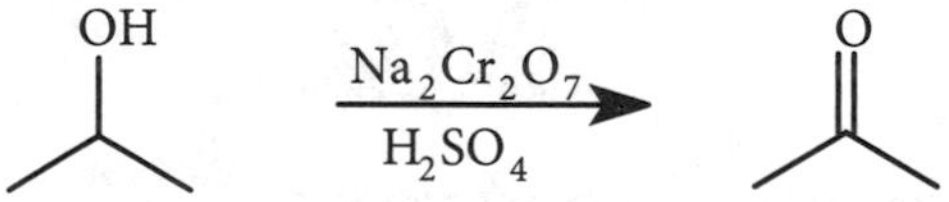

Figure 46.6

Oxidative Cleavage of Alkenes

Double bonds can be oxidatively cleaved with ozone to yield aldehydes and/or ketones (see Chapter 43, Alkenes and Alkynes).

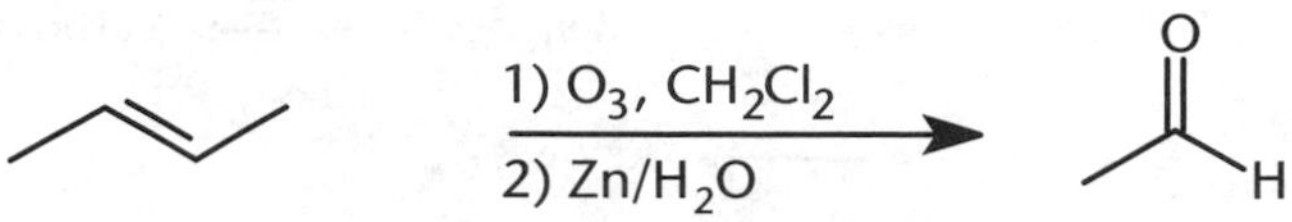

Figure 46.7

Ketones can also be synthesized by the cleavage of disubstituted alkenes with potassium permanganate:

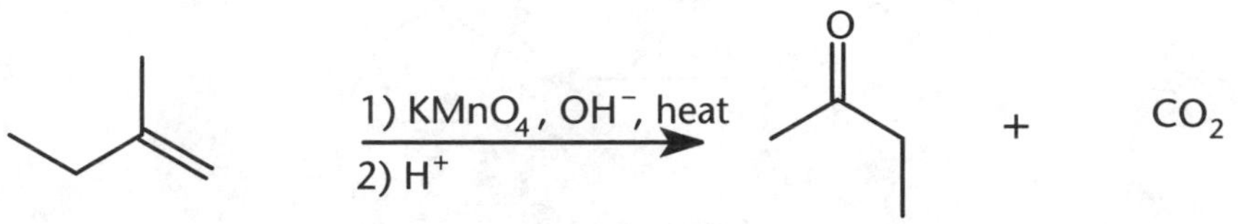

Figure 46.8

Friedel-Crafts Acylation

This reaction, discussed in Chapter 44, produces ketones of the form R–CO–Ar from benzene and an acyl halide in the presence of a Lewis acid such as $AlCl_3$.

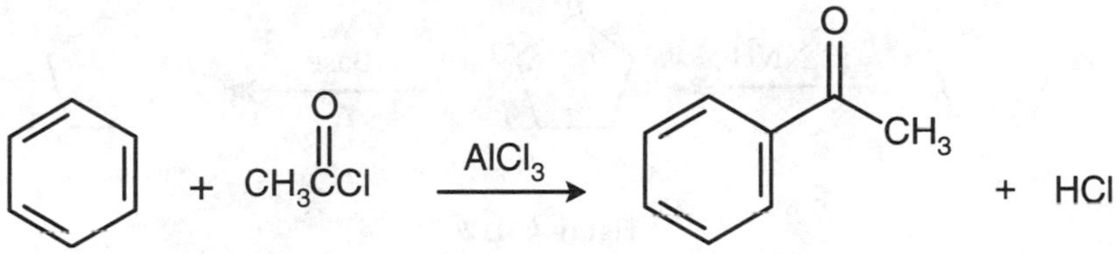

Figure 46.9

REACTIONS OF ALDEHYDES AND KETONES

Oxidation and Reduction

Aldehydes and ketones occupy the middle of the oxidation-reduction continuum. They are more oxidized than alcohols but less oxidized than carboxylic acids.

Aldehydes can be oxidized with a number of different reagents, such as $KMnO_4$, $K_2Cr_2O_7$, CrO_3, Ag_2O (Tollen's reagent), or H_2O_2. The product of oxidation of an aldehyde is a carboxylic acid. Ketones cannot undergo further oxidation unless extraordinarily harsh conditions are used to break C–C bonds.

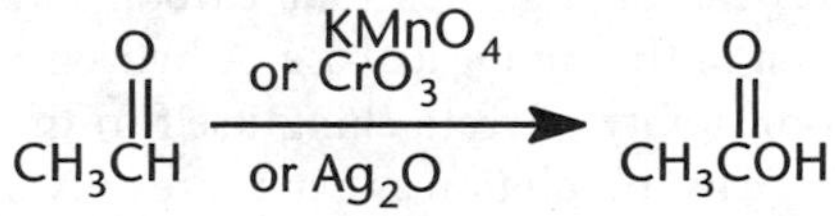

Figure 46.10

A number of different reagents will reduce aldehydes and ketones to alcohols. The two most common are lithium aluminum hydride (LAH), which is a stronger reducing agent, and sodium borohydride ($NaBH_4$), which is milder; both, however, are effective on aldehydes and ketones.

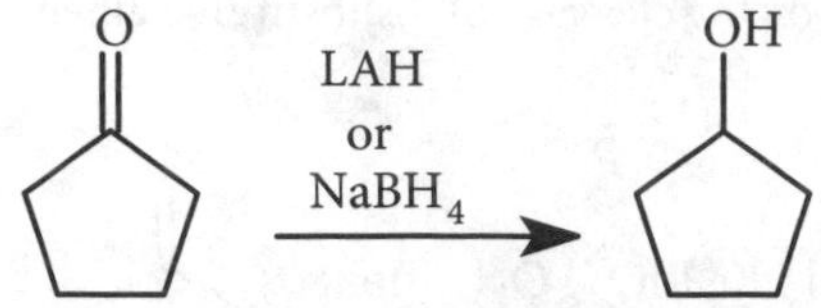

Figure 46.11

Aldehydes and ketones can be completely reduced to alkanes by two common methods. In the **Wolff-Kishner** reduction, the carbonyl is first converted to a hydrazone, which then releases molecular nitrogen (N_2) when heated and forms an alkane. The Wolff-Kishner reaction is performed in basic solution and therefore is only useful when the product is stable under basic conditions.

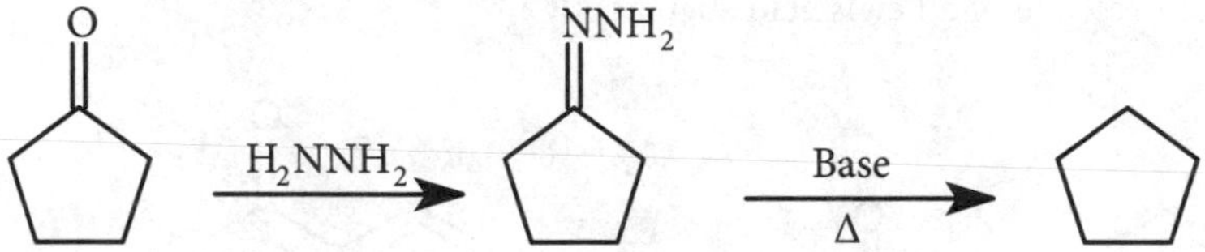

Figure 46.12

An alternative reduction to the alkane is the **Clemmensen reduction**, where an aldehyde or ketone is heated with amalgamated zinc in hydrochloric acid.

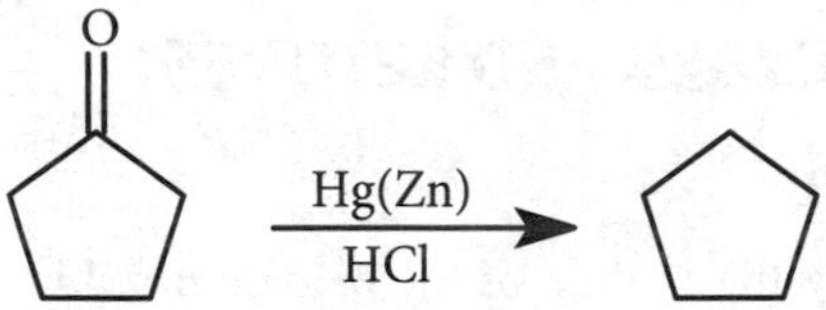

Figure 46.13

Enolization and Reactions of Enols

Aldehydes and ketones can act as nucleophiles when they undergo rearrangement to a slightly different form. Protons alpha to carbonyl groups (one carbon away) are relatively acidic ($pK_a \approx$ 20), due to resonance stabilization of the conjugate base. A hydrogen atom that detaches itself from the alpha carbon has a finite probability of reattaching itself to the oxygen instead of the carbon. Therefore, aldehydes and ketones exist in solution as a mixture of two structural isomers, the familiar **keto** form and the **enol** form, representing the unsaturated alcohol (**ene** = the double bond, **ol** = the alcohol, so **ene** + **ol** = **enol**). The two isomers, which differ only in the placement of a proton, are called **tautomers**. The equilibrium between the tautomers lies far to the keto side. The process of interconverting from the keto to the enol tautomer is called **enolization**.

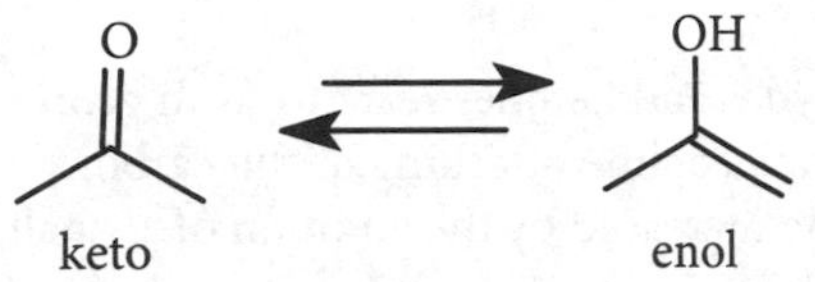

Figure 46.14

Enols are the necessary intermediates in many reactions in which aldehydes and ketones act as nucleophiles. The enolate carbanion can be created with a strong base such as lithium diisopropyl amide (LDA) or potassium hydride, KH, either of which remove the proton from the –OH group. The resulting nucleophilic carbanion will react via an S_N2 mechanism with an α,β-unsaturated carbonyl compound in a reaction called a **Michael addition**.

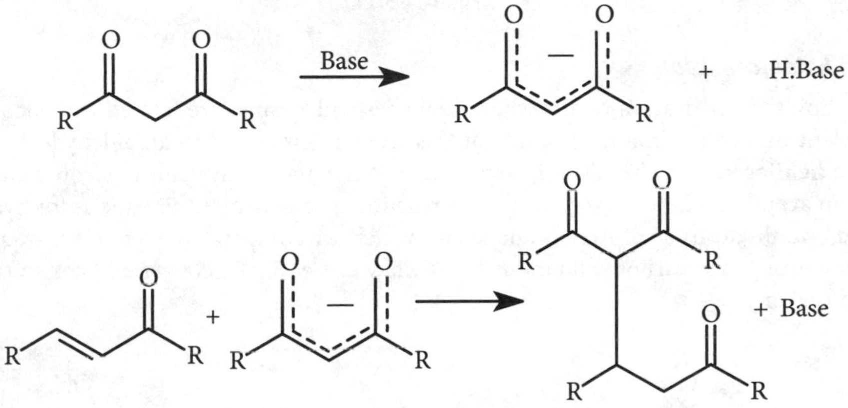

Figure 46.15

Addition Reactions

General reaction mechanism: nucleophilic addition to a carbonyl

A key property of aldehydes and ketones is the dipole created by the partially positive carbonyl carbon and the partially negative oxygen. The partial positive charge on the carbon creates a site for attack by a wide variety of electron-rich nucleophiles. Nucleophilic attack creates a tetrahedral intermediate in which the carbon-oxygen bond is reduced to a single bond and the oxygen carries a full negative charge. Because there is no good leaving group present in an aldehyde or a ketone, the carbonyl cannot re-form and an alcohol will be the end product after protonation. This general mechanism is the basis for many reactions of aldehydes and ketones that appear to be different but actually follow the same principles.

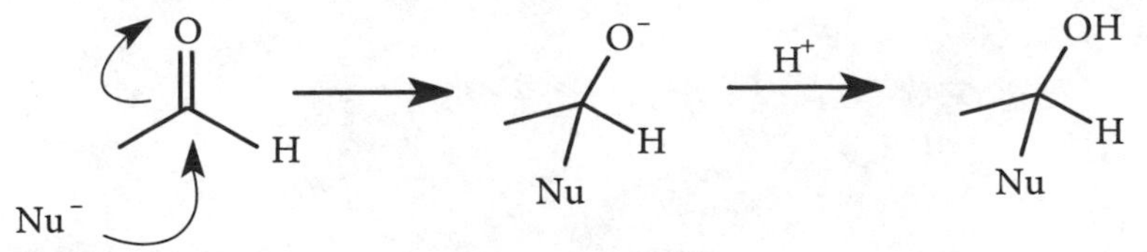

Figure 46.16

Hydration

In the presence of water, aldehydes and ketones react to form ***geminal* diols** (1,1-diols or *gem* diols). In this case, water acts as the nucleophile attacking at the carbonyl carbon. This hydration reaction proceeds slowly; the rate may be increased by the addition of a small amount of acid or base.

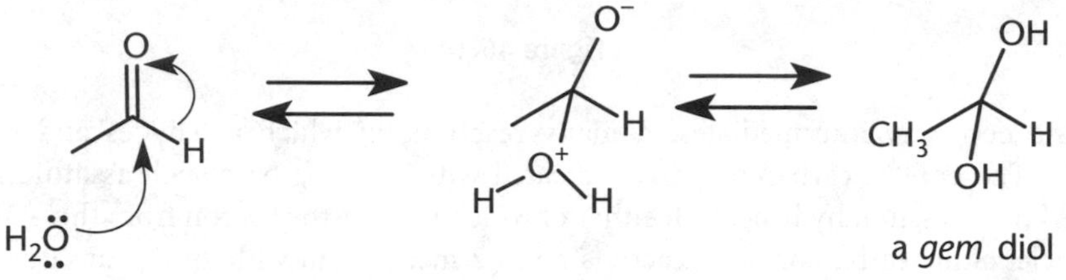

Figure 46.17

Acetal and ketal formation

A reaction similar to hydration occurs when aldehydes and ketones are treated with alcohols. When one equivalent of alcohol (the nucleophile in this reaction) is added to an aldehyde or ketone, the product is a **hemiacetal** or a **hemiketal,** respectively. When two equivalents of alcohol are added, the product is an **acetal** or a **ketal,** respectively. The reaction mechanism is the same as for hydration and is catalyzed by anhydrous acid. Acetals and ketals, which are comparatively inert, are frequently used as protecting groups for carbonyl functionalities. They can easily be converted back to the carbonyl with aqueous acid.

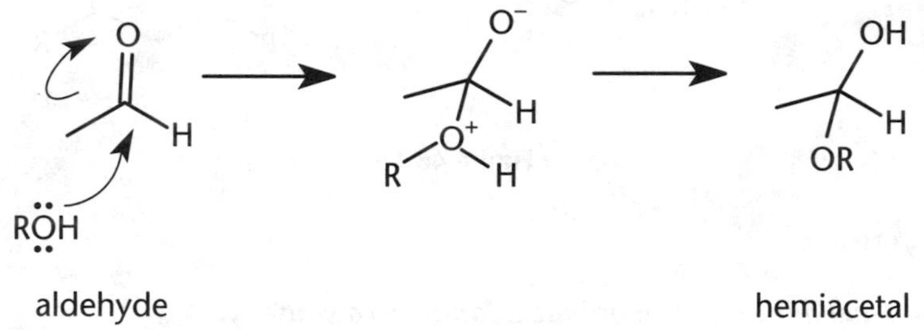

Figure 46.18

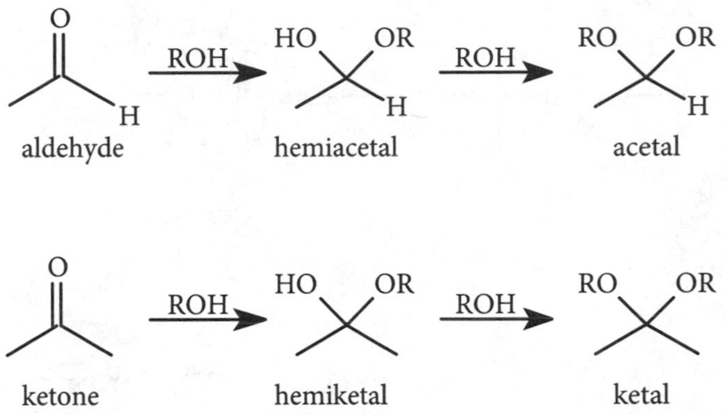

Figure 46.19

Reaction with HCN

Aldehydes and ketones react with HCN (hydrogen cyanide) to produce stable compounds called **cyanohydrins.** HCN dissociates and the strongly nucleophilic cyanide anion attacks the carbonyl carbon atom. Protonation of the oxygen produces the cyanohydrin. The cyanohydrin gains its stability from the newly formed C–C bond (in contrast, when a carbonyl reacts with HCl, a weak C–Cl bond is formed, and the resulting chlorohydrin is unstable).

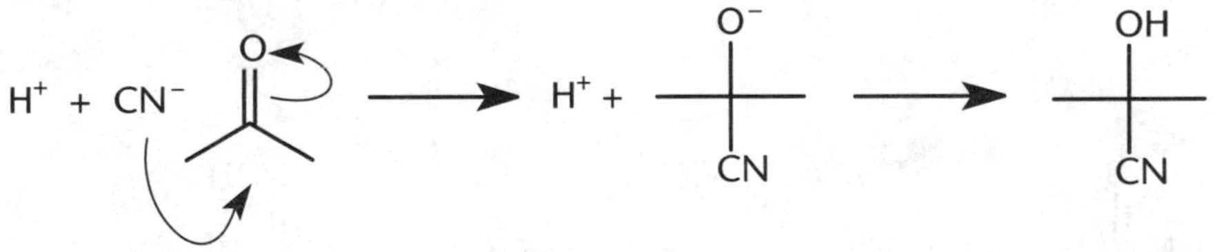

Figure 46.20

Condensations with ammonia derivatives

Ammonia and some of its derivatives are nucleophiles and can add to carbonyl compounds, but a different final product is created than in other nucleophilic attacks. In the net reaction, the C=O bond is replaced by a C=N bond. In the simplest case, ammonia adds to the carbon atom and the –OH group is protonated and lost as a molecule of water. This reaction produces an **imine,** a compound with a nitrogen atom double-bonded to a carbon atom. (A reaction in which water is lost between two molecules is called a **condensation reaction.**)

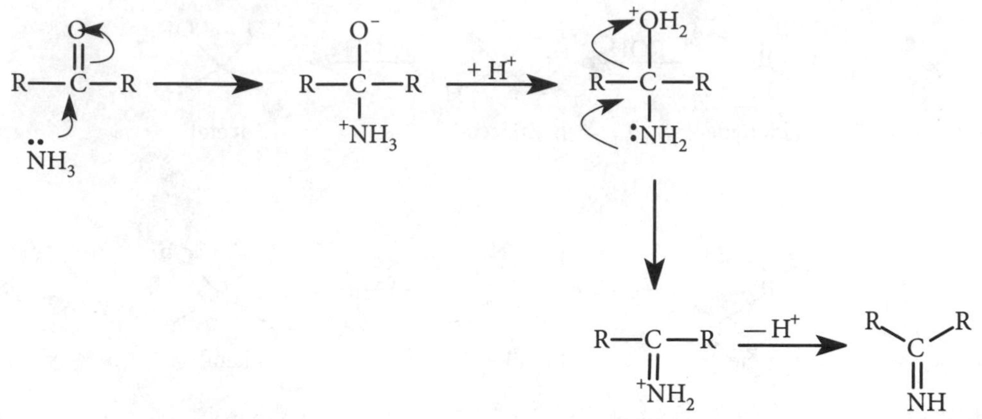

Figure 46.21

Some common ammonia derivatives that react with aldehydes and ketones are hydroxylamine (H_2NOH), hydrazine (H_2NNH_2), and semicarbazide ($H_2NNHCONH_2$); these form oximes, hydrazones, and semicarbazones, respectively.

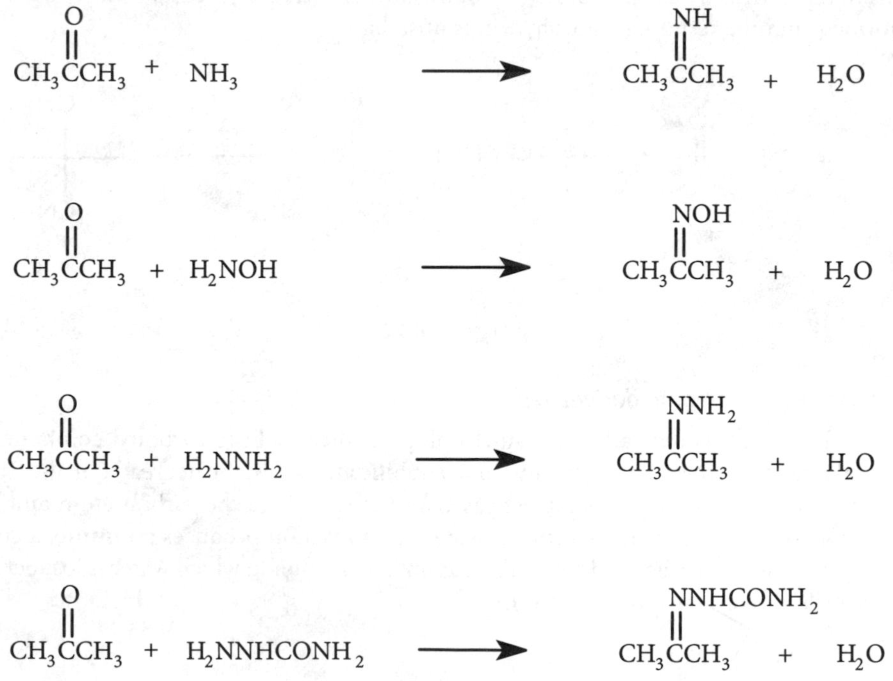

Figure 46.22

The Aldol Condensation

The aldol condensation is an important reaction that follows the same mechanism of nucleophilic addition to a carbonyl. In this case, an aldehyde acts both as nucleophile (enol form) and target (keto form). When acetaldehyde is treated with base, an enolate ion is produced. The nucleophilic enolate ion will attack the carbonyl group of another acetaldehyde molecule. The product is 3-hydroxybutanal, which contains both an alcohol and an aldehyde group. This type of compound is called an **aldol,** from **ald**ehyde and alcoh**ol.**

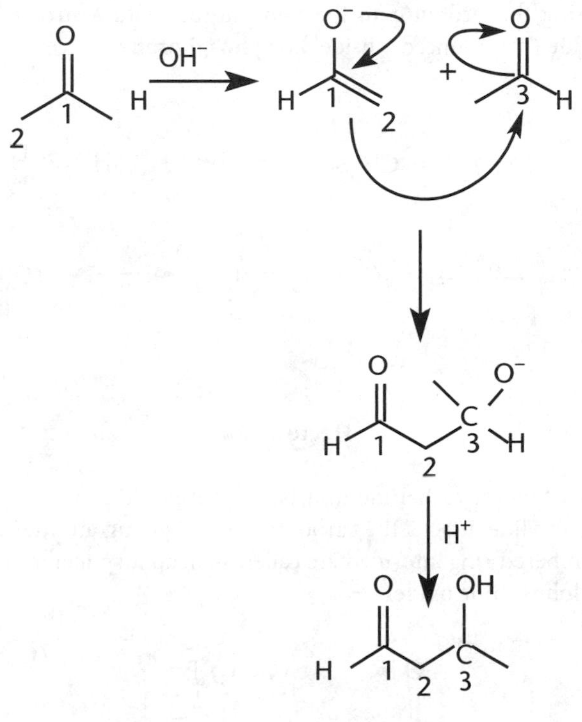

3-hydroxybutanal
(an aldol)

Figure 46.23a

When heated, this molecule can undergo elimination and lose H_2O to form a double bond, producing an α,β-unsaturated aldehyde. This type of condensation reaction is known as the **aldol condensation**.

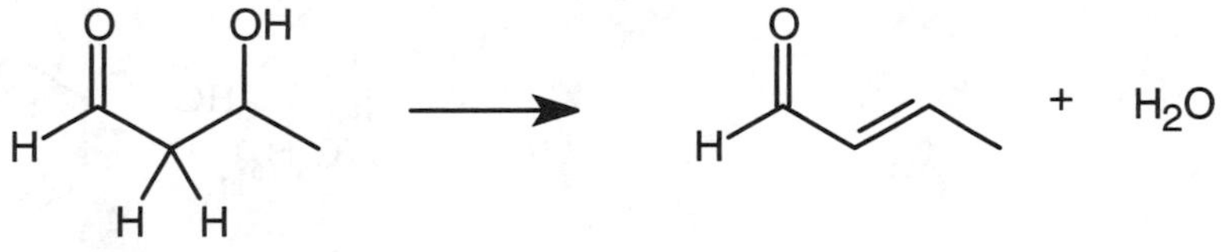

Figure 46.23b

The aldol condensation is most useful when only one type of aldehyde or ketone is present, since mixed condensations usually result in a mixture of products.

The Wittig Reaction

The **Wittig reaction** is a method of forming carbon-carbon double bonds by converting aldehydes and ketones into alkenes; in other words, the C=O bond ultimately becomes a C=C bond. The first step involves the formation of the necessary reactant: a phosphonium salt from the S_N2 reaction of an alkyl halide with the nucleophile triphenylphosphine, $(C_6H_5)_3P$. The phosphonium salt is then deprotonated (losing the proton α to the phosphorus) with a strong base, yielding a neutral compound called an **ylide** (pronounced "ill-ide") or **phosphorane**.

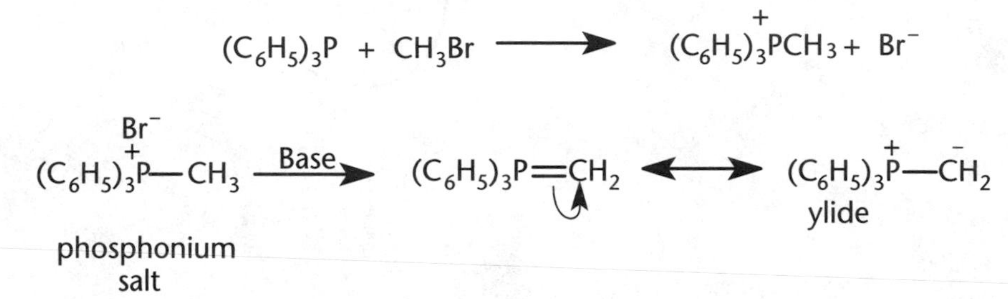

$$(C_6H_5)_3P \ + \ CH_3Br \longrightarrow (C_6H_5)_3\overset{+}{P}CH_3 + \ Br^-$$

Figure 46.24

Notice that an ylide is a type of carbanion and has nucleophilic properties. When combined with an aldehyde or ketone, an ylide attacks the carbonyl carbon, giving an intermediate called a *betaine*, which forms a four-membered ring intermediate called an oxaphosphetane. This decomposes to yield an alkene and triphenylphosphine oxide.

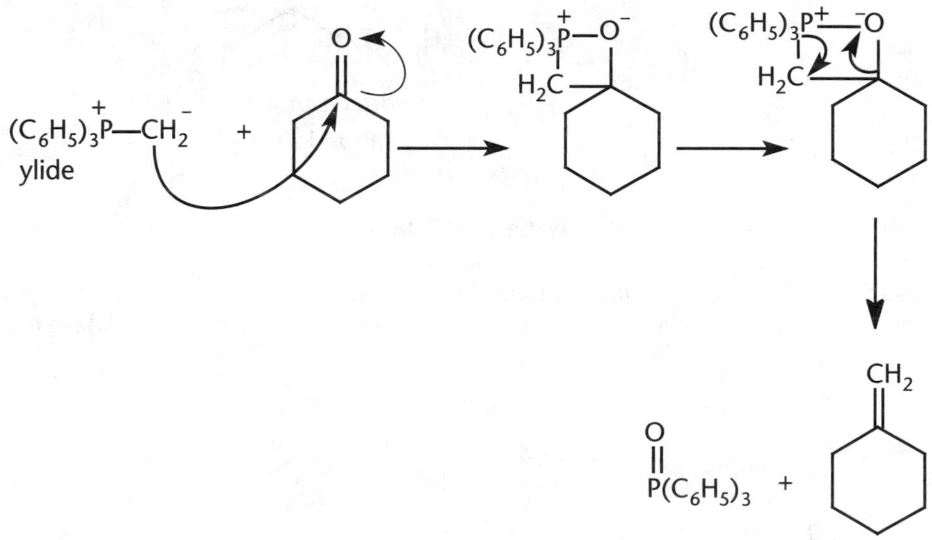

Figure 46.25

The decomposition reaction is driven by the strength of the phosphorus-oxygen bond that is formed. Although the overall mechanism has many complex steps, the net reaction is simply the substitution of a C=C bond for the original C=O bond of the cyclic ketone.

REVIEW PROBLEMS

1. The product of the reaction below is

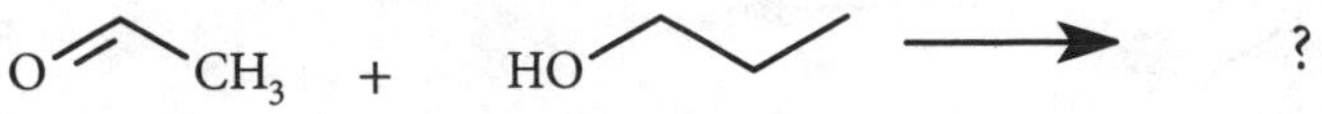

    (A)

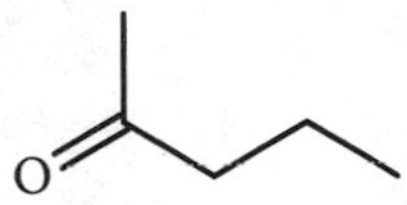

    (B)

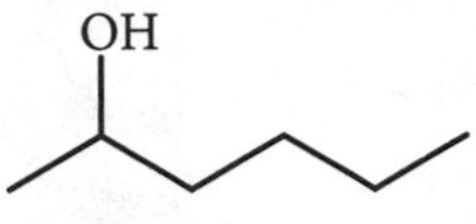

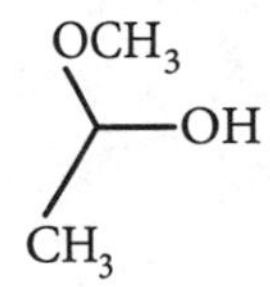

    (C)

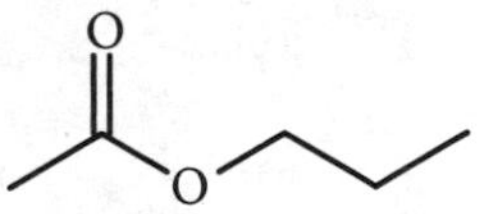

    (D)

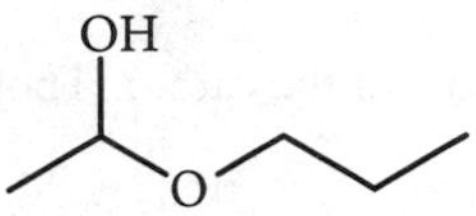

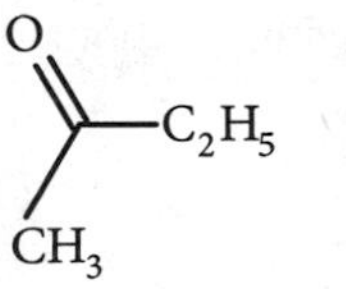

2. The major product of the reaction below is

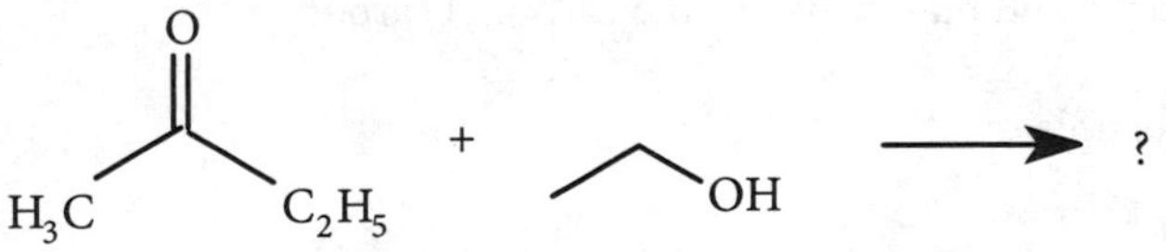

    (A) 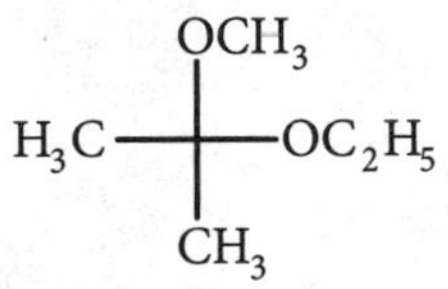 $H_3C \underset{\underset{CH_3}{|}}{\overset{\overset{OCH_3}{|}}{-}} OC_2H_5$

    (B)

    (C) 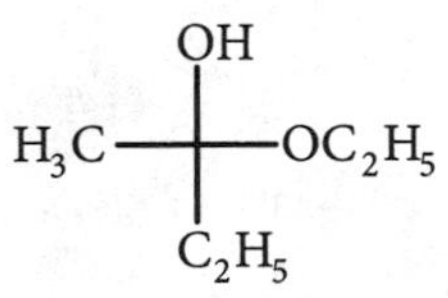 $H_3C \underset{\underset{C_2H_5}{|}}{\overset{\overset{OH}{|}}{-}} OC_2H_5$

    (D)

3. The product of the reaction below is

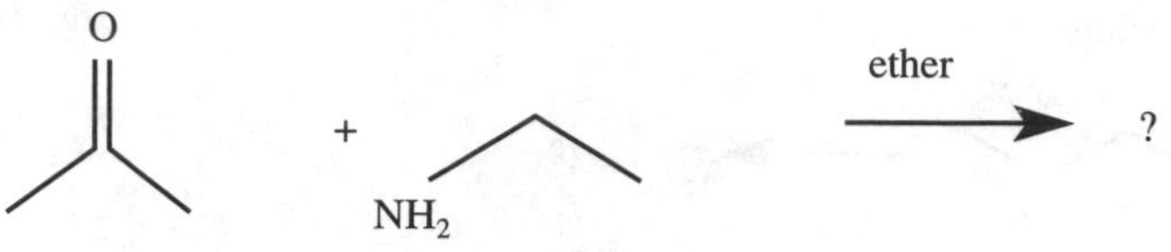

(A)

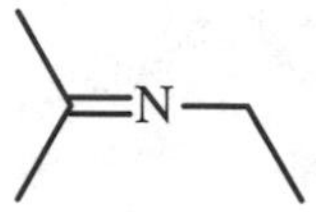

(B)

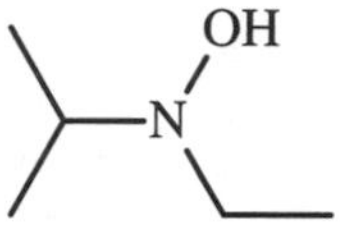

(C)

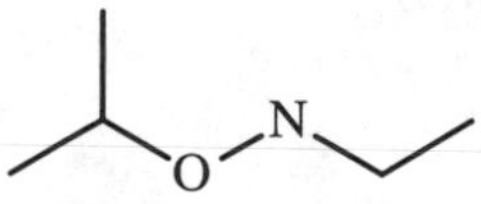

(D)

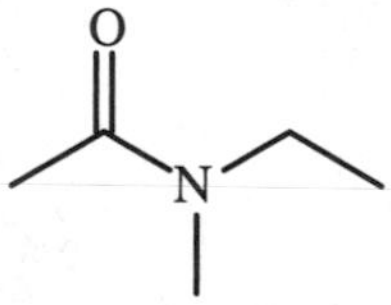

4. All of the following properties are responsible for the reactivity of the carbonyl bond in propanone EXCEPT the fact that

(A) the carbonyl carbon is electrophilic.

(B) the carbonyl oxygen is electron-withdrawing.

(C) a resonance structure of the compound places a positive charge on the carbonyl carbon.

(D) the π electrons are mobile and pulled toward the carbonyl carbon.

5. The reaction below is an example of

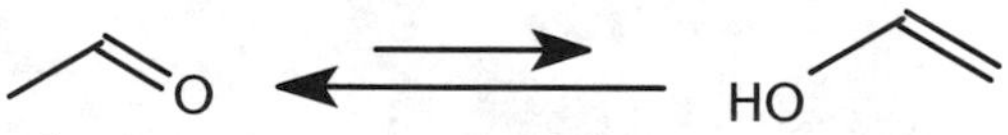

keto   enol

(A) esterification.

(B) tautomerization.

(C) elimination.

(D) dehydration.

6. Which of the following reactions produces the compound below?

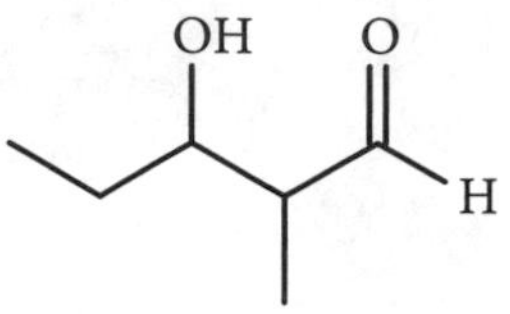

(A) $CH_3CHO + CH_3CH_2CH_2CHO$

(B) $CH_3COCH_3 + CH_3CH_2CH_2CHO$

(C) $CH_3CH_2COCH_3 + CH_3CHO$

(D) $CH_3CH_2CHO + CH_3CH_2CHO$

7. The product of the reaction below is

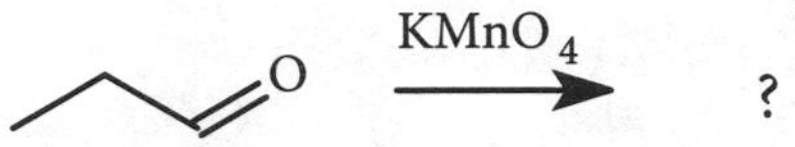

KMnO$_4$ → ?

(A) C$_3$H$_7$OH
(B) C$_2$H$_5$COOH
(C) C$_3$H$_7$CHO
(D) CH$_3$COOH

8. Heating an aldehyde with Zn in HCl produces

(A) a ketone.
(B) an alkane.
(C) an alcohol.
(D) a carboxylic acid.

9. Which hydrogen atom in the compound below is the most acidic?

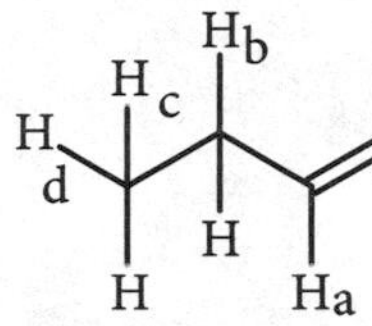

(A) a
(B) b
(C) c
(D) d

10. The product obtained in the reaction below is

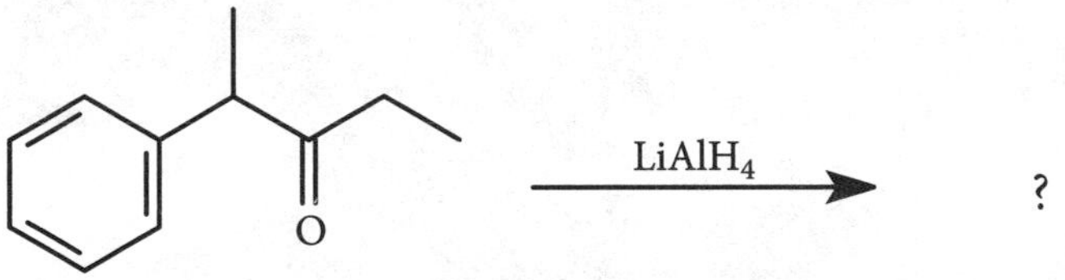

LiAlH$_4$ → ?

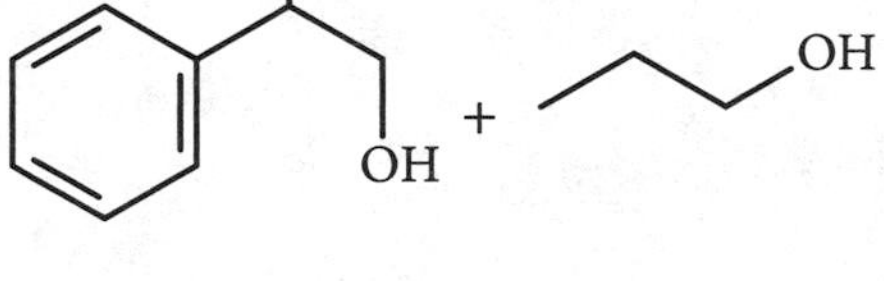

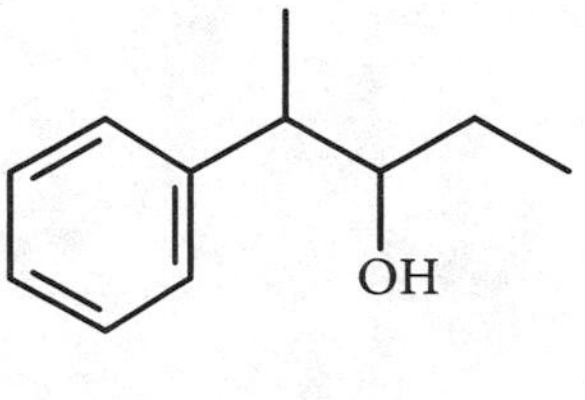

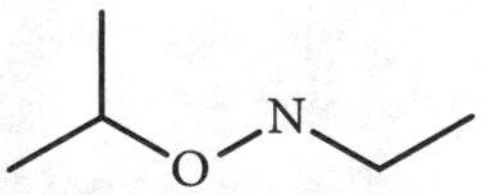

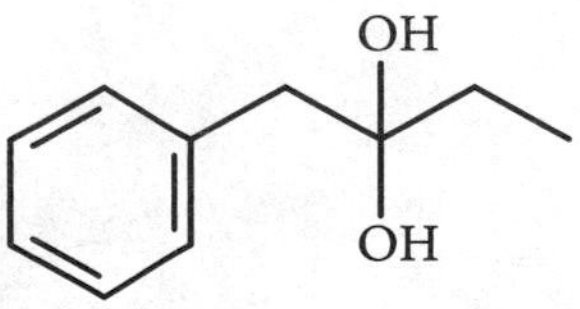

11. Draw the following compounds.

    (A) 3-Methyl-2-pentanone

    (B) 3-Hydroxypentanal

    (C) Benzyl phenyl ketone

    (D) Cyclohexane carboaldehyde

12. The product of the reaction between benzaldehyde and an excess of ethanol (C_2H_5OH) in the presence of anhydrous HCl is

(A)

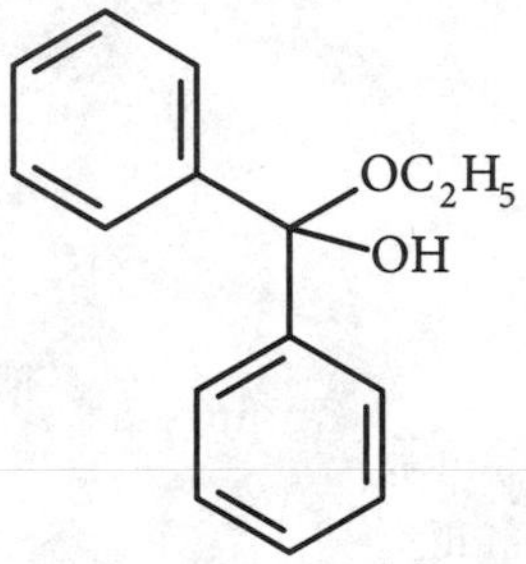

(B)

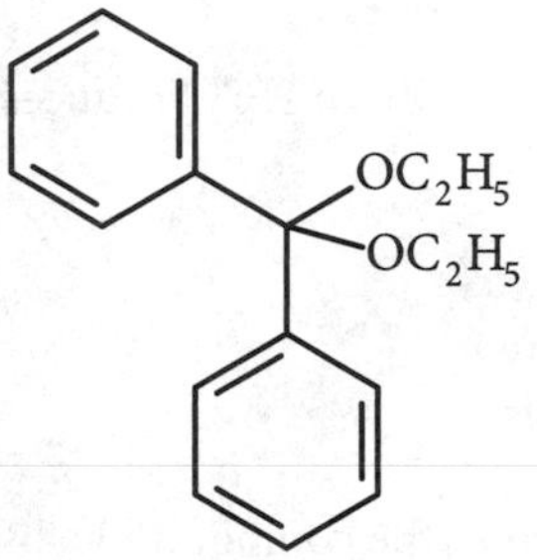

(C)

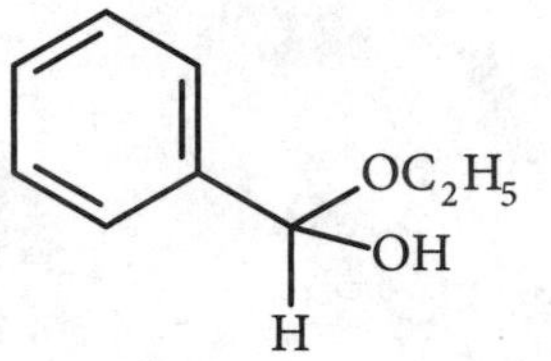

(D)

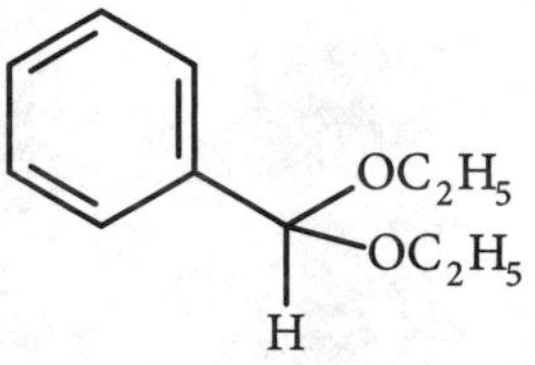

SOLUTIONS TO REVIEW PROBLEMS

1. **D** One mole of aldehyde reacts with one mole of alcohol via a nucleophilic addition reaction to form a product called a *hemiacetal*. In a hemiacetal, an –OH group, an –OR group, a H atom, and a –R group are attached to the same carbon atom.

2. **C** The reaction between one molecule of a ketone and one molecule of an alcohol produces a compound analogous to a hemiacetal called a *hemiketal*. This has an –OH group, an –OR group, and two –R groups attached to the same carbon atom. Of the given choices, only choice (C) represents a hemiketal. Choice (A) has two –OR groups and two –R groups attached to the same carbon atom; this compound is called a *ketal*. Choice (B) is a hemiacetal since it has an –OH group, an –OR group, a H atom, and a –R group attached to the same carbon atom. Choice (D) is a ketone. The correct choice, therefore, is (C). Note that a hemiketal is a very unstable compound; it reacts rapidly with a second molecule of alcohol to form a ketal.

3. **A** Aldehydes and ketones react with ammonia and primary amines to form imines (also called *Schiff bases*), compounds with a double bond between a carbon atom and a nitrogen atom.

$$(CH_3)_2C=O + H_2N - C_2H_5 \rightarrow (CH_3)_2C=NCH_2CH_3 + H_2O$$

The correct choice is (A).

4. **D** The reactivity of the carbonyl bond in propanone, and in aldehydes and ketones in general, is due to the difference in electronegativity between the carbon and oxygen atoms. The oxygen atom has higher electronegativity and is therefore electron-withdrawing. Thus, the carbonyl carbon is electrophilic and the carbonyl oxygen is nucleophilic. Choices (A) and (B) are true statements and therefore are incorrect answer choices (remember, this is an EXCEPT question; three of the answers are true and one is false). The resonance structure of propanone places a positive charge on the carbon atom, so choice (C) is also a true statement and therefore incorrect. The π electrons of the carbonyl bond are pulled toward the more electronegative element, which is oxygen, not carbon; thus, choice (D) is a false statement and the correct answer choice.

5. **B**

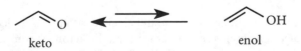

keto   enol

Esterification, choice (A), is the formation of esters from carboxylic acids and alcohols. Tautomerization, choice (B), is the interconversion of keto and enol forms of a compound. An elimination reaction, choice (C), is a reaction in which a substituent is lost and a double bond is introduced. A dehydration reaction, choice (D), is one in which a molecule of water is eliminated. The above reaction involves an interconversion of keto and enol forms of ethanal. The correct choice is therefore (B). Note that equilibrium lies to the left in the above reaction since the keto form is more stable.

6. **D**

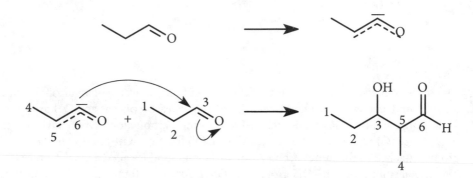

The above reaction is an example of aldol condensation. In the presence of a base, the alpha H is removed from an aldehyde, forming an enolate ion, CH_3CH^-CHO. The enolate ion then attacks the carbonyl group of another aldehyde molecule, CH_3CH_2CHO, forming the above aldol. The correct choice is (D).

7. **B** Aldehydes are easily oxidized to the corresponding carboxylic acids by $KMnO_4$. The –CHO group is converted to –COOH. In this reaction, therefore, C_2H_5CHO is oxidized to C_2H_5COOH, which is choice (B). In choice (A), the aldehyde has been reduced to an alcohol. In choice (C), a $-CH_2$ group has been added. Thus, choices (A) and (C) are incorrect. In choice (D), the –CHO group has been oxidized to –COOH, but a $-CH_2$ group has been deleted, so choice (D) is incorrect.

8. **B** Heating an aldehyde or a ketone with amalgamated Zn/HCl converts it to the corresponding alkane; this reaction is called the Clemmensen reduction. Note that aldehydes and ketones can also be converted to alkanes under basic conditions by reaction with hydrazine (the Wolff-Kishner reduction).

9. **B** The hydrogen alpha to the carbonyl group is the most acidic, since its resultant carbanion is resonance-stabilized:

10. **B** $LiAlH_4$ reduces carboxylic acids, esters, and aldehydes to primary alcohols, and ketones to secondary alcohols. In this reaction, therefore, the ketone is converted to a secondary alcohol. Thus, the correct answer is choice (B), $C_6H_5CH(CH_3)CHOHCH_2CH_3$, a secondary alcohol.

11.

(A)

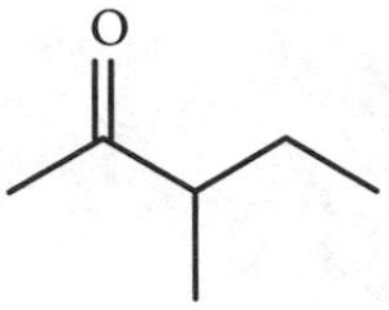

(B)

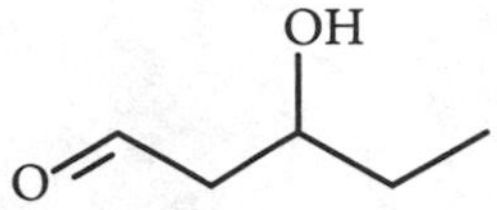

(C)

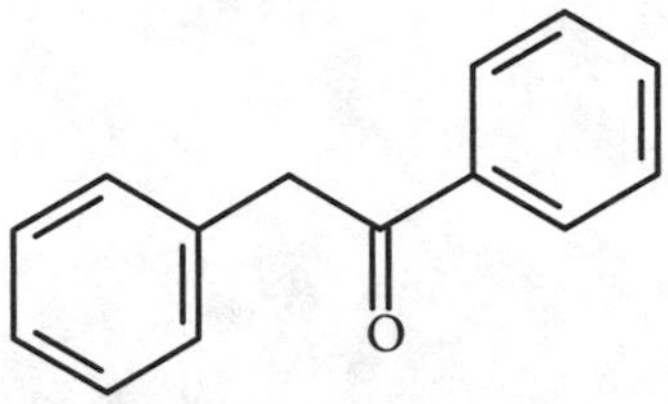

(D)

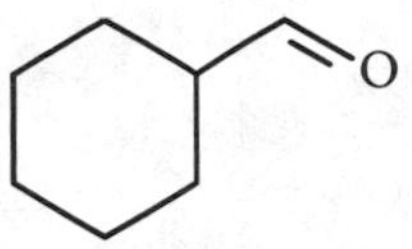

12. D This product of this reaction is an acetal: two ethoxy groups bonded to the same carbon, represented by choice (D). This question states that an excess of ethanol is present, so benzaldehyde will first be converted to a hemiacetal, having an ethoxy and a hydroxy group bonded to the same carbon. Then the hemiacetal will be converted to the acetal by another equivalent of ethanol. Choices (A) and (B) are incorrect because they show the presence of two benzene rings in the final product. Choice (C) is incorrect since this is the hemiacetal that is formed initially, which then goes on to react with excess ethanol to produce the acetal.

CHAPTER FORTY-SEVEN

Carboxylic Acids

Carboxylic acids contain a hydroxyl group (–OH) attached to a carbonyl carbon (C=O), represented by the formula –COOH. This functionality is known as a **carboxyl group,** which is always a terminal group on a molecule. Carboxylic acids are the most highly oxidized organic compounds (other than carbon dioxide). The carbonyl carbon of a carboxylic acid has three bonds to oxygen, two within the carbonyl C=O and the other to the –OH group from the same carbon.

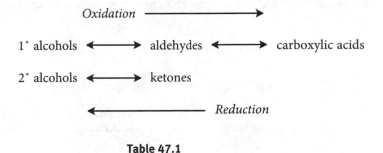

Table 47.1

The hydrogen atoms of the –OH group are highly acidic with pK_a values in the general range of 3 to 6. As with other carbonyl compounds, the C=O group is polarized with a partial positive charge on the carbon and a partial negative charge on the oxygen. Carboxylic acids occur widely in nature and are synthesized by many living organisms.

There are numerous methods of preparing carboxylic acids, but three are of particular interest: oxidation of alcohols and alkenes, carbonation with Grignard reagents, and hydrolysis of nitriles. These three mechanisms are important to study both as synthetic pathways of carboxylic acids and also as reaction pathways of other compounds.

The reactions of carboxylic acids are likewise interrelated with those of other compounds and are often driven by the dipole moment of the carbon-oxygen double bond. Carboxylic acids can be reduced to form alcohols. They can serve as the substrate for nucleophilic attack and substitution to form acyl halides, anhydrides, esters, and amides. They can decarboxylate to produce CO_2, and long-chain carboxylic acids can form soaps and micelles.

NOMENCLATURE

In the IUPAC system of nomenclature, carboxylic acids are named by adding the suffix **-oic acid** to the alkyl root. Since carboxylic acids are highly oxidized, they have very high priority in naming, and the chain is numbered so that the carboxyl group receives the lowest possible number.

2-methylpentanoic acid   4-isopropyl-5-oxohexanoic acid

Figure 47.1

Carboxylic acids were among the first organic compounds discovered. Their original names continue today in the common system of nomenclature. For example, formic acid (from Latin *formica*, meaning ant) was found in ants and butyric acid (from Latin *butyrum*, meaning butter) in rancid butter. The common and IUPAC names of the first three carboxylic acids are listed in Figure 47.2.

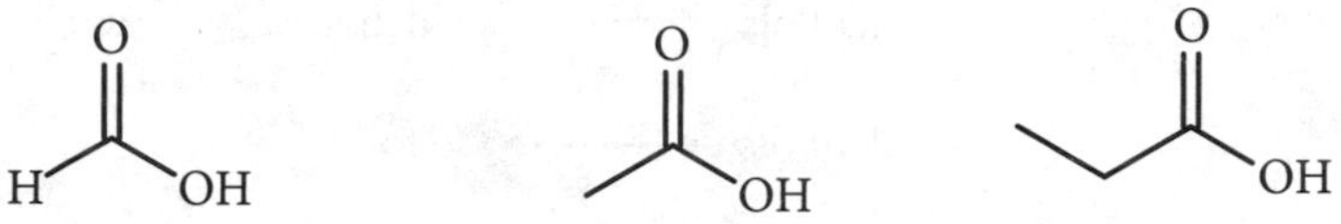

methanoic acid   ethanoic acid   propanoic acid
(formic acid)   (acetic acid)   (propionic acid)

Figure 47.2

Cyclic carboxylic acids are usually named as cycloalkane carboxylic acids. The carbon atom to which the carboxyl group is attached is numbered 1 because of the group's high priority. When a carboxylic acid is deprotonated, its name is changed to end in the suffix **-ate**. Thus, acetic acid becomes acetate when ionized and is called sodium acetate when in its sodium salt form. Typical examples are:

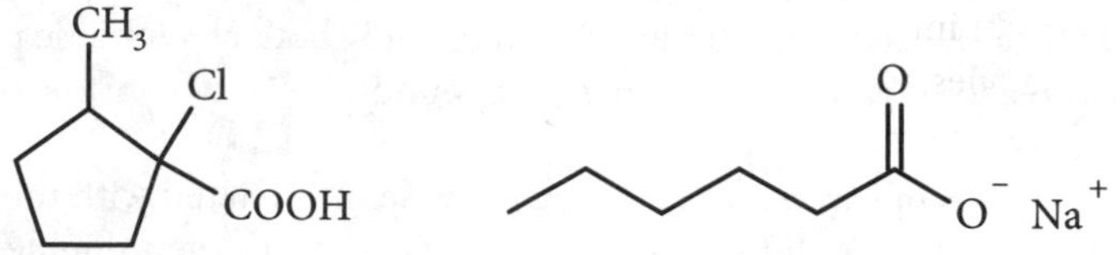

1-chloro-2-methylcyclo-   sodium hexanoate
pentane carboxylic acid

Figure 47.3

Dicarboxylic acids—compounds with two carboxyl groups—are common in biological systems. The first six straight-chain terminal dicarboxylic acids are oxalic, malonic, succinic, glutaric, adipic, and pimelic acids. Their IUPAC names are ethanedioic acid, propanedioic acid, butanedioic acid, pentanedioic acid, hexanedioic acid, and heptanedioic acid.

PHYSICAL PROPERTIES

Hydrogen Bonding

Carboxylic acids are polar and form hydrogen bonds between the –OH group of one molecule and the lone pairs of electrons on the oxygen of another molecule. As a result, carboxylic acids can form dimers: pairs of molecules connected by hydrogen bonds. The boiling points of carboxylic acids are therefore even higher than those of the corresponding alcohols. The boiling points follow the usual trend of increasing with molecular weight.

Acidity

The acidity of carboxylic acids is due to the resonance stabilization of the carboxylate anion (the conjugate base). When the hydroxyl proton dissociates from the acid, the negative charge left on the carboxylate group is delocalized and shared by both oxygen atoms.

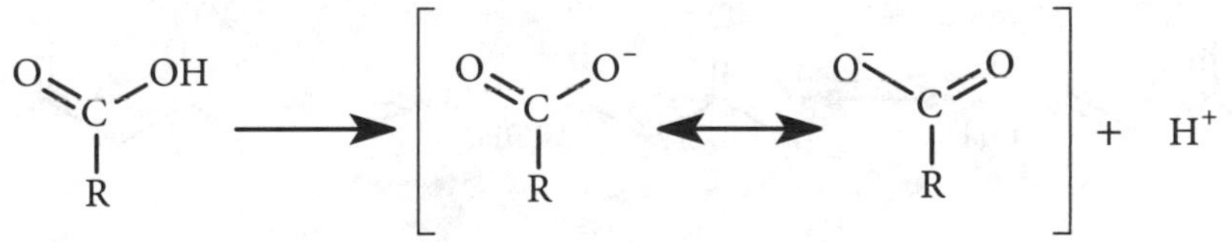

Figure 47.4

Substituents on carbon atoms adjacent to a carboxyl group can influence acidity. Electron-withdrawing groups such as –Cl or –NO_2 further delocalize the negative charge and increase acidity. Electron-donating groups such as –NH_2 or –OCH_3 destabilize the negative charge, making the compound less acidic.

In dicarboxylic acids, one –COOH group (which is electron-withdrawing) influences the other, making the first carboxyl group more acidic than the analogous monocarboxylic acid. The second carboxyl group is then influenced by the carboxylate anion. Ionization of the second group will create a doubly charged species, in which the two negative charges repel each other. Since this is unfavorable, the second proton is less acidic than that of a monocarboxylic acid.

β-dicarboxylic acids are notable for the high acidity of the α-hydrogens located between the two carboxyl groups (pK_a ~ 10). Loss of this acidic hydrogen atom produces a carbanion that is stabilized by the electron-withdrawing effect of the two carboxyl groups.

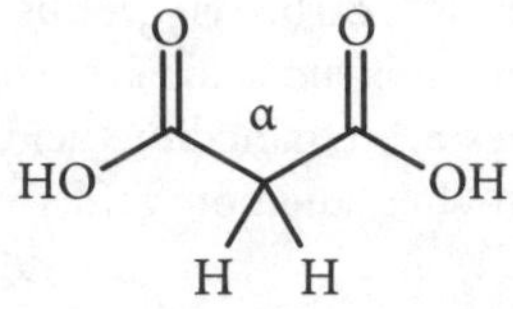

Figure 47.5

The same effect is also seen in β-ketoacids, $RC=OCH_2-COOH$. The resonance structures of the representative β-ketoacid below demonstrate the additional stability due to delocalization of the electrons from the carbonyl groups:

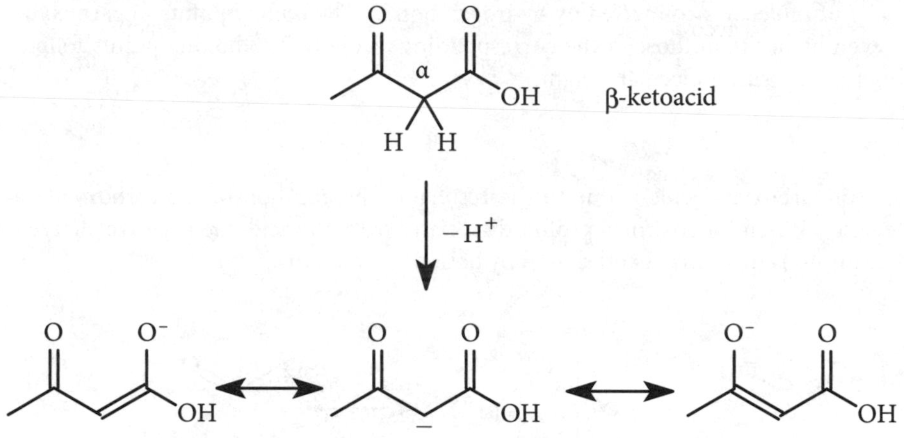

Figure 47.6

SYNTHESIS

Oxidation Reactions

Carboxylic acids can be prepared via oxidation of aldehydes, primary alcohols, and certain alkylbenzenes. Any strong oxidizing agent will create a carboxylic acid, including $KMnO_4$, $K_2Cr_2O_7$, and CrO_3. A primary alcohol can also be oxidized first with PCC to create an aldehyde and then further oxidized with Tollen's reagent to create the carboxylic acid.

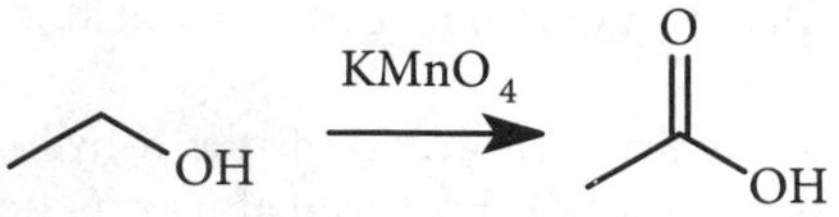

Figure 47.7

Carboxylic acids can also be prepared by the oxidative cleavage of alkenes:

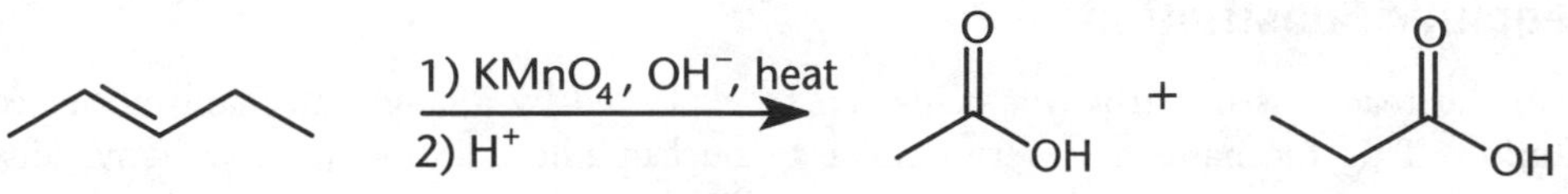

Figure 47.8

Carbonation of Organometallic Reagents

Organometallic reagents, such as Grignard reagents, react with carbon dioxide (CO_2) to form carboxylic acids. This reaction is useful for the conversion of tertiary alkyl halides into carboxylic acids, which cannot be accomplished through other methods. Note that this reaction adds one carbon atom to the chain.

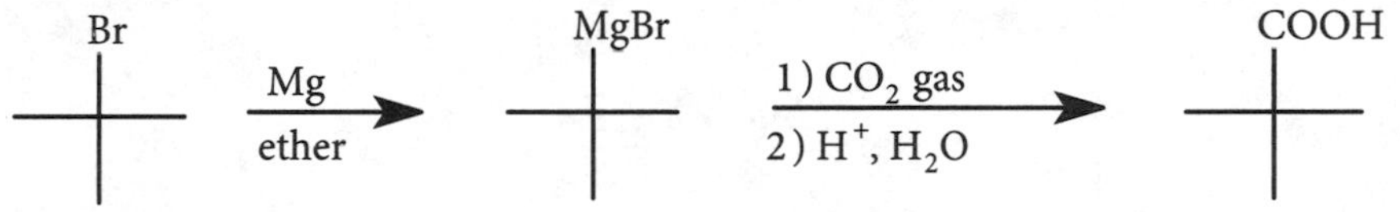

Figure 47.9

Hydrolysis of Nitriles

Nitriles, also called cyanides, are compounds containing the functional group $-C\equiv N$. The cyanide anion CN^- is a strong nucleophile and will displace primary and secondary halides in typical S_N2 fashion.

Nitriles can be hydrolyzed under either acidic or basic conditions. The products are carboxylic acids and ammonia (or ammonium salts).

Figure 47.10

This allows the conversion of alkyl halides into carboxylic acids. As in the carbonation reaction, an additional carbon atom is introduced to the carbon chain. For instance, if the desired product is acetic acid, a possible starting material would be methyl iodide.

REACTIONS

Nucleophilic Substitution

Many of the reactions of carboxylic acids can be explained by a single mechanism: nucleophilic substitution. This mechanism is very similar to nucleophilic addition to a carbonyl, discussed in Chapter 46, Aldehydes and Ketones. The key difference between the two is that nucleophilic substitution concludes with re-formation of the C=O double bond and elimination of a leaving group.

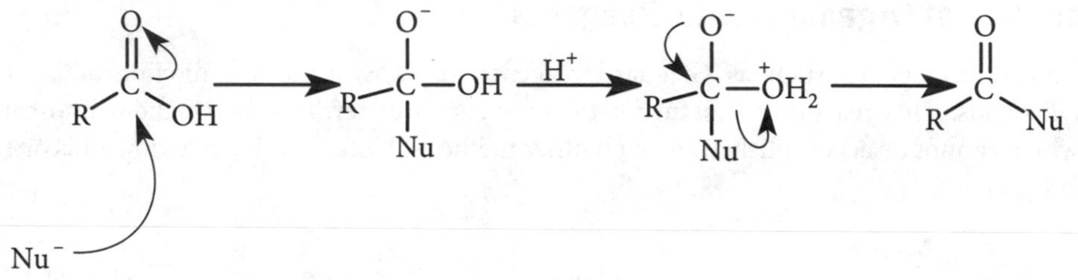

Figure 47.11

Reduction

Carboxylic acids occupy the most oxidized position of the oxidation-reduction continuum. Carboxylic acids can be reduced with lithium aluminum hydride (LAH) to their corresponding primary alcohols. Note that this reaction will not occur when the milder reducing agent $NaBH_4$ is used. Aldehyde intermediates that may be formed in the course of the reaction with LAH are also reduced to the primary alcohol. The reaction occurs by nucleophilic addition of hydride (the H^- ion) to the carbonyl group and elimination of water as a leaving group.

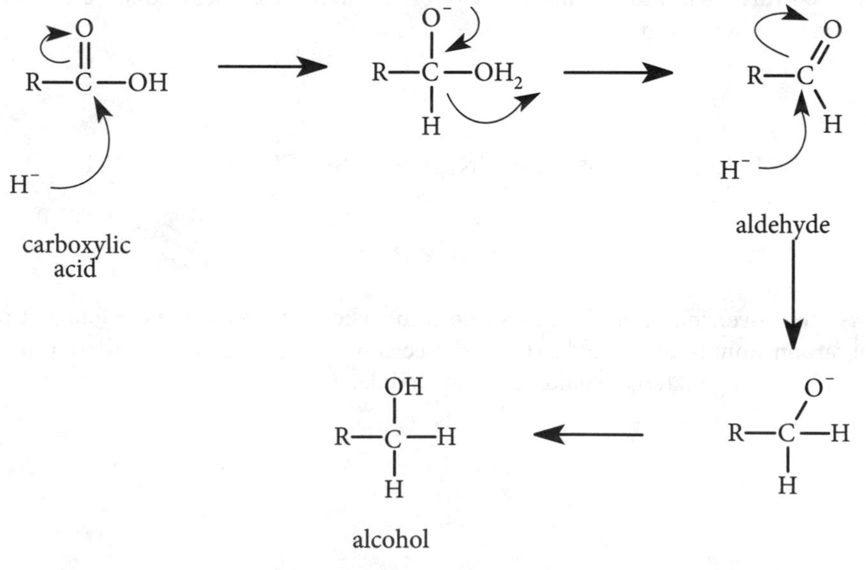

Figure 47.12

Ester formation

Carboxylic acids react with alcohols under acidic conditions to form esters and water. In acidic solution, the oxygen on the carbonyl group can become protonated. This increases the polarity of the carbon-oxygen bond, putting even more positive charge on the carbon and making it even more susceptible to nucleophilic attack. Again, water is eliminated as a leaving group, and the carbonyl re-forms. This condensation reaction occurs most rapidly with primary alcohols. Esters are discussed in more detail in Chapter 48, Carboxylic Acid Derivatives.

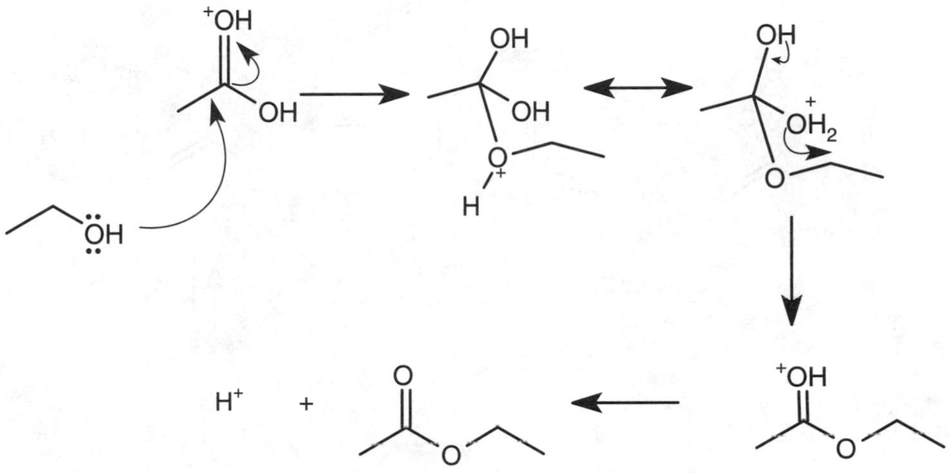

Figure 47.13

Acyl halide formation

Acyl halides, also called acid halides, are compounds with carbonyl groups bonded to halides. Several different reagents can accomplish this transformation; thionyl chloride, $SOCl_2$, is the most common.

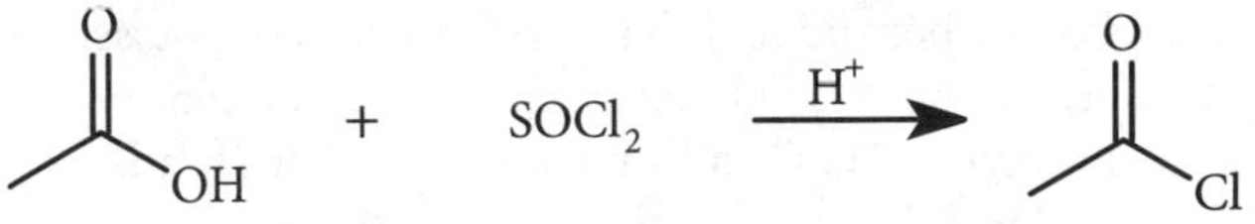

Figure 47.14

Acid chlorides are very reactive, as the greater electron-withdrawing power of the Cl^- makes the carbonyl carbon more susceptible to nucleophilic attack than the carbonyl carbon of a carboxylic acid. Also, chlorine is an excellent leaving group, making acid chlorides highly reactive. They are frequently used as intermediates in the conversion of carboxylic acids to esters and amides. Acyl halides, esters, and amides are discussed further in Chapter 48, Carboxylic Acid Derivatives.

Decarboxylation

Carboxylic acids can undergo decarboxylation reactions, resulting in the loss of carbon dioxide and thus loss of the entire carboxyl group.

1,3-dicarboxylic acids and other β-keto acids may spontaneously decarboxylate when heated. The carboxyl group is lost and replaced with a hydrogen. The reaction proceeds through a six-membered ring transition state. The enol initially formed tautomerizes to the more stable keto form as the final product.

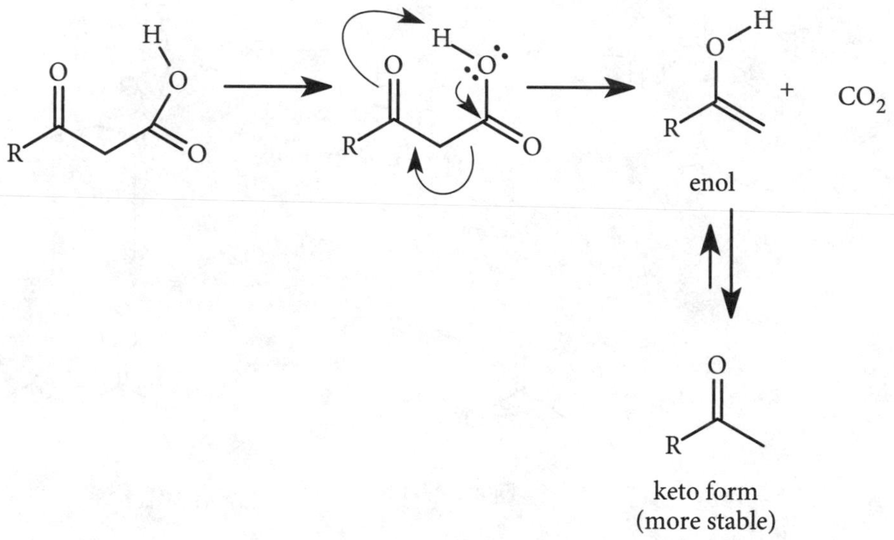

Figure 47.15

Soap Formation

When long-chain hydrocarbon carboxylic acids react with sodium or potassium hydroxide, they form salts. These salts, called soaps, are able to solubilize nonpolar organic compounds in aqueous solutions because they possess both a nonpolar "tail" and a polar carboxylate "head."

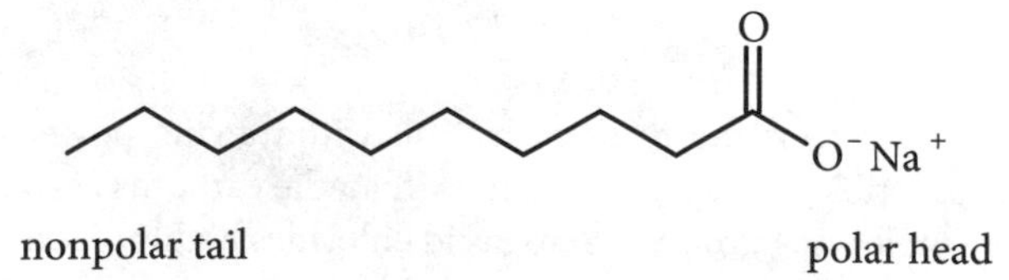

nonpolar tail   polar head

Figure 47.16

When placed in aqueous solution, soap molecules arrange themselves into spherical structures called **micelles**. The polar heads face outward, where they can be solvated by water molecules, and the nonpolar hydrocarbon chains are inside the sphere, protected from the solvent. Nonpolar molecules such as grease can dissolve in the hydrocarbon interior of the spherical micelle, while the micelle as a whole is soluble in water because of its polar shell.

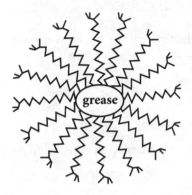

Figure 47.17

REVIEW PROBLEMS

1. Which compound in each of the following pairs is more acidic?
   (A) CH_3COOH or $CH_2ClCOOH$
   (B) $HOOCCH_2COOH$ or $HOOCCH_2COO^-$
   (C) NH_2CH_2COOH or NO_2CH_2COOH

2. Which of the following molecules could be classified as a soap?
   (A) $CH_3(CH_2)_{17}CH_2COOH$
   (B) CH_3COOH
   (C) $CH_3(CH_2)_{19}CH_2COO^-Na^+$
   (D) $CH_3COO^-Na^+$

3. Which of the following compounds would be expected to decarboxylate when heated?

   (A)

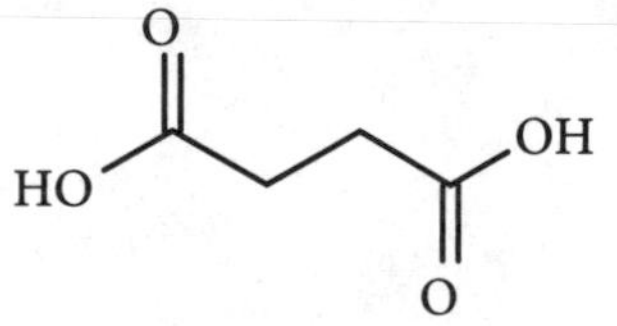

   (B)

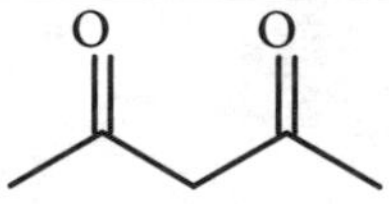

   (C)

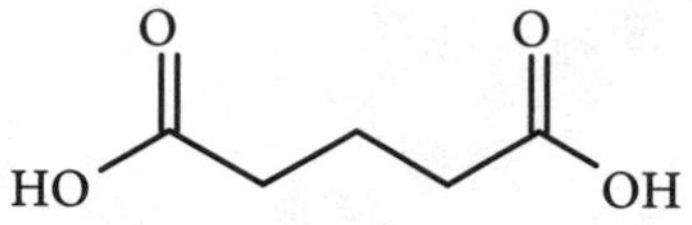

   (D)

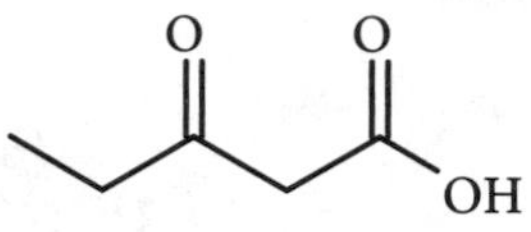

4. Oxidation of which of the following compounds is most likely to yield a carboxylic acid?
   (A) Acetone
   (B) Cyclohexanone
   (C) 2-Propanol
   (D) Methanol

5. Give the IUPAC name for each of the following carboxylic acids:

   (A)

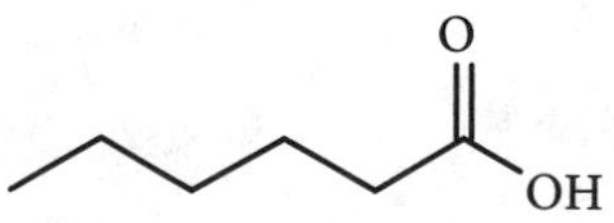

   (B)

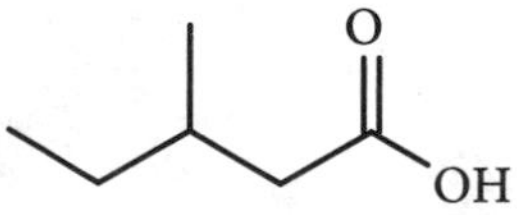

   (C)

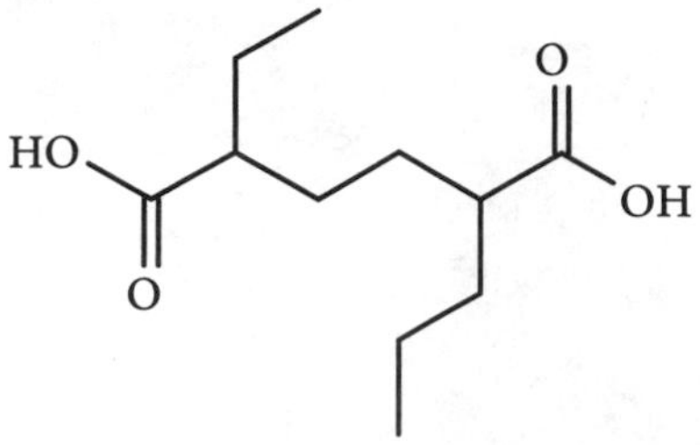

   (D)

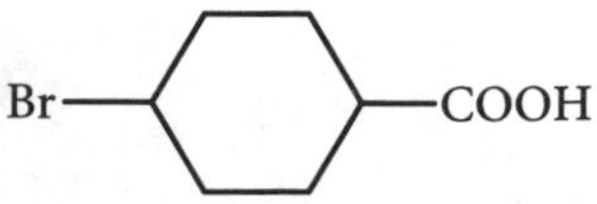

6. Draw the structures of the following carboxylic acids:

   (A) 2,3-Dimethylpentanoic acid

   (B) 3-Butenoic acid

   (C) *p*-Hydroxybenzoic acid

   (D) 4-Bromohexanoic acid

7. Carboxylic acids have higher boiling points than the corresponding alcohols because

   (A) the molecular weight of a carboyxlic acid is less than that of its corresponding alcohol.

   (B) the pH of a carboxlyic acid is lower than that of its corresponding alcohol.

   (C) acid salts are soluble in water.

   (D) hydrogen bonding is much stronger among carboxylic acids than among alcohols.

8. Which of the following carboxylic acids will be the most acidic?

   (A) $CH_3CHClCH_2COOH$

   (B) $CH_3CH_2CCl_2COOH$

   (C) $CH_3CH_2CHClCOOH$

   (D) $CH_3CH_2CH_2COOH$

9. Which of the following substituted benzoic acid compounds will be the least acidic?

   (A)

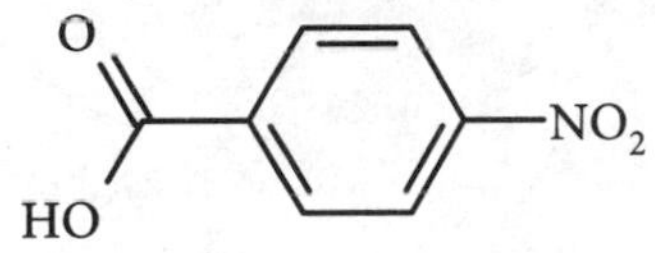

   (B)

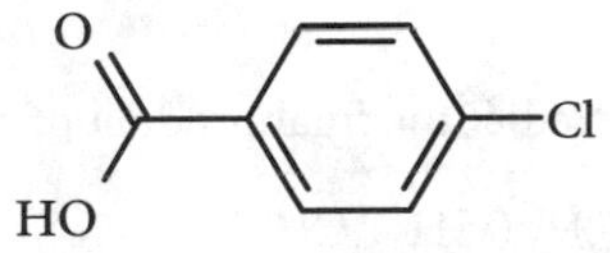

   (C)

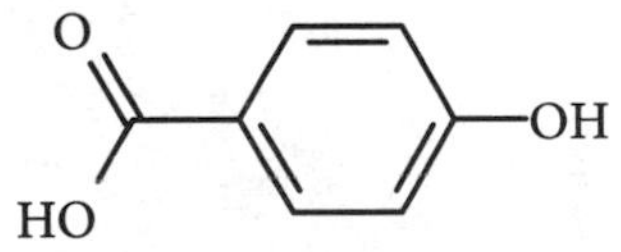

   (D)

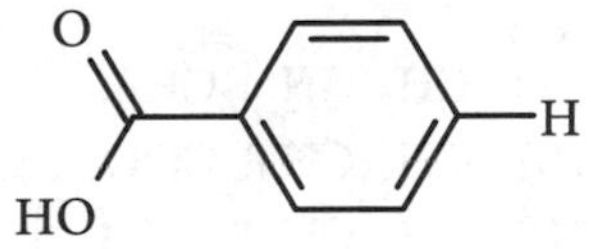

10. Rank the following compounds in order of increasing acidity.

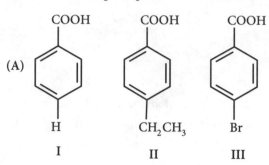

(A)

COOH	COOH	COOH
H	CH_2CH_3	Br
I	II	III

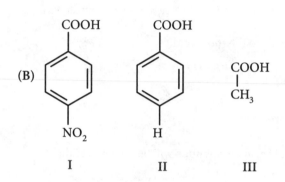

(B)

COOH	COOH	COOH
NO_2	H	CH_3
I	II	III

11. Predict the final product of the following reaction:

$$CH_3(CH_2)_4CH_2OH \xrightarrow[\text{acetone}]{CrO_3,\ H_2SO_4}$$

(A) $CH_3(CH_2)_4CHO$
(B) $CH_3(CH_2)_4COOH$
(C) $CH_3(CH_2)_4CH_3$
(D) $HOOC(CH_2)_4COOH$

12. The reduction of a carboxylic acid by lithium aluminum hydride will yield what final product?

(A) An aldehyde
(B) An ester
(C) A ketone
(D) An alcohol

SOLUTIONS TO REVIEW PROBLEMS

1. **A** CH$_2$ClCOOH

    Acetic acid is a fairly acidic compound and has a pK_a of 4.8. However, chloroacetic acid is more acidic because the chlorine atom is electron-withdrawing. This withdrawing effect stabilizes the carboxylate anion by delocalizing the charge more than the carboxyl group alone and thus facilitating the acid's dissociation.

    B HOOCCH$_2$COOH

    The maleate anion is less acidic than maleic acid because formation of a second negative charge is hindered by the presence of the first negative charge.

    C NO$_2$CH$_2$COOH

    Nitroacetic acid is more acidic than aminoacetic acid because the nitro group is electron-withdrawing while the amino group is electron-donating. The withdrawing effect delocalizes the negative charge on the anion, making it more stable. In contrast, the donating effect of the amino group concentrates the negative charge on the carboxylate group, creating a higher-energy state and destabilizing the anion.

2. **C** A soap is a long-chain hydrocarbon with a highly polar end. Generally, this polar end or head is a salt of a carboxylic acid. Choice (C) fits these criteria and is the correct answer. The remaining choices all fail one or both of the criteria and are therefore wrong. Choice (A) is not a salt. Choice (B) is acetic acid, which is not a salt and does not possess a long hydrocarbon chain. Choice (D) is sodium acetate, which is a salt but does not have a long hydrocarbon chain.

3. **D** Choice (D) is a β-keto acid: a keto group β-bonded to a carboxyl group. Decarboxylation occurs with β-keto acids and 1,3-diacids because they can form a cyclic transition state that permits simultaneous transfer of a hydrogen and loss of carbon dioxide. Choice (B) is a diketone, and this will definitely not decarboxylate. Choices (A) and (C) are 1,4- and 1,5-diacids, respectively, and will decarboxylate, but with more difficulty. The correct answer is choice (D).

4. **D** Oxidation of methanol, choice (D), will yield first formaldehyde and then formic acid; this is the correct answer. Acetone, choice (A), cannot be oxidized further unless extremely harsh conditions are used. This is because the carbonyl carbon is bonded to two alkyl groups, and further oxidation would necessitate cleavage of a carbon-carbon bond. Choice (B), cyclohexanone, is likewise limited in its options for further oxidation. Choice (C), 2-propanol, can be oxidized to acetone but no further without harsh conditions.

5. **A** Hexanoic acid
    B 3-Methylpentanoic acid
    C 5-Ethyl-2-propylhexanedioic acid
    D 4-Bromocyclohexanecarboxylic acid

6.

(A)

(B)

(C) HO—

(D)

7. **D** The boiling points of compounds depend on the strength of the attractive forces between molecules. In both alcohols and carboxylic acids, the major form of intermolecular attraction is hydrogen bonding; however, the hydrogen bonds of carboxylic acids are much stronger than those of alcohols, since the acids are much more polar than the alcohols. This makes the boiling points of carboxylic acids higher than those of the corresponding alcohols, so choice (D) is correct. Boiling points are also dependent on molecular weight, choice (A), but in this case the influence of the small difference in molecular weight is negligible compared with the effect of hydrogen bonding. Therefore, choice (A) is incorrect. Choice (B) describes the behavior of acids in solution; although this is also dependent on intermolecular forces, it is not otherwise related to the behavior of the pure acid, so choice (B) is incorrect. Choice (C) discusses the behavior of an acid's salt in solution, which is incorrect for the same reason.

8. **B** The acidity of carboxylic acids is significantly increased by the substitution of highly electronegative halogens onto the carbon chain. Their electron-withdrawing effect upon the carboxyl group increases the stability of the carboxylate anion, favoring the dissociation of the proton. This effect is especially strong for α-halogenated carboxylic acids. Among the four carboxylic acids listed, choice (D) is the only unsubstituted acid and therefore must have the lowest acidity. Choice (A) is β-halogenated, while choices (B) and (C) are α-halogenated, so (A) may be rejected. Finally, choice (B) contains 2 α-halogens and choice (C) includes only 1, so the electron-withdrawing effect in choice (B) is stronger; thus, (B) is the correct answer.

9. **C** The effects of different substituents on the acidity of benzoic acid compounds is correlated with their effects on the reactivity of the benzene ring (see Chapter 44). Activating substituents donate electron density into the benzene ring, and the ring in turn donates electron density to the carboxyl group, destabilizing the benzoate ion formed and therefore decreasing a compound's acidity. Deactivating substituents have the opposite effect: they withdraw electrons from the ring, which in turn withdraws negative charge from the carboxyl group, thus stabilizing the carboxylate anion and increasing the compound's acidity. Choice (A) contains a nitro group attached to the ring, and choice (B) has a chloride; both of these substituents have deactivating effects, so these choices may be rejected. Choice (D) is an unsubstituted benzoic acid, while choice (C) has a strongly

activating hydroxyl substituent. Thus, choice (C) will be the least acidic and is the correct answer.

10. **A II < I < III**

    An ethyl substituent has an activating and therefore electron-donating effect on the benzene ring; thus, the acidity of compound II is very low. The bromine substituent, on the other hand, has a deactivating and electron-withdrawing effect on the benzene ring, which makes compound III highly acidic. The acidity of unsubstituted benzoic acid (compound I) is somewhere in the middle. Therefore the order of increasing acidity is II, I, III.

    B III < II < I

    In this case, compound I is the strongest acid because the nitro group is a powerful deactivating and therefore electron-withdrawing substituent. On the other hand, II is a stronger acid than III because the methyl group in compound III donates electron density to the carboxyl group, decreasing the acidity of III. Here the order of increasing acidity is III, II, I.

11. **B** Jones reagent (chromium trioxide in aqueous sulfuric acid) oxidizes primary alcohols directly to monocarboxylic acids, so choice (B) is correct. This oxidizer is too strong to give an aldehyde as the final product (aldehyde will be formed but will immediately be oxidized further), so choice (A) is incorrect. Choice (D), a dicarboxylic acid, cannot form because there is no functional group "handle" on the other end of the molecule for the reagent to attack, and it cannot attack the inert alkane. Nor will it produce an alkane such as choice (C), so this is also incorrect.

12. **D** Lithium aluminum hydride is a very strong reducing agent. Its reaction with carboxylic acids yields alcohols, choice (D). Aldehydes are intermediate products of this reaction and will be further reduced to alcohols; therefore, choice (A) is incorrect. Esters are formed from carboxylic acids by reaction with alcohols, so choice (B) is incorrect. Ketones are formed by the Friedel-Crafts acylation of the acyl chloride derivatives of acids, so choice (C) is incorrect.

CHAPTER FORTY-EIGHT

Carboxylic Acid Derivatives

Carboxylic acids can be converted into several types of derivatives: **acyl halides**, **anhydrides**, **amides**, and **esters**. These are compounds in which the –OH of the carboxyl group has been replaced with **–X, –OCOR, –NH₂**, or **–OR**, respectively:

- Acyl halide: R-CO-X
- Anhydride: R-CO-O-CO-R
- Ester: R-CO-OR′
- Amide: R-CO-NH₂ or R-CO-NR₂

Carboxylic acid derivatives all have the highly polarized C=O group in which the carbon carries a partial positive charge and the oxygen has a partial negative charge. As a result, these compounds readily undergo nucleophilic substitution reactions, including hydrolysis (with H_2O as the nucleophile). They also undergo other additions and substitutions, including various interconversions between different acid derivatives. In general, the acyl halides are the most reactive of the carboxylic acid derivatives, followed by the anhydrides, the esters, and the amides.

Each of these types of carboxylic acid derivatives will be discussed in turn. Although the variety of reaction pathways can appear overwhelming, they are all closely interwoven and should be studied in relation to each other. To aid your studies, a summary of the different reactions of carboxylic acid derivatives is included at the end of this chapter.

ACYL HALIDES

Nomenclature of Acyl Halides

Acyl halides are also called **acid** or **alkanoyl halides**. The acyl group is written RCO–, and with the halide attached it is written as RCOX. Acyl halides are the most reactive of the carboxylic acid derivatives. They are named in the IUPAC system by changing the *-ic acid* ending of the carboxylic acid to **-yl halide**. Some typical examples are ethanoyl chloride (also called acetyl chloride), benzoyl chloride, and *n*-butanoyl bromide.

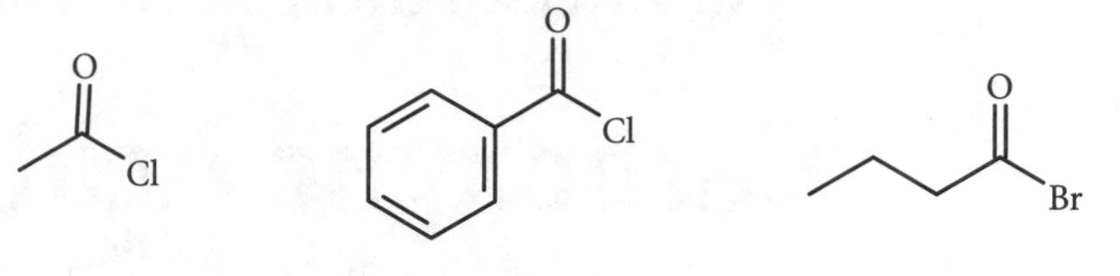

| ethanoyl chloride | benzoyl chloride | *n*-butanoyl bromide |

(acetyl chloride)

Figure 48.1

Properties of Acyl Halides

Because the –OH of the carboxyl group has been replaced by a halogen, an acyl halide is not able to form hydrogen bonds. Acyl halides are therefore less polar than comparable carboxylic acids, and demonstrate significantly lower melting and boiling points. For example, acetyl chloride boils at 51°C, compared to acetic acid which boils at 118°C.

Synthesis of Acyl Halides

The most common acyl halides are the acid chlorides, although acid bromides and iodides are occasionally encountered. Acyl chlorides are prepared by reaction of a carboxylic acid with thionyl chloride, $SOCl_2$, producing SO_2 and HCl as side products. Alternatively, PCl_3 or PCl_5 (or PBr_3, to make an acid bromide) can be used for this synthesis.

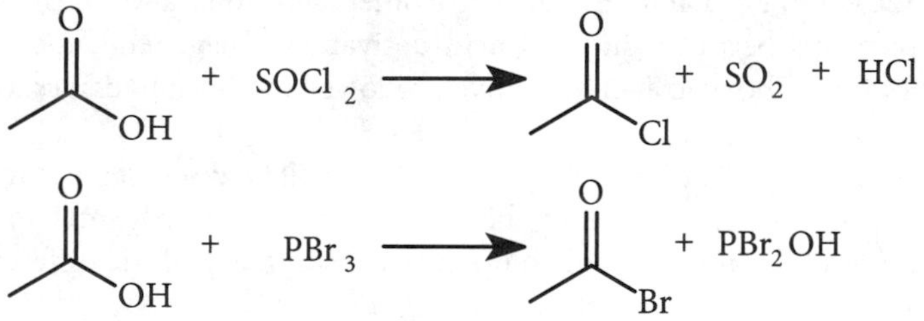

Figure 48.2

Reactions of Acyl Halides

Nucleophilic acyl substitution

Acyl halides are very reactive, as the greater electron-withdrawing power of the halogen makes the carbonyl carbon more susceptible to nucleophilic attack than the carbonyl carbon of a carboxylic acid. Because halides are excellent leaving groups, nucleophilic attack will always be followed by re-formation of the carbonyl. As a result, acyl halides readily undergo nucleophilic substitution reactions, including hydrolysis (with H_2O as the nucleophile), which produces the original carboxylic acid. Acyl halides are also frequently used as intermediates in the conversion of carboxylic acids to anhydrides, esters, and amides.

Hydrolysis

The simplest reaction of acid halides is their conversion back to carboxylic acids by classic nucleophilic attack. Acyl halides react very rapidly with water to form the corresponding acid, along with HCl, which is responsible for their irritating odor.

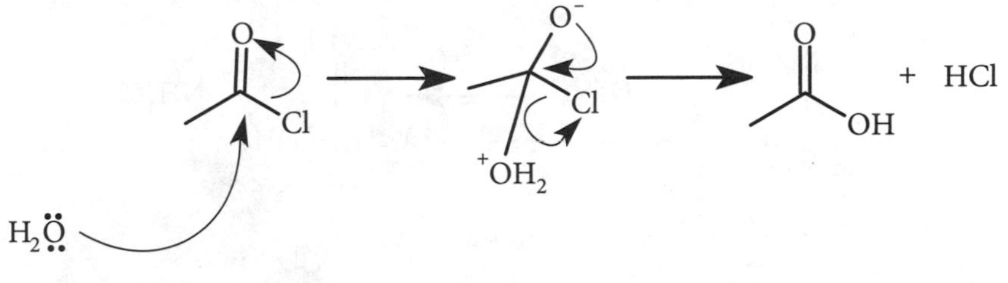

Figure 48.3

Conversion into anhydrides

Reaction of an acyl chloride with a carboxylate salt will produce an anhydride through nucleophilic attack and re-formation of the carbonyl:

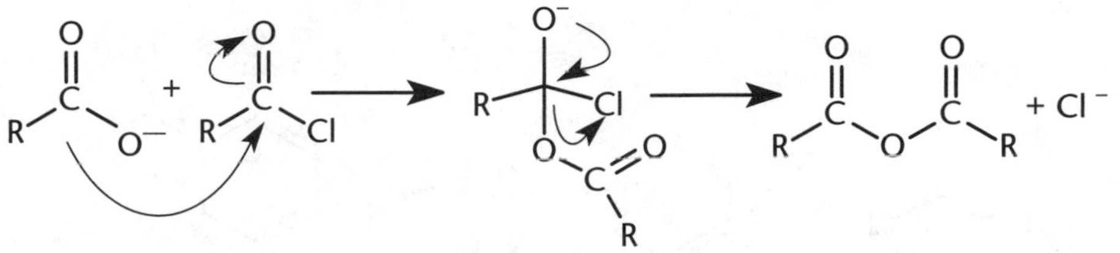

Figure 48.4

Conversion into esters

Acyl halides can be converted into esters by reaction with alcohols. The same type of nucleophilic attack found in hydrolysis leads to the formation of a tetrahedral intermediate, with the hydroxyl oxygen of the alcohol acting as the nucleophile. Chloride is displaced as the carbonyl re-forms, and HCl is released as a side-product.

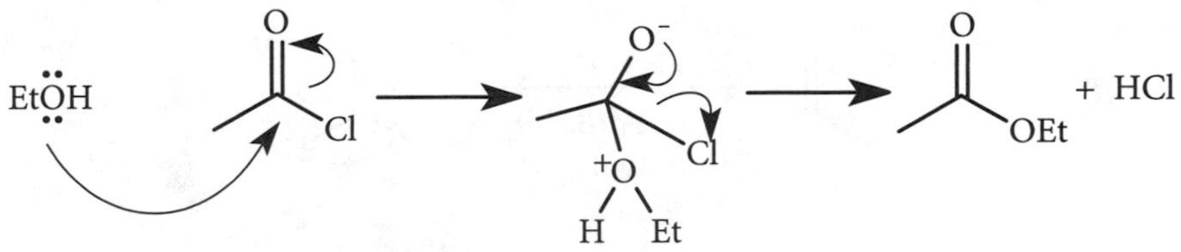

Figure 48.5

Conversion into amides

Acyl halides can be converted into amides (compounds of the general formula $RCONR_2$) by nucleophilic substitution with amines. An amine, such as ammonia, attacks the carbonyl group, displacing chloride. The side product is ammonium chloride, formed from excess ammonia and HCl. Primary and secondary amines can also be used as the nucleophile to create *N*-substituted amides.

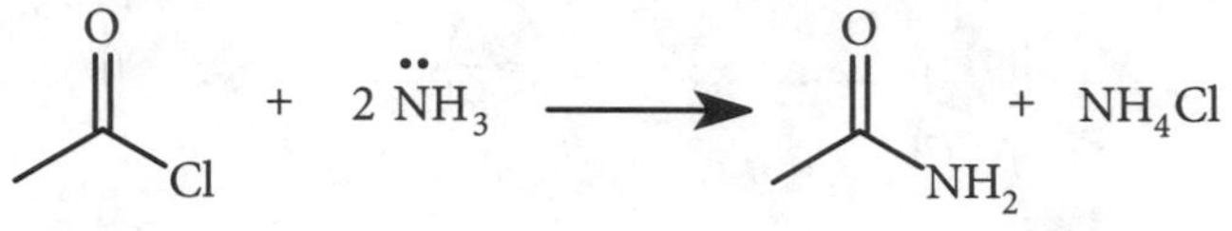

Figure 48.6

Other Reactions of Acyl Halides

Friedel-Crafts acylation

Aromatic rings can be acylated in a Friedel-Crafts reaction, as discussed in Chapter 44, Aromatic Compounds. The mechanism is electrophilic aromatic substitution, and the attacking reagent is an acylium ion, formed by reaction of an acid chloride with $AlCl_3$ or another Lewis acid. The product is an alkyl aryl ketone.

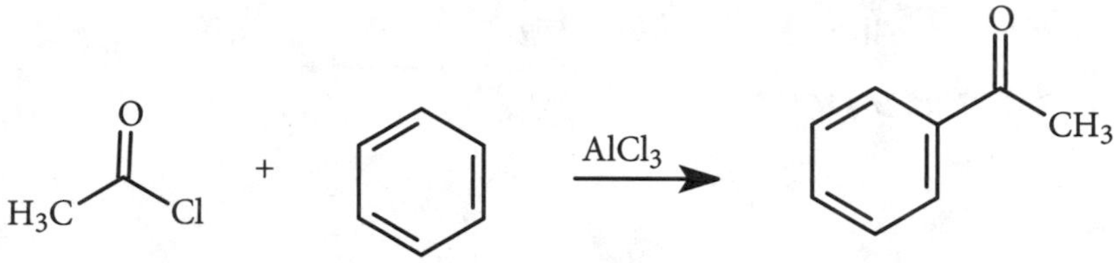

Figure 48.7

Reduction

Acid halides can be reduced to alcohols with a strong reducing agent such as LAH. They can also be selectively reduced to the intermediate aldehydes by catalytic hydrogenation in the presence of a "poison" such as quinoline, also called Lindlar's catalyst. These reaction conditions are also discussed in Chapter 43, Alkenes and Alkynes.

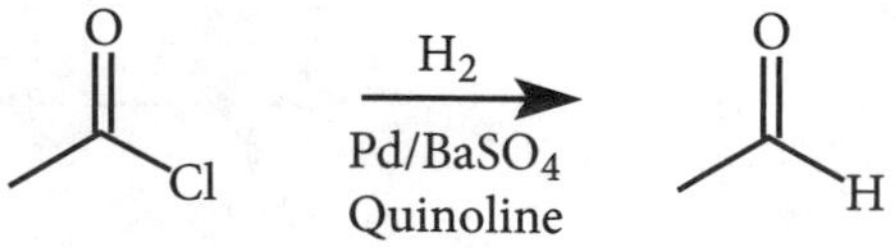

Figure 48.8

ANHYDRIDES

Nomenclature of Anhydrides

Anhydrides, also called **acid anhydrides**, are the condensation dimers of carboxylic acids, with the general formula RCOOCOR. They are named by substituting the word **anhydride** for the word *acid* in a carboxylic acid. Most anhydrides are symmetrical, although asymmetrical anhydrides exist and can be important in biological systems. The most common and important anhydride is acetic anhydride, the dimer of acetic acid. Other common anhydrides, such as succinic, maleic, and phthalic anhydrides, are **cyclic anhydrides** arising from intramolecular condensation or dehydration of diacids (Figure 48.9).

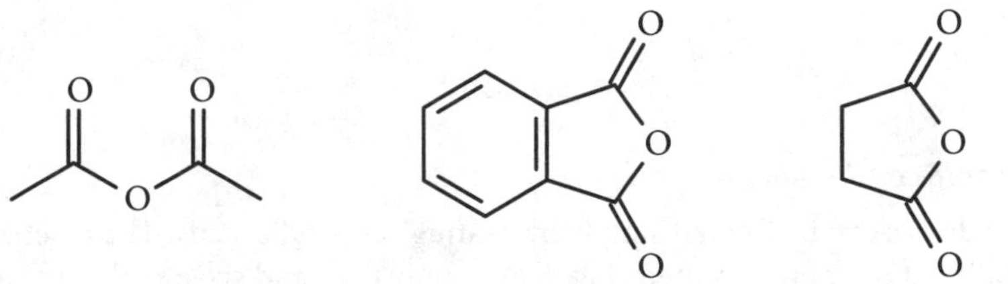

acetic anhydride

(ethanoic anhydride)

phthalic anhydride

succinic anhydride

Figure 48.9

Properties of Anhydrides

Since acid anhydrides no longer have an –OH group, they do not have the ability to form hydrogen bonds. Anhydrides therefore are less polar and demonstrate lower melting and boiling points than comparable carboxylic acids of the same molecular weight (MW). For example, ethanoic anhydride and pentanoic acid are approximately the same MW, but the anhydride boils at 140°C and the carboxylic acid at 186°C.

However, because anhydrides are often formed from the condensation of two other molecules, the product will have a higher melting or boiling point due to its larger size compared to the starting materials. For example, acetic anhydride ($CH_3CO-O-COCH_3$) boils at 140°C, compared to acetic acid (CH_3COOH) which boils at 118°C. In this case, the much larger MW of the anhydride is more influential than the effect of hydrogen bonding for the carboxylic acid.

Although anhydrides are polar, they are not considered to be soluble in water because they immediately decompose in aqueous conditions to form carboxylic acids.

Synthesis of Anhydrides

The synthesis pathways of anhydrides all involve some form of nucleophilic attack on a carboxylic acid, followed by the release of a leaving group and re-formation of the carbonyl.

Acyl chloride reaction

Anhydrides can be readily synthesized by reaction of an acyl chloride with a carboxylate salt. This is the most efficient and most commonly used method of anhydride synthesis.

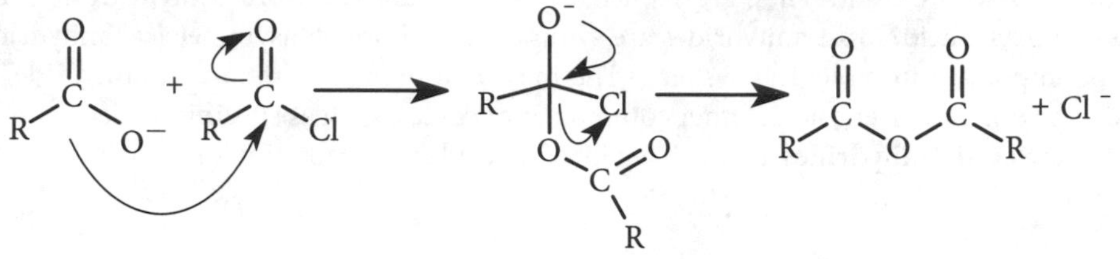

Figure 48.10

Cyclic anhydride self-condensation

Certain cyclic anhydrides can be formed simply by heating carboxylic acids. The reaction is driven by the increased stability of the newly formed ring; hence, only five- and six-membered ring anhydrides are easily made. In this case, the hydroxyl of one –COOH group acts as a nucleophile, attacking the carbonyl on the other –COOH group and releasing water.

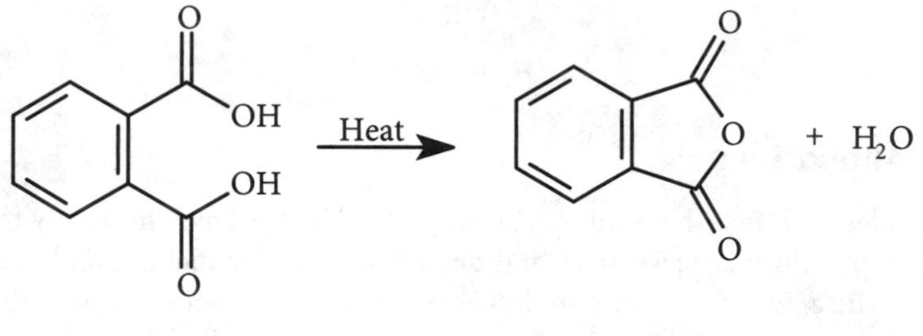

o-phthalic acid   phthalic anhydride

Figure 48.11

Condensation of two carboxylic acids

Two carboxylic acid molecules can condense to form an anhydride in a reaction releasing water; however, this reaction requires anhydrous conditions. Therefore a dehydrating reagent that will remove the water produced in the reaction is needed to prevent immediate conversion back to the carboxylic acids. Reagents such as acetic anhydride, trifluoroacetic anhydride, phosphorus pentachloride, or dicyclohexylcarbodiimide (DCC) can be used for this purpose.

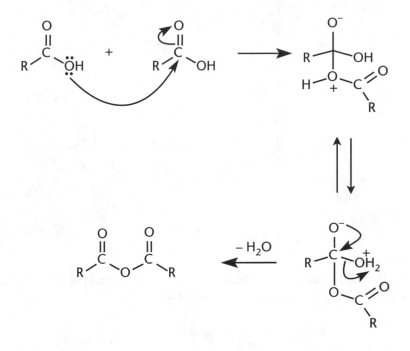

Figure 48.12

Reactions of Anhydrides

Anhydrides react under the same conditions as acid chlorides, but since anhydrides are somewhat more stable, they are less reactive. Nucleophilic attack on an anhydride is slower and produces a carboxylic acid as the side product instead of HCl. Cyclic anhydrides are also subject to these reactions, which cause ring opening at the anhydride group along with formation of the new functional groups.

Hydrolysis

Anhydrides are converted into carboxylic acids when exposed to water. Note that in this reaction, the leaving group is actually a carboxylic acid; because the anhydride is symmetrical, it produces two molecules of the same carboxylic acid.

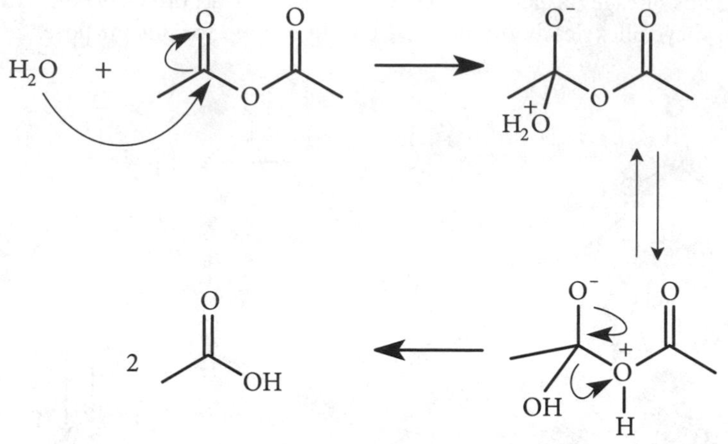

Figure 48.13

Conversion into amides

Anhydrides are cleaved by ammonia, producing an amide and a carboxylic acid. The carboxylic acid then further reacts with ammonia to form an ammonium carboxylate.

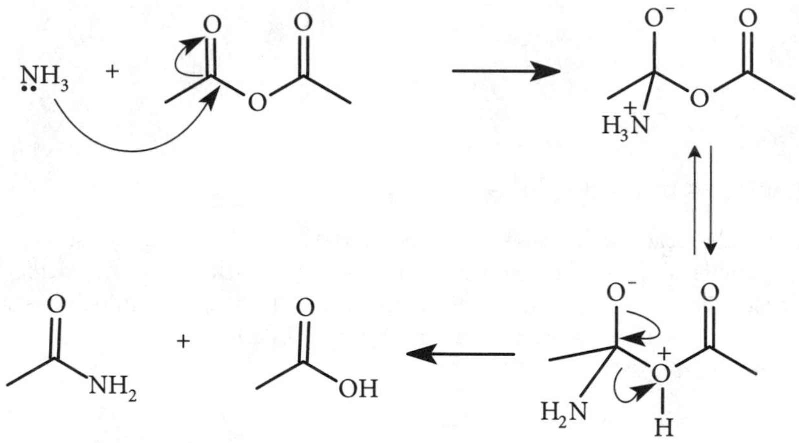

Then:

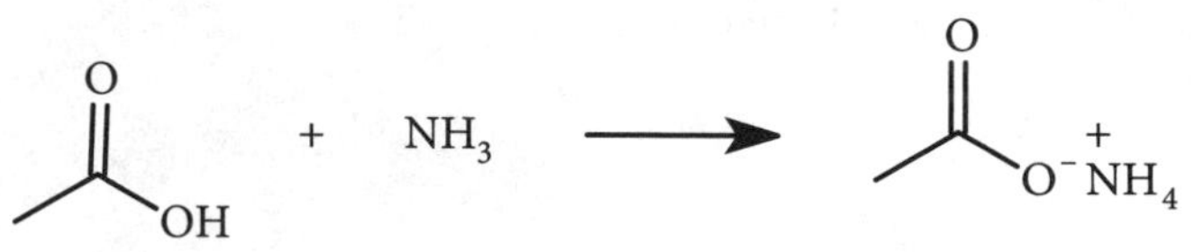

Figure 48.14

Conversion into esters and carboxylic acids

Anhydrides react with alcohols to form esters; a single anhydride molecule will produce one ester and also one molecule of carboxylic acid.

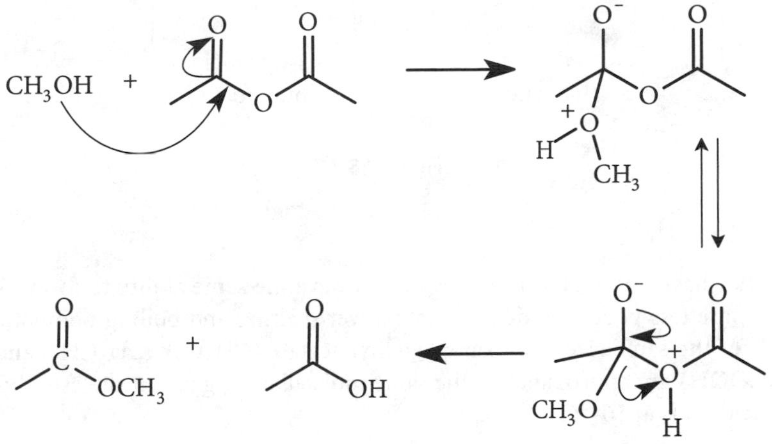

Figure 48.15

Acylation

Friedel-Crafts acylation occurs readily with anhydrides in the presence of AlCl$_3$ or other Lewis acid catalysts. This reaction produces an aryl ketone and a carboxylic acid.

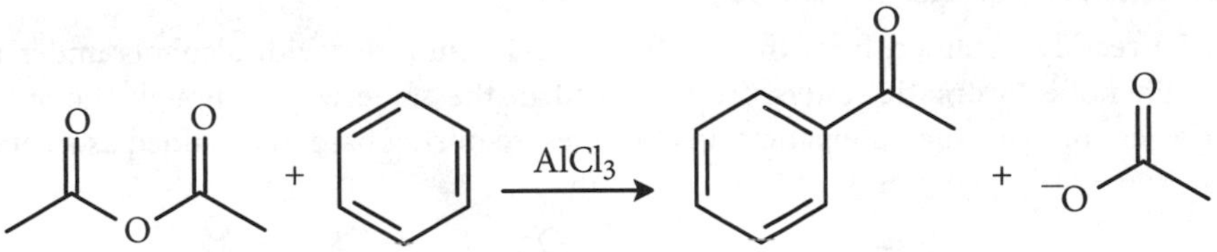

Figure 48.16

ESTERS

Nomenclature of Esters

Esters are the dehydration products of carboxylic acids and alcohols. They are commonly found in many fruits and perfumes. They are named in the IUPAC system as **alkyl** or **aryl alkanoates**. The alkyl chain attached to the non-carbonyl oxygen is named as a functional group; the carboxylic acid suffix *-oic acid* is replaced by **-oate** while retaining the carbon chain from the acid. For example, propyl acetate, derived from the condensation of acetic acid and propanol, has the structure CH$_3$COO–CH$_2$CH$_2$CH$_3$ and is called propyl ethanoate according to IUPAC nomenclature.

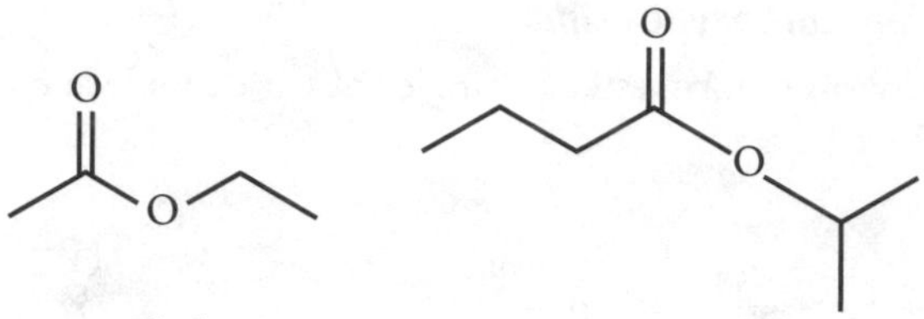

ethyl
ethanoate

isopropyl
butanoate

Figure 48.17

Properties of Esters

Since esters do not have an –OH group, they do not have the same ability to form hydrogen bonds. Esters, therefore, are less polar and demonstrate lower melting and boiling points than comparable carboxylic acids of the same size. For example, ethyl acetate ($CH_3COOCH_2CH_3$) and butanoic acid ($CH_3CH_2CH_2COOH$) are approximately the same molecular weight, but the ester boils at 77°C and the carboxylic acid boils at 164°C.

The water solubility of esters depends on the length of the hydrocarbon chain on the ester oxygen. Smaller esters have good water solubility, but as the chain becomes longer, water solubility decreases. This becomes important for very long chain esters that make up fats and oils, which are discussed in greater detail in Chapter 53, Lipids.

Synthesis of Esters

Conversion of acyl chlorides into esters

Esters can be readily obtained from the reaction of acid chlorides with alcohols under anhydrous conditions. Phenolic (aromatic) esters are produced in the same way, although the aromatic acid chlorides are less reactive than aliphatic acid chlorides, requiring base to be added as a catalyst.

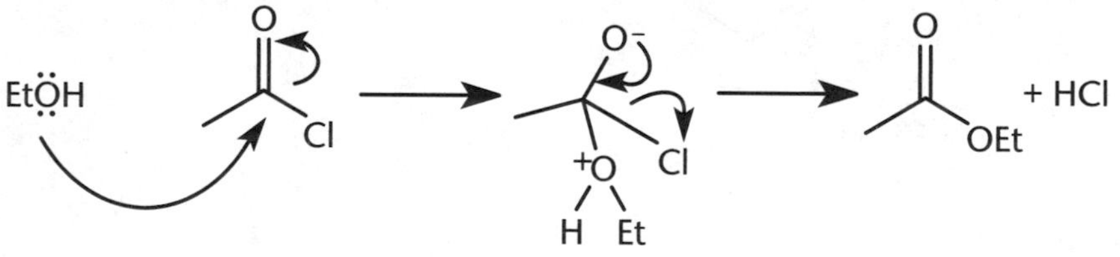

Figure 48.18

Conversion of anhydrides into esters and carboxylic acids

Anhydrides react with alcohols to form esters; a single anhydride molecule will produce one ester and also one molecule of carboxylic acid.

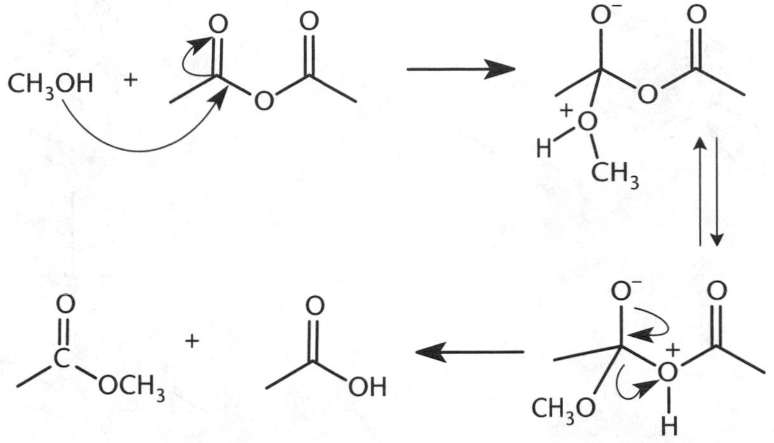

Figure 48.19

Condensation of carboxylic acids and alcohols

Mixtures of carboxylic acids and alcohols will condense into esters under anhydrous conditions, liberating water. Use of sulfuric acid as a catalyst and dehydrating reagent will drive the reaction forward:

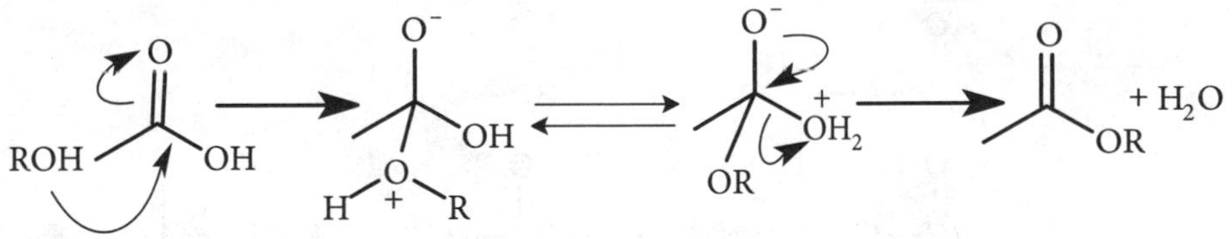

Figure 48.20

Reactions of Esters

Esters react with nucleophiles at the carbonyl carbon, although they are less reactive than acyl halides or anhydrides. Almost all reactions of esters can be recognized as nucleophilic substitutions (in which the carbonyl is retained) or nucleophilic additions (in which the carbonyl is lost).

Hydrolysis

Esters, like the other derivatives of carboxylic acids, can be hydrolyzed, yielding carboxylic acids and alcohols. Hydrolysis can take place under either acidic or basic conditions. Under acidic conditions, the first step is protonation of the carbonyl oxygen, followed by water attacking the carbonyl carbon:

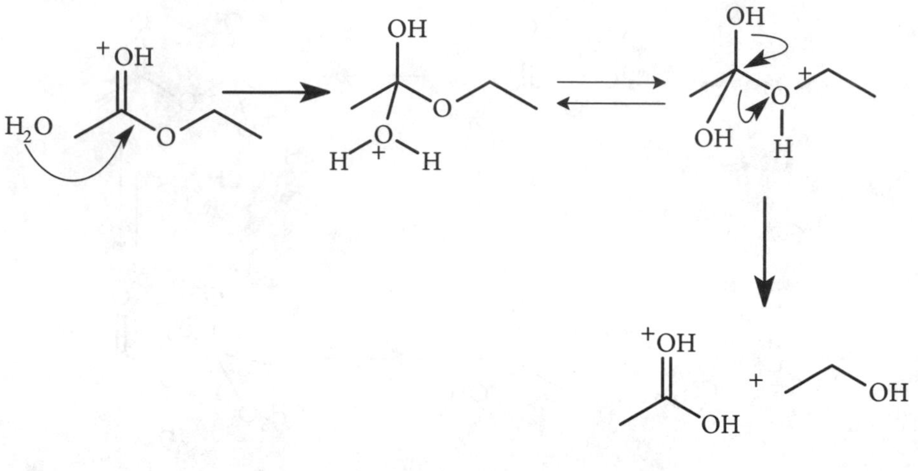

Figure 48.21

Under basic conditions, the nucleophile is OH⁻, which directly attacks the carbonyl carbon. **Triacylglycerols,** also called fats or triglycerides, are esters of long-chain carboxylic acids, often called fatty acids, and glycerol (1,2,3-propanetriol). **Saponification** is the process whereby fats are hydrolyzed under basic conditions to produce soaps. Fats are discussed in more detail in Chapter 53, Lipids.

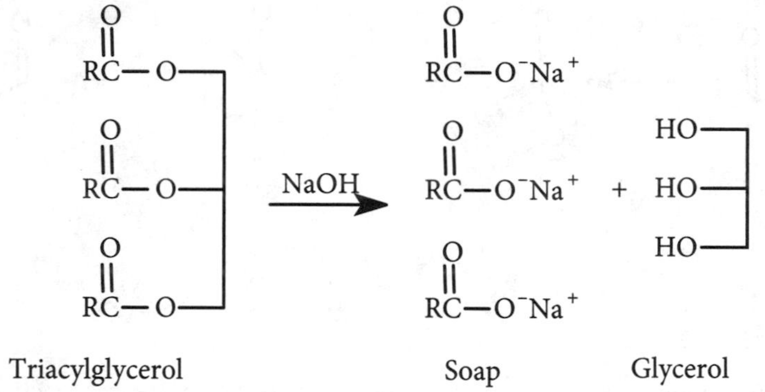

Figure 48.22

Conversion into amides

Nitrogen bases, such as ammonia, act as a nucleophile and attack the electrophilic carbonyl carbon atom, displacing the ester functional group to yield an amide and an alcohol side-product:

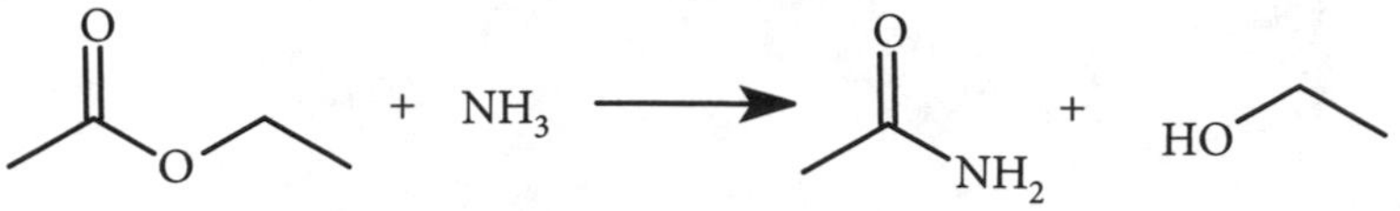

Figure 48.23

Transesterification

Alcohols can act as nucleophiles and displace the alkoxy groups on esters. This process, which transforms one ester into another, is called **transesterification**.

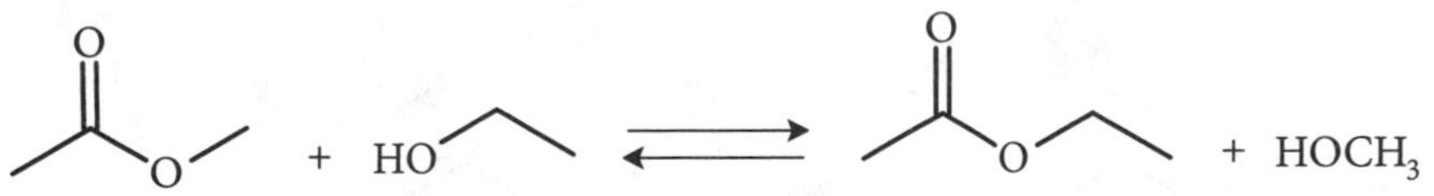

Figure 48.24

Grignard addition

Grignard reagents add to the carbonyl groups of esters to form ketones; however, these ketones are more reactive than the initial esters and are readily attacked by more Grignard reagent. Two equivalents of Grignard reagent can thus be used to produce tertiary alcohols with good yield. The intermediate ketone can be isolated only if the alkyl groups are sufficiently bulky to prevent further attack. This reaction proceeds via nucleophilic substitution followed by nucleophilic addition.

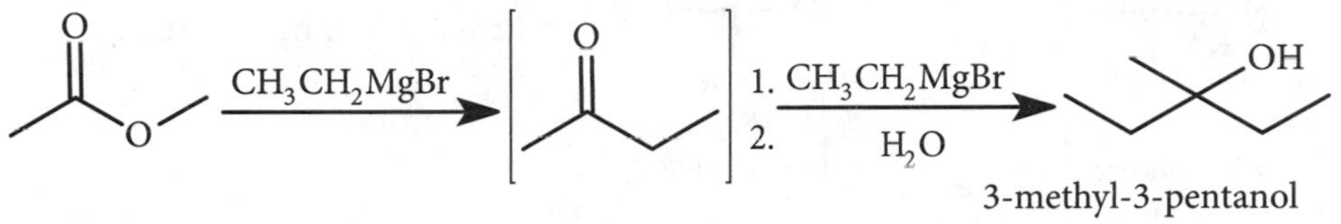

3-methyl-3-pentanol

Figure 48.25

Condensation Reactions

An important reaction of esters is the **Claisen condensation**. In the simplest case, two moles of ethyl acetate react under basic conditions to produce a β-keto ester, ethyl 3-oxobutanoate, which is also known by its common name, acetoacetic ester. (The Claisen condensation is also called the **acetoacetic ester condensation**.) The reaction proceeds by addition of an enolate anion to the carbonyl group of another ester, followed by displacement of ethoxide ion (the formation of enolate ions is discussed in Chapter 46, Aldehydes and Ketones). This mechanism is analogous to that of the aldol condensation (also covered in Chapter 46).

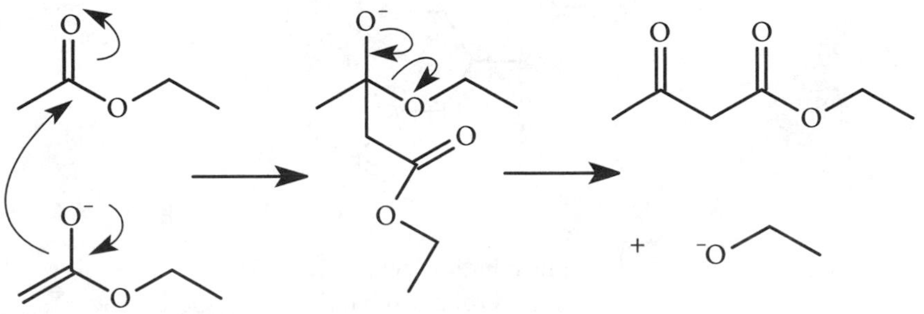

Figure 48.26

Reduction

Esters may be reduced to primary alcohols with LAH, but not with $NaBH_4$. This allows for selective reduction in molecules with multiple functional groups. Note that different alcohols are produced from the ester alkoxy functional group and the carbonyl-containing carbon chain.

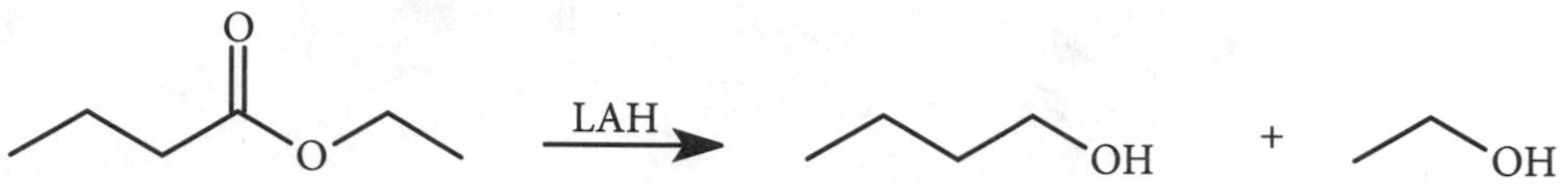

Figure 48.27

Phosphate Esters

While phosphoric acid derivatives are not carboxylic acid derivatives, they form esters with many similar properties and reactivities.

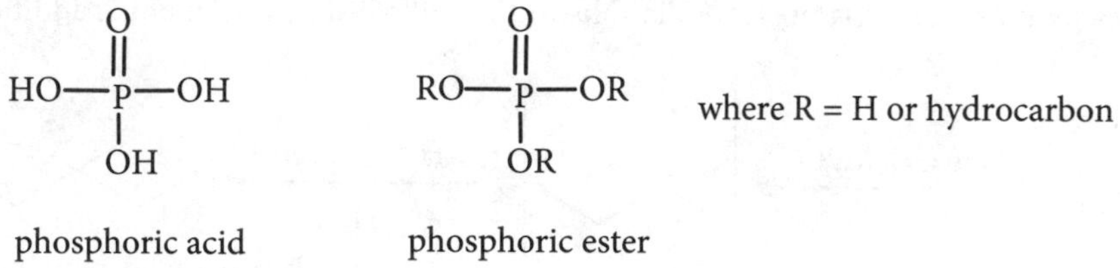

where R = H or hydrocarbon

phosphoric acid   phosphoric ester

Figure 48.28

Phosphoric acid and the mono- and diesters are acidic (more so than carboxylic acids) and usually exist as anions. Like carboxylic acid esters, under acidic conditions they can be cleaved into the parent acid (here, H_3PO_4) and alcohols.

Phosphate esters are found in living systems in the form of **phospholipids** (phosphoglycerides), in which glycerol is attached to two carboxylic acids and one phosphoric acid.

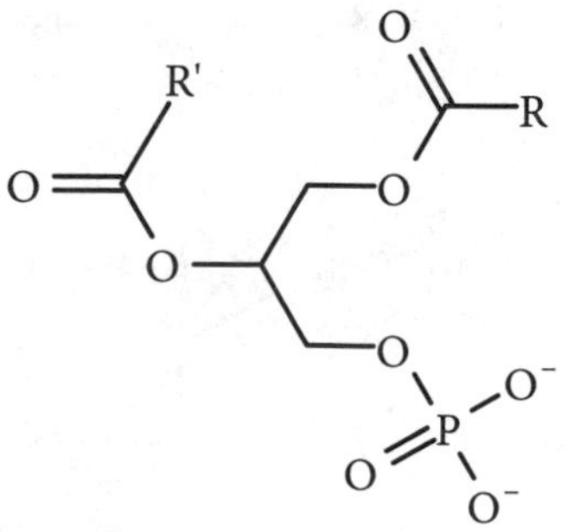

phosphatidic acid
diacylglycerol phosphate
(a phosphoglyceride)

Figure 48.29

Phospholipids are the main component of cell membranes, and phosphate/carbohydrate polymers form the backbone of nucleic acids, the hereditary material of life. The nucleic acid derivative **adenosine triphosphate (ATP)** can give up and regain one or more phosphate groups. ATP facilitates many biological reactions by releasing phosphate groups to other compounds, thereby increasing their reactivities. See Chapter 51 for more details on nucleic acids and related phosphate esters.

AMIDES

Nomenclature of Amides

Amides are compounds with the general formula $RCONR_2$, in which the R group can be either a hydrocarbon, a hydrogen, or one of each. Amides are particularly important in biological systems, as the peptide bonds that link amino acids into proteins are actually amide bonds (see Chapter 52, Proteins, for more details). Amides are named by replacing the -**oic** acid ending with -**amide**. Alkyl substituents on the nitrogen atom are listed as prefixes, and their location is specified with the letter *N*. For example, *N*-methylpropanamide has a methyl and a hydrogen as the substituents on the nitrogen and a 3-carbon chain, including the carbonyl:

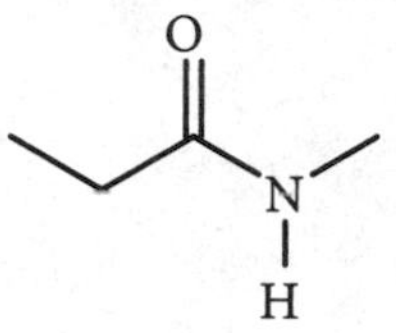

N-methylpropanamide

Figure 48.30

Properties of Amides

Although amides do not have an –OH group, those that have hydrogens as substituents on the amide nitrogen have the ability to form hydrogen bonds. In fact, when two hydrogens are present on the amide nitrogen, it has the ability to form twice as many hydrogen bonds as the corresponding carboxylic acid. As a result, amides have very high melting and boiling points, and good water solubility (with the exception of tertiary amides that have two alkyl groups on the amide nitrogen). For example, acetamide (CH_3CONH_2) boils at 221°C, while acetic acid boils at 118°C.

Synthesis of Amides

Amides are generally synthesized by the reaction of acid chlorides with amines or by the reaction of acid anhydrides with ammonia.

Conversion of acyl halides to amides

Acyl halides can be readily converted into amides by nucleophilic substitution with amines. An amine such as ammonia attacks the carbonyl group, displacing chloride. The side product is ammonium chloride, formed from excess ammonia and HCl. Primary and secondary amines can also be used as the nucleophile to create substituted amides; tertiary amines are not able to lose a hydrogen and thus cannot participate in this reaction.

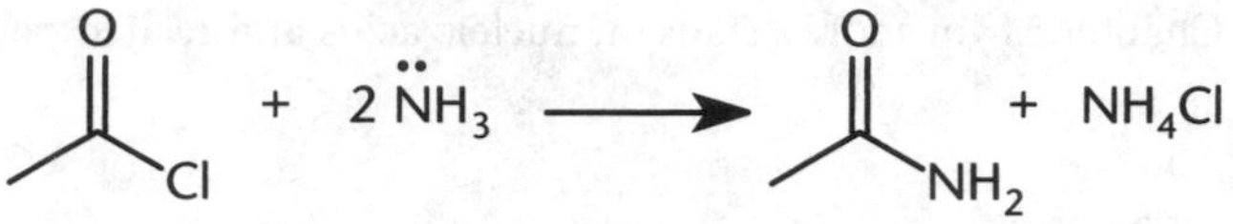

Figure 48.31

Conversion of anhydrides into amides

Anhydrides are cleaved by ammonia, producing an amide and a carboxylic acid. The carboxylic acid then further reacts with ammonia to form ammonium carboxylate.

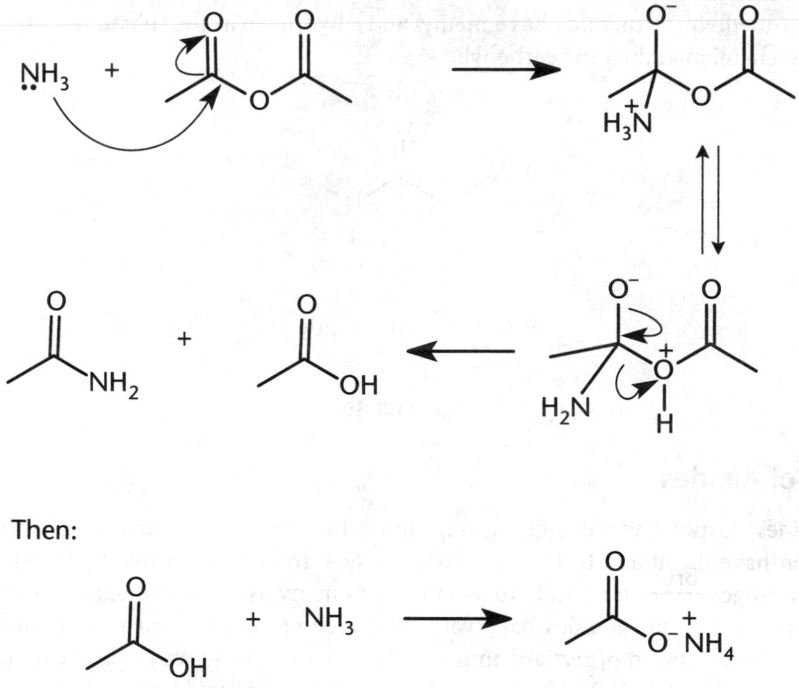

Then:

Figure 48.32

Conversion of esters into amides

Nitrogen bases such as ammonia act as nucleophiles and will attack the electrophilic carbonyl carbon atom, displacing the ester functional group to yield an amide and an alcohol side-product.

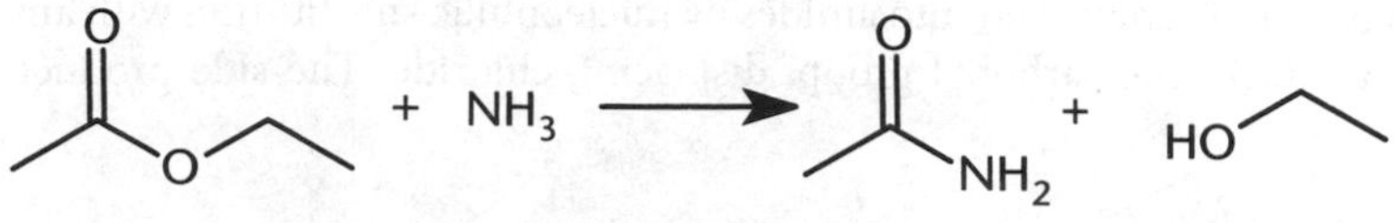

Figure 48.33

Reactions

Amides are the least reactive of the carboxylic acid derivatives but are still susceptible to nucleophilic attack as well as rearrangements and reductions.

Hydrolysis

Amides can be hydrolyzed under acidic conditions, via nucleophilic substitution, to produce carboxylic acids. Under basic conditions amides react to form carboxylates.

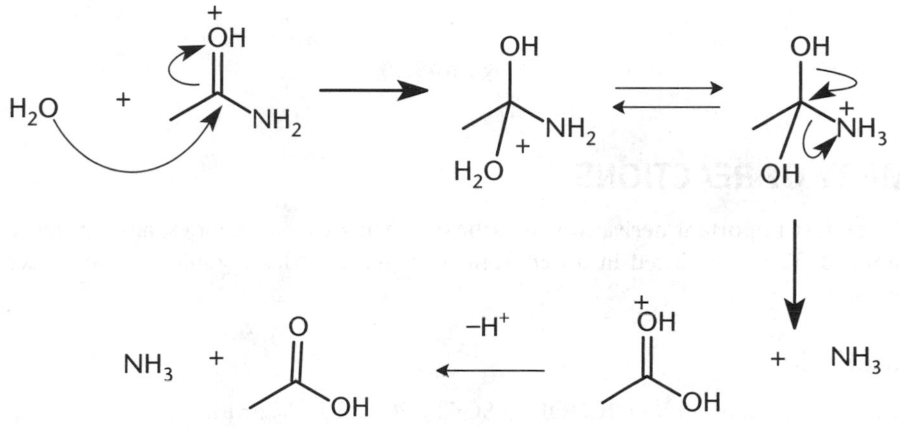

Figure 48.34

Hofmann rearrangement

The **Hofmann rearrangement** converts amides to primary amines with the loss of the carbonyl carbon as a molecule of CO_2. The mechanism involves the formation of a **nitrene**, the nitrogen analog of a carbene. The nitrene is attached to the carbonyl group and rearranges to form an **isocyanate**, which under aqueous reaction conditions is hydrolyzed to the amine.

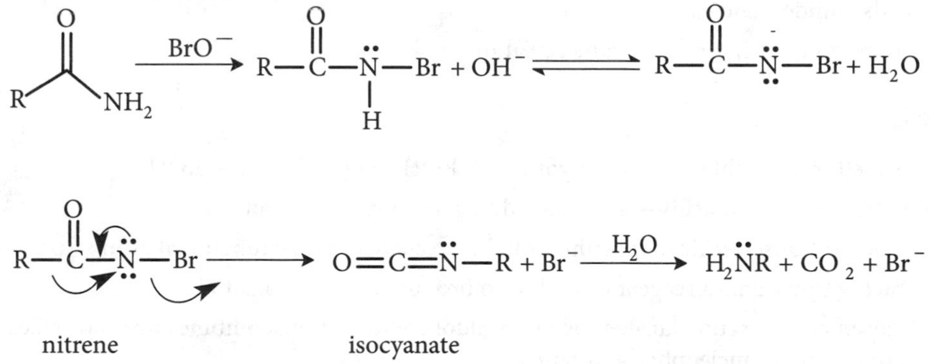

Figure 48.35

Reduction

Amides can be reduced with LAH to the corresponding amine. Notice that this differs from the product of the Hofmann rearrangement in that no carbon atom is lost. Note that, unlike with a carboxylic acid reduction with LAH, the oxygen atom is completely removed:

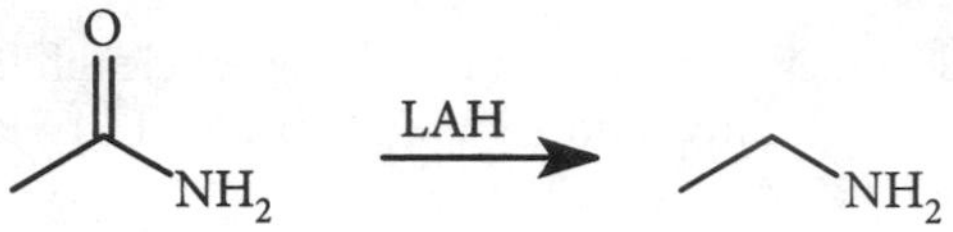

Figure 48.36

SUMMARY OF REACTIONS

- The most important derivatives of carboxylic acids are acyl halides, anhydrides, esters, and amides. These are listed in order from most reactive (least stable) to least reactive (most stable).

ACYL HALIDES:

- can be formed by adding $RCOOH + SOCl_2$, PCl_3 or PCl_5, or PBr_3
- undergo many different nucleophilic substitutions; H_2O yields carboxylic acid, while ROH yields an ester and NH_3 yields an amide
- can participate in Friedel-Crafts acylation to form an alkyl aryl ketone
- can be reduced to alcohols or, selectively, to aldehydes

ANHYDRIDES:

- can be formed by $RCOO^- + RCOCl$ (substitution) or by $RCOOH + RCOOH$ (condensation)
- undergo many nucleophilic substitution reactions, forming products that include carboxylic acids, amides, and esters
- can participate in Friedel-Crafts acylation

ESTERS:

- formed by acid chlorides or anhydrides + ROH or by $RCOOH + ROH$
- hydrolyze to yield acids + alcohols; adding ammonia yields an amide
- undergo transesterification with alcohol to exchange alkoxy functional group
- react with Grignard reagent (2 moles) to produce a tertiary alcohol
- Claisen condensation, analogous to the aldol condensation, combines two molecules of ester acting both as nucleophile and target
- very important in biological processes, particularly phosphate esters, which can be found in membranes, nucleic acids, and metabolic reactions

AMIDES:

- can be formed by acid chlorides + amines, acid anhydrides + ammonia, or ester + ammonia
- hydrolysis yields carboxylic acids or carboxylate anions
- can be transformed to primary amines via Hofmann rearrangement or reduction
- very important in formation of proteins because all amino acids are linked by amide bonds known as peptide bonds

REVIEW PROBLEMS

1. Name each of the following compounds according to the IUPAC system.

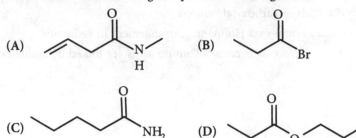

(A)   (B)

(C)   (D)

(E)

2. What would be the product of the following reaction?

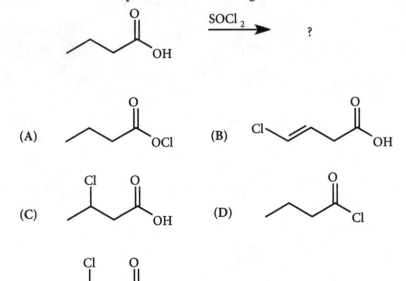

$$\xrightarrow{\text{SOCl}_2} \quad ?$$

(A)   (B)

(C)   (D)

(E)

3. During the hydrolysis of an acid chloride, pyridine (a base) is usually added to the reaction vessel. This is done because

   (A) the reaction leads to the production of hydroxide ions.
   (B) the acyl chloride is unreactive.
   (C) the hydrolysis reaction leads to the formation of HCl.
   (D) the pyridine reacts in a side-reaction with the carboxylic acid product.

4. What would be the primary product of the following reaction?

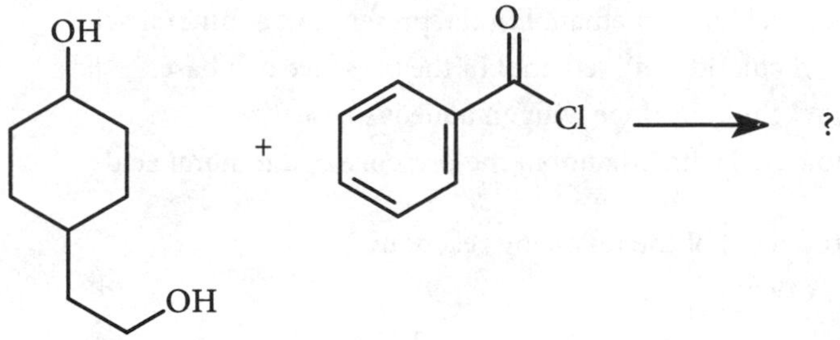

(A)

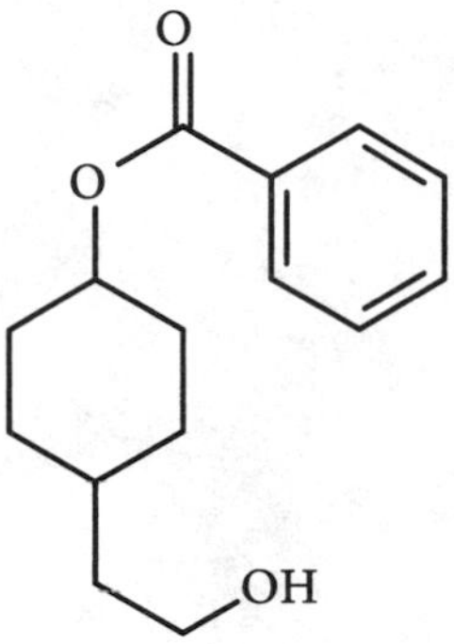

(B)

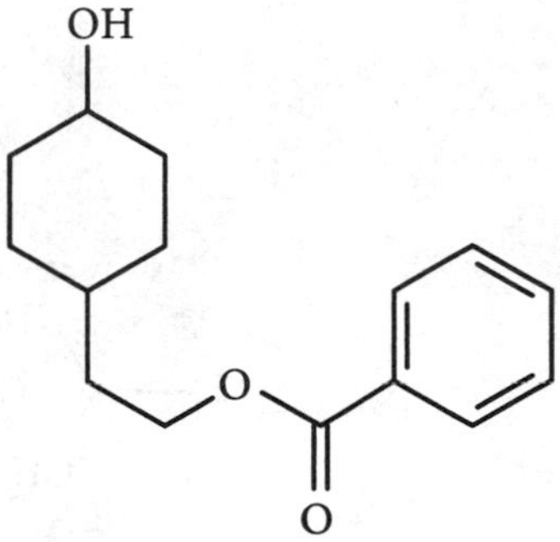

(C)

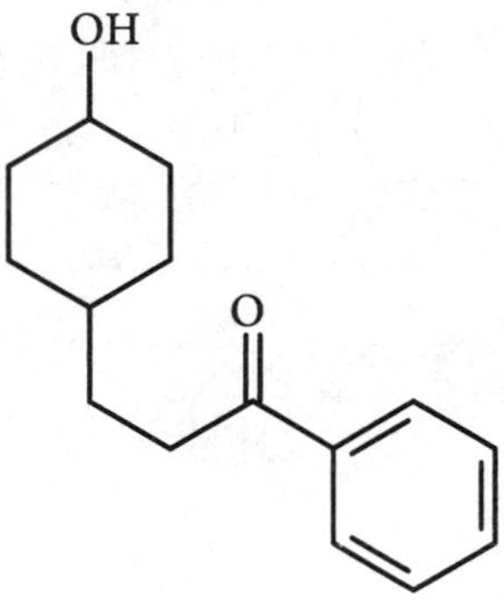

(D)

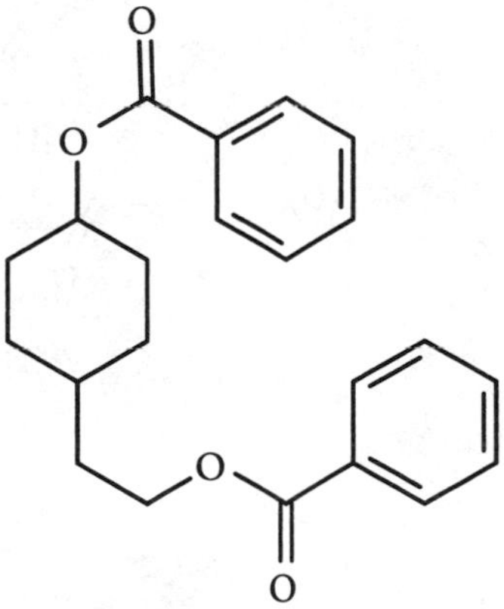

5. In order to produce a primary amide, an acid chloride should be treated with
    (A) ammonia.
    (B) an alcohol.
    (C) a primary amine.
    (D) a tertiary amine.

6. Which of the following would be the best method of producing methyl propanoate?

    (A) Reacting propanoic acid with methanol in the presence of a mineral acid
    (B) Reacting propanoyl chloride with ethanol in the presence of a base
    (C) Reacting propanoyl chloride alone with an aqueous base
    (D) Reacting propanoic acid with ethanol in the presence of a mineral acid

7. What would be the product(s) of the following reaction?

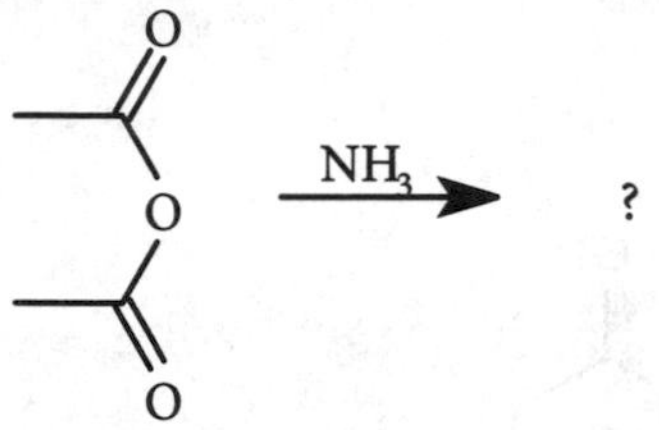

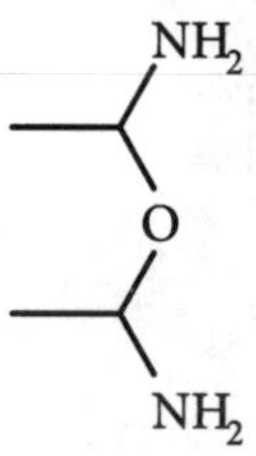

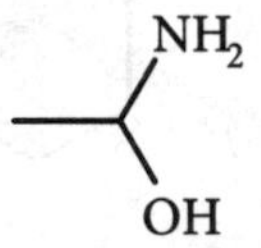

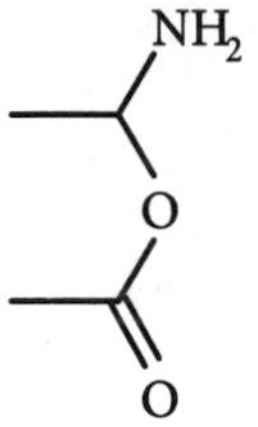

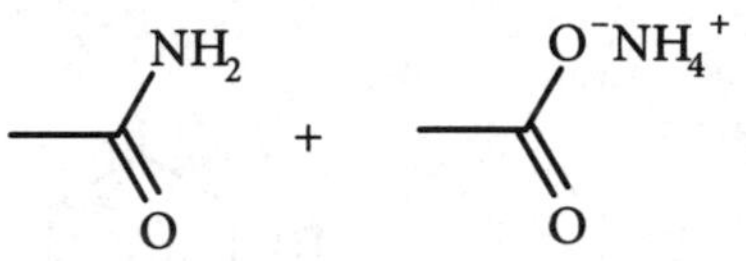

8. Which of the following correctly shows the intermediates and products of the reaction below?

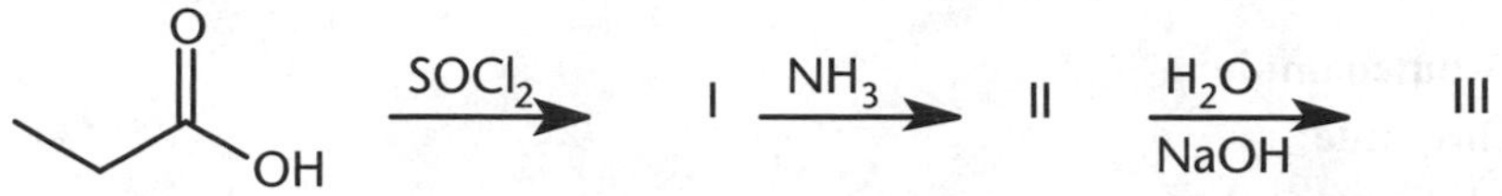

(A) 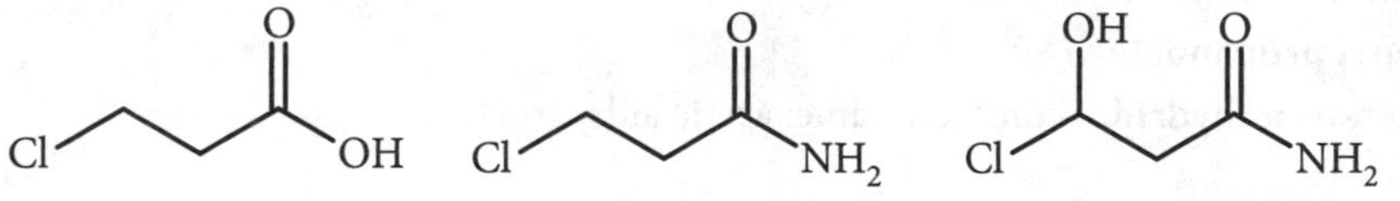

I II III

(B) 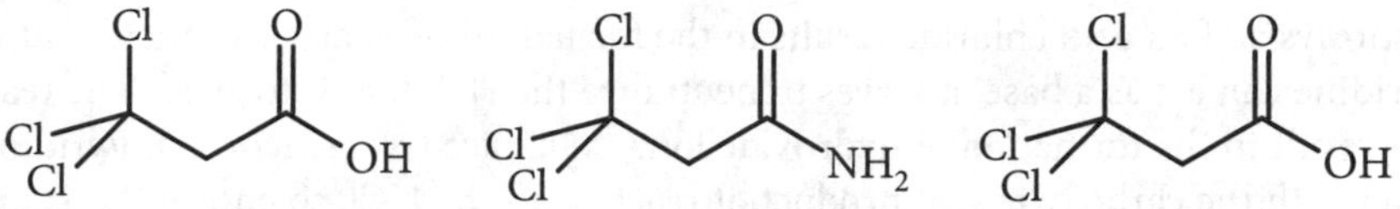

I II III

(C) 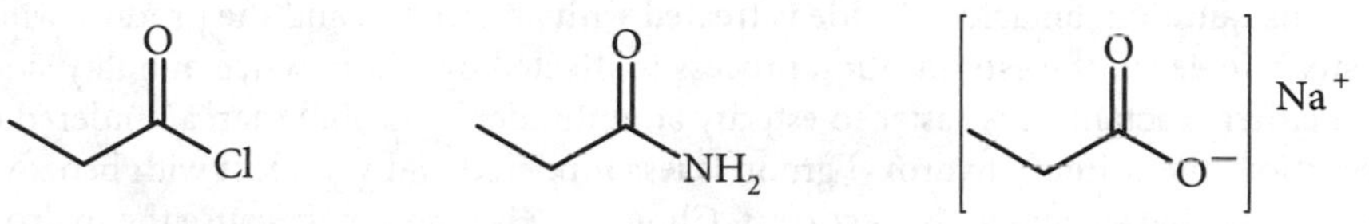

I II III

(D) 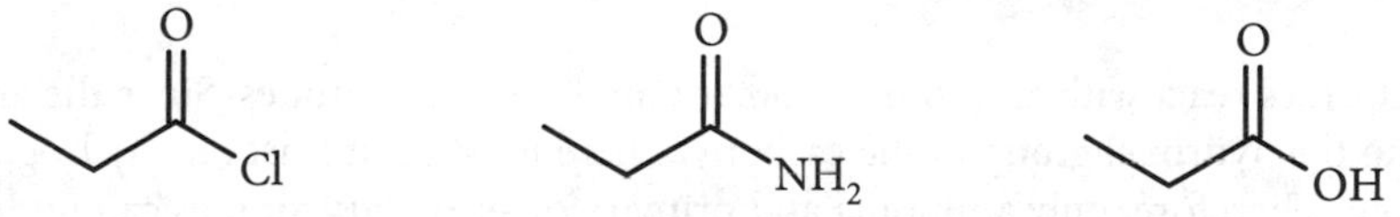

I II III

9. Prepare the following compounds from pentanoic acid. Give all reactants and reaction conditions.

(A) 1-Pentanol
(B) Pentanoyl bromide
(C) *N*-Methylpentanamide
(D) Ethyl pentanoate
(E) Pentanoic anhydride

10. What is saponification?

SOLUTIONS TO REVIEW PROBLEMS

1. **A** **N-methyl-3-butenamide**
   B **Propanoyl bromide**
   C **Pentanamide**
   D **Propyl propanoate**
   E **Ethanoic anhydride** (common name: acetic anhydride)

2. **D** Treating a carboxylic acid with thionyl chloride results in the production of an acyl chloride. In this reaction, butanoic acid is converted to butanoyl chloride, which is choice (D). Since none of the other choices are acyl chlorides, they can be eliminated.

3. **C** Hydrolysis of an acid chloride results in the formation of a carboxylic acid and HCl. Since pyridine can act as a base, it serves to neutralize the HCl that is formed. The reaction does not result in the formation of hydroxide ions, so choice (A) is incorrect. Pyridine does not react with the carboxylic acid product, it reacts with the HCl, so choice (D) is incorrect. Finally, choice (B) is incorrect because the acyl chloride is very reactive. The correct answer is choice (C).

4. **B** In this question, an acid chloride is treated with an alcohol, and the product will be an ester. However, the esterification process is affected by the presence of bulky side-chains on either reactant. It is easier to esterify an unhindered alcohol than a hindered one. In this reaction, the primary hydroxyl group is less hindered and will react with benzoyl chloride more rapidly, so choice (B) is correct. Choice (A) is incorrect because the hydroxyl group is a hindered secondary hydroxyl, and the reaction rate will be slower. Choice (C) is incorrect because it is not an ester. Choice (D) is incorrect because steric hindrance would prevent this product from being formed.

5. **A** Acid chlorides react with ammonia or other amines to form amides. Since the amine is replacing the hydroxyl group of the carbonyl, there must be at least one hydrogen on the amine. Therefore, only ammonia and primary or secondary amines can undergo this reaction. In order to obtain a primary amide, ammonia, choice (A), must be used. The reaction of an alcohol with an acid chloride produces an ester, so choice (B) is incorrect. A primary amine reacting with an acid chloride would give an *N*-substituted amide; thus, choice (C) is incorrect. Choice (D) is incorrect because tertiary amines will not react with acid chlorides.

6. **A** Methyl propanoate is an ester, which can be synthesized by reacting a carboxylic acid with an alcohol in the presence of acid: choice (A). Reacting ethanol with propanoyl chloride, choice (B), will also result in the formation of an ester, but because ethanol is used, ethyl propanoate will be formed, not methyl propanoate. This is also the case for choice (D), since ethanol is used here as well. Therefore, choices (B) and (D) are incorrect. Choice (C) is incorrect because propanoyl chloride will not form an ester in the presence of base alone. Therefore, choice (A) is the correct response.

7. **D** This question asks for the products when ammonia reacts with acetic anhydride. Recall from the text that an amide and an ammonium carboxylate will be formed. The only choice showing such a pair is (D), acetamide and ammonium acetate.

8. **C** This question gives a reaction scheme for the interconversion of propanoic acid to various derivatives, and asks what intermediate products are formed. The first reaction involves the formation of an acid chloride using thionyl chloride. Acid chlorides are made by replacing the hydroxyl group with chlorine. Thus, choices (A) and (B), which depict intact hydroxyl groups, can be eliminated. The second reaction is nucleophilic attack by ammonia on propanoyl chloride. The product should be propanamide, since ammonia will replace the chloride on the carbonyl carbon, which is correctly shown in both answer choices (C) and (D). The final reaction involves amide hydrolysis in the presence of base; therefore, the resulting carboxylic acid will exist in solution as a carboxylate salt. Thus, choice (C) is the correct answer, since it has sodium propanoate as the product of the third reaction.

9. This question asks about preparation of pentanoic acid derivatives. Where there is more than one way to make the products, the most efficient method will be given.

A **1-Pentanol**

Carboxylic acids are easily reduced by LAH to produce the corresponding primary alcohol.

B **Pentanoyl bromide**

To form pentanoyl bromide, pentanoic acid is reacted with PBr_3. The bromide replaces the hydroxyl on the carbonyl carbon.

C *N*-**Methylpentanamide**

N-Methylpentanamide can be prepared by first producing the acid chloride using thionyl chloride, and then reacting it with methylamine to yield the amide.

D **Ethyl pentanoate**

The ethyl ester of pentanoic acid can be formed by reacting it directly with ethanol in the presence of hydrochloric acid.

E **Pentanoic anhydride**

The most common method of preparing anhydrides is the reaction between an acid chloride and a carboxylate anion. To form pentanoic anhydride, one mole of pentanoic acid must be treated with thionyl chloride to yield pentanoyl chloride. This reacts with one mole of sodium pentanoate to form pentanoic anhydride.

10. Saponification is the process whereby fats are hydrolyzed under basic conditions to produce soaps.

CHAPTER FORTY-NINE

Amines

Amines are nitrogen-containing compounds of the general formula NR_3, with R representing either hydrogens, alkyl groups, or a combination of both. One of the most important features of amines is the lone pair of electrons on the nitrogen, which determines many of the chemical and physical properties of these compounds. Other nitrogen-containing compounds are similar to amines, including those with double or triple bonds between a carbon and a nitrogen (imines and nitriles), compounds with two or three nitrogens (diazides and azides), and compounds with both nitrogen and oxygen (amides, isocyanates, and nitrates).

Amines have a great deal of biological significance since they are part of amino acids, nucleic acids, and many other biomolecules (discussed in Chapters 51 and 52). They are also are important in medicine. Many nitrogen-containing compounds act as relaxants, including nitroglycerin and nitrous oxide. Nitroglycerin is given either sublingually or transdermally to relieve coronary artery spasms and angina (chest pain). Nitrous oxide is also known as laughing gas and is used as a dental anesthetic. Nitroglycerin and trinitrotoluene also have nonmedical significance as explosives due to their high reactivities.

NOMENCLATURE OF AMINES

Amines are classified according to the number of alkyl (or aryl) groups to which the nitrogen is bound. A **primary** (1°) amine is attached to one alkyl group and can be written as RNH_2; a **secondary** (2°) amine is bound to two alkyl groups and can be written as R_2NH; and a **tertiary** (3°) amine is bound to three alkyl groups and is written as R_3N. A nitrogen atom attached to four alkyl groups is called a **quaternary ammonium compound** and is written as R_4N^+; the nitrogen carries a positive charge, and these compounds generally exist as salts.

In the common naming system, amines are generally named as alkylamines. The groups are designated individually or by using the prefixes di- or tri- if they are the same. In the IUPAC system, amines are named by substituting the suffix -**amine** for the final -*e* of the name of the alkane to which the nitrogen is attached. *N* is used to label substituents attached to the nitrogen in secondary or tertiary amines. The prefix **amino**- is used for naming compounds containing a higher priority OH or a CO_2H group. Aromatic amines are named as derivatives of aniline ($C_6H_5NH_2$), the IUPAC name for which is benzenamine. Table 49.1 gives three examples of compounds named by both the common and IUPAC system:

Formula:	$CH_3CH_2NH_2$	$CH_3CH_2N(CH_3)_2$	$H_2NCH_2CH_2OH$
IUPAC:	Ethanamine	*N,N*-Dimethylethanamine	2-Aminoethanol
Common:	Ethylamine	Dimethylethylamine	2-Aminoethanol

Table 49.1

Many other nitrogen-containing organic compounds are listed in Table 49.2 with their key characteristics, and Figure 49.1 gives several example structures.

Class of compound	Characteristics
Amides	$RCONR_2$
	Discussed in Chapter 48, Carboxylic Acid Derivatives
Carbamates (urethanes)	$RNHC(O)OR'$
	Form polymers called **polyurethanes**
	Derived from isocyanates + alcohol
Isocyanates	RNCO
	Combine with alcohols to create carbamates
Enamines	$C=CH-NR_2$
	Analogous to enols
Imines	$C=NR$
Nitriles (Cyanides)	$C\equiv N$
	Named as either cyano- or -nitrile
Nitro compounds	$-NO_2$
Diazo compounds	$-N_2$
	Lose N_2 to form carbenes $R-(C:)-R'$ or $R=C:$
Azides	$-N_3$
	Readily lose N_2 to form nitrenes
Nitrenes	R-N:
	Nitrogen analog of carbenes
	Formed from azides upon loss of N_2
	Highly unstable; usually a reaction intermediate

Table 49.2

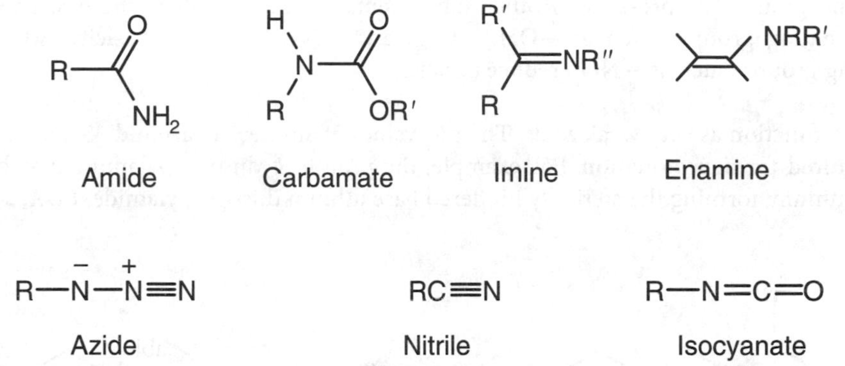

Figure 49.1

PROPERTIES OF AMINES

The boiling points of amines are between those of alkanes and alcohols. For example, methylamine (CH_3NH_2, MW = 31 g/mol) boils at $-6°C$, whereas ethane (CH_3CH_3, MW = 30 g/mol) boils at $-89°C$ and methanol (CH_3OH, MW = 32 g/mol) boils at 64.5°C. Ammonia and primary and secondary amines can form hydrogen bonds, while tertiary amines cannot; therefore, tertiary amines have lower boiling points. Since nitrogen is not as electronegative as oxygen, the hydrogen bonds of amines are not as strong as those of alcohols.

The nitrogen atom in an amine is approximately sp^3 hybridized. Nitrogen bonds to only three substituents in order to complete its octet; a lone pair occupies the last sp^3 orbital. This lone pair is very important to the chemistry of amines; it is associated with their basic and nucleophilic properties.

Nitrogen atoms bonded to three different substituents are chiral because of the geometry of the orbitals. However, these enantiomers cannot be isolated, because they interconvert rapidly in a process called **nitrogen inversion**: an inversion of the sp^3 orbital occupied by the lone pair. The activation energy for this process is only 6 kcal/mol, and only at very low temperatures is it significantly slowed or stopped.

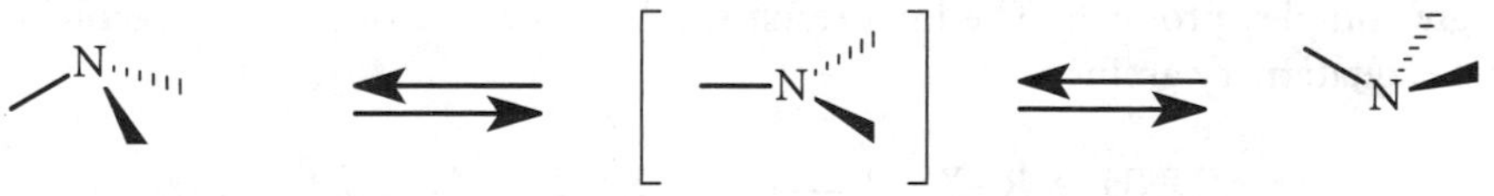

Figure 49.2

Amines are Brønsted-Lowry bases and readily accept protons to form ammonium ions; they are also classified as Lewis bases because of their ability to donate electrons (for a review of acids and bases, see Chapter 37). The pK_b values of alkyl amines are around 4, making them slightly more basic than ammonia ($pK_b = 4.76$). Aromatic amines such as aniline ($pK_b = 9.42$) are far less basic than aliphatic amines, because the electron-withdrawing effect of the ring reduces the electron-donating ability of the amino group. The presence of other substituents on the ring alters the basicity of anilines: electron-donating groups (such as $-OH$, $-CH_3$, and $-NH_2$) increase basicity, while electron-withdrawing groups (such as $-NO_2$) reduce basicity.

Amines also function as very weak acids. The pK_a values of amines are around 35, and a very strong base is required for deprotonation. For example, the proton of diisopropylamine may be removed with butyllithium, forming the sterically hindered base lithium diisopropylamide, LDA.

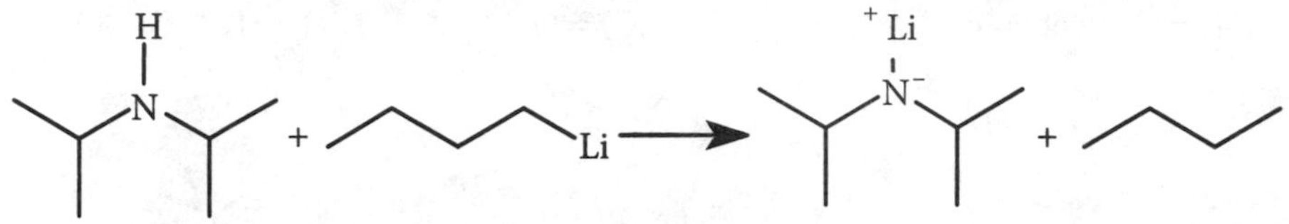

Figure 49.3

SYNTHESIS OF AMINES

Alkylation of Ammonia

Direct alkylation

Alkyl halides react with ammonia to produce alkylammonium halide salts. Ammonia functions as a nucleophile and displaces the halide atom. When the salt is treated with base, the alkylamine product is formed.

$$CH_3Br + NH_3 \longrightarrow CH_3\overset{+}{N}H_3Br^- \xrightarrow{NaOH} CH_3NH_2 + NaBr + H_2O$$

Figure 49.4

This reaction often leads to side products, because the alkylamine formed is more nucleophilic than ammonia. The alkylamine product therefore reacts with the alkyl halide faster than ammonia, leading to increasingly complex products. The final result will be a mixture of primary, secondary, tertiary and sometimes quaternary amines:

$$NH_3 + R-X \longrightarrow RNH_2 \ (1°)$$
$$RNH_2 + R-X \longrightarrow R_2NH \ (2°)$$
$$R_2NH + R-X \longrightarrow R_3N \ (3°)$$
$$R_3N + R-X \longrightarrow R_4N^+ \ (4°)$$

Gabriel synthesis

The preferred method for synthesizing amines is the **Gabriel synthesis.** This pathway converts a primary alkyl halide to a primary amine without the uncontrolled additional reactions seen in the direct alkylation of amines. The first step is the creation of phthalimide, a nitrogen source based on ammonia, but with more controlled reactivity:

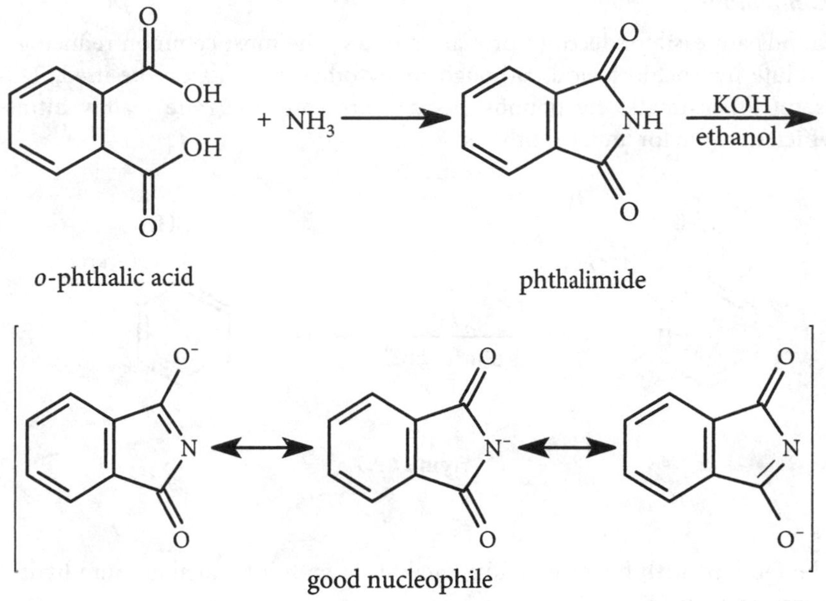

o-phthalic acid   phthalimide

good nucleophile

Figure 49.5

Phthalimide, the condensation product of phthalic acid and ammonia, acts as a good nucleophile when deprotonated. It displaces halide ions, forming *N*-alkylphthalimides, which do not further react with other alkyl halides. When the reaction is complete, the *N*-alkylphthalimide can be hydrolyzed with aqueous base to produce the alkylamine.

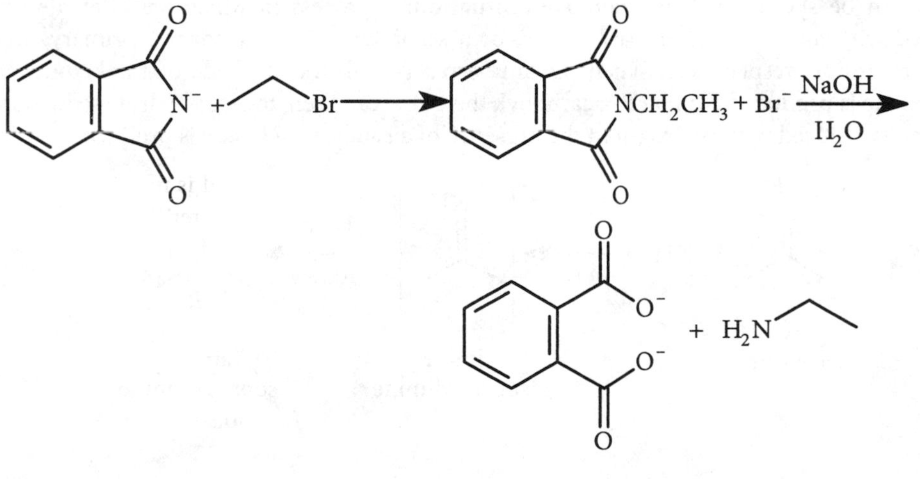

Figure 49.6

Reduction

Amines can be obtained from other nitrogen-containing functionalities through reduction reactions using typical reducing agents.

From nitro compounds

Nitro compounds are easily reduced to primary amines. The most common reducing agent is iron or zinc and dilute hydrochloric acid, although many other reagents can be used. This reaction is especially useful for aromatic compounds, because aromatic rings are readily nitrated and thus provide an efficient route for amine synthesis.

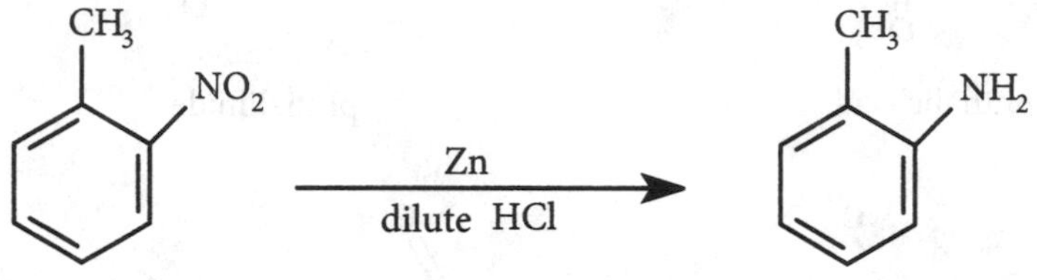

Figure 49.7

From nitriles

Nitriles can be reduced with hydrogen and a catalyst, or with lithium aluminum hydride (LAH), to produce primary amines.

$$CH_3CH_2C\equiv N \xrightarrow{\text{LAH}} CH_3CH_2CH_2NH_2$$

Figure 49.8

From imines

Amines can be synthesized by **reductive amination**: a process in which an aldehyde or ketone is reacted with ammonia, a primary amine, or a secondary amine to form a primary, secondary, or tertiary amine, respectively. When the amine reacts with the aldehyde or the ketone, an imine intermediate is produced. Similar to a carbonyl, the imine can then undergo hydride reduction. When the imine is reduced with hydrogen in the presence of a catalyst, an amine is produced.

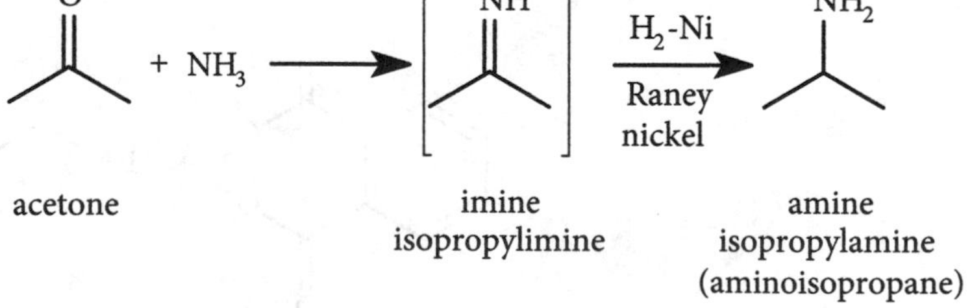

acetone   imine   amine
                 isopropylimine   isopropylamine
                                     (aminoisopropane)

Figure 49.9

From amides

Amides can be reduced with LAH to form amines (see Chapter 48, Carboxylic Acid Derivatives, to review amides).

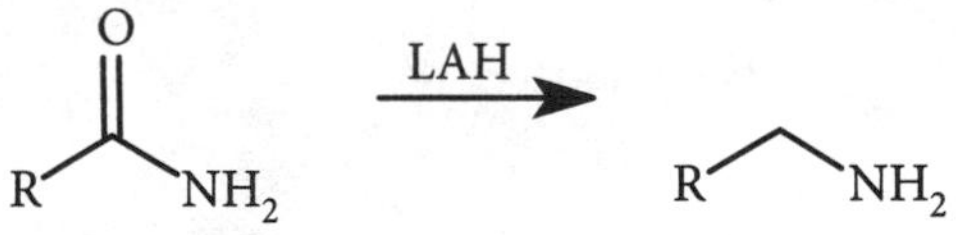

Figure 49.10

REACTIONS OF AMINES

Exhaustive Methylation

Exhaustive methylation is also known as **Hofmann elimination**. In this process, an amine is converted to a quaternary ammonium iodide salt by reacting with excess methyl iodide. Treatment with silver oxide and water converts this to the ammonium hydroxide, which, when heated, undergoes elimination to form an alkene and an amine. The predominant alkene formed is the least substituted, in contrast with normal elimination reactions, where the predominant alkene product is the most substituted.

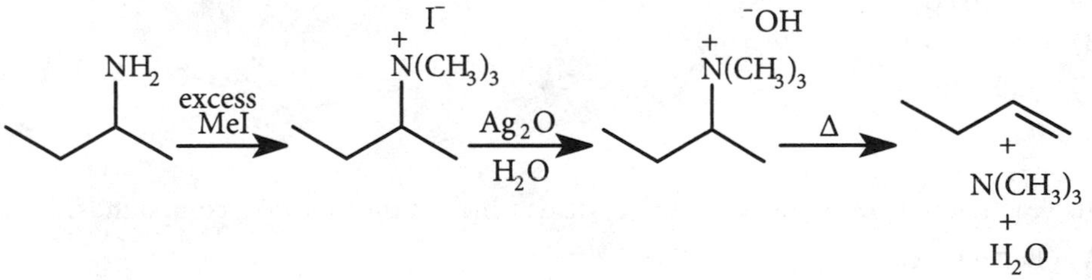

Figure 49.11

REVIEW PROBLEMS

1. A compound with the general formula $R_4N^+X^-$ is classified as a
   - **(A)** secondary amine.
   - **(B)** quaternary ammonium salt.
   - **(C)** tertiary amine.
   - **(D)** primary amine.

2. A compound with the structural formula $C_6H_5N^-N^+\equiv N$ is called
   - **(A)** a urethane.
   - **(B)** a diazo compound.
   - **(C)** an azide.
   - **(D)** a nitrile.

3. Amines have lower boiling points than the corresponding alcohols because
   - **(A)** amines have higher molecular masses.
   - **(B)** amines form much stronger hydrogen bonds.
   - **(C)** amines form weaker hydrogen bonds.
   - **(D)** amines are less dense.

4. Which of the following would be formed if methyl bromide was reacted with phthalimide and then hydrolyzed with aqueous base?
   - **(A)** $C_2H_5NH_2$
   - **(B)** CH_3NH_2
   - **(C)** $(C_2H_5)_3N$
   - **(D)** $(CH_3)_4N^+Br^-$

5. The reaction of benzamide with $LiAlH_4$ yields which of the following compounds?
   - **(A)** Benzoic acid
   - **(B)** Benzonitrile
   - **(C)** Benzylamine
   - **(D)** Ammonium benzoate

6. Suggest a method of converting $RCOOH$ to RNH_2.

7. Which of the following amines has the highest boiling point?
   - **(A)** CH_3NH_2
   - **(B)** $CH_3(CH_2)_6NH_2$
   - **(C)** $CH_3(CH_2)_3NH_2$
   - **(D)** $(CH_3)_3CNH_2$

8. If 2-amino-3-methylbutane were treated with excess methyl iodide, silver oxide, and water, what would be the major reaction products?

    (A) Ammonia and 2-methyl-2-butene

    (B) Trimethylamine and 3-methyl-1-butene

    (C) Trimethylamine and 2-methyl-2-butene

    (D) Ammonia and 3-methyl-1-butene

9. Nylon, a polyamide, is produced from hexanediamine and a substance X. This substance X is most probably

    (A) an amine.

    (B) a carboxylic acid.

    (C) a nitrile.

    (D) an alcohol.

10. A researcher wants to prepare a primary amine (RNH_2). He uses an alkyl halide (RX) and ammonia to produce an alkyl ammonium halide salt ($RNH_3^+X^-$), which he then treats with sodium hydroxide to produce the primary amine. He finds that the product is always contaminated with a secondary amine (R_2NH) and a tertiary amine (R_3N). What has he done wrong and how can he produce only the primary amine he desires?

SOLUTIONS TO REVIEW PROBLEMS

1. **B** A quaternary ammonium salt has four substituents attached to the nitrogen, resulting in a positive charge on this atom. As a result, this compound forms a salt, where X^- is usually a halide. Primary amines have the general formula RNH_2, secondary amines have the general formula R_2NH, and tertiary amines have the general formula R_3N. Therefore, choices (A), (C), and (D) are incorrect.

2. **C** This is an azide, which is unstable and readily loses nitrogen to yield a nitrene. A urethane, choice (A), has the formula RNHCOOR'. A diazo compound, choice (B), has the formula $R-N\equiv N$. A nitrile, choice (D), also called a *cyanide*, has the formula $R-C\equiv N$.

3. **C** Amines form weaker hydrogen bonds than alcohols, since nitrogen has a lower electronegativity than oxygen. The molecules are not held together as tightly and are therefore more volatile.

4. **B** The reaction between methyl bromide and phthalimide results in the formation of methyl phthalimide. Subsequent hydrolysis then yields methylamine, so answer choice (B) is the correct response. Therefore, the overall reaction is the conversion of a primary alkyl halide into a primary amine. Choice (A) is incorrect because this contains an ethyl group, not a methyl group. In order to form this compound, the initial reactant should be ethyl bromide. Choices (C) and (D) are incorrect as these are tertiary and quaternary nitrogen compounds, respectively, and the reaction only converts primary alkyl halides into primary amines.

5. **C** Lithium aluminum hydride is a good reducing agent and is used to reduce amides to amines. Reduction of benzamide will result in the formation of benzylamine, choice (C). Hydrolysis of benzamide would result in the formation of benzoic acid, so choice (A) is incorrect. Benzonitrile would be formed by the dehydration of amides, so choice (B) is also incorrect. To form ammonium benzoate, choice (D), benzamide would first have to be hydrolyzed and then reacted with ammonia, so this answer choice is also incorrect.

6. One method is transformation of the carboxylic acid to an acid chloride, followed by reaction with ammonia and then reduction with LAH (see Chapter 48, Carboxylic Acid Derivatives).

Another approach is the Curtius rearrangement:

1. $R-C(=O)-OH \xrightarrow{\text{SOCl}_2} R-C(=O)-Cl$

2. $R-C(=O)-Cl \xrightarrow{\text{NaN}_3} R-C(=O)-N-\overset{+}{N}\equiv N \xrightarrow{-\text{N}_2} O=C=N-R$

   Curtius rearrangement

3. $O=C=N-R \xrightarrow[-\text{CO}_2]{\text{H}_2\text{O}} H-N(-H)-R$

7. B As the molecular masses of comparable amines having the same degree of substitution increase, so do their boiling points. Of the choices given, choice (B), heptylamine, has the highest molecular mass (115 g/mol) and therefore the highest boiling point, 142−144°C. Choice (A), methylamine, has a mass of 31 g/mol and a boiling point of −6.3°C. Butylamine, choice (C), has a boiling point of 77.5°C, and *t*-butylamine, choice (D), has a boiling point of 44.4°C. Butylamine and *t*-butylamine have the same mass (73 g/mol), demonstrating the effect branching has on decreasing the boiling point.

8. B Treatment of an amine with excess methyl iodide, silver oxide, and water is called exhaustive methylation or Hofmann elimination. The products formed are a trisubstituted amine and an alkene. Since 2-amino-3-methylbutane is a primary amine, it will take up three methyl groups; the trisubstituted amine produced will be trimethylamine. The predominant alkene product will be the least substituted alkene, because removal of a secondary hydrogen is sterically hindered. Therefore, this reaction will produce 3-methyl-1-butene, plus trimethylamine, choice (B). Choices (A) and (D) are incorrect; ammonia cannot be a product of this reaction since the mechanism involves the addition of methyl groups. Choice (C) is incorrect because 2-methyl-2-butene, the more substituted alkene, would not be the predominant product.

9. B An amide is formed from an amine and a carboxyl group or its acyl derivatives. In this question, an amine is already given; the compound to be identified must be an acyl compound. The only acyl compound among the choices given is a carboxylic acid, choice (B).

10. The researcher gets a contaminated product because he is using a direct alkylation process, which does not stop cleanly after the first alkylation. The primary amine produced by direct alkylation is an excellent nucleophile and will react with other alkyl halides to produce secondary and tertiary amines.

$$NH_3 + R-X \longrightarrow RNH_2 \quad (1°)$$
$$RNH_2 + R-X \longrightarrow R_2NH \quad (2°)$$
$$R_2NH + R-X \longrightarrow R_3N \quad (3°)$$

Instead he should use the Gabriel synthesis, which converts an alkyl halide to a primary amine without unwanted side products. In this reaction, an imide, not ammonia, is used as the nucleophile. The product is an *N*-alkylimide, which cannot react further with alkyl halides. After the reaction is complete, the *N*-alkylimide is hydrolyzed with base to produce the primary alkylamine.

CHAPTER FIFTY

Spectroscopy

When an organic compound has been synthesized or separated from a mixture, it often must be characterized and identified. **Spectroscopy** is the process of measuring the frequencies of electromagnetic radiation (light) absorbed by a molecule. The frequencies of light that are absorbed are related to the energy levels of the molecule and different types of motion, including rotation, vibration of bonds, and electron movement. Different types of spectroscopy measure these different types of motion, allowing identification of specific functional groups and how they are connected within a molecule.

INFRARED SPECTROSCOPY

Basic Theory

Infrared (IR) spectroscopy measures molecular vibrations. The infrared spectrum of a sample is determined by passing light through the sample and recording the frequencies at which light is absorbed. These absorption frequencies correspond to the vibrations of the molecule, including **stretching, bending,** and **rotation.** The useful absorptions of infrared light occur in the frequency range from $400–4,000$ cm^{-1} (called **wavenumbers**). The wavenumber of the absorption is related to specific functional groups in a molecule, and can be used to identify these functional groups.

Bond stretching is observed in the region of $1,500–4,000$ cm^{-1}. Bending vibrations are observed in the region of $400–1,500$ cm^{-1}. Four different types of vibration that can occur are shown in Figure 50.1.

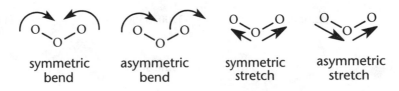

| symmetric bend | asymmetric bend | symmetric stretch | asymmetric stretch |

Figure 50.1

In addition to bending and stretching vibrations, more complex vibrations may occur. These can be combinations of bending, stretching, rotation, or motion of the whole molecule. Absorptions of these types are seen in the region of 400−1,500 cm^{-1}, known as the **fingerprint region**, which is unique to a molecule.

In order for IR light to be absorbed, the vibration of the molecule must result in a change in a bond dipole moment. Symmetrical molecules do not have a dipole moment and therefore do not absorb IR light. For example, O_2 and Br_2 do not absorb IR light, but HCl and CO do. The more complicated a molecule, the more peaks observed in its IR spectrum.

Characteristic IR Absorptions

Specific functional groups absorb at well-defined frequencies. For example, carbon-carbon single bonds absorb at around 1,200 cm^{-1}, double bonds around 1,600 cm^{-1}, and triple bonds around 2,200 cm^{-1}. Table 50.1 lists the specific absorptions of key functional groups and the vibrations that occur at those frequencies.

Functional Group	Frequency (cm^{-1})	Vibration
Alkanes	2800–3000	C—H
	1200	C—C
Alkenes	3080–3140	=C—H
	1645	C=C
Alkynes	2200	C≡C
	3300	≡C—H
Aromatic	2900–3100	C—H
	1475–1625	C—C
Alcohols	3100–3500	O—H (broad)
Ethers	1050–1150	C—O
Aldehydes	2700–2900	(O)C—H
	1725–1750	C=O
Ketones	1700–1750	C=O
Acids	1700–1750	C=O
	2900–3300	O—H (broad)
Amines	3100–3500	N—H (sharp)

Table 50.1

Some of the most useful information in an IR spectrum can often be quickly and easily determined by reviewing two key areas of absorption—from 1,700–1,750 and 3,100–3,500 cm⁻¹—to determine the presence of oxygen and nitrogen functional groups:

Functional Group	1,700–1,750 cm⁻¹	3,100–3,500 cm⁻¹
Alcohol	No	Broad peak
Aldehyde or Ketone	Yes	No
Carboxylic Acid	Yes	Broad peak
Amine	No	Sharp peak

Table 50.2

Application

A great deal of information can be obtained from an IR spectrum. Percent transmission, the inverse of absorbance, is plotted versus frequency; this gives areas of absorption the appearance of valleys on the spectrum.

Figure 50.2 shows the IR spectrum of an aliphatic alcohol. The broad peak at 3,300 cm⁻¹ is due to the hydroxyl group, while the peak at 3,000 cm⁻¹ is created by the large number of C—H bonds in the molecule.

Frequency (cm⁻¹)

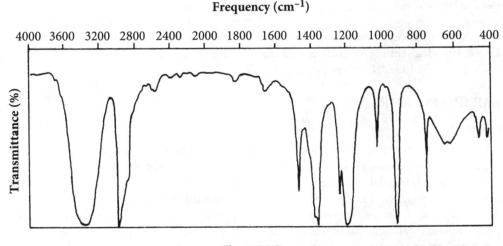

Figure 50.2

Summary of IR Spectroscopy

1. IR spectroscopy is based on the vibrations of molecules, including bending and stretching.

2. IR absorption is measured in the frequency range of 400–4,000 cm⁻¹, and is plotted as transmittance vs. wave number, with absorption appearing as "valleys" in the spectrum.

3. Different functional groups show IR absorption at different wave numbers. Some of the most useful absorption ranges to note are at 1,700 cm⁻¹ (C=O bond) and at 3,100–3,500 cm⁻¹ (O–H if broad, N–H if narrow). However, other absorption frequencies can also be important.

NUCLEAR MAGNETIC RESONANCE

Basic Theory

Nuclear magnetic resonance (NMR) spectroscopy is one of the most widely used spectroscopic tools in organic chemistry. Certain nuclei have magnetic moments that are normally oriented at random. When such nuclei are placed in a magnetic field, their magnetic moments tend to align either with or against the direction of the field. Nuclei whose magnetic moments are aligned with the field are said to be in the **α-state** (lower energy), while those whose moments are aligned against the field are said to be in the **β-state** (higher energy).

If the nuclei are then exposed to electromagnetic radiation, some in the lower energy α-state will be excited into the β-state; this transition is known as **resonating.** The absorption corresponding to this excitation occurs at different frequencies depending on the atom's environment. Other nearby atoms in the same molecule (or sometimes in the solvent) can shift the frequency at which an atom transitions between the α- and β-states. A compound may contain many nuclei that resonate at different frequencies, producing a very complex spectrum.

Since different NMR spectrometers operate at different magnetic field strengths, a standardized method of plotting the NMR spectrum has been adopted. A variable called **chemical shift**, represented by the symbol δ and with units of **parts per million** (**ppm**), is plotted on the *x*-axis. Chemical shift is compared to the standard organic molecule tetramethylsilane (TMS). TMS is always shown by a peak at 0 ppm, and the peaks of interest always appear to the left of TMS. A peak further to the left is said to be **shifted downfield**.

NMR is most commonly used to study ^1H nuclei (protons) and ^{13}C nuclei, although any atom possessing a nuclear spin (any nucleus with an odd atomic number or odd mass number) can be studied, such as ^{19}F, ^{17}O, ^{14}N, ^{15}N, or ^{31}P.

^1H NMR (Proton NMR)

Peak location

Most ^1H nuclei come into resonance between 0 and 10 δ downfield from TMS. Each distinct set of nuclei gives rise to a separate peak. The compound dichloromethyl methyl ether ($Cl_2HC-O-CH_3$) has two distinct sets of ^1H nuclei. The single proton attached to the dichloromethyl group is in a different magnetic environment compared to the three protons on the methyl group, and the two types of protons resonate at different frequencies. The three protons on the methyl group are magnetically equivalent, due to rotation about the oxygen-carbon single bond, and resonate at the same frequency. Thus, two separate peaks are seen, as shown in Figure 50.3.

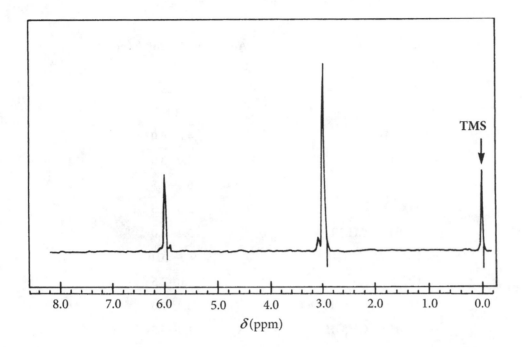

Figure 50.3

The peak at 6 ppm corresponds to the single dichloromethyl proton and the peak at 3 ppm to the three methyl protons. The size of the peaks is also significant; if the areas under the peaks are integrated, the ratio between them is 3:1, corresponding to the number of protons producing each peak. This can be roughly approximated as the relative heights of the peaks when quickly evaluating an NMR spectrum.

The single proton comes into resonance downfield from (to the left of) the methyl protons. This shift downfield is due to the electron-withdrawing effect of the chlorine atoms. The electron cloud that surrounds the ^1H nucleus ordinarily screens the nucleus from the magnetic field. The chlorine atoms pull the electron cloud away and **deshield** the nucleus, moving its resonance to the left. Conversely, electron-donating atoms **shield** the ^1H nuclei, causing them to appear further to the right. Different bonds also have different affinities for electrons. As a result, different functional groups can deshield protons in predictable ways, as shown in Table 50.3:

Type of Proton	Approximate Shift δ (ppm)
RCH_3	0.9
R_2CH_2	1.25
R_3CH	1.5
$-CH=CH$	4.6–6.0
$-C\equiv CH$	2.0–3.0
$Ar-H$	6.0–8.5
$-CHX$	2.0–4.5
$-CHOH / -CHOR$	3.4–4.0
$RCHO$	9.0–10.0
$RCHCO-$	2.0–2.5
$-CHCOOH / -CHCOOR$	2.0–2.6
$-CHOH / -CH_2OH$	1.0–5.5
$ArOH$	4.0–12
$-COOH$	10.5–12.0
$-NH_2$	1.0–5.0

Table 50.3

Peak splitting

If two magnetically different protons are within three bonds of each other, a phenomenon known as **coupling** or **splitting** occurs. Consider two protons, H_a and H_b, on the molecule 1,1-dibromo-2,2-dichloroethane (Figure 50.4).

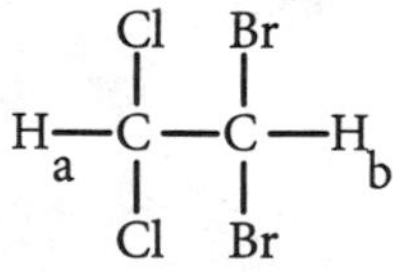

Figure 50.4

At any given time, H_a can experience two different magnetic environments, since H_b can be in either the α or the β state. These different states of H_b influence nucleus H_a, causing slight upfield and downfield shifts. Since there is a 50 percent chance that H_b will be in either state, this results in a **doublet**, two peaks of equal intensity equally spaced around the true chemical shift of H_a. H_b experiences the two different states of H_a and is likewise split into a doublet. In 1,1-dibromo-2-chloroethane (Figure 50.5), the H_a nucleus is affected by two nearby H_b nuclei, which, taken together, can be in four different states: αα, αβ, βα, or ββ.

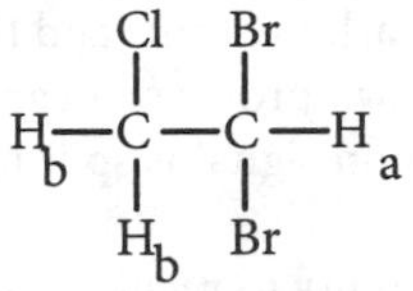

$$
\begin{array}{ccc}
& \text{Cl} & \text{Br} \\
& | & | \\
\text{H}_b\!-\!\!&\text{C}\!-\!\text{C}&\!\!-\!\text{H}_a \\
& | & | \\
& \text{H}_b & \text{Br}
\end{array}
$$

Figure 50.5

The αβ and βα states have the same net effect on the H_a nucleus, and the resonances occur at the same frequency. The αα and ββ states resonate at frequencies different from each other and from the αβ / βα frequency. The result is three peaks centered around the true chemical shift, with an area ratio of 1:2:1. The number of peaks that will appear when splitting occurs can be determined as follows: *n* hydrogen atoms couple to give *n* + 1 peaks, whose area ratios are given by Pascal's triangle, shown in Table 50.4.

Number of Adjacent Hydrogens	Total Number of Peaks	Area Ratios
0	1	1
1	2	1:1
2	3	1:2:1
3	4	1:3:3:1
4	5	1:4:6:4:1
5	6	1:5:10:10:5:1
6	7	1:6:15:20:15:6:1
7	8	1:7:21:35:35:21:7:1

Table 50.4

Summary of ¹H NMR Spectroscopy

1. NMR spectroscopy is based on the magnetic moment of nuclei, which resonate between two states.

2. Each peak in an NMR spectrum represents a single proton or a group of equivalent protons. The size of each peak represents the number of equivalent protons in a group.

3. The position of the peak (distance downfield, or to the left) is determined by the shielding or deshielding effects of other functional groups nearby.

4. The splitting of a peak is determined by the number of adjacent protons *n*, and the number of peaks is given by *n* + 1.

¹³C NMR (Carbon NMR)

¹³C NMR is very similar to ¹H NMR. Most ¹³C NMR signals, however, occur $0-200$ δ downfield from the carbon peak of TMS, so a spectrum for ¹³C NMR is easily recognized by the larger scale of the *x*-axis. Another significant difference is that only 1.1 percent of carbon atoms are ¹³C atoms. This has two effects: First, a much larger sample is needed to run a ¹³C spectrum (about 50 mg compared with 1 mg for ¹H NMR), and second, coupling between carbon atoms is generally not observed.

Coupling *is* observed, however, between carbon atoms and the protons directly attached to them. For example, if a carbon atom is attached to two protons, it can experience four different states of those protons ($\alpha\alpha$, $\alpha\beta$, $\beta\alpha$, and $\beta\beta$), and the carbon signal is split into a triplet with the area ratio 1:2:1.

An additional feature of ^{13}C NMR is the ability to record a spectrum *without* the coupling of adjacent protons. This is called **spin decoupling**, and produces a spectrum of **singlets**, each corresponding to a separate magnetically equivalent carbon atom. For example, compare the following two spectra, both of 1,1,2-trichloropropane. One (Figure 50.6) is a typical **spin-decoupled spectrum**, and the other (Figure 50.7) is spin-coupled.

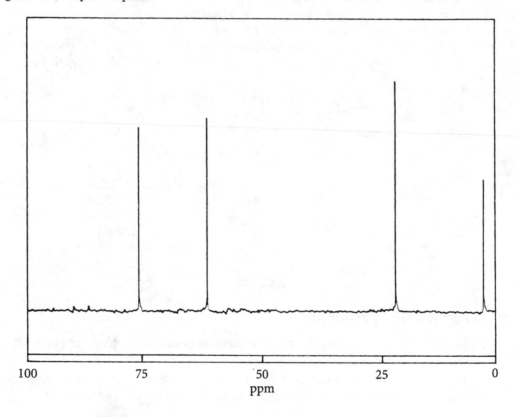

Figure 50.6

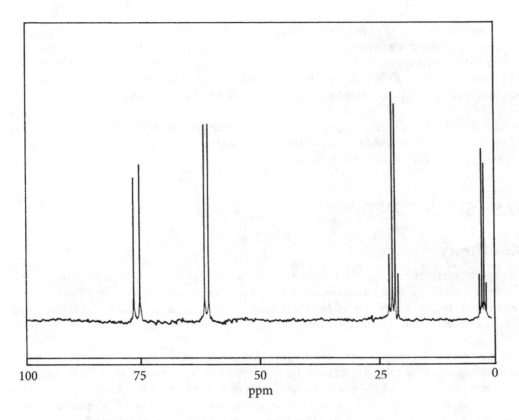

Figure 50.7

Summary of ¹H and ¹³C NMR Spectroscopy

In general, NMR spectroscopy provides information about the carbon and hydrogen skeleton of a molecule along with some suggestion of its functional groups. Specifically, NMR can provide the following types of information:

1. The number of nonequivalent nuclei, determined from the number of peaks.
2. The magnetic environment of a nucleus, determined by the chemical shift.
3. The relative numbers of nuclei, determined by integrating the peak areas.
4. The number of neighboring nuclei, determined by the splitting pattern observed (except for ¹³C in the spin-decoupled mode).

ULTRAVIOLET-VISIBLE SPECTROSCOPY

Basic Theory

Ultraviolet-visible (UV-vis) spectra are obtained by passing ultraviolet or visible light through a chemical sample (usually dissolved in an inert, nonabsorbing solvent) and plotting absorbance versus wavelength. The higher the concentration of the compound in solution, the greater the absorbance. The wavelength of absorption depends on functional groups of the molecule; in particular, conjugation leads to greater UV-vis absorption.

UV-vis spectra are often used to simply identify the presence or absence of a compound by measuring the absorbance at a characteristic wavelength for that molecule. For example, to follow the progress of an oxidation reaction using $K_2Cr_2O_7$, the absorbance of the solution at 350 nm is monitored. When large amounts of $K_2Cr_2O_7$ are present, high absorbance is recorded; when the reaction has gone to completion and the $K_2Cr_2O_7$ is no longer present, the absorption peak disappears.

Atomic absorption and emission spectra related to the energy levels of electrons are measured in the UV-vis range, and provide information on the quantum states of atoms. Atomic spectra are discussed in more detail in Chapter 27, Atomic Structure.

MASS SPECTROMETRY

Basic Theory

Mass spectrometry is a means of determining the molecular weight and structure of a molecule based on how it ionizes and decomposes under specific conditions. Mass spectrometry differs from other spectroscopic methods in two ways: No absorption of electromagnetic radiation is involved, and it is a destructive technique that does not allow the sample to be recovered and reused.

Mass spectrometers ionize the sample in a high-speed beam of electrons. The ionized sample then enters a magnetic field that deflects the ionic fragments into a detector. The net charge and mass of each particle is determined, along with the number of each type of particle (known as the **abundance**). The first ion formed is the $+1$ cation ($\mathbf{M^+}$) resulting from the removal of a single electron. This unstable ion usually decomposes rapidly into more cationic fragments. A typical mass spectrum is composed of many lines, each corresponding to a fragment with a specific **mass to charge ratio** (**m/e**, also written as **m/z**). The spectrum itself plots mass/charge on the horizontal axis and relative abundance of the various cationic fragments on the vertical axis (see Fig. 50.8).

Characteristics

The tallest peak, belonging to the most common ion, is called the **base peak**, and is assigned the relative abundance value of 100 percent; thus the amount of any other ion is a percent of the base peak. The peak with the highest m/e ratio (see Figure 50.8) is almost always the **molecular ion peak** (**parent ion peak**), $\mathbf{M^+}$, from which the molecular weight, M, can be obtained. The charge value is usually 1; hence the m/e ratio can usually be read as the mass of the fragment.

Application

Fragmentation patterns often provide information that helps identify the compound's structure. For example, while IR spectroscopy would be of little use in distinguishing between propionaldehyde and butyraldehyde, a mass spectrum would assist in identification.

Figure 50.8 shows the mass spectrum of butyraldehyde. The peak at $m/e = 72$ corresponds to the molecular cation-radical, M^+. Additional peaks represent a variety of fragments derived from the loss of groups of carbons and hydrogens.

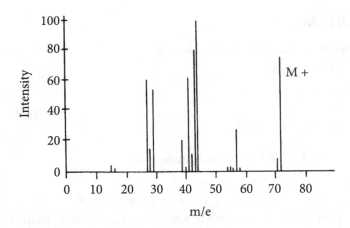

Figure 50.8

Summary of Mass Spectrometry

1. Mass spectrometry is based on the mass to charge (*m/e*) ratio of fragments of the molecule of interest.

2. Each peak in a mass spectrum corresponds to one fragment, and its height gives the relative abundance (amount) of that fragment.

3. The original molecule can be identified as the highest mass/charge ratio peak in the spectrum, as it is the +1 cation of the original compound.

4. The fragmentation pattern can give additional information about the structure of the compound.

REVIEW PROBLEMS

1. IR spectroscopy is most useful for distinguishing

   (A) double and triple bonds.
   (B) C–H bonds.
   (C) chirality of molecules.
   (D) composition of racemic mixtures.

2. Oxygen (O_2) does not exhibit an IR spectrum because

   (A) it has no molecular motions.
   (B) it is not possible to record IR spectra of a gaseous molecule.
   (C) molecular vibrations do not result in a change in the dipole moment of the molecules.
   (D) it has a molar mass less than 20 g/mol.

3. If IR spectroscopy were employed to monitor the oxidation of benzyl alcohol to benzaldehyde, which of the following would provide the best evidence that the reaction was proceeding as planned?

   (A) Comparing the fingerprint region of the spectra of starting material and product.
   (B) Noting the change in intensity of the peaks corresponding to the phenyl ring.
   (C) Noting the appearance of a broad absorption peak in the region of 3,100–3,500 cm^{-1}.
   (D) Noting the appearance of a strong absorption peak in the region of 1,700 cm^{-1}.

4. Which of the following chemical shifts would correspond to an aldehyde proton signal in a ^1H NMR spectrum?

   (A) 9.5 ppm
   (B) 7.0 ppm
   (C) 11.0 ppm
   (D) 1.0 ppm

5. The isotope ^{12}C is not useful for NMR because

   (A) it is not abundant in nature.
   (B) its resonances are not sensitive to the presence of neighboring atoms.
   (C) it has no magnetic moment.
   (D) the signal-to-noise ratio in the spectrum is too low.

6. The NMR spectra of ethanol in the presence and absence of water are shown below.

NMR spectrum of ethanol

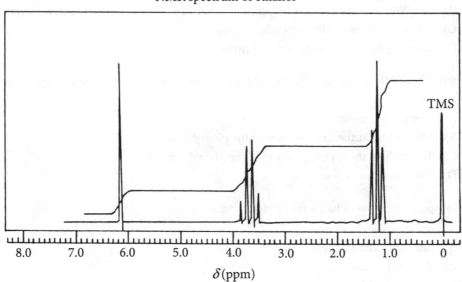

NMR spectrum of anhydrous ethanol

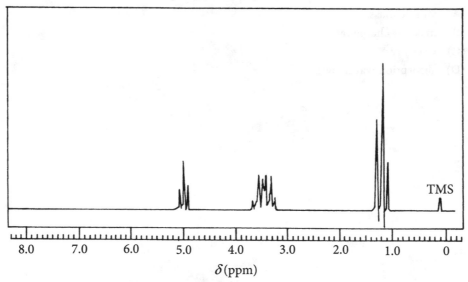

Which of the following explains the differences between the two spectra?

(A) Water also resonates, doubling the number of peaks.

(B) Carbon atoms do not couple in the presence of water.

(C) The hydroxyl proton of ethanol exchanges with protons from water, preventing it from coupling.

(D) Anhydrous ethanol forms dimers, causing the signal to split.

7. In ^{13}C NMR, splitting of spectral lines is due to

   (A) coupling between a carbon atom and protons attached to that carbon atom.
   (B) coupling between a carbon atom and protons attached to adjacent carbon atoms.
   (C) coupling between adjacent carbon atoms.
   (D) coupling between two adjacent protons.

8. In the ^{13}C NMR spectrum of methyl phenyl ketone, which carbon atom will appear the farthest downfield?

   (A) The methyl carbon
   (B) The carbon at the first position of the phenyl ring
   (C) The carbon at the *para* position of the phenyl ring
   (D) The carbonyl carbon

9. UV spectroscopy is most useful for detecting

   (A) aldehydes and ketones.
   (B) unconjugated alkenes.
   (C) conjugated alkenes.
   (D) aliphatic acids and amines.

10. Mass spectroscopy results in the separation of fragments according to

   (A) atomic mass.
   (B) mass-to-charge ratio.
   (C) viscosity.
   (D) absorption wavelength.

SOLUTIONS TO REVIEW PROBLEMS

1. A IR is most useful for distinguishing between different functional groups. Almost all organic compounds have C—H bonds (B), so that except for "fingerprinting" a compound, these absorptions are not useful. Very little information about the optical properties of a compound, such as choices (C) and (D), can be obtained by IR spectroscopy.

2. C Since molecular oxygen is a diatomic molecule with no initial net dipole, there is no net change in its dipole moment during vibration or rotation. Diatomic nitrogen and chlorine exhibit similar behavior. IR spectroscopy is based on the principle that when the molecule vibrates or rotates, there is a change in dipole moment; therefore, choice (C) is the correct answer. Choice (A) is incorrect because oxygen does have molecular motions. Choice (B) is incorrect because it is possible to record the IR of a gaseous molecule, as long as it shows a change in its dipole moment when it vibrates. Choice (D) is a false statement.

3. D In this reaction, the functional group is changing from a hydroxyl to an aldehyde. This means that a sharp peak will appear at around 1700 cm^{-1}, which corresponds to the carbonyl functionality. Therefore, choice (D) is the correct response. Choice (C) is incorrect because the reaction will be characterized by the disappearance of a peak at $3,100–3,500 \text{ cm}^{-1}$, not the appearance of one (this peak corresponds to the hydroxyl functionality). Choice (A) is possible, but the complexity of the information makes it a poor choice compared to (D). Choice (B) is the least useful, as the IR absorbance of the phenyl ring in the $675–870 \text{ cm}^{-1}$ band will not change in this reaction.

4. A The peak at 9.5 ppm corresponds to an aldehyde proton. This signal lies relatively far downfield because the carbonyl oxygen is strongly electron-withdrawing and deshields the proton. The other peaks are too upfield and represent more-shielded molecules.

5. C This isotope has no magnetic moment and will therefore not exhibit resonance. Nuclei that possess a magnetic moment are those with odd-numbered masses (^{1}H, ^{11}B, ^{13}C, ^{15}N, ^{19}F, etc.) or those with an even mass but an odd atomic number (^{2}H, ^{10}B).

6. C The normal spectrum of CH_3CH_2OH has a CH_3 group split into a triplet by the CH_2 group protons, a CH_2 group split into a quartet by the CH_3 group protons, and a hydroxyl proton singlet. This proton exchanges rapidly with the protons of water and is not able to participate in splitting. Under anhydrous conditions, this proton can couple, and it splits the neighboring quartet into a doublet such that an octet is observed. The —OH signal itself appears as a triplet due to splitting by the protons of the neighboring CH_2 group. Answer choice (A) is incorrect because it is opposite of what is true: The peaks are split in the absence of water, not its presence. Choice (B) is incorrect because the spectra are for ^{1}H NMR, not ^{13}C NMR. Answer choice (D) is incorrect because ethanol does not form dimers in solution.

7. A Coupling between adjacent carbon atoms, choice (C), is rarely seen due to the low abundance of ^{13}C. Coupling between carbon and protons on the adjacent carbon, choice (B), is never observed. Since proton coupling is only relevant to ^{1}H NMR, choice (D) is incorrect.

8. **D** The carbonyl carbon atom will be furthest downfield because of the electron-withdrawing ability of the oxygen atom. ^{13}C NMR follows the same rules of chemical shift as ^1H NMR. Choice (A), the methyl carbon, and choice (B), the carbon at position 1 of the phenyl ring, are farther from the oxygen than the carbonyl carbon and thus will not be shifted as far downfield. Choice (C), the carbon at the *para* position of the phenyl ring, is the furthest from the oxygen and will therefore be shifted downfield the least. Choice (D), the carbonyl carbon, is closest to the oxygen and therefore will experience the greatest shift and is the correct answer.

9. **C** Most conjugated alkenes, choice (C), give an intense UV absorption and are therefore most readily detected by UV spectroscopy. Aldehydes, ketones, acids, and amines, choices (A) and (D), all absorb in the UV, but other forms of spectroscopy (mainly IR and NMR) are more useful for their precise identification. Isolated alkenes, choice (B), can rarely be identified by UV.

10. **B** In mass spectrometry, a molecule is broken down into smaller charged fragments. These fragments are passed through a magnetic field and are identified according to their mass-to-charge ratios; therefore, choice (B) is the correct answer. Choice (D) is the basis for IR and NMR, not mass spectrometry, so this is incorrect. Viscosity, choice (C), doesn't form the basis for any of the spectroscopic techniques discussed, so it is also incorrect. Finally, choice (A) is incorrect because the separation of fragments does not depend solely on mass but on charge as well, and the fragments are mostly polyatomic.

Section VII

BIOCHEMISTRY

CHAPTER FIFTY-ONE

DNA and RNA

Genes are composed of **DNA** (deoxyribonucleic acid), which contains information coded in the sequence of its base pairs. This information can be transcribed into **RNA** (ribonucleic acid), which is then translated into a sequence of amino acids called a **protein**. Therefore, the DNA sequence is essentially a blueprint for protein synthesis. These proteins regulate all life functions. DNA is also able to **self-replicate**, an essential step in cell division and therefore for cell (and organism) reproduction.

DEOXYRIBOSE NUCLEIC ACID

Deoxyribose nucleic acid (DNA) is the basis for heredity. Its ability to self-replicate makes sure that the coded DNA sequence will be passed on to future generations. This concept, along with the sequences of events described above, is the **central dogma** of molecular genetics. DNA is **mutable** and can be altered under certain conditions, which similarly alters the proteins produced and therefore the organism's characteristics. Changes in DNA are often stable and are passed down from generation to generation. This provides the basis for evolution.

Central Dogma of Molecular Genetics

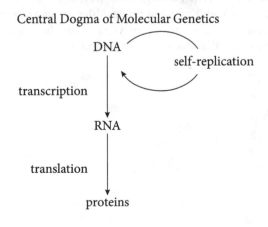

Figure 51.1

DNA Structure

The basic unit of DNA is the **nucleotide**. A nucleotide is composed of deoxyribose (a sugar) bonded to both a phosphate group and a nitrogenous base. There are two types of bases: **purines** and **pyrimidines**. Purines in DNA include **adenine** (A) and **guanine** (G); pyrimidines are **cytosine** (C) and **thymine** (T). Purines are larger in structure than pyrimidines because they possess a two-ring nitrogenous base, whereas pyrimidines have a one-ring nitrogenous base. The phosphate and sugar form a chain with the bases arranged as side groups off the chain.

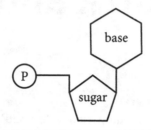

Figure 51.2

The directionality of DNA is designated by a 3′ (read as "three prime") and a 5′ (read as "five prime") end. This naming convention is based on which carbon of the sugar molecule of the DNA strand is the terminus of the helix. If the 5′ carbon is at the end of the DNA strand, then that end is referred to as the 5′ end. Similarly, if the 3′ carbon is at the end of the DNA strand, then that end is referred to as the 3′ end.

DNA is most commonly found in humans as double-stranded helices of complementary strands with the sugar-phosphate chains on the outside of the helix and the nitrogenous bases on the inside. These strands are held together by hydrogen bonds between the bases oriented toward the center. Purines pair with pyrimidines in the following pattern: T forms two hydrogen bonds with A, and G forms three hydrogen bonds with C. This pairing holds the two strands of the double helix together and links the polynucleotide chains. When arranged this way, one DNA strand has its 5' end pointing up, and the other strand has its 3' end pointing up, resulting in an **antiparallel** arrangement. This structure was discovered by James Watson and Francis Crick with the help of Rosalind Franklin and others and is therefore known as the **Watson-Crick DNA model**.

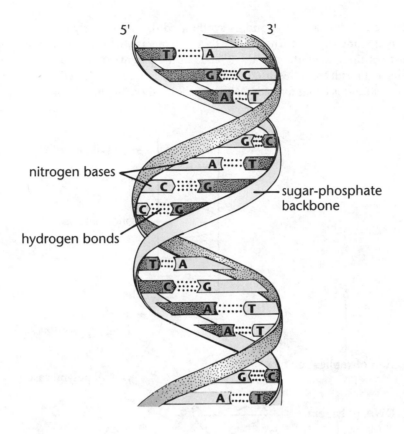

Figure 51.3

DNA Function

DNA replication

In order to replicate, the double-stranded DNA helix must unwind and separate into two single strands. This involves uncoiling the strands by **topoisomerase** and breaking the hydrogen bonds between the nitrogenous bases of each nucleotide by **DNA helicase**. The opening in the DNA molecule created by DNA helicase is known as the **replication fork**.

With their hydrogen bonds broken, each single strand can act as a template for complementary base-pairing. This allows for the synthesis of two new daughter strands. Each new daughter helix contains an intact strand from the parent helix and a newly synthesized strand, so this type of replication is referred to as **semiconservative**. The daughter strands of DNA formed from the parent strands are identical to the parent strands.

Creation of these daughter strands is a result of the action of **DNA polymerase**. DNA polymerase reads the parent DNA strand and creates a complementary, antiparallel daughter strand. DNA polymerase always reads the parent strand in the $3' \rightarrow 5'$ direction, creating a new daughter strand in the $5' \rightarrow 3'$ direction. One daughter strand is the **leading strand**, and the other is the **lagging strand**. The leading strand is continually synthesized by DNA polymerase, which attaches nucleotides to the exposed 3' end of the parent strand and follows the replication fork to the 5' end. However, the other daughter strand, the lagging strand, is synthesized discontinuously because the 5′ end of the parent strand is the one exposed. Therefore, DNA polymerase, which can only read in the 3′ → 5′ direction, must continually reattach to the 3′ ends of the parent strand being slowly exposed. The short fragments that result from this discontinuous synthesis are known as **Okazaki fragments**; as the lagging daughter strand is being formed, DNA ligase joins these fragments together.

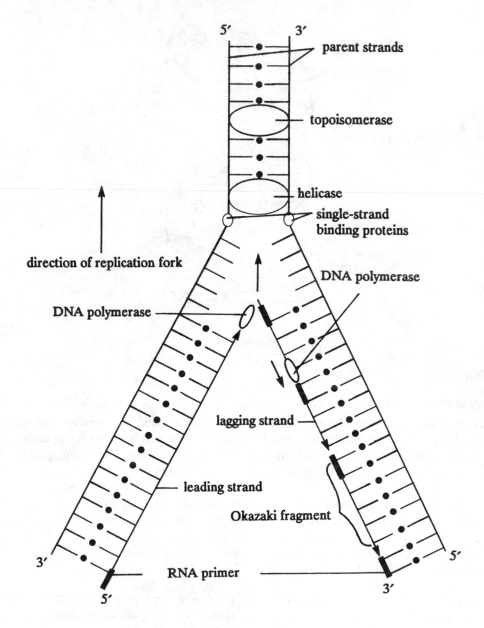

Figure 51.4

The genetic code

DNA is made up of four different nucleosides: **adenine** (A), **thymine** (T), **cytosine** (C), and **guanine** (G). In RNA, the nucleosides are identical except for thymine, which is replaced with **uracil** (U). DNA is transcribed into mRNA and arranged into **triplets** (sets of three). These triplets (also known as **codons**) are then translated from mRNA into amino acids. There are 20 amino acids that can be formed from all possible combinations of the four nucleosides. A sequence of three consecutive bases codes for a particular amino acid; e.g., the codon GGC specifies glycine, and the codon GUG specifies valine. The genetic code is universal for almost all organisms.

Given that 64 different codons are possible based on the triplet code and four possible nucleotides, and only 20 amino acids need to be coded, the code must contain synonyms. This means that most amino acids have more than one codon coding for them. This is referred to as the degeneracy or **redundancy** of the genetic code.

Second Base

First Base (5′)		U	C	A	G		Third Base (3′)
	U	UUU UUC } Phe UUA UUG } Leu	UCU UCC UCA UCG } Ser	UAU UAC } Tyr UAA UAG } Stop	UGU UGC } Cys UGA } Stop UGG } Trp		U C A G
	C	CUU CUC CUA CUG } Leu	CCU CCC CCA CCG } Pro	CAU CAC } His CAA CAG } Gln	CGU CGC CGA CGG } Arg		U C A G
	A	AUU AUC } Ile AUA AUG } Start or Met	ACU ACC ACA ACG } Thr	AAU AAC } Asn AAA AAG } Lys	AGU AGC } Ser AGA AGG } Arg		U C A G
	G	GUU GUC GUA GUG } Val	GCU GCC GCA GCG } Ala	GAU GAC } Asp GAA GAG } Glu	GGU GGC GGA GGG } Gly		U C A G

Figure 51.5

RIBONUCLEIC ACID

RNA Structure

Ribonucleic acid (RNA) is a polynucleotide that is very structurally similar to DNA with three major exceptions:

- Its sugar is ribose (instead of deoxyribose).
- It contains uracil instead of thymine.
- It is usually single stranded.

RNA can be found in both the nucleus and the cytoplasm of the cell. There are several types of RNA, all of which are involved in protein synthesis. The three major types are mRNA, tRNA, and rRNA.

Messenger RNA

Messenger RNA (mRNA) carries the complement of a DNA sequence (except that thymine is substituted with **uracil**). It transports this complement from the nucleus to the ribosomes for protein synthesis. mRNA is made from ribonucleotides complementary to the template strand of DNA. This means that mRNA has the complementary code to the original DNA. For example, because the DNA code for the amino acid valine is AAC, the mRNA sequence is the complementary UUG: A pairs with U, and C pairs with G. mRNA is monocistronic, meaning that one mRNA strand codes for one polypeptide.

Transfer RNA

Transfer RNA (tRNA) is a small RNA molecule found in the cytoplasm. It assists in the translation of mRNA's nucleotide code into a sequence of amino acids. It helps by bringing the amino acids coded for in the mRNA sequence to the ribosomes during protein synthesis. tRNA recognizes both the mRNA codon and its corresponding amino acid. This dual function is reflected in its three-dimensional structure. One end contains a three-nucleotide sequence, the **anticodon**, which is complementary to one of the mRNA codons. The other end is the site of attachment of the corresponding amino acid. Each amino acid has its own aminoacyl-tRNA synthetase, which has an active site that binds to both the amino acid and its corresponding tRNA, catalzying their attachment to form an aminoacyl-tRNA complex. There is at least one type of tRNA for each amino acid (there are approximately 40 known types of tRNA).

Ribosomal RNA

Ribosomal RNA (rRNA) is a structural component of ribosomes and is the most abundant of all RNA types. The mRNA sequence passes through two subunits of the rRNA structure and is translated into amino acids at this time. rRNA is synthesized in the nucleolus.

Transcription

Transcription is the process through which information coded in the base sequence of DNA is transcribed into a strand of mRNA that leaves the nucleus through nuclear pores. Each human chromosome is a long strand of DNA that is used to make approximately 1,000 different sequences of RNA; as such, RNA are much smaller than DNA, and only a segment of the original DNA strand is used as a template. The first step of transcription therefore occurs when RNA polymerase binds to the DNA at a **promoter region**, a short DNA sequence found upstream from the site where transcription of a specific RNA is going to take place. In humans, this is most commonly a TATA box.

Transcription factors then help **RNA polymerase** bind to the DNA molecule and initiate transcription. In a process very similar to DNA replication, the RNA polymerase surrounds the DNA molecule after it has been opened by the actions of DNA helicase and topoisomerase. The RNA polymerase then recruits and adds in complementary RNA nucleotides based on the DNA sequence. As with DNA polymerase, RNA polymerase reads in the $3' \rightarrow 5'$ direction and creates a new daughter strand in the $3' \rightarrow 5'$ direction. The RNA sequence is complementary to the original DNA sequence except that A binds with uracil (U) rather than T. RNA also uses a slightly different sugar backbone than that used in DNA: ribose (with an oxygen on C–2) instead of deoxyribose (without an oxygen on C–2).

After transcription is complete, mRNA undergoes post-transcriptional processing. RNA that has not yet been processed is known as hetero-nuclear RNA (hnRNA) or pre-RNA and contains extra nucleotides that are not necessary to create the corresponding protein. These extra sequences are called **introns**; in contrast, **exons** are the nucleotides necessary to make the protein. The introns are therefore **spliced** out (removed) by the spliceosome, leaving only the exons behind. Additionally, a **guanine cap** and a series of adenines known as a **poly-A tail** are added to the ends of the new molecule to provide protection from enzyme degradation once the RNA leaves the nucleus.

Translation

Translation is the process through which mRNA codons are translated into a sequence of amino acids. Translation occurs in the cytoplasm and involves tRNA, ribosomes, mRNA, amino acids, enzymes, and other proteins and can be divided into four distinct stages: initiation, elongation, translocation, and termination.

Initiation begins when the ribosome binds to the mRNA near its 5′ end. The ribosome scans the mRNA until it binds to a **start codon** (AUG). The initiator aminoacyl-tRNA complex, methionine-tRNA (with the anticodon 3′–UAC–5′), base pairs with the start codon.

In **elongation**, hydrogen bonds form between the mRNA codon in the A site of the ribosome and its complementary anticodon on the incoming aminoacyl-tRNA complex. A peptide bond is formed between the amino acid attached to the tRNA in the A site and the amino acid attached to the tRNA in the P site of the ribosome. After the peptide bond formation, a ribosome carries uncharged tRNA in the P site and peptidyl-tRNA in the A site.

The cycle is completed by **translocation**, in which the ribosome advances three nucleotides along the mRNA in the 5′ to 3′ direction. In a concurrent action, the uncharged tRNA from the P site is expelled, and the peptidyl-tRNA from the A site moves into the P site. The ribosome then has an empty A site ready for the entry of the aminoacyl-tRNA corresponding to the next codon.

Polypeptide synthesis undergoes **termination** when one of three special mRNA termination codons, or **stop codons** (UAA, UAG, or UGA), arrives in the A site. These codons signal the ribosome to terminate translation; they do not code for amino acids. Frequently, numerous ribosomes simultaneously translate a single mRNA molecule, forming a structure known as a **polyribosome**.

After the release of the protein from the ribosome, the protein immediately assumes its characteristic three-dimensional native conformation. This conformation is determined by the primary sequence of amino acids. Additional secondary and tertiary structural folding occurs based on the primary sequence. Furthermore, the polypeptide chains can form intramolecular and intermolecular cross-bridges with disulfide bonds. The result is a functional protein or complex of multiple proteins.

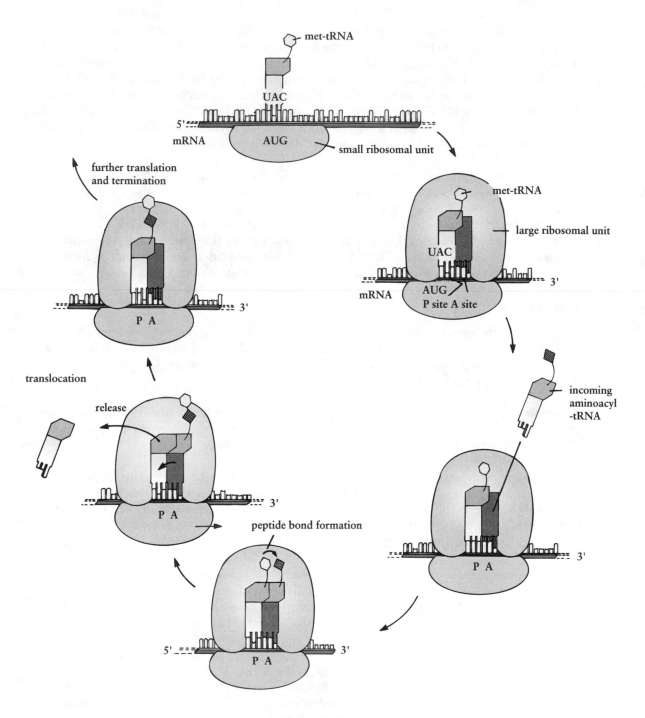

Figure 51.6

Ribosomes, where translation takes place, are composed of two subunits (consisting of proteins and rRNA), one small and one large. These bind together only during protein synthesis. As previously discussed, ribosomes also have three binding sites for tRNA: the A, P, and E sites. The **A site** (aminoacyl-tRNA complex binding site) binds to the next incoming tRNA complex. The tRNA complex is then transferred to the **P site** (peptidyl-tRNA binding site), where the tRNA contributes its amino acid to the growing polypeptide chain. Finally, having already given up its amino acid, the tRNA is released at the **E site** (exit site).

Humans and bacteria have different types of subunits that make up their ribosomes. This is another difference that drug manufacturers capitalize on when designing antibiotics. Many antibiotics target only the ribosomal structures specific to bacteria, thereby harming bacterial cells while leaving human cells unharmed.

REVIEW PROBLEMS

1. What is the central dogma of molecular genetics?

2. What of the following is NOT true about pyrimidines and purines?

    (A) Pyrimidines have a two-ring nitrogenous base
    (B) Purines have a two-ring nitrogenous base
    (C) Purines always bind to pyrimidines when a DNA helix is formed
    (D) Purines and pyrimidines make up the "rungs" of the DNA ladder

3. What is the difference between the 3′ and the 5′ ends of a DNA molecule?

4. Which model of DNA replication describes one parental strand and one new strand of DNA making up each new helix?

    (A) Semiconservative
    (B) Conservative
    (C) Dispersive
    (D) Redundancy

5. Describe the process of DNA replication, including the roles of topoisomerase and DNA helicase and the definitions of Okazaki fragments and the replication fork.

6. What is the redundancy of the genetic code?

7. What are the three major differences between RNA and DNA?

8. Distinguish between transcription and translation and describe the process that takes place within the ribosome during translation.

SOLUTIONS TO REVIEW PROBLEMS

1. The central dogma of molecular genetics states that genetic information goes from DNA to RNA to protein.

2. **A** Purines are larger molecules than pyrimidines, and each purine has a two-ring nitrogenous base, whereas each pyrimidine only has a one-ring nitrogenous base. It is true that purines and pyrimidines bind to each other when the DNA helix is formed and that they are on the inside of the helix ("rungs" of the DNA ladder), rather than the outside of the structure.

3. The 3′ end of DNA is where the carbon on the sugar molecule at the farthest end of the DNA molecule is the 3′ carbon within the ring structure. Similarly, the 5′ end is where the carbon on the sugar molecule at the DNA terminus is the 5′ carbon.

4. **A** Semiconservative replication produces two copies of DNA that each contain one parent strand and one new strand. In conservative replication there is one DNA copy with both parent strands and one with two new strands. In dispersive replication there are two copies of DNA that both have pairs of parent and new genetic material interspersed throughout the helix. Redundancy describes the multiple codons that code for the same amino acid in the genetic code.

5. DNA helicase "unzips" the DNA helix, exposing the two parent DNA strands. This opening is called the replication fork. DNA polymerase moves in a $3′ \longrightarrow 5′$ direction along both parent DNA strands, recruiting complementary nucleotides and creating the daughter strands. The leading strand is made continuously whereas the lagging strand is made discontinuously because DNA polymerase only moves in a $3′ \longrightarrow 5′$ direction. This means that on the lagging strand DNA pieces are made in short sequences rather than one long strand. The short pieces of new DNA on the lagging strand are called Okazaki fragments. Topoisomerase prevents DNA from overcoiling during replication.

6. The genetic code is redundant because more than one codon (sequence of three base pairs) codes for many amino acids. Because there are four possible nucleotides for a codon consisting of a combination of three nucleotides, 64 possible combinations of nucleotides exist to make each codon. However, since only 20 amino acids are coded for, most amino acids can be coded for by more than one sequence of nucleotides. This is referred to as the redundancy of the genetic code.

7. Three major differences between RNA and DNA are that RNA (1) contains ribose instead of deoxyribose as its sugar, (2) contains uracil instead of thymine, and (3) is usually single stranded.

8. Transcription is the process by which DNA is turned into RNA, whereas in translation RNA is turned into protein. In translation the ribosome locates a start codon near the 5′ end of the mRNA. The ribosome then reads the mRNA sequence, codon by codon, and recruits the corresponding amino acid (attached to a tRNA) encoded by the mRNA. After each codon is read, the mRNA molecule translocates within the ribosome to make room for the next codon. Once a stop codon is reached, termination occurs, and the ribosome falls off the mRNA sequence. At this point the primary structure of the protein is complete, and it assumes its three-dimensional conformation based on its primary sequence.

CHAPTER FIFTY-TWO

Proteins

Proteins are large polymers composed of many amino acid subunits. Proteins have diverse biological roles; for example, they provide structure (keratin, collagen), regulate body metabolism via hormonal control (insulin), and serve as catalysts (enzymes). Proteins are composed primarily of C, H, O, and N but may also contain phosphorus (P) and sulfur (S).

AMINO ACIDS

Amino acids contain an amine group and a carboxyl group attached to a single carbon atom (the alpha carbon atom). The other two substituents of the alpha carbon are usually a hydrogen atom and a variable side-chain referred to as the **R-group**.

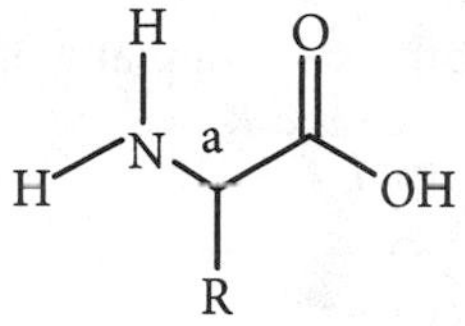

Figure 52.1

The alpha carbon is a chiral center, and thus all amino acids are optically active. The exception is glycine, the simplest amino acid, which has H as its R group and therefore does not have a chiral center and is not optically active. Almost all naturally occurring amino acids (of which there are 20) are L-enantiomers (see Chapter 40, Isomers) with the exception of those found in some bacteria that can utilize D-amino acids.

By convention, the Fischer projection for an amino acid is drawn with the amino group on the left.

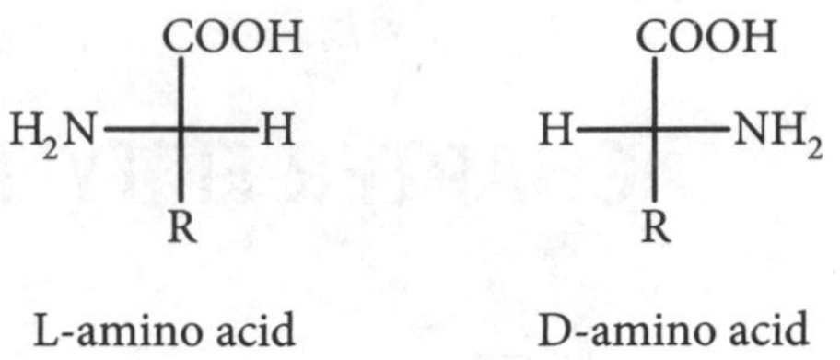

L-amino acid   D-amino acid

Figure 52.2

Acid-Base Characteristics

Amino acids have an acidic carboxyl group and a basic amino group on the same molecule. As a result, when they are in solution, amino acids sometimes take the form of neutral molecules that nevertheless contain both positive and negative charges, which are also called **zwitterions** (from German *zwitter,* hybrid).

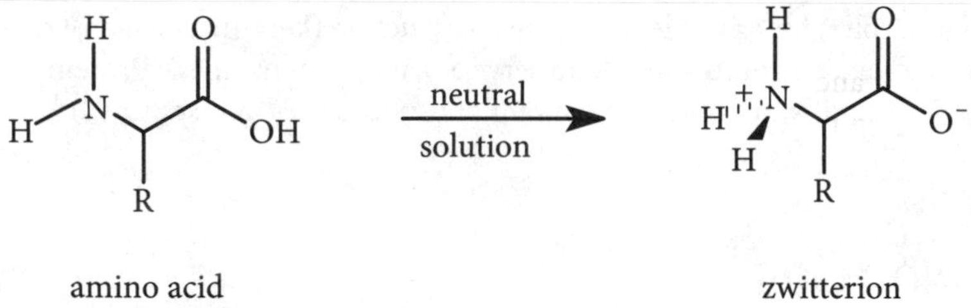

amino acid   zwitterion

Figure 52.3

Amino acids are **amphoteric**; i.e., they may act as either acids or bases depending on their environment. Amino acids in acidic solution are fully protonated. Since they have two protons that can dissociate—one from the carboxyl group and one from the amino group—amino acids have at least two dissociation constants, K_{a1} and K_{a2}.

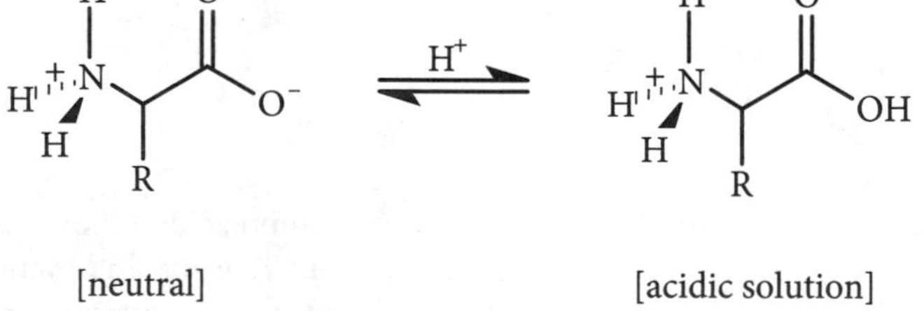

[neutral]   [acidic solution]

Figure 52.4

Amino acids in basic solution are deprotonated. They have two proton-accepting groups and, therefore, at least two dissociation constants, K_{b1} and K_{b2}.

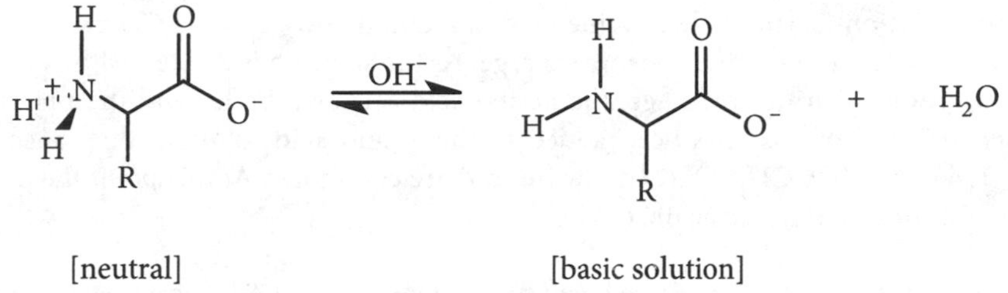

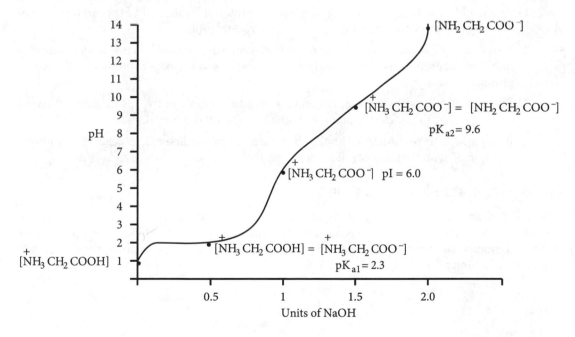

Figure 52.5

At low pH the amino acid carries an excess positive charge; at high pH, the amino acid carries an excess negative charge. The intermediate pH, at which the amino acid is electrically neutral and exists as a zwitterion, is the **isoelectric point (pI)**, or **isoelectric pH**, of the amino acid. The isoelectric pH lies between pK_{a1} and pK_{a2}.

Titration of Amino Acids

Because of their acidic and basic properties, amino acids can be titrated. The titration of each proton occurs as a distinct step resembling that of a simple monoprotic acid. The titration curve of glycine is shown below:

Figure 52.6

A 1 M glycine solution is acidic; the glycine exists predominantly as $^+NH_3CH_2COOH$. The amino acid is fully protonated and carries a positive charge. As the solution is titrated with NaOH, carboxyl groups lose a proton. During this stage, the amino acid acts as a buffer and the pH changes very slowly. When 0.5 mol of base has been added to the amino acid solution, the concentrations of $^+NH_3CH_2COOH$ and $^+NH_3CH_2COO^-$ (its zwitterion) are equimolar. At this point the pH is equal to pK_{a1}, and the solution is buffered against pH changes.

As more base is added, all of the carboxyl groups are deprotonated. The amino acid loses buffering capacity, and thus the pH rises more rapidly. When 1 mol of base has been added, glycine exists predominantly as $^+NH_3CH_2COO^-$. The amino acid is now electrically neutral; the pH is equal to glycine's pI.

Glycine passes through a second buffering stage during which pH change is slow because continued titration deprotonates its amino groups. When 1.5 mol of base have been added, the concentrations of $^+NH_3CH_2COO^-$ and $NH_2CH_2COO^-$ are equimolar, and the pH is equal to pK_{a2}.

As another 0.5 mol of base is added, all of the amino groups are deprotonated to $NH_2CH_2COO^-$; glycine is now completely deprotonated.

Certain things should be noted about the titration of amino acids:

1. When adding base, the carboxyl group loses its proton first; after all of the carboxyl groups are fully deprotonated, the amino group loses its acidic proton.

2. Two moles of base must be added in order to deprotonate one mole of most amino acids. The first mole deprotonates the carboxyl group, while the second mole deprotonates the amino group.

3. The buffering capacity of the amino acid is greatest at or near the two dissociation constants, K_{a1} and K_{a2}. At the isoelectric point, its buffering capacity is minimal.

4. It is possible to perform the titration in reverse, from alkaline pH to acidic pH, with the addition of acid; the sequence of events is reversed.

Henderson-Hasselbalch Equation

The ratio of an amino acid's ions is dependent on pH. The **Henderson-Hasselbalch equation** (previously discussed in Chapter 37, Acids and Bases) defines the relationship between pH and the ratio of conjugate acid to conjugate base and provides a mathematical expression for the dissociation constants of amino acids.

$$pH = pK_a + \log\frac{[\text{conjugate base}]}{[\text{conjugate acid}]}$$

When the pK_{a1} of glycine is known, the ratio of conjugate acid to conjugate base for a particular pH can be determined. For example, at pH 3.3, glycine, which has a pK_{a1} of 2.3, will have the ratios:

$$3.3 = 2.3 + \log\frac{[H_3N^+CH_2COO^-]}{[H_3N^+CH_2COOH]}$$

$$\log\frac{[H_3N^+CH_2COO^-]}{[H_3N^+CH_2COOH]} = 3.3 - 2.3 = 1$$

The antilog of $1 = 10$, thus: $\dfrac{[H_3N^+CH_2COO^-]}{[H_3N^+CH_2COOH]} = \dfrac{10}{1}$

So, in this example, there are ten times as many zwitterions as there are of the fully protonated form.

The Henderson-Hasselbalch equation can be used experimentally to prepare buffer solutions of amino acids. The best buffering regions of amino acids occur within one pH unit of the pK_a or pK_b. For example, the carboxyl group of glycine, which has a pK_a of 2.3, shows high buffering capacity between pH 1.3 and 3.3.

Amino Acid Side-Chains

Amino acid side-chains (R-groups) give chemical diversity to the backbone of the amino acid molecule. They also give proteins some distinguishing features. The twenty amino acids are classified according to whether their side chains are **nonpolar**, **polar** (but uncharged), **acidic**, or **basic**.

Nonpolar amino acids

Nonpolar amino acids have R-groups that are saturated hydrocarbons. The R-groups are hydrophobic and decrease the solubility of the amino acid in water. Amino acids with nonpolar side-chains are usually found buried within protein molecules, away from the aqueous cellular environment.

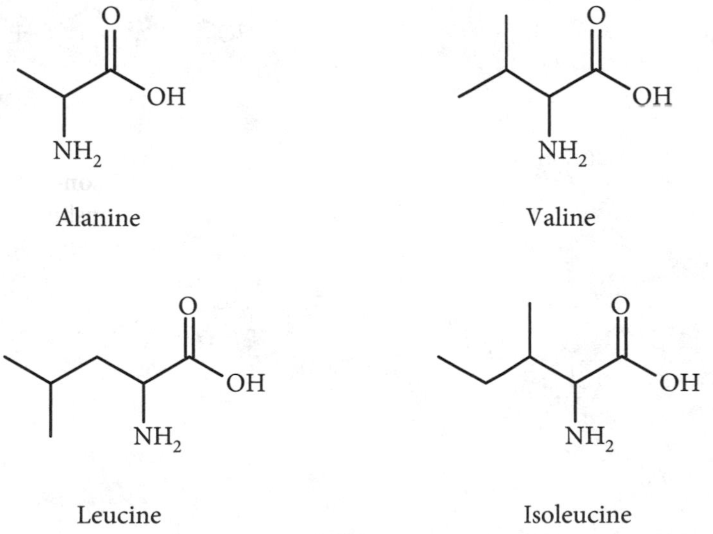

Alanine   Valine

Leucine   Isoleucine

Figure 52.7

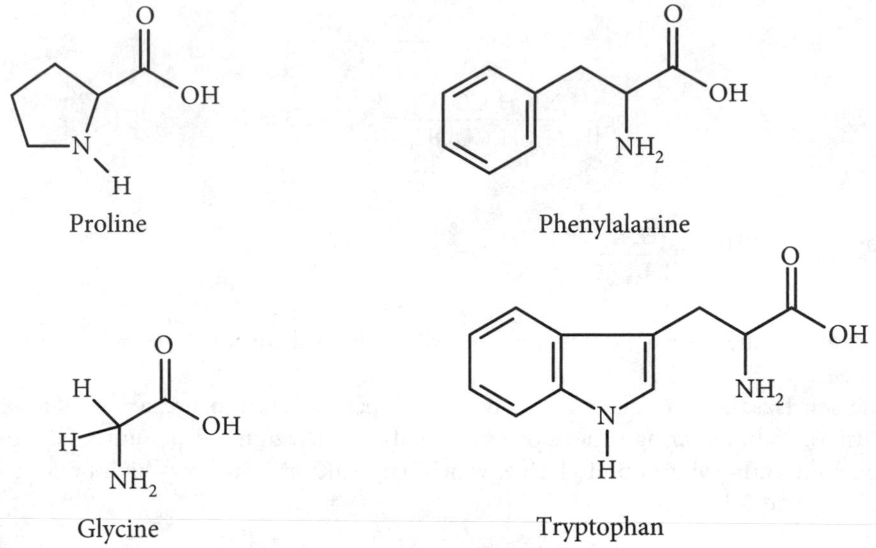

Figure 52.8

Polar amino acids

Polar amino acids have polar, uncharged R-groups that are hydrophilic, increasing the solubility of the amino acid in water. They are usually found on protein surfaces.

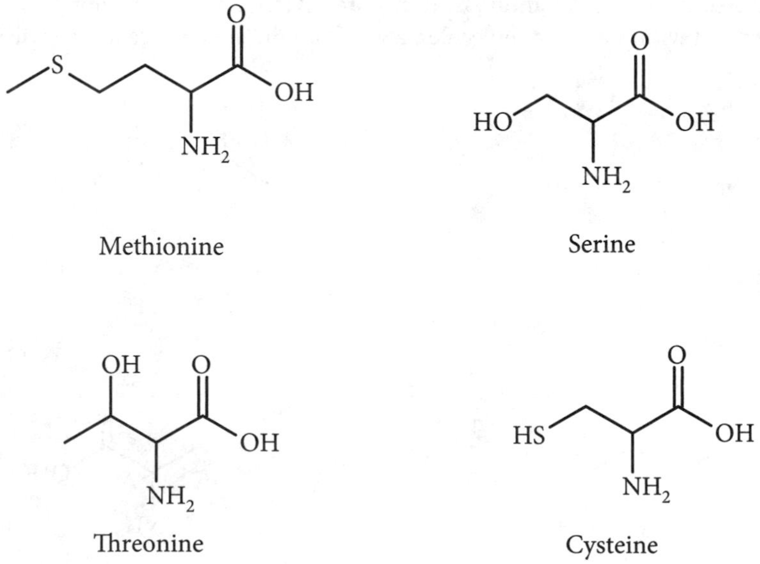

Figure 52.9

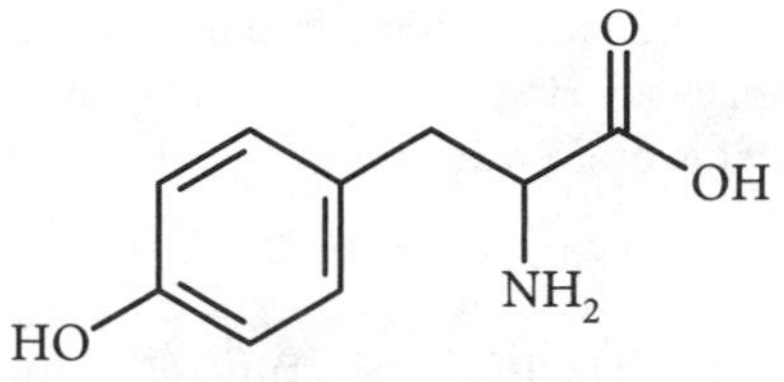

Tyrosine

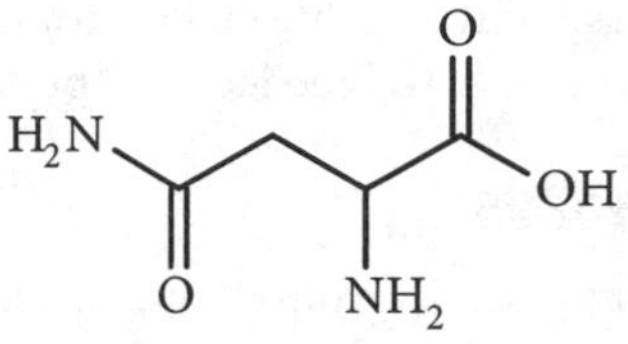

Asparagine

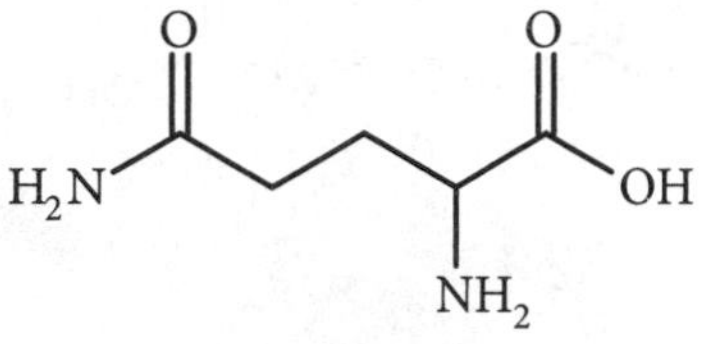

Glutamine

Figure 52.10

Acidic amino acids

Amino acids whose R-group contains a carboxyl group are called acidic amino acids. They have a net negative charge at physiological pH (pH 7.4) and exist in salt form in the body. They often play important roles in the substrate-binding sites of enzymes.

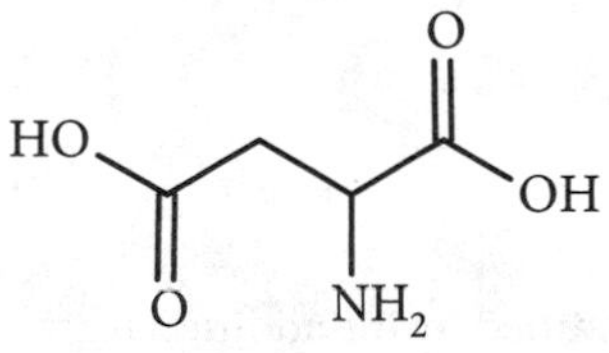

Aspartic Acid

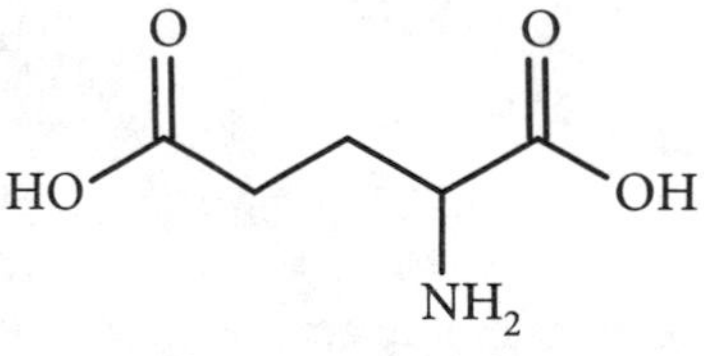

Glutamic Acid

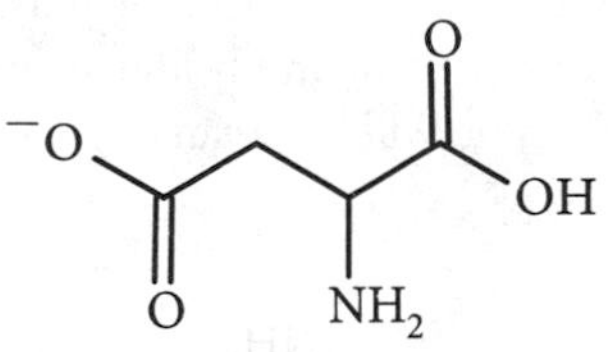

(Salt Is Aspartate)

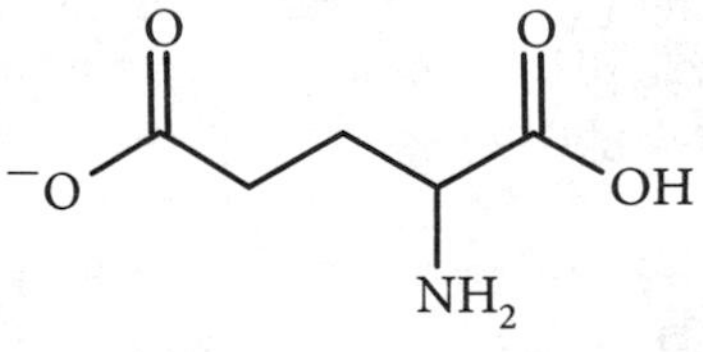

(Salt Is Glutamate)

Figure 52.11

Aspartic acid and glutamic acid each have three groups that must be neutralized during titration (two $-COOH$ and one $-NH_3^+$). Therefore, their titration curve is different from the standard curve for amino acids (exemplified by glycine). The molecule has three distinct dissociation constants—pK_{a1},

pK_{a2}, and pK_{a3}—although the neutralization curves of the two carboxyl groups overlap to a certain extent. Because of the additional carboxyl group, the isoelectric point is shifted toward an acidic pH. Three moles of base are needed to deprotonate one mole of an acidic amino acid.

Basic amino acids

Amino acids whose R-group contains an amino group are called basic amino acids and carry a net positive charge at physiological pH.

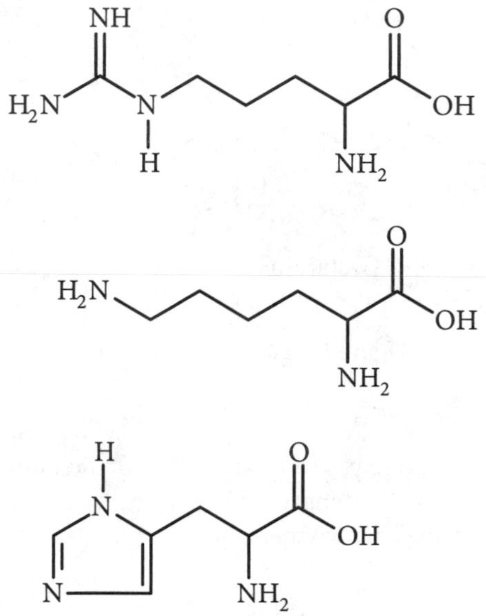

Figure 52.12

The titration curve of amino acids with basic R-groups is modified by the additional amino group that must be neutralized. Although basic amino acids have three dissociation constants, the neutralization curves for the two amino groups overlap. The isoelectric point is shifted toward an alkaline pH. Three moles of acid are needed to neutralize one mole of a basic amino acid.

Understanding titration curves and isoelectric points helps predict the charge of particular amino acids at a given pH. For example, in a mixture of glycine, glutamic acid, and lysine at pH 6.0, glycine will be neutral, glutamic acid will be negatively charged, and lysine will be positively charged.

PEPTIDES

Peptides are composed of amino acid subunits, sometimes called **residues**, linked by **peptide bonds**. Two amino acids joined together form a **dipeptide**, three form a **tripeptide**, and many amino acids linked together form a **polypeptide**.

Reactions

Amino acids are joined by **peptide bonds** (amide bonds) between the carboxyl group of one amino acid and the amino group of another. This bond is formed via a condensation reaction (a reaction in which water is lost). The reverse reaction, hydrolysis (cleavage with the addition of water) of the peptide bond, is catalyzed by an acid or base.

Certain enzymes digest the chain at specific peptide linkages. For example, **trypsin** cleaves at the carboxyl end of arginine and lysine; chymotrypsin cleaves at the carboxyl end of phenylalanine, tyrosine, and tryptophan.

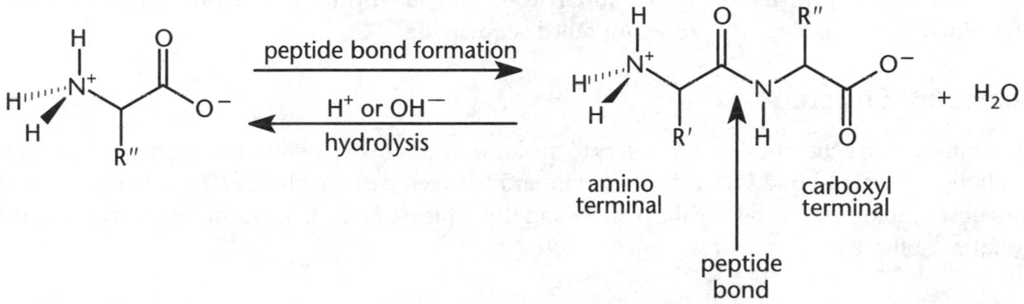

Figure 52.13

Properties

The terminal amino acid with a free alpha-amino group is known as the **amino-terminal** or **N-terminal** residue, while the terminal residue with a free carboxyl group is called the **carboxy-terminal** or **C-terminal** residue. By convention, peptides are drawn with the N-terminal end on the left and the C-terminal end on the right.

Amides have two resonance structures, and the true structure is a hybrid with partial double-bond character. As a result, rotation about the C−N bond is restricted. The bonds on either side of the peptide unit, however, have a great deal of rotational freedom.

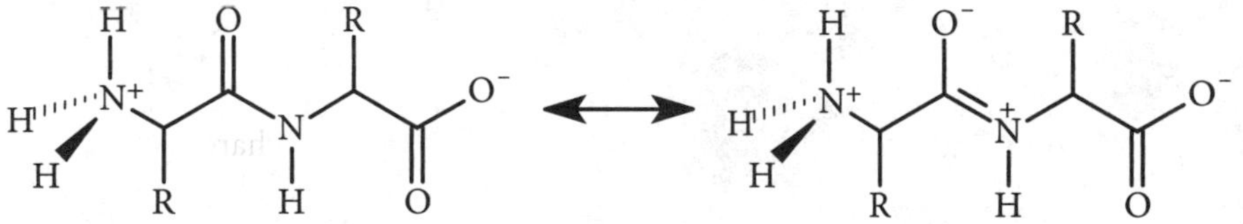

Figure 52.14

PROTEINS

Proteins are polypeptides that can range from only a few up to more than a thousand amino acids in length. Proteins serve many diverse functions in biological systems, acting as enzymes, hormones, membrane pores, receptors, and elements of cell structure. Four structural levels of protein structure—**primary**, **secondary**, **tertiary**, and **quaternary**—are described below.

Primary Structure

The primary structure of the protein refers to the sequence of amino acids, listed from the N-terminus to the C-terminus, linked by covalent bonds between neighboring residues in the chain.

The higher-level structures of a protein are dependent on the primary sequence; in other words, a protein will assume whatever secondary, tertiary, and quaternary structures are most energetically favorable given its primary structure and environment. The primary structure of a protein can be determined using a laboratory procedure called **sequencing**.

Secondary Structure

The secondary structure of a protein refers to the local structure of neighboring amino acids, governed mostly by hydrogen bond interactions within and between peptide chains. The two most common types of secondary structures are the α-**helix** and the β-**pleated sheet**. Most complex proteins contain a mixture of these two structures.

α-*Helix*

The α-helix is a rod-like structure in which the peptide chain coils clockwise about a central axis. The helix is stabilized by intramolecular hydrogen bonds between carbonyl oxygen atoms and amine hydrogen atoms four residues away. The side-chains point away from the structure's core and interact with the cellular environment. A typical protein with this structure is **keratin**, which is found in feathers and hair.

β-*Pleated sheet*

In β-pleated sheets, the peptide chains lie alongside each other in rows. The chains are held together by intramolecular hydrogen bonds between carbonyl oxygen atoms on one peptide chain and amine hydrogen atoms on another. In order to accommodate the maximum number of hydrogen bonds, the β-pleated sheet assumes a rippled, or pleated, shape. The R-groups of the amino residues point above and below the plane of the β-pleated sheet. Silk fibers are composed of β-pleated sheets.

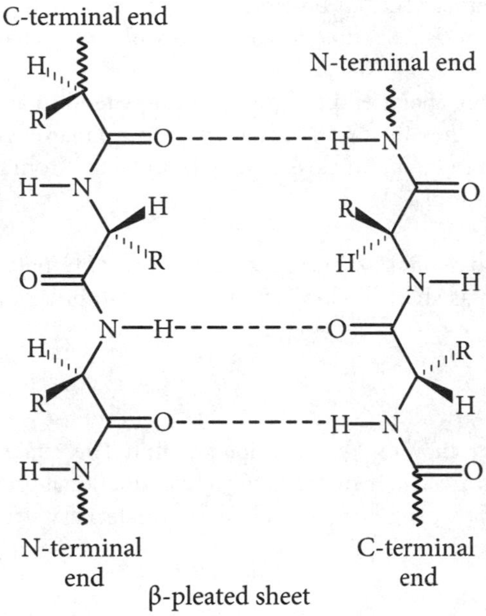

Figure 52.15

Tertiary Structure

Tertiary structure refers to the three-dimensional shape of the protein as determined by hydrophilic and hydrophobic interactions between the R-groups of amino acids that are far apart on the chain and by the distribution of disulfide bonds. In a disulfide bond, two **cysteine** molecules become oxidized to form **cystine**. Disulfide bonds create loops in the protein chain.

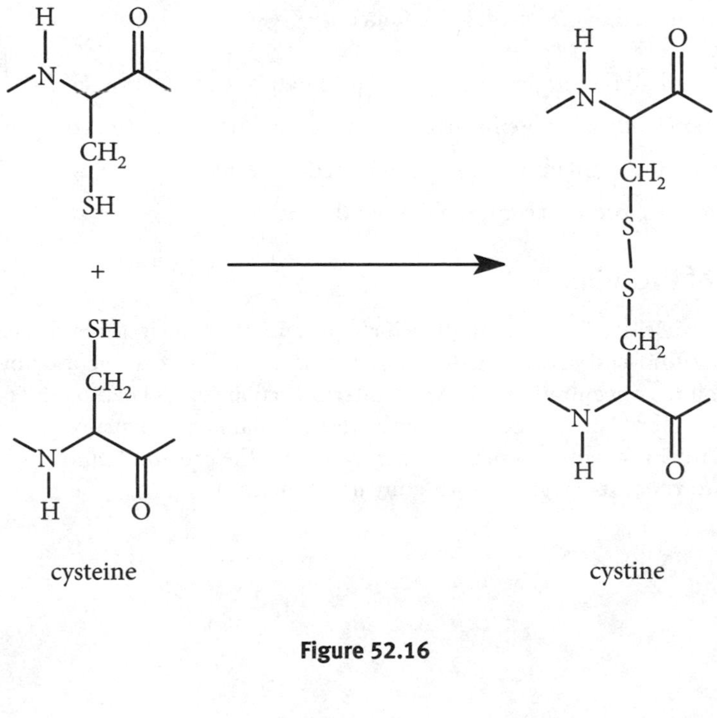

Figure 52.16

Other amino acids have significant effects on tertiary structures as well. For instance, proline, because of its shape, cannot fit into an α-helix, thereby causing a kink in the chain.

Amino acids with hydrophilic (polar and charged) R-groups tend to arrange themselves toward the outside of the protein where they interact with the aqueous cellular environment. Amino acids with hydrophobic R-groups tend to be found close together, protected from the aqueous environment by polar amino and carboxyl groups.

Proteins are divided into two major classifications on the basis of tertiary structure. **Fibrous proteins**, such as **collagen**, are found as sheets or long strands, while **globular proteins**, such as **myoglobin**, are spherical in shape.

Quaternary Structure

Some proteins contain more than one polypeptide subunit. The quaternary structure refers to the way in which these subunits arrange themselves to yield a functional protein molecule. **Hemoglobin**, which is composed of four polypeptide chains, possesses quaternary structure.

Conjugated Proteins

Certain proteins, known as **conjugated proteins**, derive part of their function from covalently attached molecules called **prosthetic groups**. This means at least one portion of their structure is not made of protein. Prosthetic groups may be organic molecules or metal ions. Many vitamins are prosthetic groups. Proteins with lipid, carbohydrate, and nucleic acid prosthetic groups are referred to as **lipoproteins**, **glycoproteins**, and **nucleoproteins**, respectively. Prosthetic groups play major roles in determining the function of the proteins with which they are associated. For example, the **heme group** carries oxygen in both myoglobin and hemoglobin. The heme is composed of an organic porphyrin ring with an iron atom bound in the center. Hemoglobin is inactive without the heme group.

Some other important conjugated proteins include:

- Albumins and globulins: primarily globular in nature and function as carriers or enzymes
- Scleroproteins: fibrous proteins that act as structural proteins (e.g., collagen)
- Chromoproteins: proteins bound to pigmented molecules
- Metalloproteins: proteins complexed around a metal ion

Denaturation of Proteins

Denaturation, or **melting**, is a process in which proteins lose their three-dimensional structure and revert to a **random-coil** state. Denaturation can be caused by detergent or by changes in pH, temperature, or solute concentration. The weak intermolecular forces keeping the protein stable and functional are disrupted. When a protein denatures, the damage is usually permanent. However, certain gentle denaturing agents do not permanently disrupt the protein. Removing the reagent might allow the protein to **renature** (regain its structure and function).

REVIEW PROBLEMS

1. If a mixture of alanine (pI = 6) and aspartic acid (pI = 3) is subjected to electrophoresis at pH 3, which of the following would you expect to occur?

   (A) Alanine will migrate to the cathode while aspartic acid migrates to the anode.
   (B) Alanine will not move while aspartic acid migrates to the cathode.
   (C) Aspartic acid will not move while alanine migrates to the cathode.
   (D) Alanine will migrate to the anode while aspartic acid migrates to the cathode.

2. In a neutral solution, most amino acids exist as

   (A) positively charged compounds.
   (B) zwitterions.
   (C) negatively charged compounds.
   (D) hydrophobic molecules.

3. What would be the charge of the following amino acid at pH 7?

   $$HOOCCH_2CH_2CHCOOH$$
   $$| \atop NH_2$$

   (A) Neutral
   (B) Negative
   (C) Positive
   (D) None of the above

4. If the following amino acid (pI = 9.74) in acidic solution is completely titrated with sodium hydroxide, what will its charge be at a pH of 3, 7, and 11?

   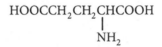

   (A) Positive, neutral, negative
   (B) Negative, neutral, positive
   (C) Neutral, positive, positive
   (D) Positive, positive, negative

5. Amino acids with nonpolar R-groups have which of the following characteristics in aqueous solution?

   (A) They are hydrophilic and found buried within proteins.
   (B) They are hydrophobic and found buried within proteins.
   (C) They are hydrophobic and found on protein surfaces.
   (D) They are hydrophilic and found on protein surfaces.

6. All of the following statements concerning peptide bonds are true EXCEPT:

   (A) Their formation involves a reaction between an amine group and a carboxyl group.
   (B) They are the primary bonds found in proteins.
   (C) They have partial double-bond character.
   (D) Their formation involves hydration reactions.

7. How many different tripeptides can be formed that contain one valine, one alanine, and one leucine?

   (A) 5
   (B) 6
   (C) 7
   (D) 8

8. Beside peptide bonds, what other covalent bonds are commonly found in peptides?

   (A) Hydrogen bonds
   (B) Ether bonds
   (C) Disulfide bonds
   (D) Hydrophobic bonds

9. Discuss primary, secondary, tertiary, and quaternary structures in proteins. What are the defining characteristics of each category?

10. α-helices are secondary structures characterized by

    (A) intramolecular hydrogen bonds.
    (B) disulfide bonds.
    (C) a rippled effect.
    (D) intermolecular hydrogen bonds.

11. Denaturation involves the loss of what types of structure?

    (A) Primary
    (B) Secondary
    (C) Tertiary
    (D) Both B and C

SOLUTIONS TO REVIEW PROBLEMS

1. **C** At pH 6, alanine will exist as a neutral, dipolar ion: The amino group will be protonated while the carboxyl group will be deprotonated. Lowering the pH to 3 will result in protonation of the carboxyl group, so the molecule will assume an overall positive charge. Alanine will, therefore, migrate to the cathode. On the other hand, aspartic acid will exist as a neutral dipolar ion at pH 3 since this is equivalent to its isoelectric point. Therefore, when it is subjected to electrophoresis, it will not move. In summary, alanine will migrate to the cathode while aspartic acid will not move, making choice (C) the correct response.

2. **B** Discussed in the section on the acid-base properties of amino acids in this chapter.

3. **B** The amino acid in question is glutamic acid, which is an acidic amino acid because it contains an extra carboxyl group. At neutral pH, both of the carboxyl groups are ionized, so there are two negative charges on the molecule. Only one of the charges is neutralized by the positive charge on the amino group, so the molecule has an overall negative charge. Thus, the answer is choice (B).

4. **D** At pH 3, the amine and carboxyl groups will be protonated to give a net positive charge. As the pH rises to 7, the proton will dissociate from the carboxyl, but both amine groups will still be fully protonated, so the charge will still be positive. At pH 11, the molecule is above its isoelectric point and will be fully deprotonated, resulting in two neutral amine groups and a negatively charged carboxylate group, so the charge at pH 11 will be negative. Therefore, the correct sequence of charges is positive, positive, negative, corresponding to choice (D).

5. **B** Nonpolar molecules or groups are those whose negative and positive centers of charge coincide. They are not soluble in water and are thus hydrophobic. Amino acids with hydrophobic R-groups are considered hydrophobic molecules; they tend to be found buried within protein molecules where they do not have to interact with the aqueous cellular environment. Choices (A) and (D) are incorrect because nonpolar R-groups cannot be hydrophilic. Choice (C) is incorrect because nonpolar molecules are seldom located on the surface of proteins, where they would interact unfavorably with the aqueous cellular environment.

6. **D** Formation of a peptide bond, which is the primary covalent bond found in proteins, involves a condensation reaction between the amine group of one amino acid and the carboxyl group of an adjacent amino acid. As a result of the carbonyl group present at the bond, the double bond resonates between C=O and C=N. This resonance gives the peptide bond a partial double-bond character and limits rotation about the bond. From this information, it can be seen that choices (A), (B), and (C) are all characteristics of the peptide bond. Choice (D) is false because the formation of the peptide bond is a condensation reaction involving the loss of water, rather than a hydration reaction, which involves the addition of water.

7. **B** The 6 tripeptides that can be formed are:

    Val-Ala-Leu, Val-Leu-Ala,

    Ala-Val-Leu, Ala-Leu-Val,

    Leu-Val-Ala, and Leu-Ala-Val.

8. **C** The key word in this question is "covalent." While hydrogen bonds and hydrophobic bonds are involved in peptide structure, they are not considered covalent bonds, since they do not involve sharing electrons. Therefore, choices (A) and (D) are incorrect. Ether bonds are covalent bonds, but they are not found in peptides. The correct answer is disulfide bonds, choice (C). Disulfide bonds are covalent bonds forming between the sulfur-bearing R-groups of cysteines. The resulting cystine molecule constitutes a disulfide bridge and often causes a loop in the peptide chain.

9. Discussed in the section on proteins in this chapter.

10. **A** When discussing secondary structure, the most important bond is the hydrogen bond. The rigid α-helices are held together by hydrogen bonds between the carbonyl oxygen of one peptide bond and the amine hydrogen of a peptide bond four residues away. This hydrogen bond is intramolecular, so choice (A) is correct. Disulfide bonds are covalent bonds usually associated with tertiary structure; therefore, choice (B) is incorrect. Choices (C) and (D) are incorrect since the rippled effect and intermolecular hydrogen bonds are both characteristic of β-pleated sheets.

11. **D** Protein denaturation involves the loss of three-dimensional structure and function. Since the three-dimensional shape of a protein is conferred by secondary and tertiary structures, denaturation disrupts these structures. Therefore, both choices (B) and (C) are correct. Denaturation does not cause a loss of primary structure since it does not cause peptide bonds to break; thus, choice (A) is incorrect.

CHAPTER FIFTY-THREE

Lipids

Lipids vary immensely in their structural organization and biological function. As a class they are characterized by insolubility in water and solubility in nonpolar organic solvents. Functionally, however, they play roles in cell structure, signaling, and energy storage, among other things. Examples of structural lipids include phospholipids and sterols, which are major components of membranes and liposomes. Lipids are also major players in signaling and function as cofactors, hormones, and intracellular messengers. In terms of energy storage, lipids store the most energy per unit weight of any molecule in the human body.

STRUCTURAL LIPIDS

Structural lipids are a major component of the phospholipid bilayer. The structure of phospholipids—hydrophilic head and hydrophobic tail—allows for bilayer formation and protects the cell from the surrounding environment. Phospholipids are **amphipathic**, meaning they have both hydrophilic and hydrophobic regions. This allows the formation of other structures in addition to the phospholipid bilayer, such as micelles and liposomes.

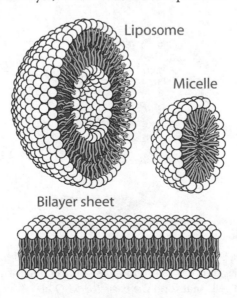

Figure 53.1

Phospholipids

Phospholipids have a polar hydrophilic head (made up of a phosphate and an alcohol) joined to a hydrophobic fatty acid tail by phosphodiester linkages. The number of fatty acid tails attached to the polar head can vary according to the type of phospholipid. Different molecules also provide the structure upon which the phospholipid is built. For example, glycerol, which is a three-carbon alcohol molecule, makes up **phosphoglycerides** and **glycerophospholipids**, whereas **sphingolipids** have a sphingosine backbone.

All lipids have a fatty acid tail. This chain can vary in both saturation and length. Fully **saturated** fatty acid tails have only single bonds (therefore, each carbon is bonded to four other atoms). These fatty acids are more stable and form solids at room temperature; these are the fatty acids found in butter. **Unsaturated** fatty acids have one or more double bonds in their structure, which create kinks in the fatty acid chains. This keeps the chains from stacking on top of each other and solidifying; therefore, these fats tend to be liquid at room temperature (e.g., olive oil). This is also why the phospholipid bilayer acts fluidly at body temperature.

Most double bonds in fatty acids are in the *cis-* configuration. *Trans-* double bonds, often referred to as *trans*-fatty acids, manifest when partially hydrogenated vegetable oils are used in production. These fatty acids decrease membrane fluidity and, along with saturated fatty acids, are associated with increased risk of atherosclerosis.

Glycerophospholipids

Glycerophospholipids are a type of phospholipid that contains a glycerol backbone. Depending on the type of glycerol in the head group, the name of the phospholipid varies. These head groups can be positively or negatively charged or they can be neutral. This polarity can dictate the glycerophospholipid's role in cell recognition, signaling, binding, and so forth. As in all phospholipids, the fatty acid chains can vary in length and saturation, introducing another variation in the lipid's structure. Glycerophospholipids are important components in membrane synthesis.

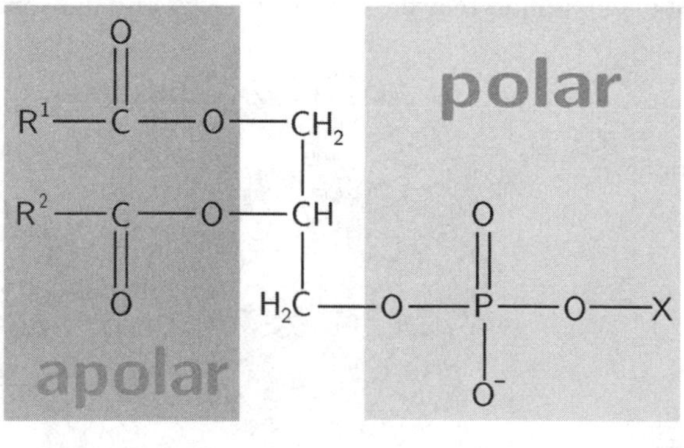

Figure 53.2

Sphingolipids

Sphingolipids have a sphingosine or sphingoid backbone and have long, nonpolar fatty acid tails and polar head groups as in other phospholipids. An example of a sphingolipid is the antigens on the surface of red blood cells that form the basis for ABO blood typing.

Waxes

Waxes consist of esters of long chain fatty acids with long chain alcohols. They form malleable solids at room temperature and function biologically as protection against the environment. In humans, waxes help prevent dehydration and provide lubrication.

SIGNALING LIPIDS

Lipids serve many roles in signaling within the body. They are coenzymes in the electron transport chain and are hormones that can carry biological signals over long distances. They also function as intracellular messengers that respond to extracellular signals. Some lipids also have conjugated double bonds that allow them to absorb light or act as pigments. Three major types of signaling lipids exist: steroids, prostaglandins, and fat-soluble vitamins.

Steroids

Steroids differ dramatically from the lipid structures described thus far. They are composed of four cycloalkane rings fused together. The functionality of steroids is determined by the oxidation status of these rings and the functional groups they carry. Because of the ring structure of these lipids (and the large number of carbons and hydrogens present), steroids are nonpolar.

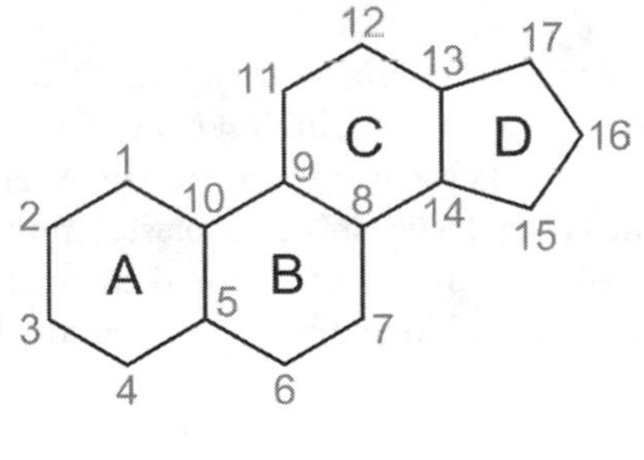

Figure 53.3

One important steroid is **cholesterol**. It is a major component of the phospholipid bilayer and helps maintain the fluidity of the bilayer. Like phospholipids, cholesterol is amphipathic and has both hydrophilic and hydrophobic parts. As a result, it can interact with both the hydrophobic tails and hydrophilic heads of phospholipids, allowing it to help maintain the fluidity of the membrane. Cholesterol also helps stabilize the cell membrane against changes in temperature. At high temperatures it keeps the membrane from becoming too permeable; at low temperatures it keeps the membrane from solidifying. It also is an important precursor to other molecules, including steroid hormones, bile acids, and vitamin D.

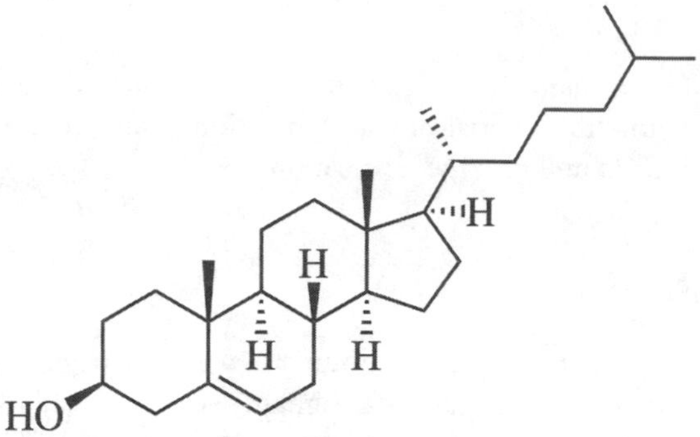

Figure 53.4

Cholesterol can be made by the body or absorbed from dietary sources. High cholesterol, or **hypercholesterolemia**, occurs when the sum of these two sources results in too much cholesterol in the body. High cholesterol is correlated with heart disease, as accumulation of cholesterol on the walls of the arteries leads to **atherosclerosis**. This is a hardening of the arterial walls caused by formation of plaques in the arteries. These plaques have the potential to dislodge from the surface of the arterial wall and subsequently lodge in another part of the body. If this occurs in the heart, it can lead to a myocardial infarction, or heart attack.

In patients with hypercholesterolemia, a common treatment is a HMG-CoA reductase inhibitor. These drugs, such as atorvastatin and simvastatin, inhibit cholesterol synthesis in the liver by blocking the action of HMG-CoA reductase, a key enzyme in the cholesterol synthesis pathway. Another treatment for hypercholesterolemia is cholestyramine. Cholestyramine induces the liver to increase its synthesis of cholesterol, thereby reducing the levels of stored cholesterol in the liver. This induces the liver to take up more cholesterol from the blood and reduces circulating cholesterol levels.

Prostaglandins

Prostaglandins are 20-carbon molecules that are also unsaturated carboxylic acids. They are derived from arachidonic acid and contain a five-carbon ring. In many tissues the function of prostaglandins is to regulate the synthesis of cyclic adenosine monophosphate (**cAMP**), a common intracellular messenger. cAMP mediates the action of many other hormones. As a result, prostaglandins can have dramatic effects on muscle function, the sleep-wake cycle, and the elevation of body temperature associated with fever and pain. Nonsteroidal anti-inflammatory drugs (NSAIDs) such as ibuprofen and naproxen inhibit the enzyme cyclooxygenase, which facilitates prostaglandin production.

Omega-3 fatty acids in the diet may be related to a decreased risk of cardiovascular disease. They replace some of the arachidonic acid in platelet membranes, thereby decreasing the ability of platelets to aggregate and resulting in a decrease in serum triglycerides.

Lipid (Fat)-Soluble Vitamins

Vitamins are essential nutrients that cannot be made in the body and therefore must be consumed in the diet. Vitamins can be categorized as either water-soluble or lipid-soluble. Water-soluble vitamins are excreted through the urine, while lipid-soluble vitamins can accumulate in stored fat. As a result, it is possible to overdose on lipid-soluble vitamins because they can accumulate to toxic levels in the body. Lipid-soluble vitamins include vitamins A, D, E, and K.

Vitamin A

Vitamin A is an unsaturated hydrocarbon that has roles in vision, growth and development, and immune function. One metabolite of vitamin A is retinal, a component of the molecular system in the eye that senses light. The storage form of vitamin A, retinol, is oxidized to retinoic acid. Retinoic acid is a hormone that regulates gene expression in epithelial development.

Vitamin D

Vitamin D, also known as **cholecalciferol**, can be consumed in this form directly or can be formed by a reaction in the skin that is driven by UV light. The liver and the kidneys convert cholecalciferol to **calcitriol**, which is the biologically active form of vitamin D. Calcitriol increases calcium and phosphate uptake in the intestines and decreases excretion of calcium in the kidneys. This promotes bone production, which is why calcium supplementation for bone health is recommended to be taken with vitamin D. Without vitamin D, calcium absorption is greatly decreased. Lack of vitamin D in children can lead to rickets, which is characterized by underdeveloped, weak long bones (such as the femur in the leg) and stunted growth.

Vitamin E

Vitamin E describes a group of closely related lipids with a substituted aromatic ring that is characteristically hydrophobic. They can be powerful antioxidants because the aromatic ring reacts with free radicals and destroys them. This prevents oxidative damage, which is an important contributor to aging and the development of cancer.

Vitamin K

Vitamin K includes a number of compounds and is vital to the formation of **prothrombin**. Prothrombin is an important clotting factor in the blood and is required to introduce calcium-binding sites on several calcium-dependent proteins. Warfarin, a commonly used anticoagulant, works by inhibiting vitamin K epoxide reductase. This is an enzyme that returns vitamin K to its reduced form after it helps carboxylate prothrombin and other blood coagulation proteins. If vitamin K cannot return to its reduced form, it cannot continue to help form blood coagulation proteins, making the patient less prone to clotting.

ENERGY STORAGE

Triacylglycerols (also called **triglycerides**) are types of lipids used specifically for energy storage. They are ideal for energy storage for two major reasons. First, the carbon atoms of fatty acids are more reduced than those of sugars, meaning that the oxidation of triglycerides gives twice as much energy per gram as carbohydrates. This makes triglycerides far more energy-dense than polysaccharides. Second, triglycerides are hydrophobic and as a result do not draw in water, thereby decreasing their weight as compared to most other organic molecules. These two factors together allow triglycerides to be both lightweight and energy-rich, making them excellent for long-term energy storage.

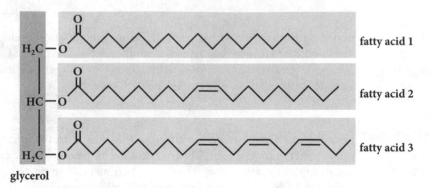

Figure 53.5

Triglyceride Structure

Triglycerides are made of three fatty acids bound to glycerol. The three fatty acids on each triglyceride are usually the same. Triglycerides are generally nonpolar and hydrophobic, making them less soluble in water. Triglyceride deposits can be found in the cytosol of cells. They are reserves of metabolic fuel that can be used when energy supplies within the cell are low. Adipocytes are special cells in animals that store large amounts of fat droplets. These are found mainly under the skin, in mammary glands, and in the abdominal cavity. As with phospholipids, the physical characteristics of triglycerides are largely determined by the saturation of their fatty acid chains.

Free Fatty Acids and Saponification

Free fatty acids circulate through the body bound to albumin. They also constitute soap, which can be produced by **saponification**. Saponification is the hydrolysis of triglycerides by using a strong base (traditionally, this base is lye).

Surfactants lower the surface tension between two solutions. Soaps can act as surfactants, functioning as a detergent or an emulsifier. This helps to combine two phases, such as oil and water, into a single phase via the formation of micelles. Micelles are aggregates of surfactant in which the hydrophobic tails are turned inward and the hydrophilic heads are on the outside. Micelles allow the surfactant to be dispersed into an aqueous solution when normally its hydrophobic tails would prevent this dispersal from occurring.

Formation of micelles allows soap to be an effective cleanser. It is also important in the absorption of fat-soluble vitamins in the body. For instance, the secretions of the gallbladder (bile salts) form micelles that allow for absorption of fatty acids, vitamins, and cholesterol in the small intestine. The pancreas also releases enzymes that degrade lipids into fatty acids and cholesterol. Once absorbed, these lipids are converted to triglycerides and packaged for storage.

REVIEW PROBLEMS

1. What does it mean when phospholipids are said to be amphipathic?

    (A) They are part of micelles.
    (B) They are a type of cholesterol.
    (C) They have both hydrophobic and hydrophilic regions.
    (D) They have a sphingosine backbone.

2. What is the difference between saturated and unsaturated fatty acids and how does this influence their structure?

3. What type of lipid is responsible for ABO blood typing?

    (A) Waxes
    (B) Glycerophospholipids
    (C) Phospholipids
    (D) Sphingolipids

4. Explain the role of cholesterol in stabilizing the cell membrane.

5. Describe the major functions of each of the fat-soluble vitamins.

6. What type of lipid is the best for energy storage?

    (A) Prostaglandins
    (B) Triglycerides
    (C) Cholesterol
    (D) Steroids

7. How are surfactants able to combine two separate phases (such as oil and water) into one phase?

SOLUTIONS TO REVIEW PROBLEMS

1. **C** Amphipathic molecules have both polar and nonpolar regions. While micelles are composed of amphipathic molecules, not all amphipathic molecules are micelles. Types of cholesterol were not discussed in this chapter. Some phospholipids that are amphipathic do have a sphingosine backbone, but that is not a requirement of an amphipathic molecule.

2. Saturated fatty acids have only single bonds (no double bonds) between their carbons, whereas unsaturated fatty acids do have double bonds. Double bonds create kinks in the fatty acid chain, which do not allow the fatty acids to pack as tightly together. This creates fats that are liquid at room temperature (e.g., oils) rather than solid at room temperature (e.g., butter).

3. **D** The antigen present on the surface of red blood cells is a type of sphingolipid, a class. This antigen determines the ABO blood type of red blood cells.

4. Cholesterol stabilizes the cell membrane by maintaining its fluidity. At high temperatures it prevents the membrane from becoming too permeable, and at low temperatures it prevents the membrane from becoming too solid. Its amphipathic nature allows it to interact with both the hydrophilic heads and the hydrophobic tails of the phospholipid bilayer.

5. Vitamin A is important in immune function, growth and development, and vision. Vitamin D is important in bone development. Vitamin E functions as an antioxidant. Vitamin K helps in the creation of prothrombin, which assists in blood clotting.

6. **B** Triglycerides are ideal for energy storage because the carbon atoms in its fatty acids are highly reduced and oxidation of these bonds provides a large amount of energy. Triglycerides are also hydrophobic and therefore do not draw in water, which decreases their weight.

7. Surfactants lower the surface tension between two solutions by forming micelles. In micelles, the hydrophobic tails are turned inward and the hydrophilic heads are on the outside, allowing the surfactanct to go into solution and create one phase.

Section VIII

READING COMPREHENSION

CHAPTER FIFTY-FOUR

Reading Critically

To do well on Reading Comprehension on Test Day, you need to read critically and understand why the author presents certain information. Preparing for this section, therefore, is an interesting task. You won't see any lengthy calculations, and you don't need to memorize complex science concepts. Instead, the best ways to study involve learning strategies, applying them to the reading you do from now until Test Day, and completing practice passages.

THE READING COMPREHENSION PASSAGE

The Reading Comprehension portion of the exam contains six short passages consisting of four to seven paragraphs and 500–600 words. Each passage pertains to natural science, social science, humanities, health, nutrition, medicine, or technology and an ethical, social, cultural, or political issue that affects it, either theoretically or in practice. The intent of the author may be to inform, persuade, or speculate, but usually the author's tone remains roughly neutral due to the nature of the content. Subtle clues may indicate an author is for or against certain ideas, but these opinions will rarely be extreme.

Outside knowledge of each field is not required to answer questions correctly in this section, and the passages are meant to cover material you do not already know. Nevertheless, rough familiarity with the general vocabulary and writing style used in each field can build your confidence and speed you up on Test Day. Reading through recent editions of journals, such as the *Journal of the American Pharmaceutical Association* and *Science*, and magazines, such as *National Geographic* and *Scientific American,* will increase your familiarity with this type of material.

Each of the six passages will be accompanied by eight questions for a total of 48 questions per section. Because you will have 50 minutes total to complete this section, allot approximately eight minutes per passage: three minutes for reading the passage and five minutes for answering the eight questions. This will give you approximately 35 seconds per question. Neither every passage nor every question should take the same amount of time due to varying difficulty and length, so use these numbers as guidelines rather than hard rules.

PCAT READING

Reading Comprehension questions are *always* about the corresponding passage. You are not necessarily looking for the answer choices that are the most factual but rather those that correspond best with the author and the passage. If you do have prior knowledge in a field, you must be careful not to apply that to the questions and instead only answer based on the information in the passage. Therefore, before you can tackle a Reading Comprehension question, you must read at least some of the corresponding passage.

There are four things you really need to know about PCAT reading:

First, you're not reading to learn anything. This is not information you need to carry with you for years, months, weeks, or even hours. You just need to use it in the next few minutes, and you will even be able to refer back to the passage when you need it.

Second, you're not reading to remember anything. If you try to remember what you read, you'll rely on memory—which is notoriously faulty—and your mind will be taken up with what you're trying to remember. That's not helpful. Your mind needs to be open and focused on the really important parts of the PCAT: the questions. Anything you think is important enough to remember will go on your map, which is discussed later in this chapter.

Third, you don't need any outside knowledge or your own leaps of logic to read the passage well. All the correct answers are supported in the passage. As stated previously, if you use what you already know, you'll be tempted to answer questions based on your own knowledge and not on the passage. That's a classic way to choose wrong answers.

And fourth, you're not reading to understand everything. After all, if there's no question on the part you didn't understand, it doesn't matter anyway. So you're not going to read and reread; you're just going to keep moving ahead and let the questions determine what you need to reread.

Considering all these points together shows that reading on the PCAT is quite different from reading almost anything else. Therefore, how you approach the passages in the Reading Comprehension section should be different from how you read anything else. Don't fall into the easy trap of approaching the passages as you would a novel or even a textbook; instead, read critically to set yourself up for success when you get to the questions. After all, answering those questions correctly is your primary goal on Test Day, so everything you do should directly serve that goal, including how you read.

Reading Critically

Ordinarily, people read for one or both of two reasons: to learn something or to pass the time pleasantly. Neither of these reasons has anything to do with the PCAT. So what do you really need to get from reading a PCAT passage that's different from everyday reading? Broadly stated, there are two primary goals in reading a PCAT passage: reading for purpose—the *why* of the text and *what* the author wants you to learn from the passage—and reading for structure— the *how* of the text and the way in which the author presents the ideas. Every PCAT Reading Comprehension question type fundamentally hinges on your ability to step back from the text and analyze *what* the author is stating, *why* the author is writing in the first place, and *how* the author puts the text together.

Notice the theme here: it's all about the author. You'll get questions about the author's ideas, her purpose, what can be inferred from her passage, and how she puts it together. If you understand little more than the author's intent, you'll still have enough to get started with the questions, so your focus as you read must always be on the author. Therefore, pay attention not only to what details are present and where they are but also why they are there. Details are the *what* of a passage, and they never exist in a vacuum; they always support an idea.

Since the majority of the Reading Comprehension question types requires only these big-picture ideas, don't get caught up in the details themselves as you read. Instead, skim over details quickly, then reread them more closely only when a question demands it. In fact, if you follow this strategy, you won't ever need to read or understand most of the details in a passage. If every question associated with a passage were a Detail question (and they won't be), each question could still generally test only one detail, meaning you would need approximately one detail per paragraph at most. Even in this extreme situation, all the other details in the passage would not be worth any points. If you spent a significant portion of your time poring over the passage to learn and memorize all the information contained within it, you would have wasted the majority of your time. Rather than spend your time on a task not directly earning you points, quickly read through the passage for main ideas and only return to specific details when necessary.

Nevertheless, although reading all the content carefully is a waste of time, don't take that too far. There's no payoff in getting through a passage with zero comprehension. Instead, know what is important in a passage and what is not. The author's ideas are important; the details can always be researched if there are questions regarding them (all it takes to find a detail in that case is for you to shift your eyes over to view the passage, which will always be on the screen next to each of its questions). Remember that the PCAT is a timed test; use your time wisely and focus on the author when reading the first time through, saving the details for a second, targeted look if a question demands it.

Using Keywords

To help you read quickly without missing important information, pay special attention to keywords, the specific words or phrases that provide structure to text. By training your eye to notice these essential words, you will be able to skim through much of each PCAT passage, slowing down to read more thoroughly only when you know an important idea is coming next. As you review the following types of keywords, add your own words to watch out for on Test Day.

Continuation keywords announce that more of the same is about to come up. Some of the most common Continuation words and phrases include:

also	*furthermore*	*in addition*	*as well as*
moreover	*plus*	*at the same time*	*equally*

Also (there's a keyword for you), the colon often does the same job: It tells you that what follows expands upon what came before, as do commas, semicolons, and dashes. When you see a Continuation keyword of any type, you can generally keep skimming if you understood what came before it since no new ideas are likely to follow.

Sequence keywords tell you there's an order to the author's ideas. Some examples are:

second (and third, fourth, etc.)	*next*
finally	*recently*

Similar to Continuation keywords, Sequence keywords show you more of the same is coming, so keep skimming.

Illustration keywords signal that an example is about to arrive. *For example* and *for instance* are very common. But think about these:

in the words of Hannah Arendt	*according to* these experts
as Maya Angelou *says*	*for* historians
to Proust	Toynbee *claims* that

In each case, what's about to follow is an example of that person's thinking. Illustration keywords also indicate you can keep skimming, but you may want to take note of any vocabulary terms or other important words that follow so you know where to return should you be required to answer a question about that detail.

Evidence keywords tell you that the author is about to provide support for a point. Here are the four most common evidence keywords:

because	*for*	*since*	*the reason is*

Although evidence keywords do show you the same point is continued, they also indicate that the author's underlying logic is coming next. If you don't have a strong grasp of the *why* behind an argument yet, you may need to pay more attention here. Otherwise, keep moving.

Contrast keywords signal an opposition or shift. There are lots of these words:

but	*however*	*although*	*not*
nevertheless	*despite*	*alternatively*	*unless*
though	*by contrast*	*yet*	*still*
otherwise	*while*	*notwithstanding*	

Contrast keywords are among the most significant in Reading Comprehension because so many passages are based on contrast or opposition. Almost certainly, something important is happening when a Contrast keyword shows up, so slow down here to ensure you follow where the argument is going next. If you are an advanced reader, you may be able to anticipate what's coming next, saving you the time of slowing down, but verify that you anticipated correctly before continuing.

Emphasis keywords may be the most welcome. Since you are reading for the author's point of view, there are no better sections to pay attention to than those where the author announces that he finds something to be important. Note these well:

above all	*most of all*	*primarily*	*in large measure*
essentially	*especially*	*particularly*	*indeed*

These words serve as great hints that the information will show up on a question, so definitely read what follows.

Conclusion keywords signal the author is about to sum up or announce the thesis. The most common is *therefore*, together with the following:

thus	*consequently*	*hence*	*in conclusion*
it can be seen	*so*	*we conclude*	*therefore*

Because these keywords have to do with the author's logic, they are especially crucial for Reading Comprehension, especially when determining the overall purpose of the passage. Slow down and read these.

THE PASSAGE MAP

To make the most of your limited reading time, take quick notes on your noteboard as you finish reading each paragraph. These notes will make up your roadmap, a literal map of the passage that shows you where to look when you need to go back and find a specific detail. Forming a roadmap also helps guide your thought processes during your first pass. You can feel confident reading quickly and focusing on the big picture ideas while ignoring most of the details because you will know exactly where to look should the need for one of those details arise.

Every passage map has four major components:

Topic: the author's basic, broad subject matter, such as *antibiotics, volcanoes,* or *the PCAT*. The passages on the PCAT will be titled according to their Topics, so you should be able to ascertain this within the first five seconds of reading.

Scope: the specific aspect of the topic that is the focus of an individual paragraph. The scope shifts throughout the passage but always relates back to the topic. For example, if the topic of a passage is *antibiotics*, the paragraphs might have scopes of *penicillins and cephalosporins, mechanisms,* and *side effects*.

Tone: the author's attitude toward the material at hand. Since PCAT passages are related to science topics, most authors attempt to maintain relatively neutral stances, but subtle clues can indicate if an author is *positive, negative,* or truly *neutral* toward the subject matter.

Purpose: the reason why the author wrote the passage or how he is trying to change your mind. The purpose is always a verb, such as to *explain, evaluate, argue,* or *compare*.

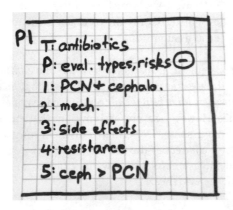

Figure 54.1

Each passage map component can convey extensive meanings, but your actual notes only need to contain enough information to help you remember the broader ideas. Make use of your own shorthand to ensure your notes for each item average approximately two to three words each. When you've finished your passage map, you should have written one overall topic, purpose, and tone for the entire passage and one scope for each individual paragraph, such as in Figure 54.1, above.

DISSECTING AN ARGUMENT

Some Reading Comprehension questions ask about the structure of a passage and the function of specific words, sentences, or paragraphs. Being able to characterize each component of the passage into such categories as supporting evidence or refutation, analogy or example, detail or inference, and fact or opinion means you not only will be able to answer questions that ask for exactly that but you will also have a deeper understanding of the passage as a whole, which is helpful for any question.

Parts of an Argument

An **argument**, in literary terms, is a set of reasons an author uses to convince you of some point. Sometimes an author is attempting to persuade you into supporting (or refuting) a theory; other times, he is simply teaching you new information. Either way, the author wants you to believe his main idea or **conclusion**. The evidence, examples, and logic the author uses to support that conclusion and prove he is correct are the **evidence**.

When the author directly states these ideas in the passage, they can be called **explicit**. However, sometimes the author doesn't include either the conclusion or all the evidence plainly in his writing and instead requires you to determine some of them on your own because the ideas are only **implied**.

If the author sets up all the evidence but forces you to realize his conclusion yourself, then you are making an **inference.** This can be a strong literary technique; if you come to a conclusion on your own rather than being told, you often are more likely to believe it. However, this does require some (minimal) work on your part, so the test makers use Inferences as one of their question types.

Assumptions, or implied evidence, are tested much less often on the PCAT. Not all possible types of evidence qualify as assumptions; instead, only the pieces of evidence required for the argument to make sense logically are classified as assumptions.

Consider the example of this statement: *Doberman Pinschers have bitten children, so no one should own any dogs.* The conclusion the speaker wants you to believe is that *no one should own any dogs;* the evidence is that *Doberman Pinschers have bitten children.* Since the conclusion is stated explicitly, you don't need to make an inference. However, several assumptions that the speaker believes to be obvious must be true for the logic to make sense: Doberman Pinschers must be representative of all dogs; otherwise, the evidence does not connect to the conclusion of *any* dog. Additionally, children being bitten must be unfavorable; if the listener actually wants children to be bitten, then the conclusion once again does not align with the evidence.

Facts and Opinions

The evidence of an argument can be further classified as fact or opinion. A **fact** is an unbiased observation or something that is irrefutable. An **opinion** interjects the author's feelings on or evaluation of a subject. To identify each, watch for the specific phrasing the author uses. Words like *should* and *seems* and phrases like in *my opinion* and *I believe* are good clues that the author is describing an opinion, but sometimes the clues are more subtle. When you need to differentiate between fact and opinion, such as in the following exercise, consider whether everyone would agree given the same data (fact) or if there could be multiple interpretations (opinion).

Practice exercise

Directions: Determine whether each statement is a fact or the author's opinion.

1. To assert that the ideal of democratic rule began with the Magna Carta is to misunderstand that the document was actually the product of a power struggle between two factions—the throne and the nobility—that were completely unconcerned about the rights of the common man.

2. Frank Lloyd Wright's designs are still held in very high regard by both the architectural community and the general public.

3. The federal government has claimed for years that reforms to make the income tax system more progressive will soon be enacted, but this seems very unlikely in light of the government's disinterest in easing the burden on low and middle-income wage earners.

4. Some scientists believe that a layer of iridium in the Earth's crust proves a comet struck the planet, wiping out the dinosaurs; others argue that this layer was formed as the result of volcanic activity.

5. Astronomers long ago established that nebulas—clouds of interstellar gas and dust—are regions of space that give birth to new starts.

6. Literary critics have rightly concluded that the interest in "ethnic inheritance" displayed by George Eliot in her novels was sparked by her inability to feel comfortable in her own surroundings.

Solutions to practice exercise

1. **Opinion:** the statement refutes a *misunderstanding* of the Magna Carta held by others.
2. **Fact:** the statement repeats a generally acknowledged truth about Frank Lloyd Wright.
3. **Opinion:** the statement takes issue with the government's claim about taxes that *seems* unlikely.
4. **Fact:** the statement describes two different views about the origins of the iridium layer.
5. **Fact:** the statement repeats a scientific observation about the birth of stars.
6. **Opinion:** the statement describes a generally accepted interpretation of George Eliot's work as *right*.

CHAPTER FIFTY-FIVE

Question Types

The PCAT test makers use the same types of questions in every Reading Comprehension section. You'll see some **comprehension** questions that test about basic facts from the passage, but you can expect other questions that test a deeper understanding of the ideas through **analysis** and **evaluation**, so it's important to be prepared for various levels of critical thinking. Although you won't earn any points directly by identifying what type each question is on Test Day, identifying question types will help you make efficient predictions and avoid wrong answers.

QUESTION TYPES

Global

Global questions test how well you understand the passage as a whole and ask for the main idea, conclusion, or thesis of a passage or paragraph. If you follow Kaplan's passage mapping strategy (see Chapter 54, Reading Critically), then you will already have determined the overall topic and purpose of the passage as well as the scope of each paragraph before reading any of the questions. When you do reach a Global question, all you need to do is predict the answer based on your written passage map. You can identify Global questions by their use of phrases such as *main purpose, title,* or *overall point.* Although each passage generally does not have more than one Global question, these can be quick points on Test Day.

Detail

Detail questions ask about statements found explicitly in the passage. These questions are often preceded by the phrase *according to the passage.* Detail questions are *not* asking about your own logic but merely about a statement directly from the passage. The best strategy for these questions is to use your notes as a literal map to show you where in the passage you should go to research the answer. You should be able to find phrasing in the passage that exactly or nearly exactly matches the correct answer choice. If you find yourself frequently missing Detail questions, ensure you are spending enough time researching; one hint is to not let yourself select the correct answer until you can point to the place in the passage that directly supports the answer choice you believe is correct.

Scattered detail

Many questions ask you to choose the one answer that is true based on the passage. Scattered detail questions reverse this and ask you to choose the one answer that is FALSE. These questions have phrasing similar to *the author mentions all of these items EXCEPT*. Three of the answer choices will appear in the passage, and one won't, so using the process of elimination is useful for these questions. Note, however, that finding three separate facts from a passage can be a slow process, so consider making quick educated guesses and saving thorough evaluation of these questions for last if you are running out of time in a section.

Tone

The author's tone or bias is rarely stated directly in a passage but is often heavily implied. Although the author of a passage may not say "I love penguins" verbatim, he may use words to describe them that indicate his opinion, such as *fascinating, remarkable, interesting,* and *superior,* to make his bias clear. Looking for these types of Opinion keywords while initially reading makes answering Tone questions straightforward, and a good prediction is one based on the overall tone of positive, negative, or neutral from your passage map. Tone questions tend to include clear indicators of their type, such as the words *tone, bias,* or *feels.*

Vocab-in-Context

Vocab-in-Context questions ask about the meanings of words or phrases in context of the passage. Unlike in the Verbal Ability section, you are not expected to know the definitions of these terms ahead of time but rather determine the meaning based on their use in the passage. When confronted with one of these questions, you should take the time to research where in the passage the phrase in question occurred and use context clues to help you determine what the author meant by including that phrase.

Many words or phrases could have multiple definitions, but only the meaning that makes sense in the context of the passage will be counted as the correct answer. For example, the word *sanction* might be used to mean "to give permission" but could also mean "to discipline or punish," so the context of its use needs to be determined to correctly evaluate its meaning. Be especially careful when a question is about a relatively common word since the usual, primary definition might not be the correct answer.

Evaluation

An extremely prevalent question type on the PCAT requires you to evaluate the way the author constructed his argument. A limited knowledge of rhetorical strategies is helpful in answering these kinds of questions. Authors might use rhetorical questions, analogies, counterexamples, or other techniques that can be asked about in Evaluation questions. There are two subtypes of Evaluation questions: Function and Structure question. As with other question types, you will want to refer back to the passage and to your map to identify the correct answer.

Structure

Structure questions are a type of Evaluation question that asks about how the author organized the passage or a part of the passage. A question might ask about the flow of the passage, requiring you to identify where the author's conclusion is within the passage and how other paragraphs relate to the author's main point. Your roadmap will be especially helpful in these kinds of questions because you'll already have an idea of how the passage was put together and can use that as your prediction. Other questions might be about specific sentences and require you to determine if the author is stating a fact or offering an opinion. When answering questions about fact versus opinion, refer back to the passage to check the context of the clause referred to in the question stem. These questions rely heavily on your ability to recognize keywords in the passage, which will frequently be sufficient to clue you in to the answer.

Function

This subtype of Evaluation question takes the task in the Structure subtype one step further. Not only do you need to recognize how the author constructed the argument using rhetorical techniques, but you need to be able to consider *why* the author did something in the passage. Function questions will ask you something like *Why did the author include X phrase?* or *What function does X serve in the passage?* To answer this kind of question, start by determining in which paragraph the detail in question occurred, then evaluate how that sentence or clause relates to the paragraph's scope, which should already be in your roadmap. If the relationship is unclear, you can find more clues by going back to the passage and looking at the sentences near the phrase in question to identify more of the context. Consider what effect the phrase has on the rest of the paragraph or overall argument. Often these questions can be answered by identifying whether a statement is the author's conclusion or supporting evidence.

Some Function questions might ask about the purpose of one paragraph and how it fits in with the rest of the passage. The question stems are usually very straightforward in these instances, asking things like *What was the purpose of paragraph X?* For this style of question, check how the paragraph's scope relates to the entire passage's purpose, both of which should already be in your roadmap. You'll likely find that these questions are fairly quick to answer.

Inference

Inference questions test your ability to use the information in the passage to draw conclusions. They may be worded in a variety of ways, such as *it can be inferred from the passage* or *the phrase X implies*. Inference questions ask you to read between the lines and find the relationships between ideas. The correct answer will be a small step from what is said directly in the passage—but only a small step. Most Inference questions have strong clues in the passage, such as a specific detail, word choice, or tone, that will help you determine just what the author is trying to convey. Although the correct answer may not be stated explicitly in the passage, you can still determine it by restating something that was stated or by combining ideas from two different sentences in the passage. Stick to the evidence in the text and avoid any answer choices that seem far-fetched.

Effectiveness

The final PCAT question type asks you to determine the effectiveness of a statement an author makes in the passage. These questions are unique in that they require you to do a bit of a critique of the passage. You can recognize these questions because they will ask things such as *Which best evaluates the effectiveness of X?* Most questions will ask about the effectiveness of evidence as support for the author's conclusion.

When faced with an Effectiveness question, your first step is to find the segment of the passage referenced and identify how it relates to the text that comes before and after. If the excerpt comes from the very beginning of a paragraph, consider how it relates to the entire previous paragraph as well. This will be enough information to formulate a strong prediction for some questions, but other problems ask you to take that knowledge one step further and evaluate how well that information supports the author's other ideas. In this case, be careful not to include too much personal opinion. Instead, find where the author has mentioned similar ideas before. If all the pieces point to the same conclusion, then these constitute strong evidence; if the pieces instead show opposite or incompatible perspectives, then the author's argument is not being strengthened. Tackling these questions in this way turns them into exercises in matching similar pieces, which is generally easier than considering one element in the abstract.

TRIAGING

Another benefit of identifying question types is that some types are answered in less time than others. The order of the question types listed above is an approximate order of difficulty. Typically, Global and Tone questions can be answered fairly quickly by referring to your map. Vocab-in-Context questions usually direct you to a specific place in the passage, and these questions tend to be less challenging questions, so you will likely find that you can answer them fairly quickly. Similarly, most Detail questions direct you to a specific place in the passage and require that you simply recognize or comprehend the detail in question. However, remember that Scattered Detail questions may be more time-consuming since they can require the process of elimination, which is slower than prediction. Evaluation, Inference, and Effectiveness questions all require higher level skills, so may be more challenging and slightly more time-consuming. You might want to answer the lower level questions first and then tackle the higher level questions when working on a passage. Often, a lower level question will help you answer a more challenging question, saving you time and earning you even more points on Test Day.

WRONG ANSWER PATHOLOGIES

Although identifying question types can help with making clear predictions of the correct answer choice, it can sometimes be just as important to know what makes an answer choice wrong as what makes one right. Wrong answer choices fall into predictable categories, and analyzing those categories allows you to get inside the mind of the test writers, which is key to maximizing your score. By identifying the common traps the test makers use, you can quickly avoid them and more easily match your predictions.

Note that many wrong answer choices correspond with multiple wrong answer pathologies. It's not important to definitively identify what makes an answer choice most wrong. Instead, as soon as you realize an answer choice is incorrect for any reason, eliminate it and keep moving. Likewise, if you have found the correct answer, don't spend time evaluating why each wrong answer choice is incorrect; in fact, evaluating all of the choices is one of the most common reasons for running out of time during a section. Instead, only use the wrong answer pathologies to aid in quickly making matches and when using the process of elimination because you are unsure of the correct answer.

Although recognizing these wrong answer pathologies is most useful in the Reading Comprehension section, the test makers use the same patterns in the other sections as well, so feel free to apply these ideas throughout the entire test!

Faulty Use of Detail

Faulty Use of Detail describes when an answer choice comes directly from the passage but does not answer the question being asked. These incorrect choices can come from a different paragraph than the one being asked about or describe ideas that are too narrow or too broad to answer the given question.

For example, Faulty Uses of Detail often are used with Global questions asking for the main idea of an entire passage. Such questions are looking for the overall topic and purpose, so any answer choices that describe only one specific scope or focus too much on only one example are incorrect. Although these specific Faulty Uses of Detail may accurately describe what is in the passage, they don't accurately reflect the main idea so are incorrect. To avoid these kinds of traps, always paraphrase and think about every question stem before tackling it to ensure you don't miss what's being asked.

Opposite

Opposite choices tend to be entirely correct except for one word, such as *not, false,* or *except,* that completely changes their meanings. Although Opposite choices are completely false as written, it can be easy to overlook that one important word in the question stem or answer choice. To avoid Opposite choices, slow down to ensure you carefully read the entire question stem and the answer you have chosen.

Distortion

Some answer choices contain parts that are correct alongside parts that are not. These often come in the form of Distortions, in which information is taken from the passage but then slightly changed to be incorrect. Similar to Opposite choices, Distortions can be wrong because of just one word, but for Distortions that word often ascribes an opinion that wasn't expressed in the passage, such as *more, better, worse,* or *preferred.*

One very common form of Distortion is the **Extreme** answer choice, which takes those ideas even further. An Extreme choice uses an idea from the passage but then adds an absolute word, such as *always, must, all, cannot,* or *never.* This tends to make a reasonable statement, such as "Most mammals bear live young," into an incorrect statement, such as "All mammals bear live young" (which is incorrect because monotremes, such as the playtpus and echidna, are mammals that lay eggs).

To avoid Distortions, ensure you have read every word of the answer choice you have chosen as correct, paraphrasing that choice to ensure it is completely right.

Out of Scope

Sometimes, an answer choice for a Reading Comprehension question describes a true statement, but that statement is not supported by information from the passage. Other times, an answer choice will seem perfectly logical but, again, is not mentioned in the passage. These are examples of Out of Scope answer choices. In the Reading Comprehension section, every correct answer must be directly supported by the passage, so using outside knowledge or even excessive reasoning can lead to choosing an incorrect answer choice. Since Out of Scope answer choices make logical sense, the best way to avoid falling into this test-maker trap is to make a strong prediction based on the passage before reading the answer choices, allowing you to bypass most choices completely since they will not match with that kind of clear prediction.

CHAPTER FIFTY-SIX

Practice Passages

PRACTICE PASSAGES

Directions: Each of the following three sets of questions is preceded by descriptive material. After reading the material, select the best answer to each question. Each passage set should take you approximately eight minutes to complete.

Relationships Between Food Resources and Population Size

One of the basic principles of ecology is that population size is to some extent a function of available food resources. Recent field experiments demonstrate that the interrelationship may be far more complex than hitherto imagined. Specifically, the browsing of certain rodents appears to trigger biochemical reactions in the plants they feed on that help regulate the size of the rodent populations. Two such examples of phytochemical regulation (regulation involving plant chemistry) have been reported so far.

Patricia Berger and her colleagues at the University of Utah have demonstrated the instrumentality of 6-methoxybenzoxazolinone (6-MBOA) in triggering reproductive behavior in the montane vole (*Microtus montanus*), a small rodent resembling the field mouse. 6-MBOA forms in young mountain grasses in response to browsing by predators such as voles. The experimenters fed rolled oats coated with 6-MBOA to nonbreeding winter populations of *Microtus*. After three weeks, the sample populations revealed a high incidence of pregnancy among the females and pronounced swelling of the testicles among the males. Control populations receiving no 6-MBOA revealed no such signs. Since the timing of reproductive effort is crucial to the short-lived vole in an environment in which the onset of vegetative growth can vary by as much as two months, the phytochemical triggering of copulatory behavior in *Microtus* represents a significant biological adaptation.

A distinct example is reported by John Bryant of the University of Alaska. In this case, plants seem to have adopted a form of phytochemical self-defense against the depredations of the snowshoe hare (*Lepus americanus*) of Canada and Alaska. Every 10 years or so, for reasons that are not entirely understood, the *Lepus* population swells dramatically. The result is intense overbrowsing of early and midsuccessional deciduous trees and shrubs. Bryant has shown that, as if in response, four common boreal forest trees favored by *Lepus* produce adventitious shoots high in terpene and phenolic resins, which effectively discourage hare browsing. He treated mature nonresinous willow twigs with resinous extracts from the adventitious shoots of other plants and placed treated and untreated bundles at hare feeding stations, weighing them at the end of each day. Bryant found that treated bundles containing even half the resin concentration of natural twigs were left untouched. The avoidance of these unpalatable resins, he concludes, may play a significant role in the subsequent decline in the *Lepus* population to its normal level.

These results suggest obvious areas for further research. For example, observational data should be reviewed to see whether the periodic population explosions among the prolific lemming (which, like the vole, is a small rodent in a marginal northern environment) occur during years in which there is an early onset of vegetative growth; if so, a triggering mechanism similar to that found in the vole may be involved.

1. The author of the passage primarily wants to

   (A) review some findings suggesting biochemical regulation of predator populations by their food sources.

   (B) outline the role of 6-MBOA in regulating the population of browsing animals.

   (C) summarize available data on the relationship between food resources and population size.

   (D) argue that earlier researchers have misunderstood the relationship between food supply and population size.

2. The passage describes the effect of 6-MBOA on voles as a "significant biological adaptation" because it

   (A) limits reproductive behavior in times of food scarcity.

   (B) leads the vole population to seek available food resources.

   (C) tends to ensure the survival of the species in a situation of fluctuating food supply.

   (D) maximizes the survival prospects of individual voles.

3. It can be inferred that the study of lemmings proposed by the author would probably

   (A) fully explain the interrelationship between food supply and reproductive behavior in northern rodent populations.

   (B) disprove the conclusions of Berger and her colleagues.

   (C) be irrelevant to the findings of Berger and her colleagues.

   (D) provide evidence indicating whether the conclusions of Berger and her colleagues can be generalized.

4. The statement "The interrelationship may be far more complex than hitherto imagined" suggests that scientists previously believed that

   (A) the amount of food available is the only food factor that affects population size.

   (B) reproductive behavior is independent of environmental factors.

   (C) food resources biochemically affect reproduction and the lifespan of some species.

   (D) population size is not influenced by available food resources.

5. The experiments described in the passage involved all of the following EXCEPT

   (A) measuring alterations in reproductive organs after a specific compound was ingested.

   (B) testing whether breeding behavior could be induced in normally nonbreeding animals by a change in diet.

   (C) measuring animals' consumption of treated and untreated foods.

   (D) measuring changes in the birth rate of test animals as opposed to control animals.

6. Bryant's interpretation of the results of his experiment depends on which of the following assumptions?

(A) The response of *Lepus* to resinous substances in nature may be different from its response under experimental conditions.

(B) The decennial rise in the *Lepus* population is triggered by an unknown phytochemical response.

(C) Many *Lepus* will starve to death rather than eat resinous shoots or change their diet.

(D) *Lepus* learns to search for alternative food sources once resinous shoots are encountered.

7. The experiments performed by Berger and Bryant BOTH study

  I. the effect of diet on reproduction in rodents.

 II. a relationship between food source and population size.

III. phytochemical phenomena in northern environments.

(A) II only

(B) III only

(C) I and II only

(D) II and III only

8. The author provides specific information to answer which of the following questions?

(A) Why does 6-MBOA form in response to browsing?

(B) Why is the timing of the voles' reproductive effort important?

(C) Are phytochemical reactions found only in northern environments?

(D) How does 6-MBOA trigger reproductive activity in the montane vole?

Foxglove

The foxglove (*Digitalis purpurea*) of the Scrophylariaceae family is a plant found in wooded areas throughout central Europe, primarily in Hungary and the Harz mountains. The botanical name *Digitalis purpurea* comes from two Latin words, *digitus* and *purpurea*. *Digitus* refers to the finger-shaped corolla of the plant. *Purpurea* refers to the purple color of the flowering part of the plant. The products derived from foxglove have been used for hundreds of years because of their remarkable effects on the heart.

Currently, *Digitalis purpurea* is commercially grown and harvested to obtain its useful by-products. The yearly crop is harvested during the months of September and October. The commercial products with therapeutic benefits are obtained only from the first year's leaves of each plant because each season after the first yields a product with decreased potency. A portion of the first season's crop is left unharvested to allow for the development of a flowering stalk, which grows in the second season. Inside the stalk are seeds, which will be cultivated into new plants each year.

At the end of each harvest, the leaves are dried and subsequently processed into therapeutic products, named cardiac glycosides. The structure of these cardiac glycosides contains a steroid nucleus with sugar moieties attached. The sugar portions of the plant products are responsible for the term *glycoside* being used. There are over 30 different glycosides processed from the first-year leaves; however, only 3 are used therapeutically: digitoxin, gitoxin, and gitaloxin. The potency and relative concentrations of each of the three glycosides may vary with each harvest depending on the environmental conditions in which the plants were grown.

Foxglove has been used for centuries to treat many different ailments. The first recorded use was by the Anglo-Saxons, who named the plant *foxes glofa*. Physicians of that time used a mixture of the plant leaves and honey to purge the body of illness. The claim of the mixture was that it aided in removing harmful obstructions from the liver and spleen. These obstructions were believed to be the cause of many illnesses and their associated sequelae, such as the aches and gastrointestinal problems of the flu. The first recorded use of foxglove for its effect on the heart was in 1775 by an English physician. He used digitoxin as a "cardiotonic" because of its stimulating effect on the heart. Digitoxin also has mild diuretic effects. This tonic was used to treat cases of "dropsy," now more commonly referred to as congestive heart failure.

Digitoxin is the glycoside obtained from foxglove currently used in the treatment of congestive heart failure and various arrhythmias. However, in treating these conditions, toxicity may occur; therefore, when using foxglove products, the individual should be under medical supervision to ensure optimal outcomes. When used properly, this natural medication may alleviate many ailments of the heart.

9. The author mentions in paragraph 3 that the potency and relative concentrations of the three glycosides may vary in order to

   (A) suggest that growers keep the amount of sunlight and water constant from season to season.
   (B) discredit the therapeutic benefits of the plant.
   (C) imply that testing the plant after each harvest is necessary to ensure that the amount of glycoside given to each person will be constant.
   (D) promote giving large doses of the plant products to each person to ensure that enough drug is given.

10. Based on the passage, it can be inferred that

   (A) foxglove may be used to treat many minor modern-day ailments.
   (B) the amount of digitoxin obtained from each leaf will be in the same proportions after each harvest.
   (C) use of foxglove may produce more harm than good if it is not used carefully.
   (D) only one glycoside obtained from foxglove has therapeutic properties.

11. Based on the passage, which of the following is TRUE?

   (A) The seeds of the first-season plants are used to grow second-season plants.
   (B) The older the plant gets, the more potent the products derived from it.
   (C) The plant's products are generally harvested in the fall season.
   (D) The plant's products, which have medical value, are obtained from the stalk.

12. Congestive heart failure is a condition in which the heart is unable to pump blood properly; therefore, digitoxin must act by

   (A) increasing the amount of blood in the body.
   (B) stimulating the heart to pump blood more effectively.
   (C) removing obstructions in the liver and spleen.
   (D) promoting the condition of dropsy.

13. Which of the following is most closely related structurally to digitoxin?

   (A) Fats
   (B) Carbohydrates
   (C) Proteins
   (D) Triglycerides

14. Based on the passage, when does foxglove normally produce flowers?

   (A) Never
   (B) Winter
   (C) First season
   (D) Second season

15. Which of the following is not mentioned in the passage as a use of foxglove?

    (A) As a proarrhythmic
    (B) Treatment of congestive heart failure
    (C) Removing obstructions from the spleen
    (D) Aid in treating gastrointestinal problems

16. The central thrust of the passage is that

    (A) foxglove products are naturally harvested medications and will have a therapeutic effect on the user.
    (B) harvesting foxglove is so difficult that it is hardly ever used even though it has many beneficial therapeutic effects.
    (C) naturally derived medications can still be used today and may be superior to synthetic medications.
    (D) only one of the foxglove products (digitoxin) is therapeutically beneficial.

Simultaneous Discovery

It is notorious that breakthroughs in science often come in tandem: the same, or almost the same, theoretical advance is made simultaneously by two or more investigators. Watson and Crick "raced" Linus Pauling to verify the helical structure of DNA; Darwin and Alfred Wallace announced the essentials of evolutionary theory simultaneously in 1858. Why should this occur? Why—to take another example—should Newton and Leibniz have worked out differential calculus independently and in isolation from one another, when they were not even working on the same sorts of problems?

Newton's work on calculus stemmed from his interest in the physical problem of the measurement of continuously changing quantities. Take, for example, the problem of determining the velocity of a freely falling body at a given instant. The body is constantly accelerating due to gravity. An approximate velocity at any time may be found by measuring the distance traveled over a very brief time interval such as a hundredth of a second; if one reduces the time interval measured until it approaches zero, the approximate velocity over the interval approaches the actual velocity at any instant as a limit. Newton's genius was to grasp how to calculate such a change over an infinitesimal time period through a mathematical operation known as differentiation.

For various reasons, Newton delayed publishing a clear account of his calculus for nearly 40 years. In the meantime, Leibniz approached calculus from a completely different standpoint, that of the formal geometric problem of determining the tangent to a curve (and later, for integral calculus, the area under a curve). However, this geometric problem was mathematically equivalent to Newton's consideration of bodies in motion, since the changing position of such a body over time can be plotted graphically as a curve in which the tangent to the curve at any point represents the velocity of the body at a given instant. Thus, Leibniz's formal geometric approach duplicated Newton's results.

This phenomenon of simultaneous discovery is surprising only to a public that views such breakthroughs as solitary acts of genius. In reality, the ground for discoveries is often thoroughly prepared in advance. In the century before Newton's birth, Europe had seen an explosion of scientific inquiry. Copernicus, Kepler, and others had formulated the laws of planetary motion and celestial mechanics. More specifically, when he began his mathematical work, Newton was already familiar with Descartes's coordinate geometry, the mathematics of infinitesimal intervals recently developed by John Wallis, and the method of finding tangents through differentiation worked out by Isaac Barrow. Thus, both the scientific problems and the conceptual tools that stimulated and facilitated Newton's astonishingly rapid development of differential calculus were already the common property of science. Given Newton's delay in publishing his work, an independent discovery of calculus by some other genius became not only possible but likely.

17. Which of the following ideas from the passage best supports the author's claim regarding why breakthroughs in science often come in tandem?

    (A) The public views such breakthroughs as solitary acts of genius.

    (B) An approximate velocity of a falling object may be found by measuring the distance traveled over a brief time interval.

    (C) Determining the tangent to a curve is mathematically equivalent to consideration of bodies in motion.

    (D) When he began his work, Newton was already familiar with Descartes's coordinate geometry.

18. The primary purpose of this passage is to

    (A) present mathematical discoveries.

    (B) clarify a recurring phenomenon in scientific history.

    (C) solve a long-standing puzzle in intellectual history.

    (D) describe a period of rapid scientific change.

19. It can be inferred from the passage that

    I. Newton based his calculus in part on the work of Descartes.

    II. Leibniz worked out differential calculus without knowing of Newton's work.

    III. Leibniz approached differential calculus from a standpoint similar to Newton's.

    (A) I only

    (B) II only

    (C) I and II only

    (D) II and III only

20. According to the author, Newton devised differential calculus in an attempt to understand

    (A) why falling bodies accelerate.

    (B) how to measure continuously varying quantities.

    (C) how to measure the area under a curve.

    (D) the relationship between average and actual speed.

21. It can be inferred that the author regards the development of calculus as

    (A) an outgrowth of previous intellectual developments.

    (B) a unique act of genius.

    (C) an achievement whose significance has been overestimated.

    (D) an unusual case of near-simultaneous discovery.

22. The passage implies that Newton and Leibniz arrived at similar results because

    (A) they used similar approaches.

    (B) they knew of each other's work.

    (C) no one had previously considered the problem of continuous motion.

    (D) the problems they considered were mathematically equivalent.

23. The author suggests that cases of simultaneous discovery

    (A) cannot really be called breakthroughs, since the important work has been done by others.
    (B) are extremely rare in science.
    (C) are made by individuals unaware of the historical influences on their thought.
    (D) seem remarkable to a public influenced by an inaccurate notion of genius.

24. In the final paragraph, the author draws connections between the work of Leibniz and Newton and the work of Copernicus and Kepler primarily to

    (A) provide support for the "great man" view of scientific history.
    (B) argue that the work of most scientific geniuses reveals unusually coincidental patterns of discovery.
    (C) expose the myth of independent scientific discovery.
    (D) describe the evolutionary nature of scientific achievement.

SOLUTIONS TO PRACTICE PASSAGES

Relationships Between Food Resources and Population Size

1. **A** *Global.* The answer to a Global question has to be broad enough to cover the entire passage without being too broad. Choice (C), for example, is incorrect because, although the author does summarize some data on the relationship between food sources and population size, it would be impossible for the passage to cover all available data on the subject. Choice (B), on the other hand, is not broad enough; 6-MBOA is discussed in only one of the paragraphs. Choice (D) is off base because the author never argues against the conclusions of earlier researchers. She just says that things are more complex than was previously thought and leaves it at that. Choice (A) summarizes the passage nicely and is the correct answer.

2. **C** *Vocab-in-Context.* This question contains a line reference that leads you to the end of paragraph 2. The biological adaptation to which the sentence is referring is the "phytochemical triggering of copulatory behavior" in voles—that is, the chemical MBOA in young mountain grasses causes voles to reproduce at just the right time, when grass is available as food. This is important because the amount of available grass varies considerably. 6-MBOA, then, ensures the survival of voles in a situation of fluctuating food supply, choice (C). 6-MBOA doesn't limit reproduction; it encourages reproduction, so (A) is incorrect. Use your common sense to eliminate choice (B): Seeking available food resources comes naturally to animals. Choice (D) is incorrect because a biological adaptation maximizes the survival of the entire species, not just individual voles.

3. **D** *Inference.* The author recommends research on the reproductive behavior of lemmings because lemmings are similar in kind and in habitat to voles. Knowing whether lemmings have a reproductive trigger mechanism similar to that of voles would allow you to determine whether Berger's findings about voles are true of other species as well. This idea is captured by choice (D). Choices (B) and (C) contradict this notion entirely. Choice (A) goes way too far; there is no way one study of lemmings could cover all there is to know about the interrelationship between food supply and reproductive behavior in northern rodent populations.

4. **A** *Inference.* Ecologists have long thought, according to the first sentence of the paragraph, that population size is a function of available food; this rules out choice (D). They just didn't realize that the interrelationship of food and population size was so complex. In other words, they thought that the amount of available food was the only food factor that affected population, choice (A). They didn't know about food that biochemically encouraged or discouraged reproduction, which eliminates choice (C). What scientists formerly thought about the link between environmental factors and reproductive behavior is not discussed, so (B) is not an option.

5. **D** *Detail.* In this All/Except question, you have to identify the choice that is not an element of either experiment. Choice (A) is mentioned in the middle of paragraph 2 as part of the mountain vole experiment. Choice (B) was part of that experiment as well, as indicated at the beginning of paragraph 2. Measuring consumption of treated and untreated foods, choice (C), was the method used in the experiment on hares. Choice (D) is the one choice that was not an element of either experiment discussed in the passage. The passage does discuss the use of a control group in the 6-MBOA experiment, but this experiment was not measuring changes in the birth rate of the animals, so (D) is the correct answer.

6. **C** *Inference.* This question asks for the assumption upon which Bryant's interpretation rests. Bryant concluded from his experiment that avoidance of unpalatable resins in the natural food source of *Lepus* may play a role in the decline in the *Lepus* population. He is assuming that hares will not eat anything at all and thus starve to death if they find resin on their food. The gist of this is captured in choice (C). Choice (A) is not an underlying assumption; Bryant's experiment would be worthless if the hares' behavior in the experiment didn't give an idea of how they behaved in nature. Choice (B) is out because Bryant's experiment does not investigate the reasons for the decennial rise in hare population. Choice (D) is incorrect because, if the hares learned to look for new sources of food once they couldn't eat the resinous shoots, their population wouldn't decrease.

7. **D** *Detail.* This Roman Numeral question is a bit reminiscent of Question 5 in that you are once again considering what was or was not part of both studies. Statement I is not true because the effect of diet on reproduction is part of Berger's study only. Both studies investigate the relationship between food source and population size, so Statement II is true. Statement III is clearly true as well, so choice (D) is the answer you want.

8. **B** *Evaluation.* This is a very general question about the passage, so let's look at the answer choices to see if some of them can be ruled out. Choices (A) and (D) are incorrect because the author does not explain why 6-MBOA forms in response to browsing or exactly how it triggers reproductive activity in the vole. Nor does he state whether phytochemical reactions can be found anywhere besides northern environments, which eliminates choice (C). That leaves choice (B), and sure enough, the importance of the timing of the voles' reproductive effort is explained in the last sentence of paragraph 2.

Foxglove

9. **C** *Evaluation.* The purpose of the author making a special note of the fact that the potency and relative concentrations of the glycosides may vary was to ensure that the reader understands that a standard extraction and distribution of the drug should not occur. The foxglove products may be very toxic if overdosed. If someone were to administer a set weight of foxglove products, the receiver would most likely receive different amounts of medication. Careful testing of each harvest needs to occur to maximize therapeutic benefit and minimize toxicity; choice (C) is correct. Choice (B) is incorrect because the entire passage is about the therapeutic effects of the plant, and (D) is incorrect because of the toxicity (see the last paragraph). In a controlled environment, choice (A) could occur; however, the plants are grown in the wild, and humans cannot control nature.

10. **C** *Inference.* Foxglove has been used for centuries to treat various ailments; however, the only current uses that are mentioned in the passage are to treat congestive heart failure and arrhythmias; choice (A) is incorrect. In supervised doses, the medication may be beneficial; however, in large doses, it can cause detrimental effects to the user. Choice (C) is correct. Three glycosides are beneficial and may vary from harvest to harvest depending on the environmental factors; choices (B) and (D) are incorrect.

11. **C** *Detail.* The foxglove products are primarily harvested in the fall months of September and October; choice (C) is correct. In harvesting the plants, the seeds of the second season are used in the next season to produce new plants; choice (A) is incorrect. The reason why new plants need to be planted each year is because with each successive season the leaves produce less potent products; choices (B) and (D) are incorrect.

12. **B** *Inference.* When treating a medical condition, the goal is usually to reverse the pathologic state. For example, in congestive heart failure, the heart is unable to effectively pump blood throughout the body; therefore, digitoxin would be used to stimulate the heart to pump blood more efficiently. This property of digitoxin is confirmed in the second-to-last sentence of paragraph 4, and choice (B) is correct. There's nothing in the passage to support the idea that digitoxin increases the amount of blood in the body or removes obstructions from the liver; choices (A) and (C) are incorrect. If dropsy was promoted, then the congestive heart failure would be worsened; choice (D) is incorrect.

13. **B** *Detail.* Digitoxin is a glycoside that is derived from plants. It has a steroid component, which has sugar moieties attached to it. Sugars are carbohydrates, so choice (B) is correct.

14. **D** *Detail.* The foxglove is harvested in the months of September and October. The first season yields the most potent products from the leaves. It is not until the second season that a flowering stalk is seen. Choice (D) is correct.

15. **A** *Detail.* Some of the older uses for the foxglove include aiding in the removal of obstructions from the spleen and liver and the treatment of gastrointestinal problems; choices (C) and (D) are incorrect. It is important to note that the previously mentioned uses were never proven effective and should not be used to treat these conditions now. Foxglove products are currently used in the treatment of congestive heart failure; choice (B) is incorrect. Any drug that is a proarrhythmic will promote arrhythmias, and foxglove products are NOT used to promote these conditions. Choice (A) is correct.

16. **A** *Global.* The main idea of the paragraph is that the foxglove is a plant that is commercially harvested to produce a product that has been used for therapeutic purposes for many years; choice (A) is correct. Choice (B) is incorrect because it suggests that the purpose of the passage is to argue that the cost of harvesting the product greatly outweighs the benefit. Choice (C) is incorrect because it references synthetic products, which are not mentioned in the passage. Choice (D) is incorrect because the passage specifically states in paragraph 3 that foxglove provides three products that provide therapeutic benefit; only digitoxin is described in detail.

Simultaneous Discovery

17. **D** *Effectiveness.* You must understand what the author's main claim is before you can evaluate what evidence supports it. The author wrote this passage to introduce the phenomenon of simultaneous discovery and explain that it happens because contemporary scientists share common knowledge. Choice (D), which illustrates Newton's (and Leibniz's) background knowledge, is the best example of that. Choice (A) is incorrect and is the idea that the author is refuting. Choices (B) and (C) are true facts but do not directly support the author's claim.

18. **B** *Global.* The opening paragraph raises the Newton-Leibniz discoveries in the context of two other examples of simultaneous discovery (DNA, evolution), something the author says happens "often." After going through the specifics in paragraphs 2–3, the author returns to the broader point in the last paragraph, stressing the dependence of great scientific breakthroughs on earlier step-by-step work. So the purpose of the whole passage is to clarify the phenomenon of simultaneous discovery, choice (B). Choices (A) and (D) omit

the broader context; the author is interested in the mathematical (choice (A)) and the scientific advances of Newton's time (choice (D)) only for how they illustrate the broader points about how great discoveries are made. The author never implies that the "puzzle" of Newton and Leibniz's simultaneous discovery is "long-standing" or that he/she is going to "solve" it, choice (C).

19. **C** *Inference.* The last paragraph states that Newton was familiar with Descartes's work, and implies that this was one of the "conceptual tools" he brought to his work on calculus (I). Paragraph 1 states that Leibniz worked "independently and in isolation" from Newton (II). Both this paragraph and paragraph 3 make it clear that Leibniz's approach was "completely different" from Newton's, contrary to III.

20. **B** *Detail.* This choice is stated explicitly in the first sentence of paragraph 2. Choice (A) is incorrect because the acceleration of falling bodies is mentioned by the author as an example of the problem of continuous motion; it is not clear that this was the specific problem Newton was working on or that Newton didn't understand "why" falling bodies accelerate. Choice (C) is mentioned as one of Leibniz's concerns (paragraph 3). Choice (D) is not mentioned at all: Paragraph 2 mentions approximate—not average—velocity; it's not implied that Newton was trying to understand the relationship between this and the actual velocity.

21. **A** *Inference.* The main question raised by the passage is: Why do simultaneous discoveries occur? The answer, given in the last paragraph, is: because the groundwork is prepared in advance. This point is made specifically in relation to Newton and Leibniz in the second sentence of paragraph 4. This idea is paraphrased in choice (A). The fact that Newton and Leibniz discovered calculus independently rules out choice (B). The author doesn't question the significance of the achievement (choice (C))—only the misconceived idea of "solitary acts of genius." The first sentence of the passage says that such cases are not unusual (choice (D)).

22. **D** *Inference.* Paragraph 3 states that although Leibniz's approach was "completely different" from Newton's, ruling out choice (A), the geometric problem he considered was "mathematically equivalent" to Newton's and "thus . . . duplicated Newton's results." Choice (D) sums this up. Leibniz and Newton worked independently, ruling out choice (B). Choice (C) is not stated and wouldn't explain their similar results anyway.

23. **D** *Inference.* Choice (D) paraphrases the first sentence of the last paragraph. Choice (A) goes too far—the author does stress the preliminary work done by others but doesn't suggest that the discovery of calculus (or similar discoveries) was not a breakthrough. Choice (B) is contradicted in the first paragraph. Choice (C) is not implied—whether or not Leibniz, Newton, Darwin, et al. were aware of their shared influences (or if they had them at all) is neither stated nor required for the author's conclusion.

24. **D** *Evaluation.* Copernicus and Kepler are mentioned in the fourth sentence of the last paragraph in the context of the series of scientific and mathematical advances that "prepared the ground" for Newton and Leibniz. So the point is that science builds on earlier work—it is evolutionary (choice (D))—even when making great advances. Of the incorrect choices, choice (C) is probably most tempting; one's first impulse is to say, "Yes, this is what the author is doing," but "expose the myth" goes too far. On reflection,

you should realize that the author doesn't think independent discovery is a myth at all. Newton and Leibniz are examples of independent discovery. Neither one, of course, was wholly "independent" of previous developments, but their discoveries were made on their own. The "great man" view in choice (A) probably refers to the misconception that breakthroughs are "solitary acts of genius" (first sentence of paragraph 4); this is not the author's view. Choice (B) is a distortion; the passage says that simultaneous discoveries occur often but not necessarily *most* of the time.

Section IX

QUANTITATIVE ABILITY

CHAPTER FIFTY-SEVEN

Quantitative Strategies

The Quantitative Ability section of the PCAT is designed to test the math skills that will be required in pharmacy school. The section contains 48 multiple-choice questions, 40 of which count toward your score. The remaining 8 questions are experimental and do not affect your score; however, you will not be able to distinguish between scored and experimental questions, so treat every question as if it will be counted.

You will have 40 minutes to complete the Quantitative Ability section, and no calculator will be provided. Scored items test Basic Math (14%), Algebra (19%), Probability and Statistics (19%), Precalculus (24%), and Calculus (24%). Each of these topics is discussed in detail in Chapters 58–62, respectively.

This chapter will introduce you to the most common Kaplan strategies that you will use for questions that require calculations on the PCAT. Although these strategies are most useful for the Quantitative Ability section, you may find them helpful throughout the test, especially with calculations in the Chemistry section. Additionally, remember that you can skip questions within a section and come back to them if you have time. Use this ability to your advantage by tackling questions that you know you can answer with relative ease and skipping questions that you know will take longer to answer.

PICKING NUMBERS

Picking Numbers is a powerful alternative to solving problems by brute force. Rather than working with unknown variables, you can pick concrete values for those variables or unknowns. In essence, you're transforming algebra or abstract math rules into basic arithmetic, giving yourself a much simpler task.

To successfully use Picking Numbers, follow these rules:

- Pick **permissible** numbers. Some problems have explicit rules such as "x is odd." Other problems have implicit rules. For example, if a word problem says, "Betty is five years older than Tim," don't pick $b = -2$ and $t = -7$; these numbers wouldn't work in the problem.

- Pick **manageable** numbers. Some numbers are simply easier to work with than others. $d = 2$ will probably be a more successful choice than $d = 492\sqrt{\pi}$, for example. The problems themselves will tell you what's manageable. For instance, $d = 2$ wouldn't be a great pick if an answer choice were $\frac{d}{12}$. (The number 12, 24, or even 120 would be much better in that case, since each is divisible by 12.)

- Once you've picked numbers to substitute for unknowns, approach the problem as basic arithmetic instead of algebra or number properties.

- Test every answer choice—sometimes certain numbers will yield a "false positive" in which a wrong answer looks right. If you get more than one "right answer," just pick a new set of numbers. The truly correct answer must work for all permissible numbers.

There are four signals that Picking Numbers will be a possible approach to the problem:

1. Variables in the answer choices
2. Percents in the answer choices
3. Answers that are fractions of an unknown value
4. Number property questions

These aren't in any particular order. You'll see many instances of each case on Test Day, so become familiar with all of them to ensure you recognize all your options on Test Day.

Picking Numbers with Variables in the Answer Choices

Whenever the answer choices contain variables, you should consider Picking Numbers. The correct answer choice is the one that yields the result that you got when you plugged the same number(s) into the question stem. Make sure that you test each answer choice, just in case more than one answer choice produces the desired result. In such a case, you will need to pick a new set of numbers and repeat the process only for the answer choices that worked out the first time.

Example: If $a > 1$, which of the following is equal to $\dfrac{2a + 6}{a^2 + 2a - 3}$?

    (A) a

    (B) $a + 3$

    (C) $\dfrac{2}{a - 1}$

    (D) $\dfrac{2a}{a - 3}$

Solution: The question says that $a > 1$, so the most manageable permissible number is 2. Then $\dfrac{2(2) + 6}{2^2 + 2(2) - 3} = \dfrac{4 + 6}{4 + 4 - 3} = \dfrac{10}{5} = 2.$

Now substitute 2 for a in each answer choice, looking for choices that equal 2 (the answer you just solved for) when $a = 2$. Eliminate choices that do not equal 2 when $a = 2$.

(A): $a = 2$. Choice (A) is possibly correct.

(B): $a + 3 = 2 + 3 = 5$. This is not 2. Discard.

(C): $\dfrac{2}{a-1} = \dfrac{2}{2-1} = \dfrac{2}{1} = 2$. Possibly correct.

(D): $\dfrac{2a}{a-3} = \dfrac{2(2)}{2-3} = \dfrac{4}{-1} = -4$. This is not 2. Discard.

You're down to (A) and (C). When more than one answer choice remains, you must pick another number. Try $a = 3$. Then $\dfrac{2(3)+6}{3^2+2(3)-3} = \dfrac{6+6}{9+6-3} = \dfrac{12}{12} = 1$.

Now work with the remaining answer choices.

Choice (A): $a = 3$. This is not 1. Discard.

Now that all three incorrect answer choices have been eliminated, you know that (C) must be correct. On Test Day, you should select (C) and move on, but just to verify right now, check to see whether (C) equals 1 when $a = 3$:

$\dfrac{2}{a-1} = \dfrac{2}{3-1} = \dfrac{2}{2} = 1$. Choice **(C)** does equal 1 when $a = 3$.

This approach to Picking Numbers also applies to many confusing word problems. Picking Numbers can resolve a lot of that confusion. The key to Picking Numbers in word problems is to reread the question stem after you've picked numbers, substituting the numbers in place of the variables.

Example: A car rental company charges for mileage as follows: x dollars per mile for the first n miles and $x + 1$ dollars per mile for each mile over n miles. How much will the mileage charge be, in dollars, for a journey of d miles, where $d > n$?

    (A) $d(x + 1) - n$
    (B) $xn + d$
    (C) $xn + d(x + 1)$
    (D) $x(n + d) - d$

Solution: Suppose you pick $x = 4$, $n = 3$, and $d = 5$. Now the problem would read like this:

A car rental company charges for mileage as follows: $4 per mile for each of the first 3 miles and $5 per mile for each mile over 3 miles. How much will the mileage charge be, in dollars, for a journey of 5 miles?

All of a sudden, the problem has become much more straightforward. The first 3 miles are charged at $4/mile. So that's $4 + $4 + $4, or $12. There are 2 miles remaining, and each one costs $5. So that's $5 + $5, for a total of $10. If the first 3 miles cost $12 and the next 2 cost $10, then the total charge is $12 + $10, which is $22.

Plugging $x = 4$, $n = 3$, and $d = 5$ into the answer choices, you get:

(A) $d(x + 1) - n = 5(4 + 1) - 3 = 22$
(B) $xn + d = 4 \times 3 + 5 = 17$
(C) $xn + d(x + 1) = 4 \times 3 + 5(4 + 1) = 37$
(D) $x(n + d) - d = 4(3 + 5) - 5 = 27$

Only (A) yields the same number you calculated when you plugged these numbers into the question stem, so (A) is the answer. There's no need for complex algebra at all.

Picking Numbers with Percents in the Answer Choices

Picking Numbers also works well on Problem Solving questions for which the answer choices are given in percents. When the answers are in percents, 100 will almost always be the most manageable number to pick. Using 100 not only makes your calculations easier, but it also simplifies the task of expressing the final value as a percent of the original.

Example: The manufacturer of Sleep-EZ mattresses is offering a 10% discount on the price of its king-size mattress. Some retailers are offering additional discounts. If a retailer offers an additional 20% discount, then what is the total discount available at that retailer?

(A) 10%
(B) 25%
(C) 28%
(D) 30%

Solution: Since the answers are in percents, pick $100 as the original price of the mattress. (Remember, realism is irrelevant—only permissibility and manageability matter.) The manufacturer offers a 10% discount: 10% of $100 is $10. So now the mattress costs $90.

Then the retailer offers an additional 20% discount. Since the price has fallen to $90, that 20% is taken off the $90 price. A 20% discount is now a reduction of $18. The final price of the mattress is $90 − $18, or $72.

The mattress has been reduced to $72 from an original price of $100. That's a $28 reduction. Since you started with $100, you can easily calculate that $28 is 28% of the original price. Choice (C) is correct.

Notice that choice (D) commits the error of simply adding the two percents given in the question stem. An answer choice like (D) will never be correct on a question that gives you information about multiple percent changes.

Picking Numbers with Answers That Are Fractions of an Unknown

Similar to when a question asks for a percent, when a question asks about any fraction of an unknown, pick numbers to represent the unknown(s) in the question stem and walk through the arithmetic of the problem using those. Look in the question stem and the answer choices for clues about what the most manageable numbers might be.

Example: Carol spends $\frac{1}{4}$ of her savings on a stereo, and then she spends $\frac{1}{3}$ less than she spent on the stereo for a television. What fraction of her savings did she spend on the stereo and television together?

(A) $\frac{1}{4}$

(B) $\frac{2}{7}$

(C) $\frac{5}{12}$

(D) $\frac{7}{12}$

Solution: Lowest common denominators of fractions in the question stem are good choices for numbers to pick. So are numbers that appear frequently as denominators in the answer choices. In this case, the common denominator of the fractions in the stem is 12, so let the number 12 represent Carol's total savings (12 dollars).

That means she spends $\frac{1}{4} \times 12$ dollars, or 3 dollars, on her stereo, and $\frac{2}{3} \times 3$ dollars, or 2 dollars, on her television. That comes out to be $3 + 2 = 5$ dollars; that's how much she spent on the stereo and television combined. You're asked what *fraction* of her savings she spent. Because her total savings was 12 dollars, she spent $\frac{5}{12}$ of her savings; (C) is correct. Notice how picking a common denominator for the variable (Carol's savings) made it easy to convert each of the fractions $\left(\frac{1}{4} \text{ and } \frac{2}{3} \times \frac{1}{4} \text{ of her savings} \right)$ to a simple integer.

A tricky part of this question is understanding how to determine the price of the television. The television does not cost $\frac{1}{3}$ of her savings. It costs $\frac{1}{3}$ *less* than the stereo; that is, it costs $\frac{2}{3}$ as much as the stereo.

By the way, some of these answers could have been eliminated quickly using basic logic. Choice (A) is too small; the stereo alone costs $\frac{1}{4}$ of her savings. Choices (D) and (E) are too large; the television costs *less* than the stereo, so the two together must cost less than $2 \times \frac{1}{4}$, or half, of Carol's savings. Although you may not be used to approaching questions using this type of broad, logical approach, you can save significant time during any section of the PCAT looking for these kinds of patterns!

Picking Numbers with Number Property Questions

Number properties deal with categorizing numbers and explaining the expected behavior of numbers based on certain rules. The most common topics you will encounter include integers/non-integers, odds/evens, positives/negatives, factors/multiples, remainders, and primes. When you see a question that asks about any of these topics and that includes any unknown values, you should immediately consider the Picking Numbers strategy. As always, remember to select permissible and manageable numbers for yourself when you pick numbers to make the math as easy as possible.

Example: If 2 is the remainder when m is divided by 5, what is the remainder when $3m$ is divided by 5?

    (A) 0

    (B) 1

    (C) 2

    (D) 3

Solution: This question tests your ability to think critically about the characteristics of remainders in division. You are told that some number, m, has a remainder of 2 when divided by 5. Pick simple, permissible numbers and apply them to the problem in the question stem.

    Since m has a remainder of 2 when divided by 5, m could be any number that is 2 greater than a multiple of 5. The simplest number to substitute for m is 7. You know that 5 goes into 7 one time with a remainder of 2. Now, apply 7 to the rest of the question stem: $3m$ divided by 5. Multiplying 3 and 7 gives you 21, and 21 divided by 5 leaves a remainder of 1. Thus, answer choice (B) is correct; no more work is required!

BACKSOLVING

Backsolving is just like Picking Numbers except, instead of coming up with the number yourself, you use the numbers in the answer choices. You'll literally work backward through the problem, looking for the answer choice that agrees with the information in the question stem. This is a good approach whenever the task of plugging a choice into the question would allow you to confirm its details in a straightforward way.

You want to Backsolve systematically, not randomly. Start with either choice (B) or (C). If the choice you pick isn't correct, you'll still often be able to figure out whether you need to try a number that's larger or one that's smaller. Since numerical answer choices will always be in ascending or descending order, you'll be able to use that information to eliminate several choices at once.

Backsolving can save you a great deal of time. It is also an exceptional approach when you have no idea how to begin a problem.

Example: Ron begins reading a book at 4:30 p.m. and reads at a steady pace of 30 pages per hour. Michelle begins reading a copy of the same book at 6:00 p.m. If Michelle started

5 pages behind the page that Ron started on and reads at an average pace of 50 pages per hour, at what time would Ron and Michelle be reading the same page?

(A) 7:00 p.m.

(B) 7:30 p.m.

(C) 8:00 p.m.

(D) 8:30 p.m.

Solution: You could perhaps set up a complex system of equations to solve this problem, but even if you knew exactly what those equations would be and how to solve them, that's not a very efficient use of your time. Backsolving would work better here. Pick an answer choice and see whether Michelle and Ron are on the same page at that time. There's no compelling reason to prefer one choice to another, so just quickly choose (B) or (C).

Let's say you choose (B). On what page is Ron at 7:30 p.m.? He started reading at 4:30 p.m., so he has been reading for 3 hours. His pace is 30 pages per hour. So he has read 30 × 3, or 90 pages. Since Michelle started 5 pages behind Ron, she would need to read 95 pages to be at the same place. She has been reading since 6:00 p.m., so she has read for 1.5 hours. At 50 pages per hour, she has read 75 pages. That's 20 short of what she needs. So (B) is not the right answer.

Since Michelle is reading faster than Ron, she'll catch up to him with more time. Therefore, they will be on the same page sometime later than 7:30 p.m., so eliminate (A) as well and try an answer choice that gives a later time. At this point, you could choose either choice (C) or (D). If (C) ends up being correct, you can choose it and move on. If (C) is too early, then (D) must be the correct answer.

Let's try out (C). At 8:00 p.m. Ron has read for 3.5 hours. At a pace of 30 pages per hour he's read 30 × 3.5, or 105 pages. Since Michelle started 5 pages behind, she'd need to read 110 pages to be at the same place. She's been reading for 2 hours at this point; at 50 pages per hour, she's read 100 pages. That's still 10 short of what she needs to catch up. So (C) is also not the right answer, and you need a later time than 8:00 p.m.—choice (D) must be correct.

As happened with this question, sometimes you may have to test more than one choice. But as you saw above, you should never have to test more than two answer choices. Stick to (B) or (C), and you'll save valuable time.

STRATEGIC GUESSING AND ESTIMATION

A well-placed guess can sometimes be the best tool you can use for a problem. Because of the severe time constraints, you need to stay on a steady pace. If you fall behind, it's a good idea to guess on the hardest problems and mark them for later rather than completing the full calculations right away. That way you'll get back lost time instead of falling further behind. And while you shouldn't be afraid to guess, you should be afraid to rush! The test makers write problems in complicated ways, and rushing almost always leads to misperception of questions (not to mention errors in arithmetic). This is a problem because the test makers base many wrong answers on the most common misperceptions. Rushing through a problem almost always guarantees a wrong answer. It's far better to guess as needed, skipping some questions and taking the time you need on others, than to rush through an entire section.

Even if you are ahead of schedule during a section, sometimes you simply will have no idea how to approach a problem. Instead of throwing away three or four minutes becoming frustrated, make a guess. If you don't know how to approach a problem, you aren't likely to choose the right answer anyway, and you can use the time you save to solve other problems that you stand a better chance of answering correctly.

Estimation can also be useful when answering questions as it can save you time and help you avoid mistakes when working through lengthy arithmetic calculations. You should consider estimation on questions that involve difficult or lengthy calculations and have answer choices that are spread fairly far apart. Once you decide to estimate, you'll want to follow a couple of general rules.

First, use scientific notation and fractions to simplify calculations. Although mastering both may take practice, you'll find the arithmetic required for either to be much simpler than leaving the number as a regular decimal. Review the rules in Chapter 58, Basic Math, if you don't feel comfortable with manipulating fractions yet; you'll need to know them to do well on certain questions anyway, so becoming adept at them now will allow you to master content and strategies at the same time.

Second, feel free to round numbers or only use powers of 10 when the answer choices vary widely. When you add or multiply numbers, round one number up and the other number down. When you subtract or divide numbers, round both numbers in the same direction. By doing so, you'll minimize the effect of rounding and arrive at a closer answer than you would if rounding randomly.

REVIEW PROBLEMS

1. Each writer for the local newspaper is paid as follows: a dollars for each of the first n stories each month and $a + b$ dollars for each story thereafter, where $a > b$. How many more dollars will a writer who submits $n + a$ stories in a month earn than a writer who submits $n + b$ stories?

   (A) $(a - b)(a + b + n)$
   (B) $a - b$
   (C) $a^2 - b^2$
   (D) $n(a - b)$

2. A crate of apples contains 1 bruised apple for every 30 apples in the crate. Three out of every four bruised apples are considered not fit to sell, and every apple that is not fit to sell is bruised. If there are 12 apples not fit to sell in the crate, then how many total apples are there in the crate?

   (A) 270
   (B) 360
   (C) 480
   (D) 600

3. Company Z spent $\frac{1}{4}$ of its revenues last year on marketing and $\frac{1}{7}$ of the remainder on maintenance of its facilities. What fraction of last year's original revenues did company Z have left after its marketing and maintenance expenditures?

   (A) $\frac{5}{14}$

   (B) $\frac{1}{2}$

   (C) $\frac{17}{28}$

   (D) $\frac{9}{14}$

4. The positive difference between Sam and Lucy's ages is a, and the sum of their ages is z. If Lucy is older than Sam, then which of the following represents Lucy's age?

   (A) $\frac{z - a}{2}$

   (B) $\frac{z + a}{2}$

   (C) $a - \frac{z}{2}$

   (D) $\frac{a - z}{2}$

5. If a bicyclist in motion increases his speed by 30 percent and then increases this speed by 10 percent, what percent of the original speed is the total increase in speed?

   (A) 40%
   (B) 43%
   (C) 64%
   (D) 140%

6. If p, q, and r are positive integers such that q is a factor of r and r is a multiple of p, which of the following must be an integer?

   (A) $\dfrac{p+q}{r}$

   (B) $\dfrac{p}{q}$

   (C) $\dfrac{r(p+q)}{pq}$

   (D) $\dfrac{r+p}{q}$

SOLUTIONS TO THE REVIEW PROBLEMS

1. **C** You are given information about the number of dollars reporters are paid to write newspaper stories. They are paid at one rate for each of a certain number of stories and another rate for each remaining story after that. You are also given information about two specific writers and the number of stories that they write. Although it is possible to complete this question using traditional math, the set up would be quite difficult. Since there are variables in the question stem and the answer choices, this is a good question to use Picking Numbers instead.

   The only permissibility rule given in the question is that $a > b$, so you could pick $a = 3$ and $b = 2$. The remaining variable is n; there are no constraints on this number, so pick a number that is easy to work with, such as 10.

   Once you have chosen your numbers, reread the question stem but mentally substitute your new numbers for the variables as this can help the problem make more sense. You want to know how much more a writer who writes $n + a = 10 + 3 = 13$ stories will make than will a writer who writes $n + b = 10 + 2 = 12$ stories.

   Start with the writer who writes 13 stories. She makes \$3 for each of the first 10 stories or \$30 total for the first ten stories. Then, she makes $a + b = 3 + 2 = \$5$ for each story after that. She wrote 3 more stories, so she earned \$15 more for the additional stories. In total, the writer earned \$45.

   Next, look at the writer who wrote 12 stories. He too will make \$3 for each of the first 10 stories or \$30 total. Then he will make \$5 for each of the remaining 2 stories, another \$10. In total, the second writer earns \$40. Therefore, the difference between the two writers' earnings is \$5. Now, plug your variables into the answer choices to find one that equals \$5:

   (A) $(3 - 2)(3 + 2 + 10) = (1)(15) = 15$. Eliminate.

   (B) $3 - 2 = 1$. Eliminate.

   (C) $3^2 - 2^2 = 9 - 4 = 5$. This could be the correct answer, but keep checking to ensure no other answer choices also calculate to 5.

   (D) $10(3 - 2) = 10(1) = 10$. Eliminate.

   Since only one answer choice yields the number 5, pick choice (C) and move on.

2. **C** This is another difficult-sounding question. Since the answer choices are all numbers, Backsolving is a great approach to use instead of traditional math. Start with choice (B). Suppose that there are 360 apples in the crate. Then $\frac{360}{30}$ apples, or 12 apples, are bruised. Then, $\frac{3}{4}$ of those 12 apples, or 9 apples, are unsellable. This is too few unsellable apples, so (B) is too small. The answer must be larger than 360, so eliminate choices (A) and (B). With only two choices remaining, you know that testing either choice will lead you to the answer. If (C) is not correct, then you'll know that (D) is the answer. If (D) is not correct, then you'll know that (C) is the answer. No matter what, you'll only have to test one more choice. Let's try choice (D). Suppose that there are 600 apples in the crate. Then $\frac{600}{30}$ apples, or 20 apples, are bruised. Of those 20, $\frac{3}{4}$ or 15, are unsalable. That's too many, so (D) is out, and choice (C) must be correct.

3. **D** Company Z spends portions of its revenues on two things. It is important to note that the answer choices are fractions and represent the fraction of last year's revenues that company Z had left after the expenses. Notice that you are given absolutely no way to know how much revenue company Z received last year, so you can use Picking Numbers to determine the total revenue. Since you must take $\frac{1}{4}$ and $\frac{1}{7}$ of the revenue, a number divisible by both 4 and 7 will be most manageable. Make the calculations as easy as possible by picking the lowest common multiple of 4 and 7: 28.

Now, "Company Z spent $\frac{1}{4}$ of its revenues last year on marketing," becomes "Company Z spent \$7 last year on marketing." The next sentence mentions "the remainder," so you need to know what that is. Since \$28 − \$7 = \$21, "Company Z spent $\frac{1}{7}$ of the remainder on maintenance," means "Company Z spent \$3 on maintenance."

What's left from \$28 after company Z spent \$7 and then \$3 is \$18. So the answer is $\frac{18}{28}$. A common factor of 2 can be canceled from both the numerator and the denominator, leaving $\frac{9}{14}$. Choice (D) is correct.

4. **B** There are two people—Sam and Lucy—whose ages are related in some way. While you could set up an algebraic equation here, notice that the answer choices all contain variables and thus allow for Picking Numbers. You are solving for Lucy's age, so be careful not to answer with Sam's age because that's likely to be one of the wrong answers.

It's easy enough to pick two numbers for a and z. But then you would still have to backtrack from those to calculate the two ages. If this happens, consider reevaluating your approach. Are there other variables you could pick first that would make things easier?

If you pick numbers for Lucy's and Sam's ages, then all you need to do to figure out the values of a and z is basic arithmetic. You might pick that Lucy is 5 years old and Sam is 3 years old. That makes a, their difference, equal to 2. And z, their sum, is equal to 8.

Plug in $a = 2$ and $z = 8$ to see which choices yield Lucy's age of 5.

(A) is $\frac{8-2}{2} = \frac{6}{2} = 3$. Eliminate.

(B) is $\frac{8+2}{2} = \frac{10}{2} = 5$. Possibly right.

(C) is $2 - \frac{8}{2} = 2 - 4 = -2$. Eliminate.

(D) is $\frac{2-8}{2} = \frac{-6}{2} = -3$. Eliminate.

Since it is the only choice that matches, (B) is correct.

5. **B** The question gives you information about two increases to the speed of a bicyclist and asks for the total percent increase in the cyclist's speed. When you encounter a percentage problem with an unknown value in the question and percentages in the answer choices, you should use the strategy of Picking Numbers and pick 100.

If the bicyclist initially rides at 100 (the units aren't mentioned in this problem, and in any case, the numbers don't need to be realistic, just permissible and manageable) and then increases his speed by 30%, he now rides at 130. He then increases this speed by 10%, so find 10% of 130, which is 13, and add it to 130. That makes his final speed 143. That is an increase of 43 over his original speed of 100. Recalling that 100 was the number you initially picked shows that 43 is 43% (or $\frac{43}{100}$) of the original speed. Answer choice (B) is correct.

6. **C** This question gives information about three variables and how they relate to each other. Since q is a factor of r, r is a multiple of q. The question stem also says r is a multiple of p. Thus, r is a multiple of both p and q. This question is very abstract and relies on your knowledge of number properties, so picking numbers that are permissible will help you make quick work of the answer choices.

Pick numbers for p, q, and r and apply them to the answer choices. Since you know r is a multiple of both p and q, start with p and q. You might pick that $p = 2$ and $q = 3$. From there, you can pick a value for r; such as $r = 6$. Now plug these values into the answer choices and eliminate any choice that does not yield an integer.

(A) is $\frac{2+3}{6} = \frac{5}{6}$. Eliminate.

(B) is $\frac{2}{3}$. Eliminate.

(C) is $\frac{6(2+3)}{2(3)} = \frac{6(5)}{6} = 5$. Possibly correct.

(D) is $\frac{6+2}{3} = \frac{8}{3}$. Eliminate.

As the only choice that fit, (C) is correct.

CHAPTER FIFTY-EIGHT

Basic Math

The test makers describe the arithmetic covered in this chapter as basic math, but that doesn't mean it's all easy to calculate, especially when you do not have access to a calculator and are under the time constraints of Test Day. Even if you once had a strong, working knowledge of number properties and how to manipulate fractions, decimals, ratios, logarithms, and means, you may find that your knowledge has deteriorated through disuse, especially if you haven't taken a math class in several years. Even if this content seems straightforward at first glance, spend some time with the practice problems and worked examples to ensure your knowledge is fresh and you won't need to waste time on Test Day recalling basic rules or formulas.

NUMBER OPERATIONS

Important terms and concepts to be familiar with for the PCAT:

- **Real number:** All numbers on the number line.
- **Integers:** All numbers with no fractional or decimal parts, including negative whole numbers and zero; multiples of 1. See the number line below.
- **Operation:** A process that is performed on one or more numbers. The four basic arithmetic operations are addition, subtraction, multiplication, and division.
- **Sum:** The result of addition.
- **Difference:** The result of subtraction.
- **Product:** The result of multiplication.
- **Reciprocal:** The result of switching the numerator and denominator of a fraction. The reciprocal of $\frac{3}{5}$ is $\frac{5}{3}$. The reciprocal of 2 is $\frac{1}{2}$ because 2 can be considered to be the fraction $\frac{2}{1}$. Multiplying any number by its reciprocal will result in 1.

Numbers and the Number Line

A number line is a straight line, extending infinitely in either direction, on which real numbers are represented as points. Decimals and fractions can also be depicted on a number line, as can numbers such as $\sqrt{2}$.

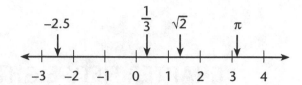

The values of numbers get larger as you move to the right along the number line. Numbers to the right of zero are **positive**; numbers to the left of zero are **negative**. **Zero** is neither positive nor negative, but it is an even integer. Any positive number is larger than any negative number. For example, 4 is larger than -300.

Laws of Operations

Commutative laws of addition and multiplication

Addition and multiplication are both **commutative**; switching the order of any two numbers being added or multiplied together does not affect the result. For example, $5 + 12 = 12 + 5$; both sums equal 17. Similarly $2 \times 6 = 6 \times 2$; both products equal 12.

$$a + b = b + a$$
$$a \times b = b \times a$$

Subtraction and division are *not* commutative; switching the order of the numbers changes the result. For instance, $3 - 2 \neq 2 - 3$; the left side yields a result of 1, whereas the right side yields a result of -1.

Similarly, $6 \div 2 \neq 2 \div 6$; the left side gives 3, whereas the right side gives $\frac{1}{3}$.

Associative laws of addition and multiplication

$$(a + b) + c = a + (b + c)$$
$$(a \times b) \times c = a \times (b \times c)$$

Addition and multiplication are both **associative**. This means that the terms can be regrouped without changing the result.

Example: $(3 + 5) + 8 = 3 + (5 + 8)$
$8 + 8 = 3 + 13$
$16 = 16$

Example: $(4 \times 5) \times 6 = 4 \times (5 \times 6)$
$20 \times 6 = 4 \times 30$
$120 = 120$

Because addition and multiplication are both commutative and associative, numbers can be added or multiplied in any order. Subtraction and division are *not* associative.

Example: $(7 - 10) - 4 = -3 - 4 = -7$, whereas $7 - (10 - 4) = 7 - 6 = 1$.
So $(7 - 10) - 4 \neq 7 - (10 - 4)$.

Example: $(24 \div 12) \div 3 = 2 \div 3 = \frac{2}{3}$, whereas $24 \div (12 \div 3) = 24 \div 4 = 6$.

So $(24 \div 12) \div 3 \neq 24 \div (12 \div 3)$.

Distributive law

The distributive law of multiplication allows you to "distribute" a factor among the terms being added or subtracted by multiplying that factor by each number in the group.

$$a(b + c) = ab + ac.$$

Example: $4(3 + 7) = (4 \times 3) + (4 \times 7)$

$4 \times 10 = 12 + 28$

$40 = 40$

Division can be distributed in a similar way, because dividing by a number is equivalent to multiplying by that number's reciprocal.

Example: $\frac{3+5}{2} = \frac{1}{2}(3 + 5) = \frac{1}{2}(3) + \frac{1}{2}(5)$

$\frac{8}{2} = \frac{3}{2} + \frac{5}{2}$

$\frac{8}{2} = \frac{3+5}{2}$

$\frac{8}{2} = \frac{8}{2}$

Don't get carried away, though. When the sum or difference is in the denominator—that is, when you're dividing by a sum or difference—no distribution is possible. $\frac{9}{4+5}$ is NOT equal to $\frac{9}{4} + \frac{9}{5}$; $\frac{9}{4+5} = \frac{9}{9} = 1$. But $\frac{9}{4}$ and $\frac{9}{5}$ are both greater than 1, so their sum can't equal 1.

Operations with signed numbers

Numbers can be treated as though they have two parts: a positive or negative sign and a number part. For example, the sign of the number -3 is negative, and the number part is 3. Numbers without any sign are understood to be positive. To add two numbers that have the same sign, add the number parts and keep the sign.

Example: What is the sum of -6 and -3?

Solution: To find $(-6) + (-3)$, add 6 and 3, and then attach the negative sign from the original numbers to the sum:

$$(-6) + (-3) = -9.$$

To add two numbers that have different signs, find the difference between the number parts and keep the sign of the number whose number part is larger.

Example: What is the sum of -7 and $+4$?

Solution: To find $(-7) + (+4)$, subtract 4 from 7 to get 3. $7 > 4$; that is, the number part of -7 is greater than the number part of $+4$, so the final sum will be negative. $(-7) + (+4) = -3$.

Subtraction is the opposite of addition. You can rephrase any subtraction problem as an addition problem by changing the operation sign from a minus to a plus and switching the sign on the second number. For instance, $8 - 5 = 8 + (-5)$. There's no real advantage to rephrasing if you are subtracting a smaller positive number from a larger positive number. But the concept comes in very handy when you are subtracting a negative number from any other number, a positive number from a negative number, or a larger positive number from a smaller positive number.

To subtract a negative number, rephrase as an addition problem and follow the rules for addition of signed numbers.

For instance, $9 - (-10) = 9 + 10 = 19$.

Here's another example: $(-5) - (-2) = (-5) + 2$. The difference between 5 and 2 is 3, and the number with the larger number part is -5, so the answer is -3.

To subtract a positive number from a negative number or from a smaller positive number, change the sign of the number that you are subtracting from positive to negative and follow the rules for addition of signed numbers.

For example, $(-4) - 1 = (-4) + (-1) = -5$.

Example: Subtract 8 from 2.

Solution: $2 - 8 = 2 + (-8)$. The difference between the number parts is 6, and the -8 has the larger number part, so the answer is -6.

Multiplying or dividing two numbers with the same sign gives a positive result.

$$(-4) \times (-7) = +28$$
$$(-50) \div (-5) = +10$$

Multiplying or dividing two numbers with different signs gives a negative result.

$$(-2) \times (+3) = -6$$
$$8 \div (-4) = -2$$

Properties of Zero, 1, and −1

Properties of zero

Adding zero to or subtracting zero from a number does not change the number.

$$x + 0 = x$$
$$0 + x = x$$
$$x - 0 = x$$

Example: $5 + 0 = 5$

$0 + (-3) = -3$

$4 - 0 = 4$

Notice, however, that subtracting a number from zero switches the number's sign. It's easier to see why if you rephrase the problem as an addition problem.

Example: Subtract 5 from 0.

Solution: $0 - 5 = -5$. That's because $0 - 5 = 0 + (-5)$, and according to the properties of zero, $0 + (-5) = -5$.

The product of zero and any number is zero.

$$0 \times z = 0$$
$$z \times 0 = 0$$

Example: $0 \times 12 = 0$

Division by zero is undefined. For practical purposes, that translates as "it can't be done." Because fractions are essentially division (that is, $\frac{1}{4}$ means $1 \div 4$), any fraction with zero in the denominator is also undefined.

Properties of 1 and −1

Multiplying or dividing a number by 1 does not change the number.

$$a \times 1 = a$$
$$1 \times a = a$$
$$a \div 1 = a$$

Example: $4 \times 1 = 4$

$1 \times (-5) = -5$

$(-7) \div 1 = -7$

Multiplying or dividing a nonzero number by −1 changes the sign of the number.

$$a \times (-1) = -a$$
$$(-1) \times a = -a$$
$$a \div (-1) = -a$$

Example: $6 \times (-1) = -6$

$(-3) \times (-1) = 3$

$(-8) \div (-1) = 8$

Order of Operations

Whenever you have a string of operations, be careful to perform them in the proper order. Otherwise, you will probably get the wrong answer.

The acronym PEMDAS stands for the correct order of operations:

> Parentheses
>
> Exponents
>
> Multiplication
>
> Division
>
> Addition
>
> Subtraction

Multiplication and division should be performed together in order from left to right, and then addition and subtraction should be performed together in order from left to right. If you have trouble remembering PEMDAS, you can think of the mnemonic phrase Please Excuse My Dear Aunt Sally.

Example: $66 \times (3 - 2) \div 11 = ?$

Solution: If you were to perform all the operations sequentially from left to right, without regard to the rules for the order of operations, you would arrive at the answer $\frac{196}{11}$. To do this correctly, however, perform the operation inside the parentheses first: $3 - 2 = 1$. Now you have:

$$66 \times 1 \div 11 = 66 \div 11 = 6$$

Example: $30 - 5 \times 4 + (7 - 3)^2 \div 8 = ?$

Solution: First perform any operations within parentheses. (If the expression has parentheses within parentheses, work from the innermost set out.)

$30 - 5 \times 4 + 4^2 \div 8$

Next, do the exponent.

$30 - 5 \times 4 + 16 \div 8$

Then, do all multiplication and division in order from left to right.

$30 - 20 + 2$

Last, do all addition and subtraction in order from left to right.

$10 + 2$

The answer is 12.

FRACTIONS

Basic Arithmetic with Fractions

$\frac{7}{8}$ $\to$ Numerator
$\to$ Denominator

Multiplying fractions: Multiply numerators by each other and denominators by each other.

$$\frac{3}{4} \times \frac{9}{7} = \frac{3 \times 9}{4 \times 7} = \frac{27}{28}$$

Dividing fractions: Flip the numerator and denominator of the fraction you're dividing by, then multiply.

$$\frac{1}{5} \div \frac{4}{11} = \frac{1}{5} \times \frac{11}{4} = \frac{1 \times 11}{5 \times 4} = \frac{11}{20}$$

Adding fractions: You can add fractions only when they have the same denominator. When you add, add only the numerators, NOT the denominators.

$$\frac{2}{3} + \frac{5}{3} = \frac{2+5}{3} = \frac{7}{3}$$

If you don't have a common denominator, you have to find one. The fastest way to get a common denominator is to multiply each fraction by a fraction whose numerator and denominator are the same as the denominator of the other fraction. (You can do this because any fraction with the same numerator and denominator is equal to 1, and multiplying any number by 1 doesn't change the value of the number.)

$$\frac{1}{3} + \frac{2}{5} = \left(\frac{1}{3} \times \frac{5}{5}\right) + \left(\frac{2}{5} \times \frac{3}{3}\right) = \frac{5}{15} + \frac{6}{15} = \frac{11}{15}$$

Subtracting fractions: This works the same way as adding fractions, except you subtract the numerators instead of adding them.

$$\frac{6}{7} - \frac{1}{2} = \left(\frac{6}{7}\right)\left(\frac{2}{2}\right) - \left(\frac{1}{2}\right)\left(\frac{7}{7}\right) = \frac{12}{14} - \frac{7}{14} = \frac{5}{14}$$

Remember, parentheses can be used to indicate multiplication instead of the "×" sign.

Reducing fractions: Whenever there is a common factor in the numerator and denominator, you can reduce the fraction by removing the factor from both parts of the fraction. You can do this because dividing the numerator and denominator by the same number doesn't change the value of the fraction as a whole. This will often make working with the fraction much easier because you'll be using smaller numbers.

$$\frac{4}{12} = \frac{1 \times 4}{3 \times 4} = \frac{1}{3} \times 1 = \frac{1}{3}$$

On Test Day, you don't actually have to write out all this math. For example, you might work like this:

$$\frac{4}{12} = \frac{1 \times 4}{3 \times 4} = \frac{1}{3}.$$

Or, even more simply, you might keep track of the multiplication operations mentally, only writing down the results. For example, if attempting to reduce $\frac{42}{28}$, you might write your work by cancelling like this:

$$\frac{{}^{6}\cancel{42}}{{}_{4}\cancel{28}} = \frac{{}^{3}\cancel{6}}{{}_{2}\cancel{4}} = \frac{3}{2}.$$

Because both 42 and 28 are divisible by 7, you can divide both the numerator (42) and the denominator (28) by 7. Thus, $\frac{42}{28}$ reduces to $\frac{6}{4}$. Because both 6 and 4 are divisible by 2, you can divide both the numerator (6) and the denominator (4) by 2. Thus, $\frac{6}{4}$ reduces to $\frac{3}{2}$.

Canceling: Whenever you have to multiply two or more fractions, you should cancel common factors before you multiply. This is a lot like reducing and has the same advantages. $\frac{1}{7} \times \frac{7}{3}$ can be canceled like this:

$$\frac{1}{\cancel{7}} \times \frac{\cancel{7}^{\,1}}{3} = \frac{1}{1} \times \frac{1}{3} = \frac{1}{3}$$

$\frac{4}{5} \times \frac{15}{12}$ can be canceled like this:

$$\frac{\cancel{4}^{\,1}}{\cancel{5}_{\,1}} \times \frac{\cancel{15}^{\,3}}{\cancel{12}_{\,3}} = \frac{1}{1} \times \frac{3}{3} = 1$$

Notice that both the 5 in the denominator of the first fraction and the 15 in the numerator of the second fraction are divisible by 5. Similarly, the 4 in the numerator of the first fraction and the 12 in the denominator of the second fraction are both divisible by 4. Simplifying fractions requires identifying these types of relationships and dividing accordingly.

Comparing Fractions

One way to compare fractions is to re-express them with a **common denominator**. $\frac{3}{4} = \frac{21}{28}$ and $\frac{5}{7} = \frac{20}{28}$. $\frac{21}{28}$ is greater than $\frac{20}{28}$ so $\frac{3}{4}$ is greater than $\frac{5}{7}$. Another way to compare fractions is to convert them both to decimals. $\frac{3}{4}$ converts to 0.75, and $\frac{5}{7}$ converts to approximately 0.714.

Mixed Numbers and Fractions

A mixed number consists of an integer and a fraction. For example, $3\frac{1}{4}$, $12\frac{2}{5}$, and $5\frac{7}{8}$ are all mixed numbers.

To convert an improper fraction (a fraction whose numerator is greater than its denominator) to a mixed number, divide the numerator by the denominator. The number of "whole" times that the denominator goes into the numerator will be the integer portion of the mixed number; the remainder will be the numerator of the fractional portion.

Example: Convert $\frac{23}{4}$ to a mixed number.

Solution: Dividing 23 by 4 gives you 5 with a remainder of 3, so $\frac{23}{4} = 5\frac{3}{4}$.

To change a mixed number to a fraction, keep the denominator of the fraction. To figure out the numerator, multiply the integer portion of the mixed number by the number in the denominator. Then add this result to the numerator of the mixed number.

Example: Convert $2\frac{3}{7}$ to a fraction.

Solution: $2\frac{3}{7} = \frac{(2 \times 7) + 3}{7} = \frac{17}{7}$

Example: Convert $5\frac{8}{9}$ to a fraction.

Solution: $5\frac{8}{9} = \frac{(5 \times 9) + 8}{9} = \frac{53}{9}$

Adding and Subtracting Mixed Numbers

Adding or subtracting mixed numbers whose fractional parts have the same denominator will probably be on the test.

Example: $3\frac{12}{17} + 4\frac{10}{17} = ?$

Solution: First, add the integer parts: $3 + 4 = 7$.

Next, add the fractional parts: $\frac{12}{17} + \frac{10}{17} = \frac{22}{17}$.

Now, $\frac{22}{17} = 1\frac{5}{17}$.

Therefore, $3\frac{12}{17} + 4\frac{10}{17} = 7 + 1\frac{5}{17} = 8\frac{5}{17}$.

Example: $4\frac{5}{8} - 2\frac{7}{8} = ?$

Solution: The wrinkle here is that the fractional part of the first number is smaller than the fractional part of the second number (i.e., $\frac{5}{8}$ is smaller then $\frac{7}{8}$). What you need to do, therefore, is borrow from the integer part of the first number to make the fractional part of the first number bigger. Borrow 1 from the integer part and add it to the fractional part (remembering that 1 can be rewritten as $\frac{8}{8}$).

So $4\frac{5}{8} = 3 + \frac{8}{8} + \frac{5}{8} = 3\frac{13}{8}$. So the problem of finding $4\frac{5}{8} - 2\frac{7}{8}$ has been replaced with the problem of finding $3\frac{13}{8} - 2\frac{7}{8}$, which is easier because the fractional part of the first number is greater than the fractional part of the second number.

Notice that all you need to do is replace $4\frac{5}{8}$ with $3\frac{13}{8}$, which is equal to $4\frac{5}{8}$. To find $3\frac{13}{8} - 2\frac{7}{8}$, first subtract the integer parts: $3 - 2 = 1$. Next subtract the fractional parts: $\frac{13}{8} - \frac{7}{8} = \frac{13-7}{8} = \frac{6}{8} = \frac{3}{4}$. So $4\frac{5}{8} - 2\frac{7}{8} = 1\frac{3}{4}$.

Example: $5\frac{1}{4} - 1\frac{3}{4} = ?$

Solution: $5\frac{1}{4} - 1\frac{3}{4} = 5 + \frac{1}{4} - 1\frac{3}{4} = \left(4 + \frac{4}{4}\right) + \frac{1}{4} - 1\frac{3}{4} = 4 + \left(\frac{4}{4} + \frac{1}{4}\right) - 1\frac{3}{4}$

$$= 4\frac{5}{4} - 1\frac{3}{4} = 3\frac{2}{4} = 3\frac{1}{2}$$

When you gain experience with this, you'll be able to skip some of the steps and do this type of problem more quickly.

Example: $8\frac{3}{25} - 4\frac{12}{25} = ?$

Solution: $8\frac{3}{25} - 4\frac{12}{25} = 7 + \frac{25}{25} + \frac{3}{25} - 4\frac{12}{25} = 7\frac{28}{25} - 4\frac{12}{25} = 3\frac{16}{25}$

RATIOS

Setting Up a Ratio

To find a ratio, put the number associated with the word *of* on top and the quantity associated with the word *to* on the bottom and reduce. The ratio of 20 oranges to 12 apples is $\frac{20}{12}$, which reduces to $\frac{5}{3}$.

Part-to-Part Ratios and Part-to-Whole Ratios

If the parts add up to the whole, a part-to-part ratio can be turned into two part-to-whole ratios by putting each number in the original ratio over the sum of the numbers. If the ratio of males to females is 1 to 2, then the males-to-people ratio is $\frac{1}{1+2} = \frac{1}{3}$ and the females-to-people ratio is $\frac{2}{1+2} = \frac{2}{3}$. In other words, $\frac{2}{3}$ of all the people are female.

Solving a Proportion

To solve a proportion, **cross-multiply**:

$$\frac{x}{5} = \frac{3}{4}$$

$$4x = 5 \times 3$$

$$x = \frac{15}{4} = 3.75$$

An Important Point About Ratios

Notice that if you are given a ratio, you can't determine how many there are of each item just from the ratio. For example, if you are told that the ratio of the number of pencils to the number of pens in a drawer is 5 to 4, you don't know that there are 5 pencils and 4 pens in the drawer. All you know is that for every 5 pencils, there are 4 pens. There might be 50 pencils and 40 pens, or there might be 10 pencils and 8 pens in the drawer.

Example: The ratio of dogs to cats in an apartment building is 3 to 2. If there are a total of 50 animals in the apartment building and all of the animals in the building are dogs or cats, how many dogs are in the building?

Solution: The fraction of animals that are dogs is $\frac{3}{3+2}$, or $\frac{3}{5}$. So the number of dogs in the building is $\frac{3}{5} \times 50$, or 30.

DECIMALS

There are two different ways to express numbers that are not integers: as fractions and as decimals. You've already seen fractions; now it's time to talk about decimals.

When a number is expressed in decimal form, it has two parts: the whole number part and the decimal fraction part. The two parts are separated by the decimal point (.). The whole number part is to the left of the decimal point; the decimal fraction part is the decimal point and the numbers to the right of the decimal point. For example, in 4.56, the whole number is 4, and the decimal fraction is 0.56.

You are certainly familiar with decimals from dealing with money: $12.45 is an example of a decimal. The part to the left of the decimal point is the whole number part: 12 in this case. The decimal fraction part is 0.45 in this case.

You can see how decimals work by looking at dollars and cents. What fraction of a dollar is 1 cent? That's 0.01 dollars. Well, there are 100 cents in a dollar, so 1 cent must represent $\frac{1}{100}$ of a dollar. So you know that the fraction $\frac{1}{100}$ is equivalent to the decimal 0.01.

Now, what fraction of a dollar is 10 cents, or 0.10 dollars? That's equal to a dime, and there are 10 dimes in a dollar, so 10 cents must be $\frac{1}{10}$ of a dollar. So you also know that $\frac{1}{10}$ is equivalent to the decimal 0.10.

Now notice this: the fraction $\frac{1}{10}$ is ten times as much as the fraction $\frac{1}{100}$. Similarly, the decimal 0.10 is ten times as much as the decimal 0.01. This should reassure you that you aren't changing the values of the fractions, only the way they're expressed.

You also can tell how each digit in a positive integer will lead to the value of that integer by the place value of that digit. For instance, in the number 27,465, the number 6 is in the tens place, so there will be $6 \times 10 = 60$ going towards the value of the integer 27,465. Each place is worth 10 times as much as the place to its right:

$$
\begin{aligned}
27,465 = 2 \times &\ 10,000 \\
+\, 7 \times &\ \ 1,000 \\
+\, 4 \times &\ \ \ \ 100 \\
+\, 6 \times &\ \ \ \ \ 10 \\
+\, 5 \times &\ \ \ \ \ \ 1
\end{aligned}
$$

Decimals work the same way. You can tell each digit in a decimal will lead to the value of that decimal by the place of that digit relative to the decimal point. The first place to the right of the decimal point is worth $\frac{1}{10}$ (thus it is called the tenths place). The second place is worth $\frac{1}{100}$ (thus it is the hundredths place). The third place is worth $\frac{1}{1,000}$ (thus it is the thousandths place). The fourth place is worth $\frac{1}{10,000}$ (thus it is the ten-thousandths place), and so on.

As before, each place is worth 10 times as much as the place to its immediate right. That's why 0.10 means $\frac{1}{10}$, and 0.01 means $\frac{1}{100}$. By the way, the decimal point is small and has a habit of getting lost (is that a decimal or a bug?); for this reason, it's best to put the 0 before the decimal. That doesn't change the value; 0.01 is the same as .01. Also, zeros to the right of the last digit of a decimal don't change its value: 0.10 is the same as 0.1; they're both $\frac{1}{10}$. Similarly, 7.59 and 7.59000 have the same value; they're both $7\frac{59}{100}$.

Changing Fractions to Decimals

To change a fraction into a decimal, divide the denominator of the fraction into the numerator.

Example: Change $\frac{415}{3,220}$ into a decimal.

Solution: First write the fraction as long division.

$$3,220\overline{)415}$$

3,220 is much bigger than 415, so add zeros to 415 to make the division work out. The only way you can do this without changing the value of 415 is by adding a decimal point after the 5. Then, change 415 to 415.00 (those zeros don't change the value of anything). Divide normally but put a decimal point in the quotient (the answer) directly above the decimal point in 415.

$$
\begin{array}{r}
.12 \\
3220\overline{)415.00} \\
\underline{322\,0} \\
93\,00 \\
\underline{64\,40} \\
28\,600
\end{array}
$$

How far you should go depends on how much accuracy you need; here, you can stop at this hundredths place because you can see the answer is going to be close to 0.13.

Changing Decimals to Fractions

How do you express 0.5 as a fraction? 0.1 represents $\frac{1}{10}$, and 0.5 is five times as much as 0.1, so 0.5 must represent 5 times $\frac{1}{10}$ or $\frac{5}{10}$.

How do you express 0.55 as a fraction? Think of it in terms of dollars and cents. $0.01 is one cent, and that's $\frac{1}{100}$ of a dollar. $0.55 is 55 cents, and that's 55 times as much, so $0.55 must be $\frac{55}{100}$ of a dollar. You can reduce this by dividing the top and bottom by 5, giving $\frac{11}{20}$. That's the fractional equivalent of 0.55.

Hopefully by this point you recognize a pattern:

$$0.1 = 1 \times \frac{1}{10} \text{ or } \frac{1}{10}$$

$$0.11 = 11 \times \frac{1}{100} \text{ or } \frac{11}{100}$$

$$0.111 = 111 \times \frac{1}{1,000} \text{ or } \frac{111}{1,000}$$

$$0.1111 = 1,111 \times \frac{1}{10,000} \text{ or } \frac{1,111}{10,000}$$

and so on.

To change decimals that are between 0 and 1 to fractions, put the digits to the right of the decimal point in the numerator. To figure out the denominator, put a 1 in the denominator and follow it with as many zeros as digits to the right of the decimal point.

Example: Change 0.564 to a fraction.

Solution: There are three digits to the right of the decimal point, so the denominator of the fraction will be 1,000 (a 1 followed by three zeros). The numerator of the fraction is 564.

$$0.564 = \frac{564}{1,000}$$

But notice that $\frac{564}{1,000}$ can be reduced. Because both 564 and 1,000 are divisible by 4, divide both the numerator and the denominator by 4; therefore, $\frac{564}{1,000} = \frac{564 \div 4}{1,000 \div 4} = \frac{141}{250}$.

Addition and Subtraction of Decimals

Add and subtract decimals the same way you add and subtract whole numbers, but make sure the decimal points are lined up before adding. In the answer, put the decimal point directly below the other decimal points.

$$0.456 + 1.234 = \begin{array}{r} 0.456 \\ + 1.234 \\ \hline 1.690 \end{array}$$

If one of the terms you are adding or subtracting is longer than another (has more digits to the right of the decimal point), add zeros to the shorter number before adding or subtracting.

$$6.97 - 3.567 = 6.970$$
$$\underline{-\ 3.567}$$
$$3.403$$

Multiplication of Decimals

As with addition and subtraction, you multiply decimals as if they were whole numbers and worry about the decimal points later. You don't need to add zeros to make the numbers the same length when you multiply, however.

$$4.5 \times 3.2 = 4.5$$
$$\underline{\times\ 3.2}$$
$$90$$
$$\underline{+\ 1350}$$
$$1440$$

To place the decimal point in the answer, count the number of digits to the right of the decimal point in each number. Here you have 1 decimal place in 4.5, and 1 in 3.2, for a total of $1 + 1$ or 2 places. Put the decimal point 2 places from the right in the answer: 14.40.

It's a good idea when you get the answer to see whether it makes sense and to check that you put the decimal point in the right place. Here the answer should be a little bigger than 4×3 or 12. So 14.40 should be about right. If you placed the decimal point incorrectly and ended up with 144, you would know that was wrong.

Division of Decimals

It's easiest to discuss division of decimals if you express the division in fractional form.

Example: $4.15 \div 32.2 = \dfrac{4.15}{32.2}$

Solution: Make both the numerator and the denominator of the fraction whole numbers; to do this, multiply both top and bottom by a sufficient power of 10. In this example, multiply by 100; this will make the denominator 3,220 and the numerator 415, leaving:

$$\frac{4.15}{32.2} = \frac{415}{3,220}$$

Now divide 3,220 into 415. You should get approximately 0.129.

Rounding Decimals to the Nearest Place

To round a decimal to the nearest place, look at the digit immediately to the right of that place. If that digit is 5, 6, 7, 8, or 9, then round up. If the digit immediately to the right of the place you are rounding to is 0, 1, 2, 3, or 4, then don't change the digit at the place you are rounding. In either case, in the rounded-off number, there will be no digits to the right of the place you are rounding.

Example: Round 0.12763 to the nearest thousandth.

Solution: The digit in the thousandths place is 7. The digit immediately to the right of the 7 is a 6. Because 6 is among the digits that are 5 or more, round up the thousandths digit from 7 to 8. So 0.12763 rounded to the nearest thousandth is 0.128.

Example: Round 0.5827 to the nearest hundredth.

Solution: The digit in the hundredths place is 8. Immediately to the right of the 8 is a 2. Because 2 is among the digits 0 through 4, keep the digit in the hundredths place the same. So 0.5827 rounded to the nearest hundredth is 0.58.

Scientific Notation

Scientific notation is a convention for expressing numbers that simplifies computation and standardizes results. To write a nonzero number in scientific notation, write the number in the form $a \times 10^n$, where n is an integer and $1 \le a < 10$ or $-10 < a \le -1$.

Example: $123 = 1.23 \times 10^2$

1.23 is the **coefficient**, and 2 is the **exponent**.

Example: $0.042 = 4.2 \times 10^{-2}$

You can obtain products and quotients of numbers expressed in scientific notation. When multiplying, one simply multiplies the coefficients and adds the exponents to find the new coefficient and exponent of the answer. Some additional conversion may be necessary so that the new coefficient a is such that $1 \le a < 10$ or $-10 < a \le -1$, as in the example below.

Example: $(1.1 \times 10^6)(5.0 \times 10^{17}) = ?$

Solution: Multiply the coefficients 1.1 and 5.0 and add the exponents 6 and 17. The answer is 5.5×10^{23}.

The quotient of two numbers expressed in scientific notation is obtained by dividing the coefficient in the numerator by the coefficient in the denominator and subtracting the exponent in the denominator from the exponent in the numerator.

Example: $\dfrac{6.2 \times 10^5}{2.0 \times 10^{-7}} = ?$

Solution: Divide 6.2 by 2.0 and subtract -7 from 5 (note that $5 - (-7) = 5 + 7 = 12$). The answer is 3.1×10^{12}.

When a number expressed in scientific notation is raised to an exponent, the coefficient is raised to that exponent, and the original exponent is multiplied by that exponent.

Example: $(6.0 \times 10^4)^2$

Solution: Square the 6.0 and multiply the exponent by 2:

$(6.0)^2 \times 10^{4 \times 2} = 36.0 \times 10^8 = 3.6 \times 10^9$

Note that when you move the decimal point one place to the left you must increase the exponent of the 10 by one, from 8 to 9.

When adding or subtracting numbers expressed in scientific notation, they must have the same exponent; when they do not, the appropriate conversion must be made first.

Example: $3.7 \times 10^4 + 1.5 \times 10^3 = ?$

Solution: First, convert 1.5×10^3 to 0.15×10^4 so both numbers have the same exponent:

$3.7 \times 10^4 + 0.15 \times 10^4 = 3.85 \times 10^4$, which can be rounded to 3.9×10^4.

PERCENTS

Percents are a special kind of ratio. Any percent can be expressed as a fraction with a denominator of 100 (*cent* means "one hundred," so *percent* means "per one hundred"). When you see the symbol %, think of it as the factor $\frac{1}{100}$. Thus, $70\% = 70\left(\frac{1}{100}\right)$.

To convert a percent to a fraction or decimal, divide the percent by 100%. Because $100\% = 1$, you are dividing the percent by 1 and are not changing the value of the percent. In the case where the percent is in the form of a decimal number followed by the percent symbol %, the shortcut is to drop the percent symbol and move the decimal point in the number two places to the left.

Percent to fraction: $78\% = \frac{78\%}{100\%} = \frac{78}{100}$

Note that in going from $\frac{78\%}{100\%}$ to $\frac{78}{100}$, the percent symbol %, which represents the factor $\frac{1}{100}$, was cancelled from the numerator and denominator.

Percent to decimal: $78\% = 0.78$

$$78\% = \frac{78\%}{100\%} = \frac{78}{100} = 0.78$$

To convert any fraction or decimal to a percent, just multiply by 100%. For decimals, just move the decimal point two places to the right and add a percent sign. For fractions, remember to reduce if you can before you multiply.

Decimal to percent: $0.29 = 0.29 \times 100\% = 29\%$

$0.3 = 0.30 \times 100\% = 30\%$

$1.45 = 1.45 \times 100\% = 145\%$

Fraction to percent: $\frac{3}{5} = \frac{3}{5} \times 100\% = \frac{3(100)}{5}\% = 3(20)\% = 60\%$

Know these common conversions. They come up frequently on the test, and you can avoid errors and save time by memorizing them instead of having to calculate them on the test.

In general, a digit with a bar over it means that the digit repeats indefinitely. In the table below, $0.3\overline{3}$ means that the 3 with the bar over it repeats indefinitely. Thus, $0.3\overline{3} = 0.3333\ldots$

Fraction	Decimal	Percent
$\frac{1}{1}$	1.0	100%
$\frac{3}{4}$	0.75	75%
$\frac{2}{3}$	$0.6\overline{6}$	$66\frac{2}{3}\%$
$\frac{1}{2}$	0.5	50%
$\frac{1}{3}$	$0.3\overline{3}$	$33\frac{1}{3}\%$
$\frac{1}{4}$	0.25	25%
$\frac{1}{5}$	0.2	20%
$\frac{1}{8}$	0.125	$12\frac{1}{2}\%$
$\frac{1}{10}$	0.1	10%
$\frac{1}{20}$	0.05	5%

The Percent Formula

The percent formula is commonly expressed in two different ways that are mathematically identical. Memorize and use whichever version of the formula you prefer. Notice how easy it is to get from one formula to the other—just multiply or divide both sides of the equation by the Whole.

$$\text{Percent} = \frac{\text{Part}}{\text{Whole}}$$

or

$$\text{Percent} \times \text{Whole} = \text{Part}$$

If the Part is 3 and the Whole is 4, then the Percent $= \frac{3}{4} = 0.75 = 75\%$.

If the Percent is 20% and the Whole is 8, then the Part $= 20\%(8) = (0.2)(8) = 1.6$.

If the Percent is 60% and the Part is 12, then $60\% \times (\text{Whole}) = 12$. So:

$$\text{Whole} = \frac{12}{60\%} = \frac{12}{\left(\frac{6}{10}\right)} = 12\left(\frac{10}{6}\right) = 20.$$

Translating

Translating percent word problems into math is relatively easy. Whenever you see the phrase "what percent *of* . . . *is* . . .?," whatever follows the word *of* is the Whole and whatever follows the verb (often *is* or *are*) is the Part.

Example: 25% of 48 is 12.

$$\frac{\text{(part)}\,12}{\text{(whole)}\,48} = 25\%$$

Example: What percent of the songbirds are cardinals?

You don't really have to know what the question is talking about to know that the Whole is the number of songbirds and the Part is the number of cardinals.

Percent Increase/Decrease

Once you understand percents, percent increase and decrease are not as difficult as they may seem.

$$\% \text{ increase} = \frac{\text{Amount of increase}}{\text{Original whole}} \times 100\%$$

$$\% \text{ decrease} = \frac{\text{Amount of decrease}}{\text{Original whole}} \times 100\%$$

$$\text{New whole} = \text{Original whole} \pm \text{Amount of change}$$

Look at the first equation above. To find a percent increase, divide the amount of increase by the original whole. Then multiply this fraction by 100%.

Example: If a number increases from 50 to 70, what is the percent increase?

Solution: The amount of increase is $70 - 50$, or 20. The original whole is 50. So the percent increase is

$$\frac{20}{50} \times 100\% = \frac{2}{5} \times 100\%.$$

What you learned about reducing fractions can help here:

$$\frac{2}{5} \times 100\% = 2 \times 20\% = 40\%$$

If the new price of an item is 130% of its previous price, then it has increased in price by 30%. If an item goes on sale at 60% of its previous price, then it has decreased in price by 40%.

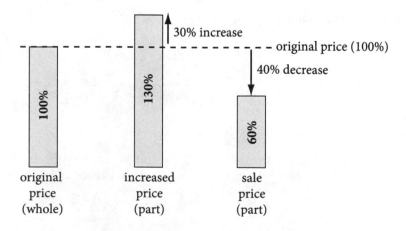

The percent increase or decrease is just the difference in percent from the whole (which is always equal to 100%).

The following table shows which formula to use—percent increase or percent decrease—when you come across different phrases in word problems:

Percent increase	Percent decrease
percent higher than	percent lower than
percent greater than	percent less than
percent gain	percent loss
percent more than	percent less than

Table 58.1

If X is $n\%$ greater than Y, then X is $(100 + n)\%$ of Y. For example, if X is 10% greater than Y, then X is 110% of Y.

If X is $n\%$ less than Y, then X is $(100 - n)\%$ of Y. For example, If X is 70% less than Y, then X is 30% of Y.

Example: If the value of a certain piece of property now is 350% of its original value when Kim purchased it, by what percent has the value of the property increased since Kim purchased it?

Solution: The percent increase is the difference from 100%. So there was a $350\% - 100\% = 250\%$ increase.

AVERAGES

Formula for Computing Averages (**Mean**)

The average formula is $\text{Average} = \dfrac{\text{Sum of the terms}}{\text{Number of terms}}$

To find the mean of a set of numbers, add them up (the sum of the terms) and divide by the number of numbers (the number of terms).

Example: To find the average of the five numbers 12, 15, 23, 40, and 40, first add them: $12 + 15 + 23 + 40 + 40 = 130$. Then divide the sum by 5: $130 \div 5 = 26$.

Using the Average to Find the Sum

$\text{Sum} = (\text{Average}) \times (\text{Number of terms})$

Example: If the average of 10 numbers is 50, then they add up to 50×10, or 500.

Finding the Missing Number

To find a missing number when you're given the average, use the sum.

Example: If the average of four numbers is 7, then the sum of those four numbers is 4×7, or 28. Suppose that three of the numbers are 3, 5, and 8. These three numbers add up to 16 of that 28, which leaves $28 - 16 = 12$ for the fourth number.

CONVERSIONS

Occasionally you will be asked to convert a quantity in a question. The quantity will be a number of units of something. Examples of quantities are 450 miles and 12 pounds. Converting a quantity means expressing the quantity in a different unit.

Example: If the distance between the city of New York and the city of London is approximately 3,500 miles, how many inches apart are these cities?

Solution: To convert from miles to inches, first convert miles to feet and then convert feet to inches:

3,500 miles (5,280 feet/1 mile)

$= 18,480,000$ feet (12 inches/1 foot)

$= 221,760,000$ feet.

Now 221,760,000 rounded to the nearest million is 222,000,000, which in scientific notation is 2.2×10^8.

Example: The moon revolves around the earth at a speed of approximately 1.02 kilometers per second. How many kilometers per hour is this approximate speed?

Solution: Since the question asks for kilometers per hour, begin by converting seconds to minutes and then converting minutes to hours.

(1.02 kilometers/1 second) (60 seconds/1minute)

$= (61.2$ kilometers/1 minute) (60 minutes/1 hour)

$= 3,672$ kilometers/hour.

LOGARITHMS

The properties of logarithms are dependent on the laws of exponents; therefore, a review of exponents is necessary before the introduction of logarithms.

In the equation: $b^c = x$

b is the base

c is the exponent

x is b raised to the exponent c, where b is positive and not equal to 1.

In the equation above, the exponent c may be an integer, a fraction, or an irrational number. The value of c may be positive, negative, or 0.

In the equation $b^c = x$, the exponent c is the exponent to which b must be raised to obtain the number x. This relationship is described by the statement "The logarithm of x to the base b," which means if $b^c = x$, then the logarithm to the base b of x is c. In other words:

The logarithm to the base b of a positive number x is equal to the exponent to which b must be raised to obtain x:

$$\text{If: } \log_b(x) = c, \text{ then: } b^c = x$$

Examples: $\log_4(16) = 2$, since $4^2 = 16$

$\log_{10}(10{,}000) = 4$, since $10^4 = 10{,}000$

$\log_{25}(5) = \frac{1}{2}$, since $25^{\frac{1}{2}} = 5$

Example: If $\log_5(x) = 3$, then $x = ?$

Solution: The expression $\log_5(x) = 3$ means that $5^3 = x$; therefore, $x = 125$.

Example: If $\log_b(36) = 2$, then $b = ?$

Solution: The expression $\log_b(36) = 2$ means that $b^2 = 36$; therefore, $b = 6$. If $b^2 = 36$, then $b = 6$ or $b = -6$. However, since you are working with a logarithm to the base b, b must be positive and not equal to 1. Thus, you cannot have $b = -6$. In this example, the only possible value of b is 6.

Example: If $\log_{10}(100) = c$, then $c = ?$

Solution: The expression $\log_{10}(100) = c$ means that $10^c = 100$. Now $100 = 10^2$. Thus, $10^c = 10^2$. Therefore, $c = 2$.

Properties of Logs

The logarithm of the product of two numbers equals the sum of the individual logarithms:

$$\log_b(s \times t) = \log_b(s) + \log_b(t)$$

The logarithm of a quotient of two numbers is the logarithm of the numerator minus the logarithm of the denominator:

$$\log_b\left(\frac{s}{t}\right) = \log_b(s) - \log_b(t)$$

The logarithm of a power with a positive base is equal to the exponent of the power multiplied by the logarithm of the base of that power:

$$\log_b(s^p) = p \times \log_b(s)$$

Log Base 10

Most commonly, logs are expressed in base 10. This means that an increase of one logarithmic unit (in base 10) corresponds to a multiplication of 10 of the actual total.

$$\log_{10}(0.1) = -1, \text{ since } 10^{-1} = 0.1$$
$$\log_{10}(1) = 0, \text{ since } 10^0 = 1$$
$$\log_{10}(10) = 1, \text{ since } 10^1 = 10$$
$$\log_{10}(100) = 2, \text{ since } 10^2 = 100$$
$$\log_{10}(1,000) = 3, \text{ since } 10^3 = 1,000$$

When working with logarithms to the base of 10, $\log_{10}(x)$ is often written $\log(x)$. For example, $\log(5.3)$ means $\log_{10}(5.3)$. When working with logarithms to the base 10, the integer of the logarithm of a number is called the **characteristic** and the decimal fraction of the logarithm of the number is called the **mantissa**. For example, consider $\log(7,435)$ (note that $\log(7,435)$ means $\log_{10}(7,435)$.) You have that $\log(7,435) = 3.87128$. In this case, for $\log(7,435)$, the characteristic is 3 and the mantissa is 0.87128. Shifting the decimal point to the right or left in a number increases or decreases the characteristic of the logarithm of that number as seen below:

Example: $\log(4.26) = \log(1 \times 4.26) = \log(10^0) + \log(4.26) = 0 + 0.62941 = 0.62941 + 0$

$\log(0.426) = \log(0.1 \times 4.26) = \log(10^{-1}) + \log(4.26) = -1 + 0.62941 = 0.62941 - 1$

$\log(0.0426) = \log(0.01 \times 4.26) = \log(10^{-2}) + \log(4.26) = -2 + 0.62941 = 0.62941 - 2$

$\log(42.6) = \log(10 \times 4.26) = \log(10^1) + \log(4.26) = 1 + 0.62941 = 0.62941 + 1$

$\log(426) = \log(10^2 \times 4.26) = \log(10^2) + \log(4.26) = 2 + 0.62941 = 0.62941 + 2$

REVIEW PROBLEMS

1. The average of 3, 15, 18, and 8 is
   (A) 5
   (B) 9
   (C) 11
   (D) 18

2. Which of the following fractions is largest?
   (A) $\frac{2}{5}$
   (B) $\frac{1}{2}$
   (C) $\frac{2}{7}$
   (D) $\frac{2}{10}$

3. $\frac{2}{7} + \frac{1}{4} =$
   (A) $\frac{1}{11}$
   (B) $\frac{3}{28}$
   (C) $\frac{15}{28}$
   (D) $\frac{7}{8}$

4. $6\frac{1}{7} - 3\frac{4}{7}$
   (A) $2\frac{3}{7}$
   (B) $2\frac{4}{7}$
   (C) $3\frac{3}{7}$
   (D) $3\frac{4}{7}$

5. Which of the following numbers is smallest?
   (A) 0.1
   (B) 0.01
   (C) 0.0407
   (D) 0.03995

6. What is the value of $5\frac{1}{4} \div 7$?

    (A) $\frac{5}{7}$

    (B) 3

    (C) $\frac{3}{4}$

    (D) $3\frac{4}{7}$

7. $16 + 0.267 + 36.78 =$

    (A) 5.347
    (B) 8.26
    (C) 52.037
    (D) 53.047

8. What is the cost of a blouse that is priced at $50.00 with a tax of 7%?

    (A) $35.00
    (B) $50.35
    (C) $53.50
    (D) $85.00

9. If a pencil costs $0.26, what is the cost of 96 pencils?

    (A) $2.49
    (B) $12.00
    (C) $24.00
    (D) $24.96

10. What is the value of $2,886 \div 37$?

    (A) 78
    (B) 708
    (C) 780
    (D) 7,008

SOLUTIONS TO REVIEW PROBLEMS

1. **C** Average $= \dfrac{\text{Sum of the terms}}{\text{Number of terms}}$

    Here, the average is $\dfrac{3+15+18+8}{4} = \dfrac{44}{4} = 11$.

2. **B** Begin by comparing choice (A), $\dfrac{2}{5}$, and choice (B), $\dfrac{1}{2}$. $\dfrac{2}{5}$ has a numerator that is less than half of its denominator, so choice (A) is less than $\dfrac{1}{2}$. Choice (A) can be eliminated. Choices (C) and (D) both have numerators that are less than half of their denominators, so these choices are also less than $\dfrac{1}{2}$ and can therefore also be eliminated. This means that choice (B), $\dfrac{1}{2}$, is the largest.

3. **C** $\dfrac{2}{7} + \dfrac{1}{4} = \left(\dfrac{2}{7} \times \dfrac{4}{4}\right) + \left(\dfrac{1}{4} \times \dfrac{7}{7}\right) = \dfrac{8}{28} + \dfrac{7}{28} = \dfrac{15}{28}$

4. **B** $6\dfrac{1}{7} - 3\dfrac{4}{7} = \left(6 + \dfrac{1}{7}\right) - 3\dfrac{4}{7} = \left(5 + \dfrac{7}{7} + \dfrac{1}{7}\right) - 3\dfrac{4}{7} = 5\dfrac{8}{7} - 3\dfrac{4}{7} = 2\dfrac{4}{7}$

5. **B** Choice (A) has a tenths digit of 1, while choices (B), (C), and (D) each have a tenths digit of 0. So choice (A) can be eliminated. Next, look at the hundredths digit: choice (B) has the smallest value at 1, so (B) is the smallest number.

6. **C** When you divide one fraction by another, you invert the second fraction and multiply.

    Think of the integer 7 as the fraction $\dfrac{7}{1}$, so that you can invert it to get the fraction $\dfrac{1}{7}$.

    Rewrite $5\dfrac{1}{4}$ as an improper fraction. $5\dfrac{1}{4} = \dfrac{5 \times 4 + 1}{4} = \dfrac{20 + 1}{4} = \dfrac{21}{4}$.

    Then $5\dfrac{1}{4} \div 7 = \dfrac{21}{4} \div \dfrac{7}{1} = \dfrac{21}{4} \times \dfrac{1}{7} = \dfrac{21 \times 1}{4 \times 7} = \dfrac{21}{28} = \dfrac{3}{4}$.

7. **D** Write the numbers in a column, making sure to align the decimal points. Write 16 as 16.000 and write 36.78 as 36.780.

    $$\begin{array}{r} 16.000 \\ 0.267 \\ +\,36.780 \\ \hline 53.047 \end{array}$$

8. **C** Add 7% of 50 to 50. 7% of 50 is $\dfrac{7}{100} \times 50 = \dfrac{7}{2} \times 1 = \dfrac{7}{2} = 3\dfrac{1}{2} = 3.5$. So the cost of the blouse is $50 + $3.50, or $53.50.

9. **D** Multiply the cost of one pencil by the number of pencils. The cost of all the pencils is $0.26 \times 96 = \$24.96$.

10. **A**
$$
\begin{array}{r}
78 \\
37\overline{)2886} \\
\underline{259} \\
296 \\
\underline{296} \\
0
\end{array}
$$

CHAPTER FIFTY-NINE

Algebra

Algebra uses the concepts of arithmetic and number properties but adds a twist: variables. **Variables** represent unknown quantities, and many algebraic questions task you with determining what numerical values variables actually represent. Variables are often defined by the rules of **equations** and **inequalities**, statements that show the relationship between two or more expressions as equal (equations) or greater than or less than each other (inequalities).

WORD PROBLEMS

Often the most challenging aspect of algebra problems is the odd way in which information is presented. Don't get frustrated; just break down the information into small pieces and take things one step at a time. Word problems can usually be translated from left to right, but this is not always the case. Say you see this sentence: "The number of stamps in George's stamp collection is twice the number that is 5 less than the number of stamps in Bill's stamp collection." Instead of trying to translate it into math all in one step, approach it piece by piece.

Whenever possible, choose letters for the variables that make sense in the context of the problem. For example, start by calling the number of stamps in George's stamp collection G and the number of stamps in Bill's stamp collection B. Now, think about the relationship between the two amounts: G is not compared to B but to 5 less than B, or $(B - 5)$. So G is twice as large as $(B - 5)$. To set them *equal* to each other, multiply $(B - 5)$ by two. The equation is $G = 2(B - 5)$.

The hardest part of word problems is the process of taking the English sentences and extracting the math from them. The actual math in word problems tends to be the easiest part. The following translation table will help you start dealing with English-to-math translation:

Word Problems Translation Table	
English	**Math**
equals, is, was, will be, has, costs, adds up to, the same as, as much as	=
times, of, multiplied by, product of, twice, double, by	×
divided by, per, out of, each, ratio	÷
plus, added to, and, sum, combined	+
minus, subtracted from, smaller than, less than, fewer, decreased by, difference between	−
a number, how much, how many, what	x, n, etc.

Table 59.1

Example: w is x less than y.

Solution: $w = y - x$

Example: Giuseppa's weight is 75 pounds more than twice Jovanna's weight.

Solution: $G = 2J + 75$

Example: In 5 years, Sandy will be 4 years younger than twice Tina's age.

Solution: $(S + 5) = 2(T + 5) - 4$

Notice here that the statement discusses the ages of Sandy and Tina *in five years*, so you must represent their ages as $(S + 5)$ and $(T + 5)$, respectively. One common mistake is to translate the right side of the equation as $2T + 5 - 4$, but that is not equivalent to $2(T + 5) - 4$.

Example: The sum of Richard's age and Cindy's age in years is 17 more than the amount by which Tim's age is greater than Kathy's age.

Solution: $R + C = (T - K) + 17$

EXPONENTS

You can't be adept at algebra unless you're completely at ease with exponents. Here's what you need to know:

Multiplying powers with the same base: To multiply powers with the same base, keep the base and add the exponents:

$$x^3 \times x^4 = x^{3+4} = x^7$$

Dividing powers with the same base: To divide powers with the same base, keep the base and subtract the exponents:

$$y^{13} \div y^8 = y^{13-8} = y^5$$

Raising a power to an exponent: To raise a power to an exponent, keep the base and multiply the exponents:

$$(x^3)^4 = x^{3 \times 4} = x^{12}$$

Multiplying powers with the same exponent: To multiply powers with the same exponent, multiply the bases and keep the exponent:

$$(3^x)(4^x) = (3 \times 4)^x = 12^x$$

Dividing powers with the same exponent: To divide powers with the same exponent, divide the bases and keep the exponent:

$$\frac{6^x}{2^x} = \left(\frac{6}{2}\right)^x = 3^x$$

Example: For all $xyz \neq 0$, $\dfrac{6x^2y^{12}z^6}{(2x^2yz)^3} = ?$

Solution: The first step is to eliminate the parentheses. Everything inside gets cubed:

$$\frac{6x^2y^{12}z^6}{(2x^2yz)^3} = \frac{6x^2y^{12}z^6}{8x^6y^3z^3}$$

The next step is to look for factors common to the numerator and denominator. The 6 on the top and the 8 on the bottom reduce to 3 over 4. The x^2 on the top cancels with the x^6 on the bottom, leaving x^4 on the bottom.

You're actually subtracting the exponents: $2 - 6 = -4$. The x^{-4} on the top is the same as $\dfrac{1}{x^4}$. The y^{12} on the top cancels with the y^3 on the bottom, leaving y^9 on the top. And the z^6 on the top cancels with the z^3 on the bottom, leaving z^3 on the top:

$$\frac{6x^2y^{12}z^6}{8x^6y^3z^3} = \frac{3y^9z^3}{4x^4}$$

ADDING, SUBTRACTING, AND MULTIPLYING POLYNOMIALS

Algebra is the basic language of mathematics, and you will want to be fluent in that language. You might not get a whole lot of questions that ask explicitly about such basic algebra procedures as combining like terms, multiplying binomials, or factoring algebraic expressions, but you will do all of those things in the course of working out the answers to more advanced questions. So it's essential that you be at ease with the mechanics of algebraic manipulations.

Combining like terms: To combine like terms, keep the variable part unchanged while adding or subtracting the coefficients:

$$2a + 3a = (2 + 3)a = 5a$$

Adding or subtracting polynomials: To add or subtract polynomials, combine like terms:

$$(3x^2 + 5x - 7) - (x^2 + 12)$$
$$= 3x^2 + 5x - 7 - x^2 - 12$$
$$= (3x^2 - x^2) + 5x + (-7 - 12)$$
$$= 2x^2 + 5x - 19$$

Multiplying monomials: To multiply monomials, multiply the coefficients and the variables separately:

$$2x \times 3x = (2 \times 3)(x \times x) = 6x^2$$

Multiplying binomials: To multiply binomials, use FOIL. To multiply $(x + 3)$ by $(x + 4)$, first multiply the First terms: $x \times x = x^2$; next the Outer terms: $x \times 4 = 4x$; then the Inner terms: $3 \times x = 3x$; and finally the Last terms: $3 \times 4 = 12$. Then add and combine like terms:

$$x^2 + 4x + 3x + 12 = x^2 + 7x + 12$$

Multiplying polynomials: To multiply polynomials with more than two terms, make sure you multiply each term in the first polynomial by each term in the second. (FOIL works only when you want to multiply two binomials.)

$$(x^2 + 3x + 4)(x + 5) = x^2(x + 5) + 3x(x + 5) + 4(x + 5)$$
$$= x^3 + 5x^2 + 3x^2 + 15x + 4x + 20$$
$$= x^3 + 8x^2 + 19x + 20$$

After multiplying two polynomials together, the number of terms in your expression before simplifying should equal the number of terms in one polynomial multiplied by the number of terms in the second. In the example above, you should have $3 \times 2 = 6$ terms in the product before you simplify like terms.

DIVIDING POLYNOMIALS

To divide polynomials, you can use long division. For example, to divide $2x^3 + 13x^2 + 11x - 16$ by $x + 5$:

$$x + 5 \overline{)2x^3 + 13x^2 + 11x - 16}$$

The first term of the quotient is $2x^2$, because that's what will give you a $2x^3$ as a first term when you multiply it by $x + 5$:

$$
\begin{array}{r}
2x^2 \\
x + 5 \overline{)2x^3 + 13x^2 + 11x - 16} \\
2x^3 + 10x^2
\end{array}
$$

Subtract and continue in the same way as when dividing numbers:

$$
\begin{array}{r}
2x^2 + 3x - 4 \\
x + 5 \overline{\smash{)}\ 2x^3 + 13x^2 + 11x - 16} \\
\underline{2x^3 + 10x^2} \\
3x^2 + 11x \\
\underline{3x^2 + 15x} \\
-4x - 16 \\
\underline{-4x - 20} \\
4
\end{array}
$$

The result is $2x^2 + 3x - 4$ with a remainder of 4.

Example: When $2x^3 + 3x^2 - 4x + k$ is divided by $x + 2$, the remainder is 3. What is the value of k?

Solution: To answer this question, start by cranking out the long division:

$$
\begin{array}{r}
2x^2 - x - 2 \\
x + 2 \overline{\smash{)}\ 2x^3 + 3x^2 - 4x + k} \\
\underline{2x^3 + 4x^2} \\
-x^2 - 4x \\
\underline{-x^2 - 2x} \\
-2x + k \\
\underline{-2x - 4} \\
k + 4
\end{array}
$$

The question says that the remainder is 3, so whatever k is, when you add 4, you get 3:

$k + 4 = 3$

$k = -1$

FACTORING

Performing operations on polynomials is largely a matter of cranking it out. Once you know the rules, adding, subtracting, multiplying, and even dividing is automatic. Factoring algebraic expressions is a different matter. To factor successfully, you have to do more thinking and less cranking. You have to try to figure out what expressions multiplied will give you the polynomial you're looking at. Sometimes that means having a good eye for the test makers' favorite factorables:

- Factor common to all terms

- Difference of squares

- Square of a binomial

Factor common to all terms: A factor common to all the terms of a polynomial can be factored out. This is essentially the distributive property in reverse. For example, all three terms in the polynomial $3x^3 + 12x^2 - 6x$ contain a factor of $3x$. Pulling out the common factor yields $3x(x^2 + 4x - 2)$.

Difference of squares: You will want to be especially keen at spotting polynomials in the form of the difference of squares. Whenever you have two identifiable squares with a minus sign between them, you can factor the expression like this:

$$a^2 - b^2 = (a + b)(a - b)$$

$4x^2 - 9$, for example, factors to $(2x + 3)(2x - 3)$.

Squares of binomials: Learn to recognize polynomials that are squares of binomials:

$$a^2 + 2ab + b^2 = (a + b)^2$$
$$a^2 - 2ab + b^2 = (a - b)^2$$

Polynomials such as those seen above can be expressed as a product of two or more polynomials of lower positive degree. Each of these polynomials is referred to as a factor of the given polynomial. Unless stated in the question otherwise, one can assume only integer coefficients for the factors of a polynomial with integer coefficients.

For example, $4x^2 + 12x + 9$ factors to $(2x + 3)^2$, and $a^2 - 10a + 25$ factors to $(a - 5)^2$.

Sometimes you'll want to factor a polynomial that's not in any of these classic factorable forms. When that happens, factoring becomes a kind of logic exercise with some trial and error thrown in. To factor a quadratic expression, think about what binomials you could use FOIL on to get that quadratic expression. For example, to factor $x^2 - 5x + 6$, think about what First terms will produce x^2, what Last terms will produce $+6$, and what Outer and Inner terms will produce $-5x$. Some common sense—and a little trial and error—will lead you to $(x - 2)(x - 3)$.

Example: For all $x \neq \pm 3$, $\dfrac{3x^2 - 11x + 6}{9 - x^2} =$

    (A) $\dfrac{2x - 3}{x + 3}$

    (B) $\dfrac{2 - 3x}{x + 3}$

    (C) $\dfrac{2x + 3}{x + 3}$

    (D) $\dfrac{3x - 2}{x - 3}$

Solution: To reduce a fraction, you eliminate factors common to the top and the bottom. So the first step in reducing an algebraic fraction is to *factor the numerator and denominator*. Here, the denominator is the difference of squares: $9 - x^2 = (3 - x)(3 + x)$. The numerator takes some thought and some trial and error. For the first term to be $3x^2$, the first terms of the factors must be $3x$ and x. For the last term of the polynomial in the numerator to be $+6$, the last terms of the binomials must be either $+2$ and $+3$, -2 and -3, $+1$ and $+6$, or -1 and -6. After a few tries, you should come up with: $3x^2 - 11x + 6 = (3x - 2)(x - 3)$. Now the fraction looks like this:

$$\frac{3x^2 - 11x + 6}{9 - x^2} = \frac{(3x - 2)(x - 3)}{(3 - x)(3 + x)}$$

In this form there are no precisely common factors, but there is a factor in the numerator that's the opposite (negative) of a factor in the denominator: $x - 3$ and $3 - x$ are opposites. Factor -1 out of the numerator and get:

$$\frac{(3x - 2)(x - 3)}{(3 - x)(3 + x)} = \frac{(-1)(3x - 2)(3 - x)}{(3 - x)(3 + x)}$$

Now $(3 - x)$ can be eliminated from both the top and the bottom:

$$\frac{(-1)(3x - 2)(3 - x)}{(3 - x)(3 + x)} = \frac{-(3x - 2)}{3 + x} = \frac{-3x + 2}{3 + x}$$

That's the same as choice (B):

$$\frac{-3x + 2}{3 + x} = \frac{2 - 3x}{x + 3}$$

Alternative: Here's another way to answer this question. Pick a number for x, and see what happens. At least one of the answer choices, the correct answer choice, will give you the same value as the original fraction, no matter what you plug in for x. However, some of the incorrect answer choices might give you the same value as the original fraction for the value that you plug in. Pick a number that's easy to work with—like 0.

When you plug $x = 0$ into the original expression, any term with an x drops out, and you end up with $\frac{6}{9}$, or $\frac{2}{3}$. Now plug $x = 0$ into each answer choice to see which ones equal $\frac{2}{3}$. Eliminate any answer choices that do not equal $\frac{2}{3}$ when $x = 0$.

When you get to (B), it works, but you can't stop there. Sometimes one or more incorrect answer choices will work for the particular value that you choose. When you pick numbers, *look at every answer choice*. All the incorrect answer choices must be eliminated when using the method of picking numbers. Choice (D) also works for $x = 0$. At least you know one of those is the correct answer, and you can decide between them by picking another value for x.

This is not a sophisticated approach, but who cares? You don't get points for elegance. You get points for right answers.

Example: Factor the following polynomial: $8xy + 18y^2$.

Solution: You can see that $2y$ is greatest common factor of each term in the polynomial. Therefore, by the distributive law, you can factor:

$8xy + 18y^2 = 2y(4x + 9y)$

In this example, $2y$ is referred to as the greatest monomial factor of the given polynomial because it is the monomial with the greatest numerical coefficient that is a factor of each term in the polynomial and each variable of the monomial is raised to the greatest exponent that is a factor of each term of the polynomial. The other factor, $4x + 9y$, cannot be reduced to a product of factors of lower positive degree and therefore is irreducible. Moreover, the greatest monomial factor of $4x + 9y$ is 1. A polynomial is said to be completely factored when it is expressed as a product of a monomial, which may or may not be a constant, and one or more irreducible polynomials, each of which has 1 as its greatest monomial factor.

THE GOLDEN RULE OF EQUATIONS

You probably remember the basic procedure for solving algebraic equations: *do the same thing to both sides.* You can do almost anything you want to one side of an equation as long as you preserve the equality by doing the same thing to the other side. Your aim in whatever you do to both sides is to get the variable (or expression) you're solving for all by itself on one side.

Example: If $\sqrt[3]{8x + 6} = -3$, what is the value of x ?

Solution: To solve this equation for x, do whatever you must to both sides of the equation to isolate x on one side. Layer by layer you want to peel away all those extra symbols and numbers around the x. First you want to get rid of that cube-root symbol. The way to undo a cube root is to cube both sides:

$$\sqrt[3]{8x + 6} = -3$$
$$\left(\sqrt[3]{8x + 6}\right)^3 = (-3)^3$$
$$8x + 6 = -27$$

Next, subtract 6 from both sides and divide both sides by 8:
$$8x + 6 = -27$$
$$8x = -27 - 6$$
$$8x = -33$$
$$x = -\frac{33}{8} = -4.125$$

The test makers have a few favorite equation types that you should be prepared to solve. Solving linear equations is usually straightforward. Generally it's obvious what to do to isolate the unknown. But when the unknown is in a denominator or an exponent, how to proceed might not be so obvious.

UNKNOWN IN A DENOMINATOR

The basic procedure for solving an equation is the same even when the unknown is in a denominator: do the same thing to both sides. In this case, you multiply to undo division.

If you wanted to solve $1 + \frac{1}{x} = 2 - \frac{1}{x}$, you would multiply both sides by x:

$$1 + \frac{1}{x} = 2 - \frac{1}{x}$$
$$x\left(1 + \frac{1}{x}\right) = x\left(2 - \frac{1}{x}\right)$$
$$x + 1 = 2x - 1$$

Now you have an equation with no denominators, which is easy to solve:

$$x + 1 = 2x - 1$$
$$x - 2x = -1 - 1$$
$$-x = -2$$
$$x = 2$$

Another good way to solve an equation with the unknown in the denominator is to *cross multiply*. That's the best way to do the following example.

Example: If $\dfrac{5}{x+3} = \dfrac{1}{x} + \dfrac{1}{2x}$, what is the value of x?

Solution: Before you can cross multiply, you need to re-express the right side of the equation as a single fraction. That means giving the two fractions a common denominator and adding them. The common denominator to use is $2x$:

$$\frac{5}{x+3} = \frac{1}{x} + \frac{1}{2x}$$

$$\frac{5}{x+3} = \frac{2}{2x} + \frac{1}{2x}$$

$$\frac{5}{x+3} = \frac{3}{2x}$$

Now cross multiply:

$$\frac{5}{x+3} = \frac{3}{2x}$$
$$(5)(2x) = (x+3)(3)$$
$$10x = 3x + 9$$
$$10x - 3x = 9$$
$$7x = 9$$
$$x = \frac{9}{7}$$

UNKNOWN IN AN EXPONENT

The procedure for solving an equation when the unknown is in an exponent is a little different. What you want to do in this situation is to re-express one or both sides of the equation so that the two sides have the same base.

Example: If $8^x = 16^{x-1}$, then $x =$

(A) $\dfrac{1}{8}$

(B) $\dfrac{1}{2}$

(C) 2

(D) 4

Solution: In this case, the base on the left is 8 and the base on the right is 16. They're both powers with bases of 2 and integer exponents, so you can re-express both sides as powers with bases of 2:

$(2^3)^x = (2^4)^{(x-1)}$

$2^{3x} = 2^{4(x-1)}$

$2^{3x} = 2^{(4x-4)}$

Thus, $2^{3x} = 2^{(4x-4)}$. When two powers have the same base, they must have equal exponents. Here, you can simply set the exponent expressions equal and solve for x:

$3x = 4x - 4$

$3x - 4x = -4$

$-x = -4$

$x = 4$

Choice (D) is correct.

Alternative: Here's another way to answer this question: Use Backsolving. Here, if you start with choice (C) and $x = 2$, you get $8^x = 8^2 = 64$ on the left side of the equation and $16^{(x-1)} = 16^{(2-1)} = 16^1 = 16$ on the right side. It's not clear whether (C) was too small or too large, so you should probably try (D) next—it's easier to work with than (B), which is a fraction (and that's also why you didn't want to start with it first). If $x = 4$, then $8^x = 8^4 = 4{,}096$ on the left side, and $16^{(x-1)} = 16^{(4-1)} = 16^3 = 4{,}096$ on the right side. No need to do any more. Choice (D) works, so it's the answer.

QUADRATIC EQUATIONS

To solve a quadratic equation, put it in the $ax^2 + bx + c = 0$ form, factor the left side (if you can), and set each factor equal to 0 separately to get the two solutions. To solve $x^2 + 12 = 7x$, first rewrite it as $x^2 - 7x + 12 = 0$. Then factor the left side:

$$x^2 - 7x + 12 = 0$$
$$(x - 3)(x - 4) = 0$$
$$x - 3 = 0 \text{ or } x - 4 = 0$$
$$x = 3 \text{ or } x = 4$$

Sometimes the left side may not be obviously factorable. You can always use the *quadratic formula*. Just plug the coefficients a, b, and c from $ax^2 + bx + c = 0$ into the formula:

$$x = \frac{-b \pm \sqrt{b^2 - 4ac}}{2a}$$

To solve $x^2 + 4x + 2 = 0$, plug $a = 1$, $b = 4$, and $c = 2$ into the formula:

$$x = \frac{-4 \pm \sqrt{4^2 - 4 \cdot 1 \cdot 2}}{2 \cdot 1}$$

$$= \frac{-4 \pm \sqrt{8}}{2} = \frac{-4 \pm 2\sqrt{2}}{2} = -2 \pm \sqrt{2}$$

For all real numbers b and c, and all nonzero real numbers a, the quadratic equation $ax^2 + bx + c = 0$ has:

- Two different real roots if $b^2 - 4ac > 0$

- One double real root if $b^2 - 4ac = 0$

- Two complex conjugate roots if $b^2 - 4ac < 0$

"In Terms Of"

So far in this chapter, solving an equation has meant finding a numerical value for the unknown. When there's more than one variable in one equation, it's generally impossible to get numerical solutions. Instead, what you do is solve for the unknown *in terms of* the other variables.

To solve an equation for one variable in terms of another means to isolate the one variable on one side of the equation, leaving an expression containing the other variable on the other side of the equation.

For example, to solve the equation $3x - 10y = -5x + 6y$ for x in terms of y, isolate x:

$$3x - 10y = -5x + 6y$$
$$3x + 5x = 6y + 10y$$
$$8x = 16y$$
$$x = 2y$$

Example: If $a = \frac{b+x}{c+x}$, what is the value of x in terms of a, b, and c?

Solution: You want to get x on one side by itself. The first thing to do is eliminate the denominator by multiplying both sides by $c + x$:

$$a = \frac{b+x}{c+x}$$
$$a(c+x) = \frac{b+x}{c+x}(c+x)$$
$$ac + ax = b + x$$

Next, move all terms with x to one side and all terms without x to the other:
$$ac + ax = b + x$$
$$ax - x = b - ac$$

Now factor x out of the left side and divide both sides by the other factor to isolate x:

$$ax - x = b - ac$$

$$x(a - 1) = b - ac$$
$$x = \frac{b - ac}{a - 1}$$

SIMULTANEOUS EQUATIONS

You can get numerical solutions for more than one unknown if you are given more than one equation. Simultaneous Equations questions take a little thought to answer. Solving simultaneous equations almost always involves combining equations, but you have to figure out the best way to combine each unique set of equations.

You can solve for two variables only if you have two distinct equations. Two forms of the same equation will not be adequate. Combine the equations in such a way that one of the variables cancels out. For example, to solve the two equations $4x + 3y = 8$ and $x + y = 3$, multiply both sides of the second equation by -3 to get $-3x - 3y = -9$. Now add the two equations; the $3y$ and the $-3y$ cancel out, leaving $x = -1$. Plug that back into either one of the original equations and you'll find that $y = 4$.

Example: If $2x - 9y = 11$ and $x + 12y = -8$, what is the value of $x + y$?

Solution: If you just plow ahead without thinking, you might try to answer this question by solving for one variable at a time. That would work, but it would take a lot more time than this question needs. As usual, the key to this Simultaneous Equations question is to combine the equations, but combining the equations doesn't necessarily mean losing a variable. Look what happens here if you just add the equations as presented:

$$
\begin{array}{r}
2x - 9y = 11 \\
+ \underline{(x + 12y = -8)} \\
3x + 3y = 3
\end{array}
$$

Suddenly you're almost there! Just divide both sides by 3 and you get $x + y = 1$.

ABSOLUTE VALUE AND INEQUALITIES

To solve an equation that includes absolute value signs, think about the two different cases. For example, to solve the equation $|x - 12| = 3$, think of it as two equations:

$$x - 12 = 3 \text{ or } x - 12 = -3$$
$$x = 15 \text{ or } 9$$

To solve an inequality, do whatever is necessary to both sides to isolate the variable. Just remember that when you multiply or divide both sides by a negative number, you must reverse the inequality sign. To solve $-5x + 7 < -3$, subtract 7 from both sides to get $-5x < -10$. Now divide both sides by -5, remembering to reverse the inequality sign: $x > 2$.

Example: What is the solution set of $|2x - 3| < 7$?

        (A) $\{x: -5 < x < 2\}$
        (B) $\{x: -5 < x < 5\}$
        (C) $\{x: -2 < x < 5\}$
        (D) $\{x: x < -5 \text{ or } x > 2\}$

Solution: What does it mean if $|2x - 3| < 7$? It means that if the expression between the absolute value bars is positive, it's less than $+7$, or if the expression between the bars is negative, it's greater than -7. If the expression between the absolute value bars is 0, its absolute value is less than 7. In other words, $2x - 3$ is between -7 and $+7$:

    $-7 < 2x - 3 < 7$
    $-4 < 2x < 10$
    $-2 < x < 5$

    Choice (C) is correct.

In fact, there's a general rule that applies here: to solve an inequality in the form $|\text{whatever}| < p$, where $p > 0$; just put that "whatever" inside the range $-p$ to p:

    $|\text{anything}| < p$ means: $-p < \text{anything} < p$
    For example, $|x - 5| < 14$ becomes $-14 < x - 5 < 14$.

And here's another general rule: to solve an inequality in the form $|\text{whatever}| > p$, where $p > 0$; just put that "whatever" outside the range $-p$ to p:

    $|\text{anything}| > p$ means: $\text{anything} < -p$ OR $\text{anything} > p$
    For example, $\left|\dfrac{3x + 9}{2}\right| > 7$ becomes $\dfrac{3x + 9}{2} < -7$ or $\dfrac{3x + 9}{2} > 7$.

REVIEW PROBLEMS

1. If $x = 3 - y^2$ and $y = -2$, what is the value of x ?
    (A) -2
    (B) -1
    (C) 1
    (D) 2

2. For all x, $2^x + 2^x + 2^x + 2^x =$
    (A) $2^{(x+2)}$
    (B) $2^{(x+4)}$
    (C) 2^{3x}
    (D) 2^{4x}

3. For all $x \neq \pm\frac{1}{2}$, $\dfrac{6x^2 - x - 2}{4x^2 - 1} =$
    (A) $\dfrac{2 - 3x}{2x + 1}$
    (B) $\dfrac{3x + 2}{2x + 1}$
    (C) $\dfrac{3x + 2}{2x - 1}$
    (D) $\dfrac{3x - 2}{2x - 1}$

4. When $3x^3 - 7x + 7$ is divided by $x + 2$, the remainder is:
    (A) -5
    (B) -3
    (C) 1
    (D) 3

5. If $\sqrt[4]{\dfrac{x+1}{2}} = \dfrac{1}{2}$, then $x =$
    (A) -0.969
    (B) -0.875
    (C) 0
    (D) 0.875

6. If $\dfrac{19}{5x + 17} = \dfrac{19}{31}$, then $x =$
    (A) 0.4
    (B) 1.4
    (C) 2.8
    (D) 3.4

7. If $(3^{x^2})(9^x)(3) = 27$ and $x > 0$, what is the value of x?

   (A) 0.27
   (B) 0.41
   (C) 0.73
   (D) 1.41

8. If $y \neq 4a$ and $x = \dfrac{y + a^2}{y - 4a}$, what is the value of y in terms of a and x?

   (A) $\dfrac{4a - 4a^2x}{x + 1}$
   (B) $\dfrac{a^2 - 4ax}{x + 1}$
   (C) $\dfrac{a^2 + 4ax}{x + 1}$
   (D) $\dfrac{a^2 + 4ax}{x - 1}$

9. If $4x + ky = 15$ and $x - ky = -25$, which of the following could be the values of x and y?

   (A) $x = -3$ and $y = -5$
   (B) $x = -2$ and $y = 3$
   (C) $x = 0$ and $y = -2$
   (D) $x = 2$ and $y = 3$

10. How many integers are in the solution set of $|4x + 3| < 8$?

    (A) None
    (B) Two
    (C) Three
    (D) Four

SOLUTIONS TO REVIEW PROBLEMS

1. **B** Substitute -2 for y into the equation $x = 3 - y^2$:

$$x = 3 - y^2 = 3 - (-2)^2 = 3 - 4 = -1$$

2. **A** The sum of 4 identical quantities is 4 times one of those quantities, so the sum of the four terms 2^x is 4 times 2^x:

$$2^x + 2^x + 2^x + 2^x = 4(2^x) = 2^2(2^x) = 2^{x+2}$$

3. **D** Factor the top and the bottom and cancel the factors they have in common:

$$\frac{6x^2 - x - 2}{4x^2 - 1} = \frac{(2x+1)(3x-2)}{(2x+1)(2x-1)}$$

$$= \frac{3x-2}{2x-1}$$

4. **B** Use long division. Watch out: The expression that goes under the division sign needs a place-holding $0x^2$ term:

$$
\begin{array}{r}
3x^2 - 6x + 5 \\
x + 2 \overline{)\,3x^3 + 0x^2 - 7x + 7} \\
\underline{3x^3 + 6x^2} \\
-6x^2 - 7x \\
\underline{-6x^2 - 12x} \\
5x + 7 \\
\underline{5x + 10} \\
-3
\end{array}
$$

The remainder is -3.

5. **B** To undo the fourth-root symbol, raise both sides to the exponent 4:

$$\sqrt[4]{\frac{x+1}{2}} = \frac{1}{2}$$

$$\left(\sqrt[4]{\frac{x+1}{2}}\right)^4 = \left(\frac{1}{2}\right)^4$$

$$\frac{x+1}{2} = \frac{1}{16}$$

Now cross multiply:

$$(x+1)(16) = (2)(1)$$
$$16x + 16 = 2$$
$$16x = -14$$
$$x = -\frac{14}{16} = -\frac{7}{8} = -0.875$$

6. **C** This might look at first glance like a candidate for cross multiplication, but that would just make things more complicated. Notice that the fractions on both sides have the same numerator, 19. If the two fractions are equal and they have the same numerator, then they must have the same denominator, so just write an equation that says that one denominator is equal to the other denominator:

$$\frac{19}{5x+17} = \frac{19}{31}$$
$$5x + 17 = 31$$
$$5x = 31 - 17$$
$$5x = 14$$
$$x = \frac{14}{5} = 2.8$$

7. **C** Watch what happens when you express everything as powers with a base of 3:

$$(3^{x^2})(9^x)(3) = 27$$
$$(3^{x^2})(3^2)^x(3^1) = 3^3$$

When you raise a power to an exponent, multiply the exponents, and keep the same base. So $(3^2)^x = 3^{2x}$:

$$(3^{x^2})(3^2)^x(3^1) = 3^3$$
$$(3^{x^2})(3^{2x})(3^1) = 3^3$$

The left side of the equation is the product of powers with the same base, so just add the exponents:

$$(3^{x^2})(3^{2x})(3^1) = 3^3$$
$$3^{x^2+2x+1} = 3^3$$

Now the two sides of the equation are powers with the same base, so you can just set the exponents equal:

$$x^2 + 2x + 1 = 3$$
$$(x+1)^2 = 3$$
$$x + 1 = \pm\sqrt{3}$$
$$x = -1 \pm \sqrt{3}$$

The positive value is $-1 + \sqrt{3}$, which is approximately 0.732.

8. **D** First multiply both sides by $y - 4a$ to clear the denominator:

$$x = \frac{y + a^2}{y - 4a}$$

$$x(y - 4a) = y + a^2$$

$$xy - 4ax = y + a^2$$

Now move all terms with y to the left and all terms without y to the right:

$$xy - 4ax = y + a^2$$
$$xy - y = a^2 + 4ax$$

Now factor the left side and divide to isolate y:

$$xy - y = a^2 + 4ax$$
$$y(x - 1) = a^2 + 4ax$$

$$y = \frac{a^2 + 4ax}{x - 1}$$

9. **B** With only two equations, you won't be able to get numerical solutions for three unknowns. But apparently you can get far enough to rule out three of the four answer choices. How? Look for a way to combine the equations that leads somewhere useful. Notice that the first equation contains $+ky$ and the second equation contains $-ky$, so if you add the equations as they are, you'll lose those terms:

$$4x + ky = 15$$
$$\underline{x - ky = -25}$$
$$5x = -10$$
$$x = -2$$

There's not enough information to get numerical solutions for k or y, but you do know that $x = -2$, so the correct answer is the only choice that has an x-value of -2.

10. **D** If the absolute value of something is less than 8, then that something is between -8 and 8:

$$|4x + 3| < 8$$
$$-8 < 4x + 3 < 8$$
$$-11 < 4x < 5$$
$$-\frac{11}{4} < x < \frac{5}{4}$$
$$-2\frac{3}{4} < x < 1\frac{1}{4}$$

There are four integers in that range: $-2, -1, 0,$ and 1.

CHAPTER SIXTY

Probability and Statistics

Questions involving probability and statistics tend to be some of the most dreaded by test takers. This isn't without good reason: The equations can appear confusing, and the questions can be time-consuming. Nevertheless, these question types can be broken down into predictable formulations that appear time and again. With good understanding of the terminology and experience with the calculations, you will find these questions to be much more manageable and possibly even a source of quick points on Test Day.

PROBABILITY

Probability is the branch of mathematics concerned with calculating the likelihood that an event will occur. This likelihood is assigned a numerical value. If p is the probability that an event will occur, then you always have that $0 \leq p \leq 1$. Thus, the probability of an event is always greater than or equal to 0 and less than or equal to 1. A probability of 0 means there is *no* chance an event will occur; while a probability of 1 means the event will *definitely* occur.

Basic Terms

While you do not need to memorize the following terms verbatim, understanding what each means is important for understanding test questions. As you read through each, consider the example of a fair die with sides numbered 1, 2, 3, 4, 5, and 6 being rolled.

Experiment: When some process is conducted, it is called an experiment. An experiment could be the process of rolling the die one time.

Outcome: One of the possible results of the experiment. An example of an outcome is the rolling of a 3.

Sample space: The set of all possible outcomes. The set of possible outcomes can be considered to be the rolling of a 1, the rolling of a 2, the rolling of a 3, the rolling of a 4, the rolling of a 5, and the rolling of a 6. Thus, the sample space in this case is {1, 2, 3, 4, 5, 6}. The probability of the sample space is always 1. Therefore, if the sample space is S, then $P(S) = 1$.

Empty set: The unique set having no elements. The empty set is often represented by ϕ, so $P(\phi) = 0$.

Event: One particular set of possible outcomes. An example of an event is the rolling of a 3 or a 5. Thus, one event, which you can call event A, is {3, 5}. So $A = \{3, 5\}$.

Elementary event: An event that is a set consisting of only one outcome, such as rolling a 4. If B is the event of rolling a 4, then $B = \{4\}$. 4 is an outcome, whereas {4} is an event. This is consistent with the definition since an event is a set of possible outcomes. Note that, as is the case with the event of rolling a 4, it is possible that the set contains just one outcome.

The sample space of an experiment can be defined in different ways, which can affect how you will need to consider outcomes and events. For example, suppose the experiment is the rolling of the die once. You can define the outcomes to be these:

One outcome is the rolling of a 1 or a 2. Define this outcome as s_1.
One outcome is the rolling of a 3. Define this outcome as s_2.
One outcome is the rolling of a 4, a 5, or a 6. Define this outcome as s_3.

In this experiment, because of how you have defined it, the only possible outcomes are s_1, s_2, and s_3. The sample space in this case is $\{s_1, s_2, s_3\}$. Under these conditions, an event could be the set consisting of s_1 and s_2. Thus, if B is the event consisting of the outcomes s_1 and s_2, then $B = \{s_1, s_2\}$.

Notation

In mathematics, the probability that event A occurs is written $P(A)$.

Describing Probability

Probability can be expressed as a percent (for example, there's a 50% chance of getting heads in a fair coin toss), as a fraction (for example, the probability of getting heads is $\frac{1}{2}$), or as a decimal (for example, there's a 0.5 chance of getting heads). What does this value mean? It's a statement of what's *likely* to happen and not a guarantee of what *will* actually happen. It's certainly possible, for example, to flip a coin 10 times and get 10 tails.

What's behind probability?

Now, how do you know that, when a fair coin is tossed, there's a 50% chance of getting heads? You figure out how many different outcomes there are for the coin toss (2: heads or tails) and then figure out how many of those outcomes give a result of heads (just 1). So 1 out of the 2 possible outcomes (or 50% of them) result in heads. That's the basic formula for probability when all the outcomes are equally likely:

$$\text{Probability} = \frac{\text{Number of desired outcomes}}{\text{Number of possible outcomes}}$$

You can see now that probability is a fraction with the number of desired outcomes on the top and the number of possible outcomes on the bottom. In other words, probability is just a way of predicting the likelihood of a specific event by figuring out what fraction of all possible outcomes have the characteristic you're looking for. Stated yet another way, probability is the fraction of all the possible outcomes that are members of the set of outcomes that is a specified event. In every probability question, your goal is to find the total number of possible outcomes and the number of desired outcomes. Keep in mind that "desired" means only that these are the outcomes that have the characteristic you're interested in, not that you necessarily want these outcomes to happen.

Example: A bag contains 10 identical balls numbered 1 through 10 inclusive. If a ball is drawn from the bag at random, what is the probability (as a percent) that it bears a number less than 4?

Solution: If there are 10 balls in the bag, and you're picking only one ball, then there are 10 possible outcomes. So you now have the bottom of our probability fraction. What you still need to do is determine the number of desired outcomes. You're interested in numbers less than 4, and the only balls that have this characteristic are 1, 2, and 3, so 3 out of the 10 balls would give us a number less than 4. That's $\frac{3}{10}$ or 30%.

So to find a probability for a single event:

1. Figure out how many outcomes are possible overall.

2. Figure out how many of the possible outcomes have the characteristic you're looking for.

3. Plug these numbers into the probability formula.

As you can see, every probability problem starts with two basic things:

1. Total possible outcomes

2. Desired outcomes

Example: A fair six-sided die with sides numbered 1, 2, 3, 4, 5, and 6 is thrown. What is the probability it lands with an even number facing up?

Solution: Desired outcomes = 3
Total possible outcomes = 6

The regular six-sided die has six numbers (1, 2, 3, 4, 5, and 6) on its faces. That gives us a total of six possible outcomes. You're interested only in the even numbers, of which there are three (2, 4, and 6). So the number of desired outcomes is three. This gives us a probability of $\frac{3}{6}$, or $\frac{1}{2}$.

Example: Of the 1,000 employees of a company, 5 employees have the job title of accountant. If one of these employees is selected at random, what is the probability this employee has the job title of accountant?

Solution: Desired outcomes = 5
Total possible outcomes = 1,000

There are 1,000 employees that could be selected. So the total number of possible outcomes is 1,000. There are 5 employees with the job title of accountant. So the number of desired outcomes here is 5. That gives a probability of $\frac{5}{1,000}$, or $\frac{1}{200}$.

Example: A certain pet store has 13 mice in a single tank. Five of the mice are white, and 8 of the mice are brown. If the store clerk reaches into the mice's tank to select a mouse at random, what is the probability that the mouse is white?

Solution: Desired outcomes = 5
Total possible outcomes = 13

If there are 13 mice total, then the number of possible outcomes is 13. Only 5 of the mice are white, so the number of desired outcomes is 5. This gives us a probability of $\frac{5}{13}$.

Probability an Event Does Not Occur

Now that you've seen how to find the probability of a single event, consider what happens when you're interested in more than one event. Let A be an event and $\overline{A}$ be the event that event A does not occur. Added together, these two events represent the entire sample set (with a probability of 1). Therefore, the probability event A does not occur is equal to 1 minus the probability that event A does occur: $P(\overline{A}) = 1 - P(A)$.

For example, suppose a fair sided die with sides numbered 1 through 6 is tossed. The probability that a 4 is rolled is $\frac{1}{6}$. Therefore, the probability that a 4 is not rolled is $1 - \frac{1}{6} = \frac{5}{6}$.

The event that a 4 is not rolled is the event that a 1, 2, 3, 5, or 6 is rolled. There are 5 desired outcomes and 6 possible outcomes. So the probability that a 4 is not rolled is $\frac{\text{Number of desired outcomes}}{\text{Number of possible outcomes}} = \frac{5}{6}$.

Multiple-Event Probability

When all the outcomes are equally likely, the probability for a single event is just $\frac{\text{Number of desired outcomes}}{\text{Number of possible outcomes}}$. But what if you're interested in the probability that *at least* one of two different events occurs? Or in the probability that two different events *both* occur? Or in the probability that one of two different events occurs and the other does *not*? In those cases, it's not enough just to determine the probabilities of the individual events; you must combine the probabilities somehow.

Probability at least one of two events will occur when both events cannot occur

Some probability questions test your ability to determine the probability of what are known technically as **mutually exclusive events**. Mutually exclusive events are those events for which the occurrence of one event eliminates the possibility of the occurrence of the other event (in other words, where the two events *exclude* each other). To find the probability that one *or* another of two mutually exclusive events will occur, you add the probabilities of the two events.

For example, what is the probability that a certain machine randomly fills a box with all pennies *or* with all dimes? If the box contains all pennies, then it can't contain all dimes. If it contains all dimes, it can't contain all pennies. So these two events are mutually exclusive in that the occurrence of one means the other can't happen at the same time. If you wanted to figure out the probability that a box contains either all pennies or all dimes, the first thing you'd need is the probabilities of the two events separately.

Say that the probability that the machine fills the box with all pennies is $\frac{1}{2}$ and the probability that the machine fills the box with all dimes is $\frac{1}{3}$. To calculate the probability that one or the other of these two events occurs, add their respective probabilities:

$$\frac{1}{2} + \frac{1}{3} = \frac{3}{6} + \frac{2}{6} = \frac{5}{6}$$

So the probability that the box contains all pennies *or* all dimes is $\frac{5}{6}$.

Remember, if two events A and B cannot both occur, then to calculate the probability that either event A *or* event B occurs (but not both), find the probabilities of A and B separately and then *add* them together.

Why do you need to add in such cases? Because with many repetitions, close to $\frac{1}{2}$ of the boxes can be expected to be filled with pennies, and close to $\frac{1}{3}$ of the boxes can be expected to be filled with dimes. Close to $\frac{1}{2} + \frac{1}{3}$ or $\frac{5}{6}$ of all the boxes will be filled with pennies or dimes, which is the same as saying that the probability that any given box contains all pennies or all dimes is $\frac{5}{6}$. Remember that a probability tells you how likely it is that something will occur.

Example: A bag contains 20 identical plastic tiles. Eleven of the tiles are marked with the numbers 1 through 11 inclusive. The remaining 9 tiles are marked with the letters A through I inclusive. If a single tile is drawn at random from the bag, what is the probability that it bears either an even number or a vowel?

Solution: To find the probability of getting either an even number *or* a vowel, you need to find the probability of each of these occurrences separately and then add them together. Start off with the even numbers. There are 20 tiles in the bag, so you know the number of total possible outcomes is 20. The even numbers in the bag are 2, 4, 6, 8, and 10, so there are five desired outcomes. The probability of withdrawing an even number is $\frac{5}{20}$ (don't reduce the fraction yet; you'll see why). Now for the vowels: The number of possible outcomes is still 20. There are three vowels in the bag (A, E, and I), so there are three desired outcomes. The probability of withdrawing a vowel is $\frac{3}{20}$. Therefore, the probability of withdrawing an even number *or* a vowel is $\frac{5}{20} + \frac{3}{20}$ (this is why you didn't want to reduce before), which sums to $\frac{8}{20}$, or $\frac{2}{5}$.

Probability Two Events Occur

So far, you have looked at the probability of one or another of two events happening, but what about the case in which *both* happen? In general, the probability that events A *and* B both occur is equal to the probability that event A occurs multiplied by the conditional probability that event B occurs given that event A occurs. You can also say that the probability that events A *and* B both occur is equal to the probability that event B occurs *multiplied* by the conditional probability that event A occurs, given that event B occurs.

Example: There are 4 blue disks and 12 green disks in a container. Two disks are to be removed from the container, one after the other. What is the probability that the first disk selected is blue and the second disk selected is green?

Solution: There are 4 blue disks and a total of $4 + 12 = 16$ disks in the container. The probability that the first disk selected is blue is $\frac{4}{16} = \frac{1}{4}$. Once a blue disk is removed from the container, there remain 3 blue disks and 12 green disks. So there are 12 green disks and $3 + 12 = 15$ disks in the container. The probability that the second disk selected is green given that the first disk selected is blue is $\frac{12}{15} = \frac{4}{5}$. Then the probability that the first disk selected is blue and the second disk selected is green is $\frac{1}{4} \times \frac{4}{5} = \frac{1}{5}$.

Independent events

Two events are said to be independent if one of these events has absolutely no effect on the probability of the other event occurring. For example, suppose a fair coin with heads and tails is tossed once and then a fair die with sides number 1, 2, 3, 4, 5, and 6 is rolled once. For the coin toss, you are interested in the event that a head is tossed (say that's event A), and for the die roll you are concerned with the event that a 1 or a 4 is rolled (say that's event B). The tossing of the coin has absolutely no effect on the rolling of the die. Thus, the event that a head results when a fair coin is tossed is independent of the event that a 1 or a 4 is tossed when a fair die is rolled.

In the case of independent events A and B, the probability that events A and B both occur is equal to the probability that event A occurs multiplied by the probability that event B occurs. Returning to the above situation, you can use that relationship to find the probability that both events A and B occur.

There are 2 possible outcomes when the coin is tossed, heads or tails. So the number of possible outcomes is 2. For the event that a head is tossed, you have one desirable outcome, heads. So the probability that, when a fair coin is tossed, the result is heads is $\frac{1}{2}$.

When the fair die is rolled, all the possible outcomes are 1, 2, 3, 4, 5, and 6. The number of possible outcomes is 6. For the event that a 1 or a 4 is rolled, there are 2 desired outcomes, which are 1 and 4. So the probability that, when the fair die is rolled, a 1 or 4 results is $\frac{2}{6} = \frac{1}{3}$.

Finally, the probability that both events A and B occur is $\frac{1}{2} \times \frac{1}{3} = \frac{1}{6}$.

Example: If the probability of finding a pearl in any given oyster is $\frac{1}{3}$ and the probability of any given pearl being black is $\frac{2}{5}$, what's the probability that if you crack open a randomly chosen oyster, you'll find a black pearl?

Solution: In $\frac{1}{3}$ of the cases when you crack open an oyster, you'll find a pearl. And in $\frac{2}{5}$ of the cases when you find a pearl, that pearl will be black. Therefore, you should find a black pearl in $\frac{2}{5}$ of $\frac{1}{3}$ of the times you open an oyster, which is $\frac{2}{5} \times \frac{1}{3}$ or $\frac{2}{15}$ of all the times you open an oyster. Therefore, the probability of finding a pearl *and* having the pearl be black is $\frac{2}{15}$.

Example: A bag contains ten identically shaped plastic tiles. Six of the tiles are red, three are blue, and one is black. If two tiles are drawn at random from the bag, without replacement, what is the probability that the first tile drawn is red and the second tile drawn is black?

Solution: First find the individual probabilities of drawing a red tile and then drawing the black tile. For the first tile drawn, there are 10 tiles in the bag, and 6 of them are red, so the probability of drawing a red tile first is $\frac{6}{10}$ or $\frac{3}{5}$. For the second tile, there are only 9 tiles left in the bag, and 1 of them is black, so the probability of getting a black tile on the second draw is $\frac{1}{9}$. Now you need to find the probability of getting a red tile on the first draw *AND* a black tile on the second draw. To do so, you multiply the individual probabilities: $\frac{3}{5} \times \frac{1}{9} = \frac{3}{45} = \frac{1}{15}$.

Probability at Least One of Two Events Occurs

Suppose you have two events A and B. You want to find the probability that at least one of the events A or B occurs. A picture of the events A and B would look like this:

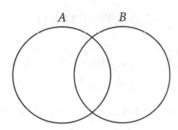

If you just add the probability that event A occurs and the probability that B occurs, the sum will include the probability of *both* events A and B occurring (the overlapping area on the Venn diagram) twice, which is included in both the probability that A occurs and the probability that B occurs. So you must subtract the probability that both events A and B occur from that sum. Remember that $P(E)$ means the probability that event E occurs. You can say that $P(A \text{ or } B) = P(A) + P(B) - P(A \text{ and } B)$.

Notice that the rule for finding the probability that at least one of events A or B occurs, $P(A \text{ or } B) = P(A) + P(B) - P(A \text{ and } B)$, also accounts for cases in which the events are mutually exclusive. If the events A and B are mutually exclusive, $P(A \text{ and } B) = 0$. So, if the events A and B are mutually exclusive, $P(A \text{ or } B) = P(A) + P(B) - P(A \text{ and } B) = P(A) + P(B) - 0 = P(A) + P(B)$.

Example: Suppose a fair coin is tossed and a fair die with sides numbered 1, 2, 3, 4, 5, and 6 is rolled. Let A be the event that the coin toss results in a head. Let B be the event that the roll of the die results in a 5. What is the probability that at least one of the events A or B occurs?

Solution: For the coin toss, $P(A) = \frac{1}{2}$. For the roll of the die, $P(B) = \frac{1}{6}$. The toss of the coin and the roll of the die are independent, so $P(A \text{ and } B) = P(A)P(B) = \frac{1}{2} \times \frac{1}{6} = \frac{1}{12}$. Then $P(A \text{ or } B) = \frac{1}{2} + \frac{1}{6} - \frac{1}{12} = \frac{6}{12} + \frac{2}{12} - \frac{1}{12} = \frac{6+2-1}{12} = \frac{7}{12}$.

Summary Comparison: And/Or

You've seen two different ways to calculate probabilities for situations involving more than one event. It's essential you understand which method to use in any given probability question. To recap:

- To find the probability of event *A or* event *B* when the events *A* and *B* are mutually exclusive, find the probability of *A* and the probability of *B* and then *add* these two probabilities. Thus, if the events *A* and *B* are mutually exclusive, $P(A \text{ or } B) = P(A) + P(B)$. (The same rule applies if you're trying to figure out the probability that *A or B or C* occurs where the events *A*, *B*, and *C* are mutually exclusive, etc.)

- For any two events *A* and *B*, to find the probability that *at least one of* event *A or* event *B* occurs, find the probability of event *A* and the probability of event *B*, *add* these two probabilities, then *subtract* from this sum the probability that both events *A* and *B* occur. Thus, for any events *A* and *B*, $P(A \text{ or } B) = P(A) + P(B) - P(A \text{ and } B)$.

- To find the probability of event *A and* event *B*, find the probability that event *A* occurs and the conditional probability that *B* occurs given that event *A* occurs, then *multiply* the probability that event *A* occurs by the conditional probability that event *B* occurs given that event *A* occurs. (The same rule applies if you're trying to figure out *A and B and C*, etc.)

MEDIAN, MODE, RANGE, AND STANDARD DEVIATION

Probability is just one way to look at statistical patterns. Using other techniques, such as determining median, mode, range, and standard deviation, also can provide equally useful information.

Median

If a group containing an odd number of terms is arranged in numerical order, the median is the middle value.

If a group containing an even number of terms is arranged in numerical order, the median is the average, or arithmetic mean, of the two middle numbers.

Example: What is the median of 4, 5, 100, 1, and 6?

Solution: First, arrange the numbers in numerical order: 1, 4, 5, 6, and 100. The middle number (the median) is 5.

Example: What is the median value of 2, 7, 8, 16, 12, and 37?

Solution: If a set has an even number of terms, then the median is the average (arithmetic mean) of the two middle terms after the terms are arranged in numerical order. Arrange the values in numerical order: 2, 7, 8, 12, 16, 37. The two middle numbers are 8 and 12. The median is the average of 8 and 12, that is, 10.

The median can be quite different from the mean (average). For instance, in the first set of numbers above, {1, 4, 5, 6, 100}, the median is 5, but the average is $\frac{1+4+5+6+100}{5} = \frac{116}{5} = 23.2$.

Mode

The mode is the number that appears most frequently in a set. For example, in the set {1, 2, 2, 2, 3, 4, 4, 5, 6}, the mode is 2.

It is possible for a set to have more than one mode. For example, in the set {35, 42, 35, 57, 57, 19}, the two modes are 35 and 57. When more than one mode exists, do not calculate the mean of these numbers but rather report each as a separate value.

Range

The range is the positive difference between the largest term in the set and the smallest term. For example, in the set {2, 4, 10, 20, 26}, the range is $26 - 2 = 24$.

Standard Deviation

Standard deviation measures the dispersion of a set of numbers around the mean. If you let σ be the standard deviation of the N values $x_1, x_2, \ldots x_N$ and let μ be the average, or arithmetic mean, of the N values $x_1, x_2, \ldots x_N$, that is, $\mu = \dfrac{x_1 + x_2 + \ldots + x_N}{N}$,

then the formula looks like this:

$$\sigma = \sqrt{\frac{1}{N}\left[(x_1 - \mu)^2 + (x_2 - \mu)^2 + \cdots + (x_N - \mu)^2\right]}$$

It can be intimidating, so it helps to break up the process into the following steps:

1. Find the arithmetic mean of the set.
2. Subtract the mean of the set from each term in that set.
3. Square each result.
4. Take the mean of those squares.
5. Calculate the positive square root of that average.

Fortunately, you will only very rarely be required to apply this formula and only on the most difficult questions. When standard deviation is tested, all you will generally need to understand is the basic concept: Standard deviation represents how close or far the terms in a set or list are from the average. Thus, standard deviation is a measure of how widely dispersed the terms of a list are, or how widely dispersed the members of a set are.

Thus, {1, 2, 3} and {101, 102, 103} have the same standard deviation since they both have one term on the mean and two terms exactly one unit away from the mean. Quickly sketching number lines can confirm this:

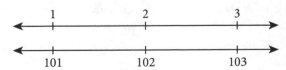

The set {1, 3, 5} will have a smaller standard deviation than {0, 3, 6}. Both sets have a mean of 3, but the first has terms 2, 0, and 2 units from the average, while the second has terms 3, 0, and 3 units from the average. Again, you can confirm this by quickly sketching number lines:

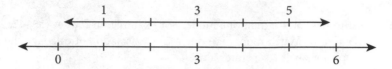

You could also calculate the standard deviation for the sets {1, 3, 5} and {0, 3, 6} to confirm:

$\{1, 3, 5\}$
mean = 3

$$\sigma = \sqrt{\frac{1}{3}\left[(1-3)^2 + (3-3)^2 + (5-3)^2\right]}$$
$$= \sqrt{\frac{1}{3}\left[(-2)^2 + 0^2 + 2^2\right]}$$
$$= \sqrt{\frac{1}{3}(8)}$$
$$= \sqrt{\frac{8}{3}}$$

$\{0, 3, 6\}$
mean = 3

$$\sigma = \sqrt{\frac{1}{3}\left[(0-3)^2 + (3-3)^2 + (6-3)^2\right]}$$
$$= \sqrt{\frac{1}{3}\left[(-3)^2 + 0^2 + 3^2\right]}$$
$$= \sqrt{\frac{1}{3}(9+0+9)}$$
$$= \sqrt{\frac{1}{3}(18)}$$
$$= \sqrt{6}$$

Since 6 is larger than $\frac{8}{3}$, the standard deviation of the second, more widely spaced set of numbers is larger than that of the first set.

Below are the key concepts to remember about median, mode, range, and standard deviation.

- When the numbers in a list with an odd number of numbers is arranged in ascending or descending order, the median is the middle number.
- When the numbers in a list with an even number of numbers is arranged in ascending or descending order, the median is the average of the two middle numbers.
- The mode of a list of terms is the term that appears most frequently. Having more than one mode is possible.
- The range is the positive difference between the largest term in the list and the smallest term.
- Standard deviation measures the dispersion of a set of numbers around the mean. You will rarely be required to apply the formula for standard deviation. Instead, use critical thinking and quick sketches of number lines to determine how close the terms in a list are from the mean.

COMBINATIONS AND PERMUTATIONS

Some questions ask you to count the number of possible ways to select a small subgroup from a larger group. If the selection is **unordered**, then it's a combination question. But if the selection is **ordered**, it is a permutation question.

For example, if a question asks you to count the possible number of different slates of officers who could be elected to positions in class government, then order matters—President Joseph and Vice President Rose is a different slate than President Rose and Vice President Joseph. You would use the permutations formula in this scenario. But if you had to count the number of possible pairs of flavors of jelly beans, you are solving a combinations question; cherry and lemon is the same pair as lemon and cherry, so order does not matter (that is, you wouldn't count those as two different pairs).

The very first thing you need to do is use critical thinking to figure out whether a given question calls for an ordered or an unordered selection; otherwise, you won't know which formula to use.

Combinations

The combinations formula is used when solving for the number of k unordered selections one can make from a group of n items where $k \leq n$. This is usually referred to as $_nC_k$, which is said as "n choose k." It is often helpful to say it this way to yourself because that's what making combinations is: an act of choosing small groups from a larger group.

Here's the formula, in which $n!$, or n-factorial, is the product of n and every positive integer smaller than n (for example, $5! = 5 \times 4 \times 3 \times 2 \times 1$), where n is a positive integer:

$$_nC_k = \frac{n!}{k!(n-k)!}$$

Example: A company is selecting 4 members of its board of directors to sit on an ethics subcommittee. If the board has 9 members, any of whom may serve on the subcommittee, how many different selections of members could the company make?

Solution: Since the order in which you select the members doesn't change the composition of the committee in any way, this is a combinations question. The size of the group from which you choose is n, and the size of the selected group is k. So $n = 9$ and $k = 4$.

$$_9C_4 = \frac{9!}{4!(9-4)!}$$

$$= \frac{9!}{4!5!}$$

$$= \frac{9 \times 8 \times 7 \times 6 \times 5 \times 4 \times 3 \times 2 \times 1}{4 \times 3 \times 2 \times 1 \times 5 \times 4 \times 3 \times 2 \times 1}$$

Save yourself some work. There's rarely a need to multiply out factorials since many of the factors can quickly be canceled.

$$_9C_4 = \frac{9 \times 8^2 \times 7 \times 6 \times 5 \times 4 \times 3 \times 2 \times 1}{4 \times 3 \times 2 \times 1 \times 5 \times 4 \times 3 \times 2 \times 1}$$

$$= 9 \times 2 \times 7 = 126$$

Sometimes the problems will be more complicated and will require multiple iterations of the formula.

Example: County X holds an annual math competition to which each county high school sends a team of 4 students. If school A has 6 boys and 7 girls whose math grades qualify them to be on their school's team, and competition rules stipulate that the team must consist of 2 boys and 2 girls, how many different teams might school A send to the competition?

Solution: The order of selection doesn't matter here, so you can use the combinations formula. But be careful … if you lump all the students together in a group of 13 and calculate $_{13}C_4$, you'd wind up including some all-boy teams and all-girl teams. The question explicitly says you can only select 2 boys and 2 girls. So you aren't really choosing 4 students from 13 but rather choosing 2 boys from 6 and 2 girls from 7. Multiply the two combinations together to get the answer.

$$_6C_2 \quad \text{and} \quad _7C_2$$

$$\frac{6!}{2!4!} \times \frac{7!}{2!5!} =$$

$$\frac{6 \times 5 \times 4 \times 3 \times 2 \times 1}{2 \times 1 \times 4 \times 3 \times 2 \times 1} \times \frac{7 \times 6 \times 5 \times 4 \times 3 \times 2 \times 1}{2 \times 1 \times 5 \times 4 \times 3 \times 2 \times 1} =$$

$$\frac{\cancel{6}^3 \times 5 \times \cancel{4 \times 3 \times 2 \times 1}}{\cancel{2} \times 1 \times \cancel{4 \times 3 \times 2 \times 1}!} \times \frac{7 \times \cancel{6}^3 \times \cancel{5 \times 4 \times 3 \times 2 \times 1}}{\cancel{2} \times 1 \times \cancel{5 \times 4 \times 3 \times 2 \times 1}} =$$

$3 \times 5 \times 7 \times 3 = 315$ possible teams consisting of 2 boys and 2 girls.

Permutations

If the order of selection matters, use the permutation formulas instead:

Number of permutations (arrangements) of n items $= n!$

Number of permutations of k items selected from n items $= {_nP_k} = \dfrac{n!}{(n-k)!}$

Example: How many ways are there to arrange the letters in the word ASCENT?

Solution: Order matters here since ASCENT is different from TNECSA. There are 6 letters in the word, so you must calculate the permutations of 6 items:

$$6! = 6 \times 5 \times 4 \times 3 \times 2 \times 1 = 720$$

Another way to solve this question is to draw a quick sketch of the problem with blanks for the arranged items, then write in the number of possibilities for each blank in order. Finally, multiply the numbers together. Many high-difficulty permutation questions resist formulaic treatment but are easier to complete with the *draw blanks* or *slot filling* approach.

Here's how you would use this technique to solve the ASCENT problem:

ASCENT has 6 letters, so you need 6 blanks:

$$\_\_ \times \_\_ \times \_\_ \times \_\_ \times \_\_ \times \_\_$$

There are 6 letters you might place in the first blank (A, S, C, E, N, or T):

$$\underline{6} \times \_\_ \times \_\_ \times \_\_ \times \_\_ \times \_\_$$

No matter which letter you placed there, there will be 5 possibilities for the next blank:

$$\underline{\ 6\ } \times \underline{\ 5\ } \times \underline{\ \ } \times \underline{\ \ } \times \underline{\ \ } \times \underline{\ \ }$$

There will be 4 for the next, 3 thereafter, 2 after that, and just 1 letter left for the last:

$$\underline{\ 6\ } \times \underline{\ 5\ } \times \underline{\ 4\ } \times \underline{\ 3\ } \times \underline{\ 2\ } \times \underline{\ 1\ } = 720$$

Notice that you wind up reproducing the arrangements formula, $n!$. It's quite possible to solve most permutation problems without knowing the right formulas ahead of time, although knowing the formulas can save you time on Test Day.

Example: There are 6 children at a family reunion, 3 boys and 3 girls. They will be lined up single-file for a photo, alternating genders. How many arrangements of the children are possible for this photo?

Solution: You may not be sure how to approach this with a formula, so draw a picture. You know you'll have 6 blanks, but you don't know whether to begin with a boy or with a girl. It could be either one. So try both:

bgbgbg or *gbgbgb*

$$\underline{\ \ } \times \underline{\ \ } \times \underline{\ \ } \times \underline{\ \ } \times \underline{\ \ } \times \underline{\ \ } + \underline{\ \ } \times \underline{\ \ } \times \underline{\ \ } \times \underline{\ \ } \times \underline{\ \ } \times \underline{\ \ }$$

Any of the three boys could go in the first spot, and any of the three girls in the second:

$$\underline{\ 3\ } \times \underline{\ 3\ } \times \underline{\ \ } \times \underline{\ \ } \times \underline{\ \ } \times \underline{\ \ } + \underline{\ \ } \times \underline{\ \ } \times \underline{\ \ } \times \underline{\ \ } \times \underline{\ \ } \times \underline{\ \ }$$

The next spot can be filled with either of the remaining two boys; the one after by either of the two remaining girls. Then the last boy and the last girl take their places:

$$\underline{\ 3\ } \times \underline{\ 3\ } \times \underline{\ 2\ } \times \underline{\ 2\ } \times \underline{\ 1\ } \times \underline{\ 1\ } + \underline{\ \ } \times \underline{\ \ } \times \underline{\ \ } \times \underline{\ \ } \times \underline{\ \ } \times \underline{\ \ }$$

That's the boy-first possibility. The same numbers of boys and girls apply to the girl-first possibility, and so you get:

$$\underline{\ 3\ } \times \underline{\ 3\ } \times \underline{\ 2\ } \times \underline{\ 2\ } \times \underline{\ 1\ } \times \underline{\ 1\ } + \underline{\ 3\ } \times \underline{\ 3\ } \times \underline{\ 2\ } \times \underline{\ 2\ } \times \underline{\ 1\ } \times \underline{\ 1\ }$$

$$9 \times 4 \times 1 + 9 \times 4 \times 1$$

There are $36 + 36 = 72$ possible arrangements of 3 boys and 3 girls, with alternating genders.

Hybrids of Combinations and Permutations

Some questions involve elements of both ordered and unordered selection.

Example: How many ways are there to arrange the letters in the word ASSETS?

Solution: Earlier you saw that the rearrangement of ASCENT was a permutation. But what about ASSETS? The order of the E, the A, the T, and the Ss matter, but the order of the three Ss themselves does not.

Think about it this way: Put a tag on the Ss … $AS_1S_2ETS_3$. If you just calculated 6! again, you'd be counting $AS_1S_2ETS_3$ and $AS_3S_1ETS_2$ as different words, even though with the tags gone, you can see they aren't (ASSETS is the same as ASSETS). So you'll need to eliminate all the redundant arrangements from the 6! total.

For each specification of the positions of the different letters A, E, and T, there are 3! ways to permute 3 distinguishable Ss, like S_1, S_2, and S_3. For each specification of the positions of the different letters A, E, and T, there is just one way to permute 3 indistinguishable Ss. So the total number of permutations, for 6 distinguishable letters, which is 6!, must be divided by 3! because of the 3 indistinguishable Ss.

So instead of 6! arrangements, as there were for ASCENT, the word ASSETS has $\frac{6!}{3!}$ arrangements.

$$\frac{6!}{3!} = \frac{6 \times 5 \times 4 \times 3 \times 2 \times 1}{3 \times 2 \times 1} = 6 \times 5 \times 4 = 120$$

The same logic would apply to the arrangements of ASSESS … $\frac{6!}{4!}$.

And if two letters repeat, you need two corrections to eliminate the counting of redundant arrangements. For instance, the number of arrangements of the letters in the word REASSESS is $\frac{8!}{4!2!}$.

Some tricky problems boil down to the same logic as this rearranging letters problem.

Example: A restaurant is hanging 7 large tiles on its wall in a single row. How many arrangements of tiles are possible if there are 3 white tiles and 4 blue tiles?

Solution: This problem essentially asks for the arrangements of *WWWBBBB*. Although there are 7 total tiles to arrange, all the white tiles are indistinguishable from one another, as are the blue tiles. Therefore, you will need to divide out the number of redundant arrangements from the 7! total arrangements:

$$\frac{7!}{3!4!} = \frac{7 \times 6 \times 5 \times 4 \times 3 \times 2 \times 1}{3 \times 2 \times 1 \times 4 \times 3 \times 2 \times 1} = 7 \times 5 = 35$$

Did you notice that $\frac{7!}{3!4!}$ is the same as $_7C_3$? This is also the same as $_7C_4$, $\frac{7!}{4!3!}$.

Whether you consider "rearrange *WWWBBBB*" to mean "choose 3 of the 7 tiles to be white (the rest will be blue)," or consider "rearrange *WWWBBBB*" to mean "choose 4 of the 7 tiles to be blue (the rest will be white)," the result is the same. As you'll soon see, many probability questions involve just this kind of calculation.

REVIEW PROBLEMS

1. A certain school has 50 students assigned to five distinct classes so that the numbers of students in the classes are consecutive and each student is assigned to only one class. What is the probability that a student selected at random from the 50 students is in one of the two largest classes?

    (A) 38%
    (B) 42%
    (C) 46%
    (D) 48%

2. A certain machine produces toy cars in a repeating cycle of blue, red, green, yellow, and black. If a string of six consecutively produced cars is selected at random from all the possible strings of six consecutively produced cars, what is the probability that, in the string selected, two of the cars are red?

    (A) $\frac{1}{6}$

    (B) $\frac{1}{5}$

    (C) $\frac{1}{3}$

    (D) $\frac{2}{5}$

3. A certain circular stopwatch has exactly 60 second marks and a single hand. If the hand of the watch is randomly set to one of the marks and allowed to count exactly 10 seconds, what is the probability that the hand will stop less than 10 marks on either side of the 53-second mark?

    (A) $\frac{1}{6}$

    (B) $\frac{19}{60}$

    (C) $\frac{1}{3}$

    (D) $\frac{29}{60}$

4. A certain board game is played by rolling a pair of fair six-sided dice and then moving one's piece forward the number of spaces indicated by the sum showing on the dice. A player is "frozen" if her opponent's piece comes to rest in the space already occupied by her piece. If player *A* is about to roll and is currently six spaces behind player *B*, what is the probability that player *B* will be frozen after player *A* rolls?

    (A) $\frac{1}{36}$

    (B) $\frac{5}{36}$

    (C) $\frac{1}{6}$

    (D) $\frac{1}{3}$

5. A machine is made up of two components, *A* and *B*. Each component either works or fails. The failure or nonfailure of one component is independent of the failure or nonfailure of the other component. The machine works if at least one of the components works. If the probability that each component works is $\frac{2}{3}$, what is the probability that the machine works?

   (A) $\frac{1}{9}$

   (B) $\frac{4}{9}$

   (C) $\frac{1}{2}$

   (D) $\frac{8}{9}$

6. In the list 3, 4, 5, 5, 5, 5, 7, 11, 21, what fraction of the data is less than the mode?

   (A) $\frac{2}{9}$

   (B) $\frac{1}{3}$

   (C) $\frac{2}{3}$

   (D) $\frac{7}{9}$

7. Amanda goes to the toy store to buy 1 ball and 3 different board games. If the toy store is stocked with 3 types of balls and 6 types of board games, how many different selections of the 4 items can Amanda make?

   (A) 20
   (B) 23
   (C) 40
   (D) 60

8. A code is to be made by arranging 7 letters. Three of the letters used will be the letter A, two of the letters used will be the letter B, one of the letters used will be the letter C, and one of the letters used will be the letter D. If there is only one way to present each letter, how many different codes are possible?

   (A) 42
   (B) 210
   (C) 420
   (D) 5,040

SOLUTIONS TO THE REVIEW PROBLEMS

1. **C** The correct answer is 46%. To find the probability, you need possible outcomes and desired outcomes. The possible outcomes here are just the total number of students you have to choose from. The desired outcomes are the number of students in the two largest classes. How can you find that, though? The key to this problem is the fact that the numbers of students in the classes are consecutive. Whenever you see *consecutive* in a math problem, it's there for a specific reason. It tells you that each number in the series is separated from the next by a fixed amount. Consecutive integers are separated by 1, consecutive even integers by 2, etc. So here you know that if you add up the numbers of students in all the classes, you'll get 50. You also know that the numbers of students in the classes are separated by 1. So let's call the number of students in the smallest class x. The next largest class would have $x + 1$ students, then $x + 2$ students, $x + 3$ students, and $x + 4$ students. If you add these up, you get $5x + 10 = 50$. Now you can solve for x: subtract 10 from both sides to get $5x = 40$, then divide both sides by 5 to get $x = 8$. So the smallest class has 8 students, and the two largest classes then will have $8 + 3$ and $8 + 4$ students respectively, which gives a total of 23 students in the two largest classes. So the probability is $\frac{23}{50} = \frac{23}{50} \times \frac{2}{2} = \frac{46}{100} = 46\%$.

2. **B** The correct answer is $\frac{1}{5}$. You need to find the number of possible and the number of desired outcomes. You're going to be randomly selecting a possible string of six consecutively produced cars, and you want to know what the probability is that the string will contain two red cars. How many different possible strings of six consecutive cars are there? You have five colors, so any one of them could be the first in the string of six that you choose. That gives five different strings of six, so 5 is the number of possible outcomes here. What about desired outcomes? You need to know how many of those five strings have two red cars. What does getting two red cars depend on? It depends on the color of the first car of the string of six. For example, if blue is the first car of the string, then you'd get blue, red, green, yellow, black, and then blue again. So, the only way to get two red cars is if the first car of the string is red because then you'd have red, green, yellow, black, blue, and then red again as the sixth car. So one out of the five strings will contain two red cars, and that's a probability of $\frac{1}{5}$.

3. **B** The correct answer is $\frac{19}{60}$. There's a watch with a single hand and 60 second marks. Say you randomly spin the hand so it points to one of those marks and then you let the watch count 10 seconds. What are the chances that the hand will end up pointing to a mark that's less than 10 marks from the 53-second mark? What would it depend on? It would depend on the mark the hand began counting from. How many marks are less than 10 marks from 53 seconds? This is a good question for scrap paper. If you jot down 53 and then count 9 in either direction (remember, you need less than 10, so you don't want to count 10), you start with 44 seconds and count all the way past 53 seconds to the mark that is 2 seconds after the minute mark, with the minute mark also being the 0-second mark. This gives 19 marks that are less than 10 marks from 53 seconds. To end up less than 10 marks from 53 seconds, you need to end on one of those 19 marks. Each one of those 19 marks corresponds to another mark that's exactly 10 seconds earlier than it, which would be marks 34–52. If the hand begins counting from any of the 19 marks that go from 34 to 52, it will end up on a mark between 44 and 02. So there are 19 marks that have the characteristic you're looking for. That's 19 out of 60, or $\frac{19}{60}$.

4. **B** The correct answer is $\frac{5}{36}$. In this game, a player is "frozen" whenever another player lands on the spot where the first player already has her piece. The question asks for the probability that player *B* will be frozen by player *A*, who's six spaces behind. What does it depend on? It depends on whether player *A* gets a roll of exactly 6 on the dice. So what's the probability of getting 6 on the dice? First, figure out the total possible outcomes for the roll. Since there are six numbers on each die, the total number of possible rolls is 6 × 6, or 36. So there are 36 possible rolls. How many of them would allow player *A* to move exactly six spots? Any roll that adds up to 6 will. So you could have (1, 5), (2, 4), and (3, 3). But since there are two dice, there are two ways to get (1, 5) and (2, 4) because either die could get the 1 or the 5, etc. So there's (1, 5), (5, 1), (2, 4), (4, 2), and (3, 3). That's five possible rolls that add up to exactly 6. So 5 out of the 36 possible rolls would allow player *A* to freeze player *B*, which gives a probability of $\frac{5}{36}$.

5. **D** The fastest way to do this is to find the probability that neither component works and subtract that from 1. Since the probability of a component working is $\frac{2}{3}$, the probability of a component not working is $1 - \frac{2}{3} = \frac{1}{3}$. Therefore, the probability that neither component works is $\frac{1}{3} \times \frac{1}{3} = \frac{1}{9}$, and the probability that the machine works is $1 - \frac{1}{9} = \frac{8}{9}$.

6. **A** This question can be answered by using the definitions of mode and fraction. Determine the mode, the total number of items in the list, and the number of items in the list less than the mode. The mode of any list of numbers is the number that appears most frequently in the list. In this case, the mode is 5. The total number of items in the list is 9. Finally, the number of items in the list less than the mode, or 5, is 2. So the final fraction is $\frac{2}{9}$.

7. **D** Amanda is buying 1 ball and 3 different board games from a selection of 3 balls and 6 types of board games. You need to find the number of different selections of 4 items that Amanda can make. Amanda is choosing 3 board games from a total of 6, so you can use the combination formula (since a different arrangement of the same board games is not considered a different selection) to find the number of combinations of board games:

$$_nC_k = \frac{n!}{k!(n-k)!}$$

$$_6C_3 = \frac{6!}{3!(6-3)!}$$

$$_6C_3 = \frac{6 \times 5 \times 4 \times 3!}{3! \times 3!}$$

$$_6C_3 = 20$$

Amanda has 20 ways to choose 3 board games from a total of 6. For each of those 20 ways, Amanda can choose 1 of 3 balls, so there are 20 × 3 = 60 different ways for Amanda to choose 1 ball and 3 games from 3 balls and 6 games.

8. **C** You need to make a seven-letter code, but some of the letters are repeated. You have three *As*, two *Bs*, one *C*, and one *D*. Calculate the number of different permutations, remembering to take the repeated letters into account. To calculate the number of permutations where some of the elements are indistinguishable, divide the total number of permutations (here, 7!) by the factorial of the number of indistinguishable elements. So you have $\dfrac{7!}{3!2!} = \dfrac{(7 \times 6 \times 5 \times 4 \times 3 \times 2 \times 1)}{(3 \times 2 \times 1)(2 \times 1)} = 420$.

CHAPTER SIXTY-ONE

Precalculus

Precalculus bridges the gap between algebra and calculus. The material presented in different schools' courses varies widely, so ensure you understand all the material PCAT test makers consider to be precalculus: graphing and manipulating functions, complex numbers, and vectors.

GRAPHING EQUATIONS

When graphing an equation, it's best to identify a few key parameters initially to get an overall sense of the function. Doing these in order provides a repeatable way to tackle almost any equation:

1. **Determine what type of function is presented.**

    Equations can be linear, absolute value, quadratic, polynomial, radical, and piecewise. Knowing what general category the equation or function falls under gives you an idea as to what the graph should look like.

    - **Linear:** These come in one of two general forms:
        - The graph of the equation $y = mx + b$ is a straight line where $m =$ slope and $b = y$-intercept.
        - The graph of the equation $x =$ constant is a vertical line. This is not a function.
    - **Absolute Value:** The graph of the equation $y = |ax + b|$, where a and b are constants and $a \neq 0$, has a V-shape.
    - **Quadratic:** The graph of the equation $y = ax^2 + bx + c$, where $a \neq 0$, is a parabola.
    - **Polynomial:** The graph of the equation $y = p(x)$, where $p(x)$ is a polynomial, can take on any squiggly-line shape. When $p(x) = ax^2 + bx + c$, where $a \neq 0$, $p(x)$ is a quadratic polynomial.
    - **Radical:** The radical function cannot take a negative value under the radical.
    - **Piecewise:** These have no general form because they can be continuous or discontinuous functions that may take on the characteristic shapes of other general functions over certain ranges.

2. **Identify the *y*-intercepts and the *x*-intercepts.**

Obvious points on the graph of an equation are points where the graph in question crosses the *x*- and *y*-axes. A *y*-intercept is the *y*-coordinate of a point where the graph crosses the *y*-axis. An *x*-intercept is the *x*-coordinate of a point where the graph crosses the *x*-axis. At a *y*-intercept, $x = 0$. At an *x*-intercept, $y = 0$. You find the *y*-intercept or *y*-intercepts by letting $x = 0$ and find the *x*-intercept or *x*-intercepts by letting $y = 0$.

3. **Identify the zeros of functions.**

Find the zeros of the function *f* by finding the *x*-intercepts of the graph of the equation $y = f(x)$.

4. **Find the domain.**

The domain of a function defines all the values that *x* can have for the function.

5. **Determine the range.**

The range of a function defines all the values that *y* can have for the function.

The following examples illustrate these five steps.

Example: Graph $y = 3x + 2$.

Solution: 1. This is a nonvertical straight line.

2. The *y*-intercept (where $x = 0$) is $y = 2$. The *x*-intercept (where $y = 0$) is $x = -\frac{2}{3}$.

3. If the function is *f*, where $f(x) = 3x + 2$, then there are no other zeros for this function.

4. The domain is all real numbers because *x* can be any real number.

5. The range is all real numbers because *y* can be any real number.

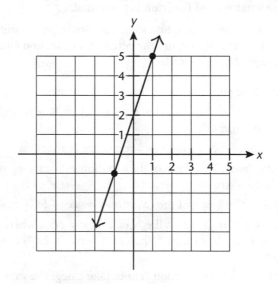

Example: Graph $y = |x+1|$.

Solution: 1. This is an absolute value and fits in the general form of the equation $y = |ax + b|$, so it should have a V-shape.

2. The y-intercept is $y = 1$. The x-intercept is $x = -1$.

3. There are no other zeros for the function $f(x) = |x+1|$.

4. The domain is all real numbers.

5. The range is $[0, \infty)$. This means y can be any value from 0 to ∞, including 0.

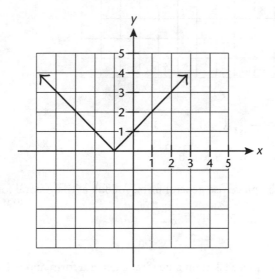

Example: Graph $y = \sqrt{2x - 5}$.

Solution: 1. This is a radical. The graph of this particular equation is part of a parabola.

2. When $x = 0$, $y = \sqrt{-5}$. That means the graph never crosses the y-axis. The x-intercept is $x = \dfrac{5}{2}$.

3. There are no other zeros for the function $f(x) = \sqrt{2x - 5}$.

4. The domain for this function is $\left[\dfrac{5}{2}, \infty\right)$.

5. The range for this function is $[0, \infty)$.

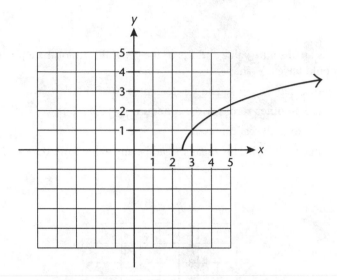

Example: Graph $y = \dfrac{2x-6}{x^2-9},\ x \le 0,\ x \ne -3$

$$= x^2 - 6x + 5,\ x > 0$$

Solution: 1. This fits the piecewise general form, so look at the general form of each piece.

$$\frac{2x-6}{x^2-9} = \frac{2(x-3)}{(x+3)(x-3)} = \frac{2}{x+3}.$$

The first piece is $y = \dfrac{2}{x+3},\ x \le 0,\ x \ne -3$.

The second piece takes on a quadratic general form and will be part of a parabola.

2. The only y-intercept is $y = \dfrac{2}{3}$. The x-intercepts are $x = 1$ and $x = 5$.

3. The vertical asymptote has the equation $x = -3$, and the horizontal asymptote has the equation $y = 0$.

4. The domain is $(-\infty, -3) \cup (-3, \infty)$. This means x can be any number but -3.

5. The range is all real numbers.

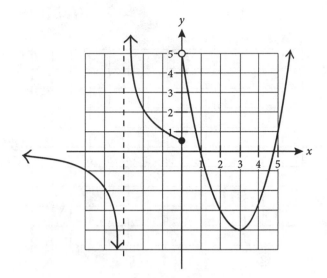

COMPLEX NUMBERS

All of the above examples used only real numbers. However, imaginary numbers are also tested on the PCAT. Real numbers are all numbers that are positive, negative, or zero. Imaginary numbers are those that contain $i = \left(\sqrt{-1}\right)$.

Complex numbers are composed of both real and imaginary numbers and take on the following general form:

$$z = x + yi, \text{ where } z \text{ refers to the complex number.}$$

These can be plotted a graph, just like with functions, where the x-axis deals with real numbers and the y-axis deals with imaginary numbers.

Graphing Complex Numbers

Complex numbers define a point on a graph of real and imaginary numbers. Although this plot looks very similar to the regular graphs from the discussions of functions earlier in this chapter, there are some subtle differences. First, because both real and imaginary numbers are present, the graph is plotted on a complex plane. This leads to the second difference: All y values on the y-axis have a number followed by i to illustrate that the y-axis refers to the imaginary part of the complex number. Finally, complex numbers are usually assigned new variables like "z" or "w" to help distinguish them from variables normally used in real number sets only. This can be seen with the following example.

Example: Graph the following complex numbers:

       1. $z = 6 + 4i$

       2. $w = -3 - 5i$

       3. $v = 8 - 2i$

Solution:

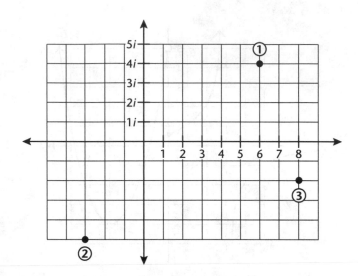

Mathematical Operations on Complex Numbers

Just like with functions, you can perform mathematical operations on complex numbers.

Adding and subtracting complex numbers

To add and subtract complex numbers, you simply combine all the real parts and all the imaginary parts separately.

Example: Given the following complex numbers, find the sum.

$t = 3 + 4i$
$s = 0$ (yes, 0 is a complex number)
$u = 4i$
$v = 3$

Solution: $t + s + u + v = (3 + 4i) + (0) + (4i) + (3)$

x (the real part) $= 3 + 0 + 0 + 3 = 6$
y (the imaginary part) $= 4i + 0i + 4i + 0i = 8i$
Therefore, the sum $= 6 + 8i$.

There is a special trait about the sum of two complex numbers. If you plot 0, z, w, and $z + w$, you generally get four points that define the vertices of a parallelogram. This is known as the **Parallelogram Rule**. You can see this when you plot the above complex numbers because $t = u + v$ and $s = 0$.

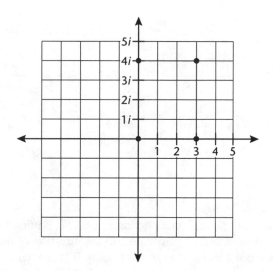

Note that the parallelogram will not always be a rectangle although it is in this case.

Multiplying complex numbers

To multiply complex numbers, use the same strategy as for multiplying polynomials: Multiply the coefficients of each real and imaginary part separately.

Example: Given the following complex numbers, find the product.

$$z = -5 + 6i$$
$$w = 3 - 2i$$

Solution: $z \times w = (-5 + 6i) \times (3 - 2i) = (-5 \times 3) + (-5 \times -2i) + (6i \times 3) + (6i \times -2i)$

$$= -15 + 10i + 18i - 12i^2 \text{ (remember } i^2 = -1)$$
$$= -15 + 10i + 18i - 12(-1)$$
$$= -15 + 10i + 18i + 12$$
$$= -3 + 28i$$

Dividing complex numbers

Division is more complex because of complex conjugates. The conjugate of a complex number $a + bi$ is simply defined as $a - bi$. They are important because any complex number times its conjugate gives only a real answer; the imaginary part goes away. This is important because, when dividing complex numbers, you only want to have real numbers in the denominator. Multiplying by complex conjugates is the way to get only real numbers in the denominator.

Example: Using the two complex numbers above, find the value of $\frac{z}{w}$.

Solution: $\dfrac{z}{w} = \dfrac{-5+6i}{3-2i} = \dfrac{-5+6i}{3-2i} \times \dfrac{3+2i}{3+2i}$ (Remember, this is the same as multiplying by 1.)

$$= \frac{(-5 \times 3) + (-5 \times 2i) + (6i \times 3) + (6i \times 2i)}{(3 \times 3) + (3 \times 2i) + (-2i \times 3) + (-2i \times 2i)} = \frac{(-15) + (-10i) + (18i) + \left(12i^2\right)}{(9) + (6i) + (-6i) + \left(-4i^2\right)}$$

$$= \frac{-15 - 10i + 18i + (12(-1))}{9 + 6i - 6i + (-4(-1))} = \frac{-15 + 8i - 12}{9 + 4}$$

$$= \frac{-27 + 8i}{13} = -\frac{27}{13} + \frac{8}{13}i$$

VECTORS

While complex numbers define a point, vectors define a line. This is important to remember because now you have to keep in mind both the magnitude and the direction of the line when dealing with vectors. Vectors start at one point and end at another point. It is convenient to describe vectors that start at the origin (denoted O) and end at a point (denoted P). The point that has the arrow defines the direction.

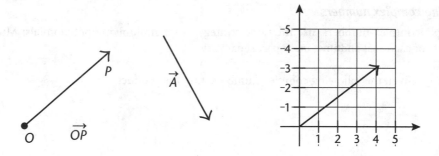

Vectors can be denoted as $\overline{OP}$ or $\overrightarrow{OP}$. Typically, vectors are denoted simply as a single variable, such as $\vec{A}$ or **A**.

Vectors that start at the origin and end at another point can be described simply as coordinates. This is known as the rectangular form. An example is $4i + 3j$. The "i" in vectors is not the same "i" from complex numbers, but vectors in this form are graphed in the same way. In this case, the i part is a unit vector in the positive x direction, and the j part is a unit vector in the positive y direction. The origin of the axes also serves as the origin for the vector. You may also see them defined as a magnitude and an angle only, like 5, 45°. This is known as the polar form and tells you the magnitude (or length) of the vector is 5 units at an angle of 45°. Get used to seeing vectors in both the rectangular form and the polar form because both of these forms are prevalent.

Mathematical Operations on Vectors

Similar to complex numbers, you can perform mathematical operations on vectors.

Adding and subtracting vectors

The sum or difference of vectors is called a **resultant** because it's the vector that is the result of adding or subtracting vectors. To be able to find the resultant:

1. Break down each vector into its components in the x- and y-directions using the following equations:
   i. $Ax = A \times \cos \theta$
   ii. $Ay = A \times \sin \theta$

2. Combine all the x components and then all the y components.

3. Resolve the resultant into a magnitude and direction.

Example: Find the resultant $\vec{R} = \vec{A} + \vec{B}$, in both rectangular and polar form, of the following two vectors: $\vec{A} = 3, 30°$ and $\vec{B} = 5, 60°$, given that $\cos 60° = \frac{1}{2}$ and that $\sin 60° = 0.87$.

Solution: 1. $A_x = A \times \cos \theta = 3 \times \cos 30° = 3 \times \sin 60° = 3 \times 0.87 = 2.61$

$A_y = A \times \sin \theta = 3 \times \sin 30° = 3 \times \cos 60° = 3 \times \frac{1}{2} = 1.5$

$B_x = B \times \cos \theta = 5 \times \cos 60° = 5 \times \frac{1}{2} = 2.5$

$B_y = B \times \sin \theta = 5 \times \sin 60° = 5 \times 0.87 = 4.35$

2. $A_x + B_x = 2.61 + 2.5 = 5.11$

$A_y + B_y = 1.5 + 4.35 = 5.85$

In rectangular form, the resultant is $\vec{R} = 5.11i + 5.85j$.

3. $R = \sqrt{5.11^2 + 5.85^2} \approx \sqrt{26.11 + 34.22} \approx 7.77$

$\theta_R = \tan^{-1}\left(\frac{A_y + B_y}{A_x + B_x}\right) = \tan^{-1}\left(\frac{5.85}{5.11}\right) \approx 48.86°$

In polar form, the resultant is $\vec{R} \approx 7.77, 48.86°$.

Multiplying vectors

Vector multiplication has many meanings. Conceptually, it is not very straightforward, and you need to understand what the vectors represent to understand what type of multiplication you will want to use. The two most common types of multiplication of vectors are briefly covered below.

Dot Product: Let $\vec{X}$ and $\vec{Y}$ be vectors and let θ be the angle between these vectors. The dot product of the vectors $\vec{X}$ and $\vec{Y}$ is found using the following equation:

$$\vec{X} \bullet \vec{Y} = \left|\vec{X}\right|\left|\vec{Y}\right|\cos\theta$$

Because the dot product results in a number, or a magnitude, it is often referred to as the scalar product. Let $\vec{Y}$ be a nonzero vector. Then $\dfrac{\vec{Y}}{\left|\vec{Y}\right|}$ is a unit vector in the direction of $\vec{Y}$. The dot product of $\vec{X}$ and $\dfrac{\vec{Y}}{\left|\vec{Y}\right|}$ is the magnitude of the component of the vector $\vec{X}$ In the direction of the vector $\vec{Y}$.

Therefore: $\vec{X} \bullet \dfrac{\vec{Y}}{\left|\vec{Y}\right|} = \dfrac{\vec{X} \bullet \vec{Y}}{\left|\vec{Y}\right|} = \dfrac{\left|\vec{X}\right|\left|\vec{Y}\right|\cos\theta}{\left|\vec{Y}\right|} = \left|\vec{X}\right|\cos\theta$.

Example: Find the dot product of the two vectors $\vec{A}$ and $\vec{B}$ from the previous example.

Solution: $\vec{A} \bullet \vec{B} = \left|3\right|\left|5\right|\cos 30° \approx 3 \times 5 \times 0.87 = 13.05$

Cross Product: The cross product allows you to find a new vector that is perpendicular to the plane of the two vectors being multiplied. Because you are finding a vector, this is also referred to as the vector product. Use the following equation to find the cross product:

$$\vec{A} \times \vec{B} = \left|\vec{A}\right|\left|\vec{B}\right|\sin\theta\ \mathbf{n}$$

Here, θ represents the smaller angle between the two vectors and $\mathbf{n}$ is a unit vector perpendicular to the plane formed by the vectors $\vec{A}$ and $\vec{B}$. The magnitude of $\vec{A} \times \vec{B}$ is $\left|\vec{A}\right|\left|\vec{B}\right|\sin\theta$. The direction of $\vec{A} \times \vec{B}$ is determined by the right hand rule. The right hand rule says that when you rotate the right hand from $\vec{A}$ to $\vec{B}$ through the smaller angle between $\vec{A}$ and $\vec{B}$, then your thumb points in the direction of $\vec{A} \times \vec{B}$. This is the direction of the unit vector $\mathbf{n}$.

Example: Given the vectors $\vec{A}$ and $\vec{B}$ from the previous two examples, find the cross product.

Solution: $\vec{A} \times \vec{B} = \left|3\right|\left|5\right|\sin 30°\,\mathbf{n}\ = 3 \times 5 \times 0.5\ \mathbf{n} = 7.5\ \mathbf{n}$

The magnitude of $\vec{A} \times \vec{B}$ is 7.5. Here, $\mathbf{n}$ represents the unit vector in the positive z direction. Remember, $\vec{A} \times \vec{B}$ is a vector in the plane perpendicular to the plane of vectors $\vec{A}$ and $\vec{B}$. The right hand rule says that $\vec{A} \times \vec{B}$ is in the positive z direction. So $\vec{A} \times \vec{B}$ is 7.5 units long in the positive z direction.

CHAPTER SIXTY-TWO

Calculus

Calculus and precalculus together constitute approximately fifty percent of the Quantitative Ability section, so be sure to spend sufficient time studying and practicing the material to feel confident on Test Day. Although you may remember completing lengthy calculations using obscure rules as part of your undergraduate coursework, the test makers do not require extensive knowledge of how to integrate the most difficult functions but rather only expect you to know the basics. Remember also that the PCAT is a multiple-choice test, so use the Quantitative Strategies discussed in Chapter 57 whenever they would be advantageous—for example, finding a derivative tends to be much easier than finding an integral, so using Backsolving can be a great approach for avoiding some lengthy calculations!

LIMITS & CONTINUITY

A limit is a value that a function approaches at a certain point. Not all functions have limits, but many do.

Intuitive Definition: Let $y = f(x)$ be a function. Suppose a and L are numbers such that:

- When x is close to but not equal to a, $f(x)$ is close to L;
- As x gets closer and closer to but not equal to a, $f(x)$ gets closer and closer to L;
- $f(x)$ can be made as close to and remain as close to L as you want by making x close to but not equal to a.

Then you can say that the **limit** of $f(x)$ as x approaches a is L and write:

$$\lim_{x \to a} f(x) = L$$

The formal definition of a limit is quite a bit more complicated: If the limit of $f(x)$ as x approaches a is L, for each positive number ε there is a positive number δ such that, if $|x - a| < \delta$ and $x \neq a$, $|f(x) - L| < \varepsilon$.

To understand what this means, work out the following example:

Example: A function $f(x) = x + 4$. At $x = 5$, $f(x) = 9$. Does $f(x)$ stay close to 9 if x stays close to 5?

Solution: To determine if $f(x)$ stays close to 9, evaluate $f(x)$ at numbers x close to 5.

x	$f(x)$
5.1	9.1
5.01	9.01
5.001	9.001
5.0001	9.0001
4.9	8.9
4.99	8.99
4.999	8.999
4.9999	8.9999

As x gets closer to 5 without equaling 5, $f(x)$ gets closer to 9.

Some functions won't allow for certain values, and yet the limit of a function as x approaches such a value still exists.

Example: The function f is such that $f(x) = \dfrac{x^2 - 1}{x - 1}$. At $x = 1$, the function is undefined, so $x \neq 1$. What is the limit of this function?

Solution: Make x close to but not equal to 1:

x	$f(x)$
1.1	2.1
1.01	2.01
1.001	2.001
1.0001	2.0001
0.9	1.9
0.99	1.99
0.999	1.999
0.9999	1.9999

This example fits the definition of a limit. As x gets closer to 1, $f(x)$ gets closer to 2, but x can never equal 1. The limit can therefore be written as:

$$\lim_{x \to 1} f(x) = 2$$

Evaluating Limits

When the $\lim_{x \to a} f(x) = L$, $f(x)$ is the **limit expression**. When evaluating limits, incorporate the methods you learned to factor polynomials to simplify the limit expression, then plug in the a value for x and solve to find the limit of the function.

Example: Find the limit of $\dfrac{x^2 - 1}{x - 1}$ as x approaches 1; that is, find $\lim_{x \to 1} \dfrac{x^2 - 1}{x - 1}$.

Solution: First factor the polynomial, recognizing you have the difference of two squares in the numerator.

$$\lim_{x \to 1} \frac{x^2 - 1}{x - 1} = \lim_{x \to 1} \frac{(x + 1)(x - 1)}{x - 1}$$

Then, simplify the expression:

$$\lim_{x \to 1} \frac{(x + 1)(x - 1)}{x - 1} = \lim_{x \to 1} (x + 1)$$

Now plug in the a value (in this case 1) and evaluate.

$$\lim_{x \to 1} (x + 1) = 1 + 1 = 2$$

Remember that this is the value of the limit and not the value of the given function at $x = 1$ because, by definition, the function cannot have a value at $x = 1$.

Example: Find the limit of $\dfrac{x^2 - x - 12}{x^2 + x - 6}$ as x approaches -3; that is, find $\lim_{x \to -3} \dfrac{x^2 - x - 12}{x^2 + x - 6}$.

Solution: When it's not immediately apparent you need to simplify the expression to find the limit, do a quick check to see if the expression can be evaluated at the a value. However, even if it cannot, note that a limit could still exist.

At $x = -3$, $x^2 + x - 6$ equals 0:

$$(-3)^2 + (-3) - 6 = 9 - 3 - 6 = 0$$

In this case, the denominator equals 0 at $x = -3$, so you must simplify to check if a limit exists.

Follow the step-by-step approach of finding a limit to get:

$$\lim_{x \to -3} \frac{x^2 - x - 12}{x^2 + x - 6} = \lim_{x \to -3} \frac{(x - 4)(x + 3)}{(x - 2)(x + 3)} = \lim_{x \to -3} \frac{x - 4}{x - 2} = \frac{-3 - 4}{-3 - 2} = \frac{-7}{-5} = \frac{7}{5}$$

If $x \to \infty$ or $-\infty$, however, things work differently. Terms like x and x^2 will go to infinity, but, the higher the power of x, the faster that term increases (when x is 100, x^2 is 10,000, and x^3 is 1,000,000). So, if you must take the limit of a fraction at infinity, divide all terms by the highest power of x. By definition, the limit of 1 divided by any positive integer power of x as x goes to infinity equals 0: $\lim\limits_{x \to \infty} \dfrac{1}{x^n} = 0$, where n is any integer greater than 1.

Example: Find $\lim\limits_{x \to \infty} \dfrac{x^2 - x - 12}{x^2 + x - 6}$.

Solution:
$$\lim_{x \to \infty} \frac{x^2 - x - 12}{x^2 + x - 6} = \lim_{x \to \infty} \frac{\dfrac{x^2 - x - 12}{x^2}}{\dfrac{x^2 + x - 6}{x^2}} = \lim_{x \to \infty} \frac{1 - \dfrac{1}{x} - \dfrac{12}{x^2}}{1 + \dfrac{1}{x} - \dfrac{6}{x^2}} = \frac{1 - 0 - 0}{1 + 0 - 0} = \frac{1}{1} = 1$$

Note that the PCAT distinguishes between a limit of infinity and no limit at all. A **limit of infinity** (∞ or $-\infty$) means f increases or decreases without bound as x approaches its target. For example: $\lim\limits_{x \to 0} \dfrac{1}{x^2} = \infty$ because $\dfrac{1}{x^2}$ gets larger and larger as $x \to 0$ from both sides.

On the other hand, saying a function has **no limit** means the function does not converge on any one value as it approaches a. For example, $\lim\limits_{x \to \infty} \sin x$ has no limit because $\sin x$ is constantly oscillating between $+1$ and -1. Similarly, $\lim\limits_{x \to 0} \dfrac{1}{x}$ has no limit because it approaches ∞ from the right but $-\infty$ from the left.

CONTINUITY

You can use limits to determine whether or not a function is continuous. All polynomial functions are continuous; that is, small changes in the input result in small changes in the output. But not all functions are continuous, instead oscillating around a set range (such as some trigonometric functions) or stopping and starting somewhere else (such as some compound functions). It is easiest to see if a function is continuous or discontinuous by analyzing it graphically:

Continuous for all x Discontinuous at $x = 0$

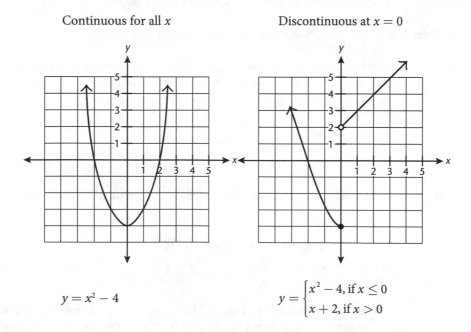

$y = x^2 - 4$

$$y = \begin{cases} x^2 - 4, \text{if } x \leq 0 \\ x + 2, \text{if } x > 0 \end{cases}$$

For a function to be continuous at $x = a$, the following three criteria must be met:

1. For a given function $f(x)$, $f(a)$ must be defined.
2. $\lim\limits_{x \to a} f(x)$ has a finite value.
3. $\lim\limits_{x \to a} f(x) = f(a)$

Example: Determine whether the following function is continuous at $x = 1$.

$$f(x) = \begin{cases} 3x^2 - 5, & \text{if } x \neq 1 \\ 2, & \text{if } x = 1 \end{cases}$$

Solution: Check to see if the criteria are met:

1. $f(1)$ is defined:

$$f(1) = 2$$

2. The limit is finite:

$$\lim_{x \to a} f(x) = \lim_{x \to 1}(3x^2 - 5) = 3(1^2) - 5 = 3(1) - 5 = 3 - 5 = -2$$

3. However, $\lim\limits_{x \to 1} f(x) \neq f(1)$:

$$\lim_{x \to 1} f(x) = \lim_{x \to 1}(3x^2 - 5) = -2$$

$$f(1) = 2$$

Therefore, this function is not continuous at $x = 1$.

Example: Is the function $f(x) = \dfrac{x^2 - 3x - 4}{x^2 + 4x + 3}$ continuous at $x = 2$?

Solution: The denominator factors into:

$$x^2 + 4x + 3 = (x + 3)(x + 1)$$

so $f(x)$ is discontinuous at $x = -3$ and at $x = -1$ because it fails to meet the first criterion for those values of x. However, the question asks if the function is continuous at $x = 2$, so plug in 2 and check all the criteria:

1. $f(2)$ is defined:

$$f(2) = \frac{2^2 - 3(2) - 4}{2^2 + 4(2) + 3} = \frac{4 - 6 - 4}{4 + 8 + 3} = \frac{-6}{15} = \frac{-2}{5}$$

2. The limit is finite:

$$\lim_{x \to 2} f(x) = \lim_{x \to 2}\frac{x^2 - 3x - 4}{x^2 + 4x + 3} = \lim_{x \to 2}\frac{(x - 4)(x + 1)}{(x + 3)(x + 1)}$$

$$= \lim_{x \to 2}\frac{x - 4}{x + 3} = \frac{2 - 4}{2 + 3} = \frac{-2}{5}$$

3. $\lim\limits_{x \to a} f(x) = f(a)$, which in this case is $\lim\limits_{x \to 2} f(x) = f(2)$:

$$\lim_{x \to 2} f(x) = \frac{-2}{5}$$

$$f(2) = \frac{-2}{5}$$

Therefore, the function is continuous at $x = 2$. Because the function is a fraction whose numerator and denominator are both polynomials, it is continuous everywhere the denominator $\neq 0$.

DERIVATIVES

A **derivative** describes the slope of the line tangent to a curve. Derivatives are formally defined as:

$$f'(x) = \lim_{h \to 0} \frac{f(x+h) - f(x)}{h}$$

$f(x)$ is a **function** of x. Examples are $f(x) = x^2$ or $f(x) = 3x^3 + 3$. Another way to write this is: $y = f(x)$, such as $y = x^2$ or $y = 3x^3 + 3$. The derivative of a function can be notated in several ways:

$$f'(x), \frac{df(x)}{dx}, \text{ or } \frac{dy}{dx}$$

For functions that involve x being raised to an exponent, you can find the derivative using the rule:

$$\text{If } f(x) = x^n, \text{ then } f'(x) = nx^{n-1}$$

Similarly, if $f(x) = x^n$, then $\frac{df(x)}{dx} = nx^{n-1}$, and if $y = x^n$, then $\frac{dy}{dx} = nx^{n-1}$.

For $f(x)$, $f'(x)$ is called the first derivative of the function $f(x)$ with respect to x.

The process of finding a derivative is called **differentiation**.

Derivative of a number: When $f(x) = c$, where c is a number, then $f'(x) = 0$.

Example: $f(x) = 4x^3 + 2x + 1$. What is $f'(x)$?

Solution: To find the derivative of the sum of a number of functions, find the derivative of each function separately and then add them together.

$$\frac{d}{dx}(4x^3) = 4(3x^2) = 12x^2$$

$$\frac{d}{dx}(2x) = 2(1x^0) = 2x^0 = 2$$

$$\frac{d}{dx}(1) = \frac{d}{dx}(x^0) = 0x^{-1} = 0$$

So $f'(x) = 12x^2 + 2 + 0 = 12x^2 + 2$.

Although this basic system works for simple functions, more complex functions require additional steps:

The **product rule** is used when two functions are multiplied together:

$$\frac{d}{dx}(f(x)g(x)) = f(x)\frac{dg(x)}{dx} + g(x)\frac{df(x)}{dx}$$

Note that the derivative here is not simply the product of the two derivatives.

The **quotient rule** is used to find the derivative when one function is divided by another:

$$\frac{d}{dx}\frac{f(x)}{g(x)} = \frac{g(x)f'(x) - f(x)g'(x)}{[g(x)]^2}$$

Watch out for the order of terms here—it matters! Also, the quotient rule is time consuming, so look for alternative ways to solve a problem (for example, if the fraction is $\frac{x^9}{x^2}$, you're better off converting that to x^7.

Finally, for a "function of a function," use the **chain rule**:

$$\frac{d}{dx}f(g(x)) = \frac{df}{dg}\frac{dg}{dx} = f'(g)g'(x)$$

This means treat g as a variable to find the derivative of f with respect to g, then find the derivative of g with respect to x. Finally, multiply those two results together.

Evaluating the Derivative at a Point

For $f(x)$, $f'(a)$ is $f'(x)$ evaluated when $x - a$.

Example: What is the derivative of $f(x) = 4x^2 + 2$ at $x = 3$?

Solution: $f'(x) = 4(2x) + 0 = 8x$

$f'(3) = 8(3) = 24$

First find an expression for the derivative and then plug in the value of x.

Graphical interpretation of a first derivative

Understanding the practical meaning of the first derivative can helpful for answering many questions. If y is a function of x such that $y = f(x)$, then the derivative of y with respect to x is the slope of the curve $y = f(x)$ at any given point. Thus, the derivative at a point tells you the slope of the curve at that point.

Take a parabola, as shown below, for example:

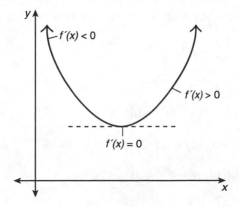

For points on the curve to the left of the point where the slope is 0, the slope is negative. This means the first derivative, $f'(x)$, is negative. At the bottom of the curve, the slope is horizontal with a slope of zero, and so $f'(x) = 0$. For points on the curve to the right of the point where the slope is 0, the slope is positive, and so $f'(x) > 0$. A positive slope indicates that the function is increasing, whereas a negative slope indicates that the function is decreasing. Therefore:

$\dfrac{dy}{dx} > 0$: Positive slope, function is *increasing*.

$\dfrac{dy}{dx} < 0$: Negative slope, function is *decreasing*.

$\dfrac{dy}{dx} = 0$: Zero slope (horizontal).

$\dfrac{dy}{dx} =$ undefined: No slope (vertical).

Example: What is the slope of the curve $y = 3x^2 + 2$ at $x = 5$?

Solution: $f'(x) = \dfrac{dy}{dx} = 3(2x) + 0 = 6x$

$f'(x) = 6x$

$f'(5) = 6(5) = 30$

The slope is 30 at $x = 5$.

Rate interpretation of a first derivative

The slope of a function $y = f(x)$ tells you how fast y changes with respect to x. If a line has a large slope, y changes rapidly with small changes in x. For a line with zero slope, a large change in x produces no change in y. Because the first derivative is the slope of a function at a point, the derivative tells you the rate of change of y with respect to x. For instance, a large, positive $f(x)$ means that $f(x)$ is increasing quickly, whereas a small, positive $f'(x)$ means $f(x)$ is increasing slowly. If $f'(x) = 0$, this means $f(x)$ is not changing at that point.

Higher Order Derivatives

$f'(x)$ is the first derivative of $f(x)$, but the process can be repeated to determine higher order derivatives. These are called the second derivative, third derivative, fourth derivative, and so on. The second derivative is the derivative of the first derivative. The second derivative of a function is found by taking the derivative of the first derivative of that function. The second derivative of $f(x)$ is written $f(x)$ where the number of apostrophes indicates the *order* of the derivative.

For $y = f(x)$, $\dfrac{dy}{dx} = f'(x)$ and $\dfrac{d^2y}{dx^2} = f''(x)$.

Example: If $f(x) = 4x^4 + 2x^3 + 3x$, what is $f''(x)$?

Solution: $f'(x) = 4(4x^3) + 2(3x^2) + 3(1) = 16x^3 + 6x^2 + 3$

$f''(x)$ is the derivative of $f'(x)$:

$f''(x) = 16(3x^2) + 6(2x) + 0 = 48x^2 + 12x$

Graphical interpretation of a second derivative

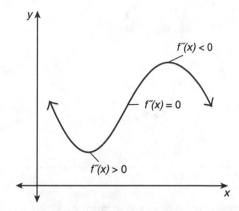

The first derivative tells you whether the function at that particular point is increasing or decreasing. The second derivative tells you whether the first derivative is increasing or decreasing. In other words, if $f''(x)$ is positive, the slope of the function is increasing. If $f''(x)$ is negative, the slope is decreasing. A **point of inflection** is a point where the slope changes from increasing to decreasing or vice versa and so $f''(x) = 0$ as it changes from positive to negative. However, just because $f''(x) = 0$ does not necessarily mean the point is a point of inflection. For example, if $f(x) = x^6$, then $f'(x) = 6x^5$ and $f''(x) = 6(5x^4) = 30x^4$. At $x = 0$, $f''(0) = 0$, yet there is no point of inflection at $x = 0$.

The second derivative of a function is said to be related to the concavity of the function:

$f''(x) > 0$ (positive): Concave up (like the letter U); slope is *increasing*.

$f''(x) < 0$ (negative): Concave down; slope is *decreasing*.

Rate interpretation of a second derivative

The first derivative tells you the rate of change of y with respect to x. The second derivative tells you how fast the first derivative (or slope) changes as x changes. For instance, a large, positive $f''(x)$ means that the slope of $f(x)$ is increasing quickly, whereas a small, positive $f''(x)$ means that the slope of $f(x)$ is increasing slowly. If $f''(x) = 0$, this means the slope is not changing at this point.

In practical terms, this is often seen in the context of moving bodies. If a function is graphing the position of an object in motion versus time, the first derivative shows the rate of change of position, also known as the velocity. The second derivative, then, shows the rate of change of the velocity, which is the acceleration. So a large, positive second derivative indicates a large, positive acceleration, and therefore the object is speeding up (increasing velocity), and the original function would show an exponentially increasing change in position.

Minimum and Maximum Values

The first and second derivatives of a function can be used to find the maximum and minimum values of that function. A valley in the graph of a function is called a **local minimum**. A peak in the graph of a function is called a **local maximum**. The word *local* is used because the value may not be the largest or smallest in the entire graph, but there is a localized peak or valley around that point. See the graph below for an example:

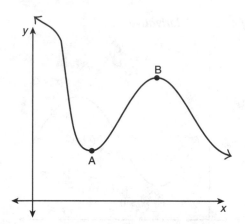

Point *A* is a local minimum, and point *B* is a local maximum. Point *B* is not the highest point on the graph, nor is point *A* the lowest point on the graph.

Note that at points *A* and *B*, the first derivative of the function, that is, the slope, is zero. Thus, if $f'(x) = 0$, that point can be a local minimum point or a local maximum point.

To find out more, find the second derivative of the function. Note that at point *A*, the function is concave up, with $f''(x) > 0$. At point *B*, the function is concave down, with $f''(x) < 0$. Thus, $f''(x) > 0$ and $f'(x) = 0$ indicate a local minimum, and $f''(x) < 0$ and $f'(x) = 0$ indicate a local maximum.

There is another possibility to note. Consider the case when the first derivative is zero but the point is neither a local minimum nor a local maximum:

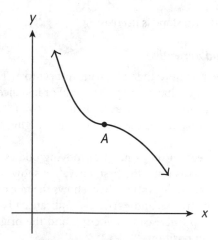

The slope at point *A* is zero, but this point is neither a peak nor a valley. The function is decreasing everywhere as shown. Thus, to be a local minimum or maximum, the function must be decreasing on one side of point *A* and increasing on the other side.

To find local maxima/minima:

1. Find all points where $f'(x) = 0$.

2. Find the value of $f''(x)$ at these points.

3. If $f''(x) > 0$: The point is a local minimum.

   If $f''(x) < 0$: The point is a local maximum.

Example: What is the smallest possible value of $f(x)$ for $f(x) = 4x^2 + 2x - 2$?

Solution: Find $f'(x)$: $f'(x) = 4(2x) + 2(1) - 0 = 8x + 2$

Solve $f'(x) = 0$ for x: $8x + 2 = 0$

$$8x = -2$$
$$x = \frac{-2}{8}$$
$$x = -\frac{1}{4}$$

Find $f''(x)$: $f''(x) = 8(1) = 8$ for all x.

Check the sign of $f''(x)$: $f''(x) > 0$

Because $f''(x) > 0$, $x = -\frac{1}{4}$ is a local minimum. Since $f''(x) > 0$ for all x, at $x = -\frac{1}{4}$ $f(x)$ attains its smallest possible value.

Plug $-\frac{1}{4}$ in for x in the expression $4x^2 + 2x - 2$:
$$4\left(-\frac{1}{4}\right)^2 + 2\left(-\frac{1}{4}\right) - 2 = 4\left(\frac{1}{16}\right) + 2\left(-\frac{1}{4}\right) - 2$$
$$= \frac{1}{4} - \frac{1}{2} - 2$$
$$= -\frac{9}{4}$$

The smallest possible value for the function is $-\frac{9}{4}$, which occurs when $x = -\frac{1}{4}$.

Trigonometric and Transcendental Functions

Trigonometric and transcendental functions have derivatives, too.

$\frac{d}{dx}(\sin x) = \cos x$	$\frac{d}{dx}(\cos x) = -\sin x$
$\frac{d}{dx}(\tan x) = \sec^2 x$	$\frac{d}{dx}(\cot x) = -\csc^2 x$
$\frac{d}{dx}(\sec x) = \sec x \tan x$	$\frac{d}{dx}(\csc x) = -\csc x \cot x$

To remember these derivatives, first note that all the "co-" functions (cosine, cotangent, cosecant)—and only those functions—have negative signs in their derivatives. Second, each pair of functions (sin/cos, tan/cot, sec/csc) uses the same basic formula.

Similarly, you can take the derivatives of the exponential function and the natural logarithm as well:

$$\frac{d}{dx}(e^x) = e^x \qquad \frac{d}{dx}(\mathrm{l}x) = \frac{1}{x}$$

The exponential function e^x is its own derivative, while the derivative of the natural logarithm is $\frac{1}{x}$. Thus, as x gets larger, the slope of $\ln x$ gets smaller.

INTEGRALS

Indefinite Integrals

Integration is the inverse operation (opposite) of differentiation. When you **integrate** a function, you find the **integral** of that function.

The integral of $f(x)$, with respect to x, is written $F(x) = \int f(x)\,dx$.

If $f(x) = \frac{dF(x)}{dx}$, then $f(x)$ is the derivative of $F(x)$, and $F(x)$ is an antiderivative of $f(x)$.

The rule for integrating powers of x is very similar to that for differentiation:

If $f(x) = x^n$, $F(x) = \int x^n dx = \frac{x^{n+1}}{n+1} + C$ (for $n \neq -1$).

Integral of a number: When dealing with functions with no variables, remember that $f(x) = 5$ can be written $f(x) = 5x^0$. So the integral of 5 is $\int 5\,dx = \int 5x^0\,dx = 5\left(\frac{x^{0+1}}{0+1}\right) + C = 5x + C$.

Meaning of the constant, C: The C in the above formula is an unknown constant (often called the **constant of integration**) and is often ignored when calculating integrals because it is cumbersome to carry through many steps of algebra. However, it is important to understand why this constant is present. Consider the function $f(x) = x^4 + x^3 + 2$. The derivative of this function is $f'(x) = 4x^3 + 3x^2$. However, if you were given that $f'(x) = 4x^3 + 3x^2$ and asked to find $f(x)$, all you could say for sure is that $f(x) = x^4 + x^3 + C$. C could be 0 or 2 or $\frac{17}{5}$ or any other number. $f'(x)$ ends up the same regardless of the value of C. So, whenever you integrate a function, to be completely accurate, you must include an unknown constant.

Example: Find $\int 3x^3 dx$.

Solution: $\int 3x^3 dx = 3\int x^3 dx = 3\left(\frac{x^{3+1}}{3+1}\right) + C = 3\left(\frac{x^4}{4}\right) + C = \frac{3}{4}x^4 + C$

To show that integration and differentiation are inverse operations, consider the function $f(x) = x^2$:

The derivative of $f(x)$ is $f'(x) = 2x$.

Now, take the integral of $f'(x)$:

$$\int 2x\,dx = 2\int x\,dx = 2\left(\frac{x^{1+1}}{1+1}\right) + C = 2\left(\frac{x^2}{2}\right) + C = x^2 + C$$

The integral of the derivative of $f(x)$ is $f(x) + C$.

To find the integral of the sum of a number of functions, find the integral of each function and then add them together:

$$F(x) = \int [f(x) + g(x)]\,dx = \int f(x)\,dx + \int g(x)\,dx$$

Example: Find $\int \left(x^2 + 2x^{-2} + 1\right)dx$.

$$\int \left(x^2 + 2x^{-2} + 1\right)dx = \int x^2\,dx + \int 2x^{-2}dx + \int 1\,dx$$

$$= \int x^2\,dx + \int 2x^{-2}dx + \int x^0\,dx$$

$$= \frac{x^{2+1}}{2+1} + 2\left(\frac{x^{(-2)+1}}{(-2)+1}\right) + \frac{x^{0+1}}{0+1} + C$$

$$= \frac{x^3}{3} + 2\left(\frac{x^{-1}}{-1}\right) + \frac{x^1}{1} + C$$

$$= \frac{x^3}{3} - 2x^{-1} + x + C$$

Definite Integrals

The indefinite integral of a function is another function. The definite integral is a number. To find the definite integral you need to know the **limits of integration**. The limits of integration are two numbers written at the top and bottom of the integral sign:

$$\int_a^b f(x)\,dx$$

This is the definite integral of $f(x)$ from $x = a$ to $x = b$. Here, you are integrating $f(x)$ from a to b. Finding the definite integral involves first finding the indefinite integral, using the process outlined above, and then evaluating this integral at the points $x = a$ and $x = b$. The value of the definite integral is the value of an antiderivative at $x = b$ minus the value of that antiderivative at $x = a$. There is some notation to be familiar with here:

If $F(x)$ is an antiderivative of $f(x)$, $\int_a^b f(x)\,dx = F(x)\big|_a^b = F(b) - F(a)$.

The vertical line to the right of $F(x)$ indicates that $F(x)$ is to be evaluated from $x = a$ to $x = b$, which means $F(b) - F(a)$.

Note that C, the constant of integration, is present in both $F(b)$ and $F(a)$, so it cancels out of $F(b) - F(a)$. Finding the definite integral thus eliminates the unknown constant.

Example: $\int_{-3}^{3}(3x^2 - 2x)dx = ?$

Solution:
$$\int_{-3}^{3}(3x^2 - 2x)dx = \left(\frac{3x^3}{3} - \frac{2x^2}{2}\right)\Big|_{-3}^{3}$$

$$= (x^3 - x^2)\Big|_{-3}^{3}$$

$$= [(3)^3 - (3)^2] - [(-3)^3 - (-3)^2]$$

$$= (27 - 9) - (-27 - 9)$$

$$= 18 - (-36)$$

$$= 18 + 36$$

$$= 54$$

Graphical interpretation of integrals

Graphically, if f is a function such that $f(x) \geq 0$ for $a \leq x \leq b$, then the integral of the function f from $x = a$ to $x = b$ is the area under the curve $y = f(x)$ and above the x-axis from $x = a$ to $x = b$.

Example: Find the area under the line $y = 2x$ from $x = 3$ to $x = 7$.

Solution: $\int_{3}^{7} 2x \, dx = 2\left(\frac{x^2}{2}\right)\Big|_{3}^{7} = x^2\Big|_{3}^{7} = (7^2) - (3^2) = 49 - 9 = 40$

The area under $y = 2x$ from $x = 3$ to $x = 7$ is 40.

Consider the graph of this function:

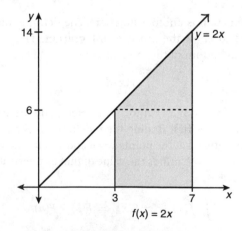

$f(x) = 2x$

The shaded area is the area under the line. The shaded area consists of a triangular area and a rectangular area. The area of the triangle is $\frac{1}{2} \times$ base $\times$ height $= \frac{1}{2}(7 - 3)$ $(14 - 6) = \frac{1}{2}(4)(8) = 16$. The area of the rectangle is the product of the lengths of the two sides: $(7 - 3)(6) = 24$. The total area is $16 + 24 = 40$.

Now, it may seem simpler to find the area geometrically. This is true for simple, linear functions but not for curves.

Example: Find the area under the curve $y = x^2$ between $x = 1$ and $x = 3$.

Solution: $\int_1^3 x^2 \, dx = \left.\frac{x^3}{3}\right|_1^3 = \frac{3^3}{3} - \frac{1^3}{3} = \frac{27}{3} - \frac{1}{3} = 9 - \frac{1}{3} = 8\frac{2}{3}$

The graph of the function is shown below:

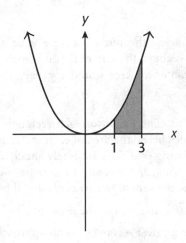

The shaded area is the area under the curve from $x = 1$ to $x = 3$. There is no simple geometric way to calculate the area under this curve, which is precisely the reason calculus was invented!

Theory of integration

Integration is a process of addition. In the same way that multiplication is a faster version of many steps of addition, integration is a faster way to perform many steps of addition and multiplication.

Consider the previous example again:

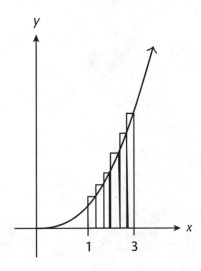

Suppose you want to determine the area under the curve from $x = 1$ to $x = 3$. For simplicity, work with rectangles whose heights are the maximum value of $f(x)$ in each interval. To approximate the area under the curve, one method would be to add up the areas of all of the rectangles shown. However, this would not be completely accurate because the rectangles overshoot the curve slightly and some of the area of each rectangle is not under the curve.

The total area of the rectangles equals: (Area of rectangle 1) + (Area of rectangle 2) + (Area of rectangle 3) + ⋯

The smaller you make the rectangles, the more accurate your approximation becomes because less of the area of the rectangles is above the curve. If you somehow had an enormous number of tiny rectangles, your approximation of the area would approach the *actual* area. This is the idea of integration!

Call the width of each rectangle dx. The height of each rectangle is $f(x)$. The area of each of the rectangles is the width times the height. So the area of each rectangle is $f(x)dx$. Now here comes the trick: In an integral, you are assuming that dx is infinitely small, and there are an infinite number of rectangles. Mathematically speaking, as the greatest rectangle width approaches 0, the number of rectangles approaches infinity, and the sum of the areas of all of these rectangles approaches the true area under the curve. So $\int_a^b f(x)\,dx$ is the sum of the areas of all of the rectangles from point $x = a$ to point $x = b$, assuming that the greatest rectangle width approaches 0. This is the practical value of calculus: being able to find the area under and between curves. So watch out for questions on the PCAT asking for exactly that!

REVIEW PROBLEMS

1. Find the area under the curve $f(x) = -3x^2 + 3$ from $x = -1$ to $x = 1$.

2. What is the slope of the curve $y = 4x^5 + 3x^2 + 1$ at $x = 2$?

3. Find $\dfrac{dy}{dx}$ if $y = 4x^5 + 7x^4 + 10x^3 + 7x^{-1} + 5$.

4. What is area under the curve $y = 4x^3 + 6x$ from $x = 2$ to $x = 3$?

5. If $f(x) = 2x^4 + 10x$, what is the value of $f'(-2)$?

6. Find the value of $\displaystyle\int_1^3 \left(2x - 3 + \frac{24}{x^2}\right) dx$.

SOLUTIONS TO REVIEW PROBLEMS

1.   This problem is asking you to find the definite integral $\int_{-1}^{1} (-3x^2 + 3)\, dx$ because when the function is nonnegative, the definite integral, evaluated between two points, is the area under the curve between those two points. Here, $-3x^2 + 3 = 3(1 - x^2)$ and $3(1 - x^2) \geq 0$ for $-1 \leq x \leq 1$. Integrate:

$$\int_{-1}^{1} (-3x^2 + 3)\, dx = \left(-3\left(\frac{x^3}{3}\right) + 3\left(\frac{x^1}{1}\right)\right)$$

$$= (-x^3 + 3x)\Big|_{-1}^{1}$$

$$= [-(1^3) + 3(1)] - [-(-1^3) + 3(-1)]$$

$$= [-1 + 3] - [-(-1) + 3(-1)] = [2] - [1 - 3] = 2 - (-2) = 2 + 2 = 4$$

The area under the curve from $x = -1$ to $x = 1$ is 4.

2.   To find the slope of the curve, find the first derivative of the function $y = f(x) = 4x^5 + 3x^2 + 1$.

$f'(x) = 4(5x^4) + 3(2x^1) + 0 = 20x^4 + 6x.$

To find the slope at $x = 2$, find $f'(2)$:

$f'(2) = 20(2^4) + 6(2) = 20(16) + 12 = 320 + 12 = 332.$

The slope at $x = 2$ is 332.

3.   If $y = x^n$, $\dfrac{dy}{dx} = nx^{n-1}$.

The derivative of a sum is the sum of the derivatives.

Here, $y = 4x^5 + 7x^4 + 10x^3 + 7x^{-1} + 5$.

$$\frac{dy}{dx} = 4(5x^4) + 7(4x^3) + 10(3x^2) + 7(-1x^{-2}) + 0$$

$$= 20x^4 + 28x^3 + 30x^2 - 7x^{-2}$$

4.   Since $4x^3 + 6x > 0$ for $2 \leq x \leq 3$, the area under the curve $y = 4x^3 + 6x$ from $x = 2$ to $x = 3$ is $\int_{2}^{3} (4x^3 + 6x)\, dx$.

To find $\int_{2}^{3} (4x^3 + 6x)\, dx$, first find an antiderivative of $4x^3 + 6x$.

If $n \neq -1$, then $\int x^n dx = \dfrac{x^{n+1}}{n+1} + C$, where C is a constant.

The indefinite integral of a sum is the sum of the indefinite integrals.

Now $\int (4x^3 + 6x)\, dx = 4\left(\dfrac{x^{3+1}}{3+1}\right) + 6\left(\dfrac{x^{1+1}}{1+1}\right) = 4\left(\dfrac{x^4}{4}\right) + 6\left(\dfrac{x^2}{2}\right) = x^4 + 3x^2.$

Thus, $\int (4x^3 + 6x)\,dx = x^4 + 3x^2 + C$, where C is a constant.

Then

$$\int_2^3 (4x^3 + 6x)\,dx = \left(x^4 + 3x^2\right)\Big|_2^3$$

$$= [3^4 + 3(3^2)] - [2^4 + 3(2^2)]$$

$$= [81 + 3(9)] - [16 + 3(4)]$$

$$= (81 + 27) - (16 + 12)$$

$$= 108 - 28$$

$$= 80$$

The area under the curve $y = 4x^3 + 6x$ from $x = 2$ to $x = 3$ is 80.

5. If $y = x^n$, $\dfrac{dy}{dx} = nx^{n-1}$.

The derivative of a sum is the sum of the derivatives.

Here, $f(x) = 2x^4 + 10x$.

$f'(x) = 2(4x^3) + 10(1x^0) = 8x^3 + 10$

To find $f'(-2)$, substitute -2 for x in $f'(x)$.

$f'(-2) = 8(-2)^3 + 10$

$\qquad = 8(-8) + 10$

$\qquad = -64 + 10$

$\qquad = -54$

6. To find $\int_1^3 \left(2x - 3 + \dfrac{24}{x^2}\right)dx$, first find an antiderivative of $2x - 3 + \dfrac{24}{x^2}$.

If $n \neq -1$; then $\int x^n dx = \dfrac{x^{n+1}}{n+1} + C$, where C is a constant.

The indefinite integral of a sum is the sum of the indefinite integrals:

$$\int \left(2x - 3 + \frac{24}{x^2}\right)dx = \int \left(2x - 3 + 24x^{-2}\right)dx$$

$$= 2\left(\frac{x^{1+1}}{1+1}\right) - 3\left(\frac{x^{0+1}}{0+1}\right) + 24\left(\frac{x^{-2+1}}{-2+1}\right)$$

$$= 2\left(\frac{x^2}{2}\right) - 3\left(\frac{x^1}{1}\right) + 24\left(\frac{x^{-1}}{-1}\right)$$

$$= x^2 - 3x - 24x^{-1}$$

$$= x^2 - 3x - \frac{24}{x}$$

Thus:

$$\int \left(2x - 3 + \frac{24}{x^2}\right) dx = x^2 - 3x - \frac{24}{x} + C, \text{ where } C \text{ is a constant.}$$

Therefore:

$$\int_1^3 \left(2x - 3 + \frac{24}{x^2}\right) dx = \left(x^2 - 3x - \frac{24}{x}\right)\Big|_1^3$$

$$= \left(3^2 - 3(3) - \frac{24}{3}\right) - \left(1^2 - 3(1) - \frac{24}{1}\right)$$

$$= (9 - 9 - 8) - (1 - 3 - 24)$$

$$= -8 - (-26)$$

$$= -8 + 26$$

$$= 18$$

Index

A

Abdominal cavity, 353, 381
ABO blood groups, 259, 342
Absolute configuration, 587–588
Absolute refractory period, 330
Absolute value and inequalities, 889
Absolute zero, 519
Absorption, definition, 239
Acetals, 682–683
Acetoacetic ester condensation, 723
Acetylcholine, 317
Acetylene (ethyne), 572, 637
Achiral molecules, definition, 585
Acid-base disorders, 364
Acid-base indicators, 533
Acid chlorides, from carboxylic acids, 701
Acid halides. *See* Acyl halides
Acidosis, 364
Acids
    acid-base indicators, 533
    acid dissociation constant (K_a), 537, 537–539
    acid equivalents, 540–541
    amphoteric species, 541
    Arrhenius definition, 533–534
    Brønsted-Lowry definition, 534
    buffer solutions, 543
    conjugate acid/base pairs, 534, 537, 537–538,
        539–540, 543
    equivalence points, 541–542, 544
    equivalent weight, 541
    Henderson-Hasselbalch equation, 543, 782–783
    Lewis definition, 432, 534
    neutralization reactions, 472, 539
    nomenclature, 534
    normality (N), 540–541
    pH, 535–536
    pH meters, 541
    polyprotic acids, 544
    polyvalence, 540–541
    properties, 533, 535–539
    salt formation, 539–540
    strong acids and bases, 536–537
    titration, 541–544
    water dissociation constant (K_w), 535, 538
    weak acids and bases, 537–538
    See also Bases; Titration
Acquired characteristics, 271
Acquired immunodeficiency syndrome
    (AIDS), 303
Acquired or specific immunity, 305
Acromegaly, 369
Acrosomal process, 383
Acrosome, 381
ACTH-releasing factor (ACTH-RF), 371
Actin, 224, 329, 331
Actinides, 411
Action potentials, 309, 310–311
Activated complexes, 485
Activation energy (E_a), 485
Active immunity, 294, 304

Actual yield, 453–454
Acyl halides (acid halides, alkanoyl halides)
    conversion into amides, 714, 725–726
    conversion into anhydrides, 713
    conversion into esters, 713
    formation, 701
    Friedel-Crafts acylation, 679, 714, 728
    hydrolysis, 713
    nomenclature, 711–712
    nucleophilic acyl substitution, 712
    properties, 712
    reactions, 712–714, 728
    reduction, 714
    synthesis, 712
Adaptive immunity, 305
Adaptive radiation, 274
Adenine, 768, 771
Adenosine triphosphate (ATP)
    and muscle contraction, 330, 332
    from glucose catabolism, 239, 240–244
    gain and loss of phosphate groups, 725
Adrenal cortex, 368, 369, 373
Adrenal glands, 368
Adrenal medulla, 340, 368, 387
Adrenocortical steroids, 368
Adrenocorticotropic hormone (ACTH), 368, 369
Aerobic respiration, development of, 279
Aerobic respiration, waste products, 359
Afferent neurons, 314
Airways, 344
Alcohol fermentation, 242
Alcohols
    common names, 573, 659–660
    dehydration reactions, 664
    diols (or glycols), 573, 635, 682
    elimination reactions, 664
    geminal diols (carbonyl hydrates), 573, 682
    hydrogen bonds, 660–661
    hydroxyl group, 659, 660–661
    nomenclature, 573, 659–660
    oxidation reactions, 665–666, 678
    phenols, 660, 661, 663, 665, 666, 668
    physical properties, 660–661
    reaction mechanisms, 661–662
    substitution reactions, 664–665
    synthesis by addition reactions, 662
    synthesis by reduction reactions, 663
    synthesis by substitution reactions, 663
    vicinal diols, 573, 635
Aldehydes
    acetal formation, 682–683
    addition reactions, 681–684
    aldol condensation, 684–685
    Clemmensen reduction, 680
    common names, 575, 675–676
    condensation with ammonium derivatives,
        683–684
    cyanohydrin formation, 683
    enol form, 680–681
    enolization, 680–681

    hemiacetal formation, 682–683
    hydration to form geminal diols, 682
    keto form, 680–681
    Michael addition, 681
    nomenclature, 573–574, 675–676
    nucleophilic addition to carbonyl, 681
    overview, 677–678
    oxidation reactions, 679
    physical properties, 677
    reduction reactions, 679–680
    synthesis, 678–679
    Wittig reaction, 686
    Wolff-Kishner reduction, 680
Aldol condensation, 684–685
Aldosterone, 363, 368, 373, 374
Algebra
    absolute value and inequalities, 889
    differences of squares, 882
    equations, definition, 877
    exponents, operations, 878–879
    factor common to all terms, 882
    factoring, 881–883
    FOIL for multiplying binomials, 880
    golden rule of equations, 884
    inequalities, definition, 877
    polynomials, adding, subtracting, or
        multiplying, 879–880
    polynomials, dividing, 880–881
    quadratic equations, 886–888
    quadratic formula, 887
    simultaneous equations, 888
    squares of binomials, 882
    unknown in a denominator, 884–885
    unknown in an exponent, 885–886
    word problems, 867–868, 877–878
Aliphatic compounds (alkyl compounds), 648
Alkali metals (Group IA), 416
Alkaline earth metals (Group IIA), 413, 416
Alkanes
    branched-chain alkanes, 568–570
    combustion reactions, 622–623
    common names, 570
    disproportionation, 623
    free radical substitution reactions, 621–622
    nomenclature, 567–570, 615–616
    prefixes for number of carbon atoms, 567, 615
    primary (1°) carbon atoms, 615
    pyrolysis (cracking), 623
    quaternary (4°) carbon atoms, 615–616
    secondary (2°) carbon atoms, 615
    straight-chain alkanes, 567, 616
    substitution reactions, 616–622
    tertiary (3°) carbon atoms, 615
    See also Nucleophilic substitution reactions
Alkenes
    addition of H_2O, 634, 662
    addition of HX (hydrogen halide), 634
    addition of X_2 (halogens), 633
    anti-Markovnikov addition, 634
    cis-trans isomers, 584, 629

Alkenes (*Continued*)
  common names, 571, 629–630
  (*E*) isomers, 584
  electrophilic addition reactions, 633–634
  free radical additions, 634
  hydroboration, 634–635
  Markovnikov addition, 633, 634
  nomenclature, 570–571, 629–630
  oxidation with ozone, 635, 678
  oxidation with peroxycarboxylic acids, 635, 668
  oxidation with potassium permanganate, 635–636, 679
  ozonolysis, 636
  polymerization, 637
  reactions, 632–637
  reduction by hydrogen, 632
  synthesis, 630–632
  (*Z*) isomers, 584
Alkyl halides (haloalkanes)
  elimination reactions, 630–631
  from alcohols, 669
  from electrophilic addition reactions, 633
  from free radical substitution reactions, 620
  in Williamson ether synthesis, 668
  nomenclature, 573
  nucleophilic substitution reactions, 617
Alkynes
  anti-Markovnikov addition, 639
  electrophilic addition reactions, 639
  free radical additions, 639–640
  hydroboration, 640
  Markovnikov addition, 639
  nomenclature, 573, 637
  overview, 629
  oxidation, 641
  physical properties, 637
  reactions, 638–641
  reduction, 638–639
  synthesis, 638
Allantois, 387
Alleles, definition, 253
Allosteric inhibition, 249
Alpha decay, 556–557
Alpha particle (α-particle), 556–557
Alternative solution task in writing, 31
Amber, 276
Amides
  conversion into amines, 726
  from acyl halides, 714, 724–725
  from anhydrides, 719, 726
  from esters, 726
  Hofmann rearrangement, 727
  hydrolysis, 727
  nomenclature, 725
  properties, 725
  reactions, 727–728, 728
  reduction, 728
  synthesis, 725–726
Amines
  exhaustive methylation, 743
  from amides, 726, 728, 743
  from direct alkylation of ammonia, 741
  from Gabriel synthesis, 741–742
  from reduction of nitriles, 742
  from reduction of nitro compounds, 742
  from reductive amination of imines, 742
  Hofmann elimination, 743
  nitrogen inversion, 739
  nomenclature, 737–738
  primary (1°) amines, 737
  properties, 739–740
  quaternary ammonium compounds, 737
  reactions, 743
  secondary (2°) amines, 737

  synthesis, 740–743
  tertiary (2°) amines, 737
Amino acids
  acid-base characteristics, 780–783
  acidic amino acids, 785–786
  alpha carbon, 779
  amphoteric molecules, 780
  and genetic code, 771
  basic amino acids, 786
  Fischer projections, 779–780
  Henderson-Hasselbalch equation, 782–783
  isoelectric point (pI) or isoelectric pH, 781
  nonpolar amino acids, 783–784
  oxidative deamination, 246
  peptide bonds, 786–787
  polar amino acids, 784–785
  R-groups (side chains), 779, 783–786
  structure, 779–780
  titration, 781–782
  transamination reactions, 246
  transport by circulatory system, 343
  zwitterions, 780, 783
  See also Peptides; Proteins
Aminopeptidases, 354
Ammonia, toxicity, 246
Amnion, 385, 387
Amorphous solids, 506
Amphipathic molecules, 795
Amphiprotic species, 541
Amphoteric species, 541, 780
Amylase, 352, 355
Anabolic reactions, 239
Anaerobic conditions, 242
Analogies
  Antonym bridges, 98
  Association bridges, 98
  bridge types, 97, 97–100
  building good bridges, 100–101
  Characteristic bridges, 99
  Classification bridges, 99–100
  parts of speech in the question, 102
  Part/Whole bridges, 99
  prompt words in analogy questions, 95
  stem words in analogy questions, 95
  Stop-Think-Predict-Match strategy, 95–97
  Synonym bridges, 97–98
  trap error choices, 102–103
  working backward, 102
Analogous structures, 277
Anaphase, 229, 233
Androgens, 368
Angiotensin, 368, 373
Angular momentum, 398
Anhydrides (acid anhydrides)
  acylation, 719
  conversion into amides, 718, 726
  conversion into esters and carboxylic acids, 719, 719–720
  cyclic anhydrides, 715, 716, 717
  from acyl chloride reaction, 714, 715
  from condensation of two carboxylic acids, 715
  hydrolysis, 717–718
  nomenclature, 715
  properties, 715
  reactions, 717–719, 728
  self-condensation of cyclic anhydrides, 716
  synthesis, 712, 715–717
Anions, 415
Anterior pituitary, 369, 370–371
Antibacterial agents, 294
Antibodies (immunoglobulins), 303, 304
Antibonding orbitals, 436
Anticholinesterases, 314
Anticodons, 772

Anti conformation, 591
Antidiuretic hormone (ADH; vasopressin), 363, 370
Antifungal agents, 295
Antigens, 300, 342
Anti-Markovnikov addition, 634, 639
Antiparallel arrangement of strands, 768
Antiparasitic agents, 295
Antiporters, 226
Antiseptics, 293
Antiviral agents, 294–295
Anus, 352
Aorta, 337
Apostrophes, 60–62
Appendicular skeleton, 326
Aqueous solutions, 462, 465
Arginine, 787
Arguments. *See* Dissecting an argument
Aromatic compounds
  aryl compounds or arenes, 648
  benzyl group, 648
  catalytic reduction, 652
  common names, 648, 649–650
  conjugated bonds, 647–648
  electrophilic aromatic substitution, 650–652, 665, 714
  Friedel-Crafts acylation, 651, 679
  halogenation, 650
  Hückel's rule, 647
  meta- or *m-* disubstituted benzenes, 649, 652
  nitration, 651
  nomenclature, 648–650
  ortho- or *o-* disubstituted benzenes, 649
  para- or *p-* disubstituted benzenes, 649, 652
  phenols, 660, 661, 663, 665, 666, 668
  phenyl group (Ph), 648
  polycyclic and heterocyclic aromatic compounds, 649–650
  properties, 650
  reactions, 650–652
  substituent effects, 651–652
  sulfonation, 651
Arrhenius acids and bases, 533–534
Arteries, 337, 340
Arterioles, 337
Aspartic acid, 785
Assimilation, 239
Associative laws of addition and multiplication, 852–853
Assortive mating, 276
Asymmetric (chiral) carbon atoms, 585
Atherosclerosis, 796, 798
Atomic absorption spectra, 400, 758
Atomic emission spectra, 399, 758
Atomic mass unit (amu or u), 395
Atomic number (*Z*), 395, 397, 411, 553
Atomic orbitals, 400, 435–436, 605–606
Atomic radii, 412
Atomic structure
  atomic absorption spectra, 400
  atomic emission spectra, 399
  atomic number (*Z*), 395, 397, 553
  atoms, definition, 395
  Aufbau principle, 402
  Avogadro's number, 397
  azimuthal (angular momentum) quantum number, 401, 435–436
  Balmer series, 399
  Bohr's model of hydrogen atom, 397–400
  compounds, definition, 395
  dalton (Da), 395
  Dalton's atomic theory, 395
  electron configuration, 402–403
  electrons, 396

elements, definition, 395
energy states, 400
frequency, 399
ground state, 398
Heisenberg uncertainty principle, 400
Hund's rule, 403
isotopes, 395, 396, 397
isotopic notation, 553
line spectra, 399
Lyman series, 399
magnetic quantum number, 401
mass number (*A*), 397, 553
mole, 397
molecular weight, 397
neutrons, 396
nucleus, 395
orbital filling, 402–403
orbital radius, 398
orbitals, 400, 435–436
paired electrons, 401
parallel spins, 401
Pauli exclusion principle, 400
Planck's constant, 398, 399
principal quantum number, 400–401
protons, 395–396
quanta, 397–398
quantized energy, 398
quantum mechanical model of atoms, 400–404
quantum numbers, 400–402, 605
quantum theory, 397, 398–399
Rydberg constant, 398
shells, 401, 605
spin quantum number, 401
standard atomic weight, 397
subatomic particles, 395–396
unified atomic mass unit (amu or u), 395
valence electrons, 396, 403–404
Atoms, definition, 395
ATP and muscle contraction, 329, 331, 332
Atria, 338
Atrioventricular (AV) node, 339
Atrioventricular valves, 339
Attenuated pathogens, 294
Aufbau principle, 402
Autolysis, 224
Autonomic ganglia, 387
Autonomic nervous system (ANS), 317–318, 340
Autosomes, 259
Autotrophic aerobes, 279
Autotrophic anaerobes, 279
Autotrophs, definition, 290
Average molecular speeds, 525
Averages (mean)
arithmetic mean (μ) in statistics, 904, 905
finding missing number, given sum, 870
formula for computing, 869
using to find the sum, 869
Avogadro's number, 397, 448
Avogadro's principle, 520
Axial skeleton, 326
Axons, 309
Azimuthal (angular momentum) quantum number, 401

B

Backsolving strategy, 842–843
Bacteria
asexual reproduction, 262, 286
bacillus bacteria, 286
binary fission, 262
coccus bacteria, 285
Gram negative bacteria, 286
Gram positive bacteria, 286

lawn (plated bacteria culture), 287
spirillum bacteria, 286
Bacterial genetics
antibody resistance genes, 263
bacterial genome, 262
bacteriophages and, 263–264, 287
conjugation, 262–263, 286
corepressors, 265
F factor, 263
gene regulation, 264–266
genetic variance, 262
Hfr (high frequency of recombination) cells, 263
inducers, 264
inducible systems, 264, 265
operator region, 264
operons, 265
plasmids, 260, 262
promoter regions, 264, 772
recombination, 264
regulation of transcription, 264
regulator genes, 265
replication, 262
repressible systems, 264, 265
repressor binding sites, 264
sexual mating, 262–263
structural genes, 264
transduction, 263–264, 286
transformation, 262, 286
See also Genetics
Bactericidal agents, 294
Bacteriophages, 263–264, 287
Bacteriostatic agents, 294
Base dissociation constant (K_b), 535, 537–539
Base equivalents, 540–541
Basement membrane, 299
Bases
acid-base indicators, 533
amphoteric species, 541
Arrhenius definition, 533–534
base dissociation constant (K_b), 535, 537–539
base equivalents, 540–541
Brønsted-Lowry definition, 534
buffer solutions, 543
conjugate acid/base pairs, 534, 537, 537–538, 539–540, 543
equivalence points, 541–542
equivalent weight, 541
Henderson-Hasselbalch equation, 543
Lewis definition, 432, 534
neutralization reactions, 472, 539
normality (*N*), 540–541
pOH, 535–536
polyprotic bases, 544
properties, 533, 535–539
salt formation, 539–540
strong acids and bases, 536–537
titration, 541–544
weak acids and bases, 537–538
See also Acids; Titration
Basic math
averages (mean), finding missing number, 869
averages (mean), formula for computing, 869
averages (mean), using to find the sum, 869
conversions of units, 870
logarithms, 870–872
part-to-part and part-to-whole ratios, 860
percents, 866–869
ratios, 860–861
See also Decimals; Fractions; Numbers and number operations
Basophils, 302
Bending vibration, 749–750
Benzyl group, 648
Beta decay, 557–558

Beta particle (β-particle), 556–557
β-pleated sheets, 788–789
Bile, 92, 355, 359, 373
Bimolecular elimination (E2) reactions, 631–632
Bimolecular nucleophilic substitution (S_N2) reactions, 619–621, 631
Binding energy, 553, 554–555
Biology section of PCAT
timing requirements and tips, 24
Birth, 389
Blastocoel, 386–387
Blastula, 386
Blastulation, 386–387
Blood
ABO blood groups, 259, 342
clotting, 343–344
clotting cascade, 343
deoxygenated blood, 338
diastole, 339
donor and recipient blood types in transfusions, 342
erythrocytes (red blood cells or RBCs), 341–342
leukocytes (white blood cells), 301–303, 341
oxygenated blood, 338
plasma, 341
platelets, 341
Rh factor, 342–343
serum, 343
transport of gases, 343
transport of nutrients and wastes, 343
type AB as universal recipient, 342
type O as universal donor, 342
See also Circulatory system
Blood serum, 343
Blood vessels, 337, 340–341
B lymphocytes (B cells), 303
Boat conformation, 592
Body-centered cubic unit cells (crystals), 507
Bohr's model of hydrogen atom, 397–400
Boiling point, 508
Boiling-point elevation (ΔT_b), 510
Boltzmann constant (k), 525
Bolus, 352
Bond energy, 426
Bonding. *See* Chemical bonding
Bonding orbitals, 436
Bond length, 426
Bond order, 426
Bone, 325–326
Bone formation, 326
Bone marrow, 326, 342
Botulinum toxin, 314
Bowman's capsule, 360, 361
Boyle's law, 517–518
Brain, 315–316
Brainstem, 316
Broad-spectrum antimicrobials, 296
Brønsted-Lowry acids and bases, 534
Brownian movement, 227
Buffer solutions, 543
Bundle of His (AV bundle), 339

C

Calcitonin, 372
Calculus
constant of integration, 938
continuity, 930–932
definite integrals, 939–942
functions, 932
graphical interpretation of integrals, 940
integral of a number, 938
integral of the sum of a number of functions, 939
integrals of functions, 938
limits, evaluating, 929–930

Calculus (*Continued*)
  limits of integration, 939
  limits, overview, 927–929
  theory of integration, 941–942
  See also Derivatives
Capillaries, 337, 340
Carbohydrates
  and respiration, 240
  as fuel molecules in cells, 240, 244, 245
  glucose catabolism, 240–244
  simple sugars, transport by circulatory system, 343
  synthesis by autotrophs, 279
Carbon-carbon bonds, 438
Carbon cycle, 290
Carbon dioxide as waste product, 359
Carbon group (Group IVA), 417
Carboxylic acid derivatives
  summary of reactions, 728–729
  See also Acyl halides; Amides; Anhydrides; Esters
Carboxylic acids
  acidity, 697–698
  acyl halide (acid halide) formation, 701
  common names, 576, 696
  decarboxylation reactions, 702
  dicarboxylic acids, 697, 702
  ester formation, 701
  from anhydrides, 719, 719–720, 720–721
  from carbonation of organometallic reagents, 695, 698
  from hydrolysis of nitriles, 698
  from oxidation reactions, 695, 698–699
  hydrogen bonding, 697
  nomenclature, 696–697
  nucleophilic substitution, 700–701
  physical properties, 697–698
  reactions, 695, 700–703
  reduction, 700
  soap formation, 702
  synthesis, 695, 698–699
  See also Fatty acids
Cardiac contraction, 339–340
Cardiac muscle, 331, 332
Cardiac output, 339
Cardiovascular system
  arteries, 337, 340
  blood, 341–343
  blood vessels, 337, 340–341
  heart, 338–340
  lymphatic system, 301, 341
  pulmonary circulation, 338
  respiratory system, 344–347
  systemic circulation, 338
  See also Circulatory system
Cartilage, 325
Cascade effects, 374–375
Catabolic reactions, 239
Catalysts, 487
Catecholamines, 368
Cations, 415
Cell division
  anaphase, 229, 233
  and cell cycle, 228
  and chromosomes, 228–233
  centrioles, 229
  centromere, 228, 229, 233
  chromatin, 228, 231
  cleavage furrow, 229
  crossing over, 231
  cytokinesis, 228, 229
  diploid number, 229
  disjunction, 233
  G1 phase, 228

G2 phase, 228
haploid (1*N*) cells, 231, 233
interphase, 228, 231
karyokinesis (nuclear division), 228
kinetochore, 229, 233
meiosis, 231–233
metaphase, 229, 233
metaphase plate, 229
microtubules, 229
mitosis, 228–230
M phase, 228
nondisjunction, 233
nuclear division (karyokinesis), 228
primary sex cells, 231
prophase, 229, 231
sister chromatids, 228–229, 231, 233
S phase, 228
synapsis, 231
telophase, 229, 233
Cell-mediated immunity, 301, 301–303
Cell membrane, 222–223, 226–227
Cell nucleus, 223
Cell structure
  cell membrane, 222–223
  centrioles, 224
  cilia, 224
  cytoplasm, 224
  cytoskeleton, 224
  endoplasmic reticulum (ER), 223, 227
  flagella, 224
  fluid mosaic model, 222–223
  Golgi apparatus, 223
  lysosomes, 224
  microfilaments, 224
  microtubules, 224, 229
  mitochondria, 224
  nucleolus, 223
  nucleus, 223
  ribosomes, 223, 775
  vacuoles and vesicles, 224
Cell theory, 221
Cellular biology, 221–237
Cellular respiration, 242–244
Cellular transport
  active transport, 226
  antiporters, 226
  Brownian movement, 227
  cyclosis or streaming, 224, 227
  diffusion (extracellular transport), 227, 239
  endocytosis, 226, 227
  endoplasmic reticulum role, 227
  exocytosis, 227
  extracellular transportation, 227
  facilitated diffusion (passive transport), 226, 311
  intracellular transportation, 227
  osmosis, 225–226
  phagocytosis, 226
  pinocytosis, 226
  pumps, 226, 311
  simple diffusion, 225–226
Central dogma of molecular genetics, 767
Central nervous system (CNS), 309, 315–317
Centrioles, 224, 229
Centromere, 228, 229, 233
Cerebellum, 316
Cerebral cortex, 315
Cervix, 381
Chain reactions (nuclear), 555–556
Chair conformation, 592
Chalcogens (nitrogen family, Group VIA), 417
Characteristic of a logarithm, 872
Charles's law, 518–519
Chemical bonding
  antibonding orbitals, 436

atomic orbitals, 435–436, 605–606
bond energy, 426
bonding electrons, 427
bonding orbitals, 436
bond length, 426
bond order, 426
carbon-carbon bonds, 438
chemical bonds, overview, 425
coordinate covalent bonds, 432
covalent bonds, notation, 426
covalent bonds, overview, 426, 605
covalent bonds, properties, 426
covalent bonds, types of, 431–432
dipole-dipole interactions, 436, 437
dipole-ion interactions, 436
dipole moment, 432, 434–435
double covalent bonds, 426, 607
formal charges, 428–429
hybrid orbitals, 607–609
hydrogen bonding, 436, 437
intermolecular forces, 425, 436–437
ionic bonds, 425–426, 605
Lewis acids as electron acceptors, 432, 534, 633
Lewis bases as electron donors, 432, 534, 633
Lewis dot symbols, 427
Lewis structures, 427–431
London dispersion forces (LDF), 436, 437
lone electron pairs, 427
molecular geometry of covalent molecules, 432–434
molecular orbitals, 436, 606–607
nodes, 605
nonbonding electrons, 427
nonpolar covalent bonds, 432
octet rule, 425
octet rule exceptions, 431
pi (π) bonds, 436, 607
polar covalent bonds, 431–432
polar molecules, 432, 434–435
resonance, 429–431
resonance hybrids, 429
resonance structures, 429–431
sigma (σ) bonds, 436, 607
single covalent bonds, 426, 606–607
sp^2 hybrid orbitals, 608–609
sp^3 hybrid orbitals, 607–608, 608
sp hybrid orbitals, 609
triple covalent bonds, 426, 607
valence shell electron-pair repulsion (VSEPR) theory, 432–434
van der Waals forces, 436
Chemical digestion, 352
Chemical equations, balancing, 451–452
Chemical kinetics
  activated complexes, 485
  activation energy (E_a), 485
  catalysts, 487
  collision theory of chemical kinetics, 484–485
  concentration and reaction rates, 486
  endothermic reactions, 485
  energy barriers, 485
  enthalpy change (ΔH), 485
  enzymes as catalysts, 487
  exothermic reactions, 485–486
  first-order reactions, 483–484
  intermediates, 479, 485
  medium, effect on reaction rates, 486
  mixed-order reactions, 484
  potential energy diagrams, 485
  rate constants, 480–482
  rate-determining step, 479, 480
  rate laws, 480–482
  reaction coordinate, 485
  reaction mechanisms, 479

reaction orders, 480–481, 482–484
reaction rates, 480–487
second-order reactions, 484
temperature and reaction rates, 486
transition states, 485
transition state theory, 485–486
zero-order reactions, 482–483
Chemical reactions
balancing redox reactions, 474–476
combination reactions, 471, 476
decomposition reactions, 471, 476
double displacement reactions, 472
electrolysis, 471
half-reaction method (ion-electron method), 474–476
ionic equations, 472
metathesis reactions, 472
net ionic equations, 472
neutralization reactions, 472
nuclear *vs.* chemical reactions, 553–554
oxidation, definition, 473
oxidation numbers, 473–474
oxidation-reduction (redox) reactions, 473–476
oxidizing agents, 473
products of chemical reactions, 472
reactants, 471
reducing agents, 474
reduction, definition, 473
single displacement reactions, 472, 477
spectator ions, 472
Chemistry section of PCAT
timing requirements and tips, 24
Chirality, 585–590
Chiral molecules, definition, 585
Cholecystokinin (CCK), 354, 373
Cholesterol, 797–798
Chorion, 385, 387
Chromatin, 228, 231
Chromosomal breakage, 261
Chromosomes
and cell division, 228–233
and genes, 253
autosomes, 259
chromosomal breakage, 261
crossing over, 231, 256
nondisjunction, 233, 260–261
replication, 262
See also Genetics
Chrondrocytes, 325
Chylomicrons, 341
Chyme, 353, 354, 355, 373
Chymotrypsin, 355, 787
Cilia, 285, 381, 391
Circadian rhythms, 373
Circulatory system
ABO blood groups, 259, 342
and autonomic nervous system, 340
and vagus nerve, 340
aorta, 337
arteries, 337, 340
arterioles, 337
atria, 338
atrioventricular (AV) node, 339
atrioventricular valves, 339
blood, 341–343
blood serum, 343
blood vessels, 337, 340–341
bone marrow, 342
bundle of His (AV bundle), 339
capillaries, 337, 340
cardiac contraction, 339–340
cardiac output, 339
chylomicrons, 341
clotting, 343–344

clotting cascade, 343
deoxygenated blood, 338
diastole, 339
donor and recipient blood types in transfusions, 342
erythrocytes (red blood cells or RBCs), 341–342
extracellular transport, 227
fibrin, 343
fibrinogen, 343
functions of, 343
heart, 338–340
heartbeat, 339
heart rate, 339
heart rate regulation, 339–340
hemoglobin, 341, 343
interstitial fluid, 341
lacteals, 341
leukocytes (white blood cells), 301–303, 341
lymph, 301, 341
lymph nodes, 301, 341
lymph vessels, 301, 341
mitral valve, 339
oxygenated blood, 338
oxyhemoglobin, 341
plasma, 341
platelet plug, 343
platelets, 341
prothrombin, 343
pulmonary arteries, 340
pulmonary capillaries, 346
pulmonary circulation, 338
pulmonary veins, 340
Purkinje fibers, 339
Rh factor, 342–343
semilunar valves, 339
sinoatrial (SA) node (the pacemaker), 339
stroke volume (left ventricle), 339
systemic circulation, 338
systole, 339
thrombin, 343
thromboplastin, 343
transport of gases, 343
transport of nutrients and wastes, 343
tricuspid valve, 339
type AB blood as universal recipient, 342
type O blood as universal donor, 342
veins, 337, 340
ventricles, 338
venules, 337
See also Cardiovascular system
cis isomers, 584, 630
Citric acid cycle (Krebs cycle), 243, 244
Claisen condensation, 723
Cleavage, 385–386
Cleavage furrow, 229
Clemmensen reduction, 680
Clichés, avoiding, 41
Clotting (blood), 343–344
Clotting cascade, 343
Coacervate droplets, 279
Coccus bacteria, 285
Codominance, 258–259
Codons, 261, 771, 772, 773
Coefficients
complex numbers, 923
polynomials, 880, 882, 883
quadratic formula, 887
scientific notation, 865
stoichiometric coefficients, 451–452, 474, 480, 496
Coenzymes, 243, 246, 249, 797
Collagen, 343, 790
Colligative properties
boiling-point elevation (ΔT_b), 510

freezing-point depression (ΔT_f), 509–510
molality (m), 510
osmotic pressure (Π), 510
Raoult's law, 509, 511
vapor pressure lowering, 509, 511
Collision theory of chemical kinetics, 484–485
Colloquialisms, 52–53
Colons, 57–58
Color-blindness, 260
Combination reactions, 471, 476
Combinations (statistics), 906–909, 909–911
Combustion reactions of alkanes, 622–623
Commas, 55–57
Common ion effect, 500–501
Commonly misused words, 67–70
Commutative laws of addition and multiplication, 852
Compact bone, 325
Comparative anatomy, 277
Comparative biochemistry (physiology), 277
Comparative embryology, 277
Complex ions, 418
Complex numbers
adding and subtracting, 922
dividing, 923–924
graphing, 921–922
imaginary numbers, 921
multiplying, 923
parallelogram rule, 922–923
Composite score, PCAT, 8
Compounds, definition, 395, 447
Comprehension questions, 813
Concentrated solutions, 462
Concentration units (solutions), 462–464
Concentric contraction, 330
Concise writing
junk phrases, avoiding, 36
needless qualification, avoiding, 37–38
redundancy, avoiding, 37
unnecessary sentences, avoiding, 38
Conclusion keywords, 808–809
See also Usage and style
Conclusion task in writing, 31
Condensation, 507
Condensation reactions, definition, 683
Condensed phases, 505
Configuration, definition, 586
Conformational isomers, 590–593
Conjugate acid/base pairs, 534, 537, 537–538, 539–540, 543
Conjugation (bacteria), 262–263, 286
Constitutional isomers, 583–584
Context, vocabulary exercises, 181, 186, 191, 196
Continuation keywords, 110, 807
Contrast keywords, 110, 808
Convergent evolution, 273
Conversions of units, 870
Coordinate covalent bonds, 432
Cori cycle, 331
Corona radiata, 382
Corpus luteum, 369, 382, 383
Correctness in writing, 35–36, 43
See also Grammar and form; Usage and style
Cortical reaction, 383
Corticosteroids, 368
Cortisol, 368
Cortisone, 368
Covalent bonding
carbon-carbon bonds, 438
coordinate covalent bonds, 432
double covalent bonds, 426
molecular geometry, 432–434
nonpolar covalent bonds, 432
notation, 427

Covalent bonding (*Continued*)
  polar covalent bonds, 431–432
  properties of covalent bonds, 426
  single covalent bonds, 426
  triple covalent bonds, 426
  types of covalent bonds, 431–432
  valence shell electron-pair repulsion (VSEPR)
    theory, 432–434
Cracking (pyrolysis) of alkanes, 623
Creatine phosphate, 332
Cretinism, 371
Critical point, 509
Crossing over, 231, 256
Crystalline solids, 506
Crystallization, 462
Curare, 314
Cyanohydrins, 683
Cyclic adenosine monophosphate (cyclic AMP),
  373–374, 798
Cycloalkanes, 570, 592–593
Cycloalkenes, nomenclature, 571
Cyclohexane
  boat conformation, 592
  chair conformation, 592
  cyclic conformations, 592–593
  disubstituted, 593
  monosubstituted, 592–593
  twist boat conformation, 592
  unsubstituted, 592
Cyclosis or streaming within cells, 224, 227
Cysteine, 789
Cystine, 789
Cytokinesis, 228, 229
  See also Cell division
Cytoplasm, 224
Cytoplasmic inheritance, 260
Cytosine, 768, 771
Cytoskeleton, 224
Cytotoxic T (TC) cells (CD8+ T cells), 302

D
Dalton (Da), 395
Dalton's atomic theory, 395
Dalton's law of partial pressures, 524
Darwin's finches of the Galápagos islands, 274,
  278
Darwin's theory of natural selection, 271–272
Dashes, 59
Daughter isotopes, 556
DDT-resistant insects, evolution of, 272
Deamination reactions, 246, 359
Debye, 432
Decimals
  addition and subtraction, 863–864
  changing decimals to fractions, 863
  changing decimals to percents, 866–867
  changing fractions to decimals, 862
  changing percents to decimals, 866
  coefficients and scientific notation, 865
  division, 864
  exponents and scientific notation, 865–866
  multiplication, 864
  rounding to the nearest place, 864–865
  scientific notation, 865–866
  See also Fractions
Decomposition reactions, 471, 476
Definitions
  vocabulary, 137–177
  vocabulary exercises, 179–180, 184–185,
    189–190, 193–195, 199–200
Dehydrogenation, 240
Demes, 273
Dendrites, 309
Dendritic cells, 302

Denominator, 855
Density of gases, 521–522
Density of water, 464
Deposition, 508
Derivatives
  chain rule, 933
  definition. *See also* Calculus
  derivative of a number, 932
  evaluating at a point, 933–934
  functions, 932
  graphical interpretation of second derivative,
    935
  graphical representation of first derivative,
    933–934
  local maximum and minimum values,
    935–937
  point of inflection, 935
  product rule, 932
  quotient rule, 933
  rate interpretation of first derivative, 934
  rate interpretation of second derivative, 935
  trigonometric and transcendental functions,
    937–938
Dermis, 299
Detail questions, 813–814, 816
Dextrorotatory compounds, 588
Diabetes mellitus, 372
Diastereomers, 589–590
Dictionary (vocabulary list), 137–177
Diction errors, 67
Diencephalon, 315
Difference (numbers), 851
Diffusion
  cellular transport, 225–226, 227, 239
  facilitated diffusion (passive transport), 226,
    311
  gas exchange, 337, 346
  Graham's law of diffusion and effusion, 525–526
  osmotic pressure, 510
Digestion, definition, 239, 351
Digestive system
  absorption in small intestine, 353
  amylase from pancreas, 355
  anus, 352
  bile, 92, 355, 359, 373
  bolus, 352
  chemical digestion, 352
  cholecystokinin (CCK), 354, 373
  chyme, 353, 354, 355, 373
  digestion, definition, 239, 351
  digestion hormones, 354, 373
  digestive tract, overview, 352–353
  duodenum, 353, 354
  esophagus, 352, 352–353
  extracellular digestion, definition, 351
  gallbladder, 352, 354
  gastrin, 354, 373
  ileum, 353
  intracellular digestion, definition, 351
  intrinsic factor, 353, 354
  jejunum, 353
  large intestine, 352, 355
  liver, 352, 353, 354, 355
  lower esophageal (cardiac) sphincter, 353
  mastication, 352
  mechanical digestion, 352
  mucus secretion, 353
  oral cavity, 352
  pancreas, 352, 354, 355
  pepsin, 353
  peristalsis, 353
  pharynx, 352
  pyloric sphincter, 353
  rectum, 355

  saliva, 352
  salivary amylase (ptyalin), 352
  salivary glands, 352
  secretin, 354, 373
  small intestine, 352, 353–354
  stomach, 352, 353
  trypsin, 355
  villi in small intestine, 353
Dihybrid cross, 256–257
Dihydroxyacetone phosphate, 241
Dilute solutions, 462
Dilution, 464–465
Diploid number, 229
Dipole-dipole interactions, 436, 437
Dipole-ion interactions, 436
Dipole moment, 432, 434–435
Disaccharidases, 354
Disjunction, 233
Dispersion forces, 436, 437
Dissecting an argument
  argument, definition, 810
  assumptions, 810
  conclusion, 810
  evidence, 810
  explicit ideas, 810
  facts and opinions, 810–811
  implied ideas, 810
  inferences, 810
  parts of an argument, 810
  See also Reading Comprehension section of
    PCAT
Dissolution, 461
Distributive laws of multiplication and division,
  853
Diuretics, effect in kidneys, 363
Divergent evolution, 273
Dizygotic (fraternal) twins, 385
DNA (deoxyribonucleic acid)
  adenine, 768, 771
  antiparallel arrangement of strands, 768
  central dogma of molecular genetics, 767
  codons (triplets), 771
  cytosine, 768, 771
  double helix, 768
  genetic code, 771
  guanine, 768, 771
  lagging strand in replication, 769–770
  leading strand in replication, 769–770
  nucleotides, definition and structure, 768
  Okazaki fragments, 770
  promoter regions, 264, 772
  purines, 768
  pyrimidines, 768
  redundancy of genetic code, 771
  regulation of transcription, 223, 264–265, 373
  replication, 769–770
  replication fork, 769
  semiconservative replication, 769
  structure, 768–769
  thymine, 768, 771
  transcription to RNA, 772–773
  Watson-Crick DNA model, 768, 768–769
  See also Genetics; RNA
DNA helicase, 769
DNA ligase, 770
DNA polymerase, 769–770, 773
Dorsal root ganglia, 316
Double displacement reactions, 472
Double helix, 768
Down syndrome, 260–261
Drosophila melanogaster, 257–258, 260
Duodenum, 353, 354
Dwarfism, 369
Dynamic contraction, 329–330

E

E1 (unimolecular elimination) reactions, 631
(*E*) isomers, 584
E2 (bimolecular elimination) reactions, 631–632
Eccentric contraction, 330
Eclipsed conformation, 591
Ectoderm, 386, 387
Ectopic pregnancy, 386
Effectiveness questions, 815–816, 816
Effective nuclear charge (Z_{eff}), 412
Effector cells, 313
Efferent neurons, 314
Effusion, 525–526
Ejaculatory duct, 380
Electrolysis, 471
Electrolytes, 462
Electron affinity, 413–414
Electron capture, 559
Electron configuration, 402–403
Electronegativity, 414
Electrons
    bonding electrons, 427
    lone electron pairs, 427
    nonbonding electrons, 427
    paired electrons, 401
    parallel spins, 401
    valence electrons, 396, 403–404, 411
Electron transport chain (ETC), 240, 243
Electrophilic addition reactions, 633–634, 639
Electrophilic aromatic substitution, 650–652, 665, 714
Elements, definition, 395
Elimination, definition, 359
Elimination reactions
    alcohols, 664
    alkene synthesis, 630–632
    alkyl halides, 630–631
    E1 (unimolecular elimination) reactions, 631
    E2 (bimolecular elimination) reactions, 631–632
    Hofmann elimination, 743
    Zaitsev's rule, 632
Embryology
    allantois, 387
    amnion, 385, 387
    autonomic ganglia, 387
    birth, 389
    blastocoel, 386–387
    blastula, 386
    blastulation, 386–387
    chorion, 385, 387
    cleavage, 385–386
    comparative embryology, 277
    dizygotic (fraternal) twins, 385
    early developmental stages, 385–387
    ectoderm, 386, 387
    ectopic pregnancy, 386
    endoderm, 386
    fertilization, 379–380, 383–384
    first trimester of pregnancy, 388
    gametogenesis, 379, 387
    gastrula, 277, 386
    gastrulation, 386
    gestation, 388–389
    growth of organs, 387
    labor, 389
    mesoderm, 386, 387
    monozygotic (identical) twins, 385
    morula, 386
    neural crest cells, 387
    neural tube, 387
    neurulation, 387
    notochord, 387
    organogenesis, 387

placenta, 294, 305, 343, 374, 383, 385, 387–388
placental development, 387–388
second trimester of pregnancy, 388
sensory ganglia, 387
third trimester of pregnancy, 389
umbilical cord, 387, 389
yolk sac, 387
See also Reproductive system
Emphasis keywords, 110, 808
Empirical formulas, 449
Emulsions, 506
Enantiomers, definition, 585
Endochondral ossification, 326
Endocrine system
    acromegaly, 369
    ACTH-releasing factor (ACTH-RF), 371
    adrenal cortex, 368, 369, 373
    adrenal glands, 368
    adrenal medulla, 340, 368, 387
    adrenocorticotropic hormone (ACTH), 368, 369
    aldosterone, 363, 368, 373, 374
    androgens, 368
    anterior pituitary, 369, 370–371
    antidiuretic hormone (ADH; vasopressin), 363, 370
    calcitonin, 372
    catecholamines, 368
    cholecystokinin (CCK), 354, 373
    corpus luteum, 369, 382, 383
    cortical sex hormones, 368
    cortisol, 368
    cortisone, 368
    cretinism, 371
    diabetes mellitus, 372
    direct pituitary hormones, 369
    dwarfism, 369
    endocrine glands, overview, 367
    endorphins, 369
    epinephrine (adrenaline), 340, 368
    erythropoietin (EPO), 342, 373
    estrogens, 369, 374, 382
    follicle stimulating hormone (FSH), 369, 382
    gastrin, 354, 373
    gastrointestinal hormones, 373
    gigantism, 369
    glucagon, 372
    glucocorticoids, 368, 369, 372
    gonadotropin releasing hormone (GnRH), 382
    growth hormone (GH, somatotropin), 369
    hyperthyroidism, 371
    hypothalamus, 369, 370–371
    hypothyroidism, 371
    insulin, 372
    islets of Langerhans, 372
    kidneys, 373
    luteinizing hormone (LH), 369, 382
    mechanism of hormone action, 373–374
    melanocyte-stimulating hormone (MSH), 369
    melatonin, 373
    mineralocorticoids, 368
    neurosecretory cells of the hypothalamus, 369, 371
    norepinephrine (noradrenaline), 317, 368
    oxytocin, 369, 371
    parathyroid glands, 372
    parathyroid hormone (PTH), 372
    peptide hormones, 373–374
    pineal gland, 373
    pituitary gland, 369–370
    posterior pituitary (neurohypophysis), 369–370
    prolactin, 369

renin, 373
second messenger, 373–374
secretin, 354, 373
specific receptors for hormones, 373
steroid hormones, 374
testes, 367, 368, 369, 374
thyroglobulin, 371
thyroid, 371–372
thyroid-stimulating hormone (TSH), 369
thyroxine (T4), 371
transcortins, 368
triiodothyronine (T3), 371
tropic pituitary hormones, 369
Endocytosis, 226, 227
Endoderm, 386
Endoplasmic reticulum (ER), 223, 227
Endorphins, 369
End point (titration), 541
Energy-independent carriers, 226
Energy states, 400
Enolization, 680–681
Enthalpy change (ΔH), 485
Envelope conformation, 592
Enzymes
    active sites, 246
    allosteric inhibition, 249
    and coenzymes, 243, 246, 249, 796
    as catalysts, 246, 487
    competitive inhibition, 249
    hydrolysis reactions, 249
    induced fit theory, 247
    in the mouth, 300
    lactase, 249
    lipases, 249
    lock and key theory, 247
    noncompetitive inhibition, 249
    proteases, 249
    reaction types, 249
    specificity and reaction rates, 247–248
Eosinophils, 302
Epidermis, 299
Epinephrine (adrenaline), 340, 368
Epoxides, 574, 669–670
Equilibrium
    and pressure or volume changes, 497–498
    and temperature changes, 498
    common ion effect, 500–501
    definition, 495
    equilibrium constant (K_{eq}), 495–497, 538
    gas-liquid equilibrium, 507–508
    gas-solid equilibrium, 508
    Gibbs functions for equilibria, 508
    ion product (Q_{sp}) of a compound in solution, 499
    law of mass action, 495–496
    Le Châtelier's principle, 497–498
    liquid-solid equilibrium, 508
    phase equilibria, 507–508
    reaction quotient (*Q*), 496
    reversible reactions, 495, 498, 507
    solubility product constant (K_{sp}), 499–500
    solution equilibria, 498–501
Equivalence points, 541–542
Equivalents, 448–449
Equivalent weight, 541
Erythroblastosis fetalis, 343
Erythrocytes (red blood cells or RBCs), 341–342
Erythropoietin (EPO), 342, 373
Esophagus, 352, 352–353
Esters
    Claisen condensation (acetoacetic ester condensation), 723

Esters (*Continued*)
conversion into amides, 722, 726
from acyl chlorides, 714, 720
from anhydrides, 719, 720–721
from carboxylic acids and alcohols, 720
Grignard addition, 723
hydrolysis, 721–722
nomenclature, 719
phosphate esters, 724–725
properties, 720
reactions, 721–724, 728
reduction, 724
synthesis, 720–721
transesterification, 723
Estimation strategy, 843–844
Estrogens, 369, 374, 382
Ethers
cleavage, 669–670
common names, 573, 666–667
cyclic ethers, 574, 667, 668
epoxides, 574, 669–670
hydrogen bonds, 667
nomenclature, 573–574, 666–667
oxiranes, 574, 636, 667, 668
peroxide formation, 669
physical properties, 667
reactions, 669–670
synthesis, 667–668
Williamson ether synthesis, 668
Ethyne (acetylene), 572, 637
Evaluation questions, 814–815, 815
Evaporation, 507
Evidence keywords, 808
Evolution
acquired characteristics, 271
adaptive radiation, 274
aerobic respiration, development of, 279
amber, 276
analogous structures, 277
assortive mating, 276
autotrophic aerobes, 279
autotrophic anaerobes, 279
autotrophs, development of, 279
coacervate droplets, 279
comparative anatomy, 277
comparative biochemistry (physiology), 277
comparative embryology, 277
competition, 272
components of evolution, 272–276
convergent evolution, 273
Darwin's finches of the Galápagos islands, 274, 278
Darwin's theory of natural selection, 271–272
DDT-resistant insects, evolution of, 272
demes, 273
divergent evolution, 273
early evolution of life, 278
evidence of evolution, 276–278
evolutionary history, 273–274
fitness, 271
fossil casts, 276
fossil imprints, 276
fossil molds, 276
fossil record, 276–277
founder effect, 276
gene flow, 272–273, 276
genetic drift, 276
geographic barriers, 278
heterotroph hypothesis, 278–279
heterotrophic aerobes, 279
heterotrophic anaerobes, 279
homologous structures, 277
imprints, 276
inheritance (transmission) of variations, 272

intraspecific competition, 278
isolated populations, 273
Lamarckian evolution, 271
marsupials, 278
microevolution, 275–276
migration of populations, 274, 278
mutation, 276
natural selection, 271–272, 276
new species, evolution of, 272
niches, 274
organic synthesis (Stanley L. Miller experiment), 279
origin of life, 278–279
overpopulation, 272
parallel evolution, 273
petrification, 276
phylogeny, 273
population genetics, 274–275
primitive cell formation, 279
primordial soup, 278
reducing and oxidizing atmosphere, 279
reproductive isolation, 273, 278
sexual selection, 276
speciation, 272–273
Excess reactants, 453
Excretion, definition, 239
Excretory system
aldosterone, 363, 368, 373, 374
antidiuretic hormone (ADH; vasopressin), 363, 370
aquaporins (water channels), 363
Bowman's capsule, 360, 361
collecting duct (kidney), 360, 362–363, 370
concentrated urine formation, 362–363
cortex (kidney), 360, 363
counter-current-multiplier system, 363
distal convoluted tubule, 360, 362–363
effect of diuretics, 363
excretion, definition, 239
filtration (kidney), 361
glomerulus, 360, 361
hyperosmolar regions of kidney, 363
liver, 359
loop of Henle, 360, 362–363
lungs, 359
medulla (kidney), 360, 363
metabolic wastes, 359
nephron structure, 360–362
osmolarity gradient (kidney), 362, 363
osmosis, 363
passive and active transport, 361
peritubular capillaries, 361
pH maintenance, 363–364
proximal convoluted tubule, 360, 362
reabsorption of water and nutrients, 363, 368
renal pelvis, 360
secretion of waste (kidney), 362
selective permeability of nephrons, 362, 363
skin, 359
structure (kidney), 360–362
urethra, 360
urinary bladder, 360
urine formation, 361–362
Exhalation, 345
Exocrine glands, 367, 372, 373
Exocytosis, 227
Exons, 773
Exothermic reactions, 485–486
Expiratory reserve volume, 347
Explanation task in writing, 31
Exponential decay, 560–561
Exponents
and logarithms, 870–871
chemical rate laws, 480–481

order of operations, 856
p-scale values, 535
scientific notation, 865–866
unknown in, 885–886
Extension (joints), 327
Extracellular digestion, definition, 351
Extrapyramidal system, 327

F

Face-centered cubic unit cells (crystals), 507
Factoring, 881–883
Fats as fuel molecules in cells, 245–246
Fatty acids
enzymatic synthesis, 248
free fatty acids, 800
in phospholipids, 796
in triacylglycerols (fats or triglycerides), 722
metabolism, 246
omega-3 fatty acid, 798
saturated fatty acids, 796–797
trans-fatty acids, 796
unsaturated fatty acids, 796–797
See also Carboxylic acids; Lipids
Faulty parallelism, 46–48
Female reproductive system, 381–385
Fermentation, 242
Fertilization, 379–380, 383–384
Fertilization membrane, 383–384
Fever, 301
Fibrin, 343
Fibrinogen, 343
Fibrous proteins, 790
First ionization energy (IE), 412–413
First-order reactions, 483–484
First trimester of pregnancy, 388
Fischer projections, 586
Fission reactions, 553, 555–556
Fitness (evolution), 271
Flagella, 224, 285
Flexion (joints), 327
"Flight or fight" responses, 317
FOIL for multiplying binomials, 880
Follicles, 381
Follicle stimulating hormone (FSH), 369, 382
Follicular phase, 382
Forceful writing
clichés, avoiding, 41
jargon, avoiding, 41–42
needless self-reference, avoiding, 39, 43
passive voice, avoiding, 39–40
vague language, avoiding, 40–41
weak openings, avoiding, 40
See also Usage and style
Forebrain (prosencephalon), 315
Formal charges, 428–429
Formula mass, 447
Fractions
adding fractions, 857
basic arithmetic with, 856–858
canceling fractions, 858
changing decimals to fractions, 863
changing fractions to decimals, 862
changing fractions to percents, 866–867
changing percents to fractions, 866
comparing fractions, 858
denominator, 855
dividing fractions, 857
mixed numbers, adding and subtracting, 859–860
mixed numbers and fractions, conversions, 858–859
multiplying fractions, 857
numerator, 857
reducing fractions, 857–858

subtracting fractions, 857
See also Basic math; Decimals
Free radical additions to alkenes, 634
Free radical additions to alkynes, 639–640
Free radical substitution reactions, 621–622
Freezing, 508
Freezing point, 508
Freezing-point depression (ΔT_f), 509–510
Frequency, 399
Friedel-Crafts acylation, 651, 679, 714, 719, 728
Fruit fly (*Drosophila melanogaster*), 257–258
Functional groups
  characteristic IR absorptions, 750
  nitrogen-containing organic compounds, 738–739
  summary, 577
Function questions, 815
Fungi
  diploid phase, 288
  fission (asexual reproduction), 288–289
  haploid phase, 288
  spores, 289
Fusion or melting, 508
Fusion reactions, 553, 555

G

G1 phase (cell cycle), 228
G2 phase (cell cycle), 228
Gabriel synthesis, 740–741
Gallbladder, digestive function, 352, 354
Gametes, production by meiosis, 231, 233
Gametogenesis, 379, 387
Gamma decay, 558–559
Ganglia, 315
Gas constant (*R*), 510, 520–521
Gases, properties, 505–506
Gas exchange (lungs), 337, 344, 346
Gas laws
  absolute zero, 519
  Avogadro's principle, 520
  Boyle's law, 517–518
  Charles's law, 518–519
  Dalton's law of partial pressures, 524
  density and ideal gas law, 521–522
  gas constant (*R*), 510, 520–521
  Graham's law of diffusion and effusion, 525–526
  ideal gases, 517–523
  ideal gas law, 520–523
  Kelvin temperature (K), 517
  kinetic molecular theory of gases, 524–526
  molar mass and ideal gas law, 522–523
  pressure units, 517
  real gases, 523
  volume units, 517
Gas-liquid equilibrium, 507–508
Gas-solid equilibrium, 508
Gastrin, 354, 373
Gastroesophageal reflux disease (GERD), 353
Gastrula, 277, 386
Gastrulation, 386
Gauche conformation, 591, 592
Genetic code, 771
Genetics
  ABO blood groups, 259
  alleles, definition, 253
  autosomes, 259
  central dogma of molecular genetics, 767
  chromosomal breakage, 261
  codominance, 258–259
  codons, 261, 771
  color-blindness, 260
  corepressors, 265
  crossing over, 231, 256

cytoplasmic inheritance, 260
dihybrid cross, 256–257
Down's syndrome, 260–261
Drosophila melanogaster, 257–258, 260
environmental factors, 260
filial or F generations, 254
frameshift mutation, 261
gene, definition, 253
gene mutation, added, deleted, or substituted bases in, 261
gene regulation, 264–266
genetic problems, 260–262
genotype, definition, 253
hemophilia, 260
heterozygous, definition, 253
homozygous, definition, 253
incomplete dominance, 258
inducers, 264
inducible systems, 264, 265
Mendel's first law (Law of Segregation), 253–256
Mendel's Law of Dominance, 253–254
Mendel's second law (Law of Independent Assortment), 256–258
missense mutation, 261
monohybrid crosses, 254
monosomy, 260–261
mutations, 261–262
nondisjunction, 233, 260–261
non-Mendelian inheritance patterns, 258–260
nonsense mutation, 261
operator region, 264
operons, 265
parental or P generation, 254
phenotype, definition, 253
phenylketonuria (PKU), 262
point mutation, 261
promoter regions, 264, 772
Punnett square diagrams, 254–255
recessive alleles, definition, 253
regulation of transcription, 223, 264–265, 373
regulator genes, 265
repressible systems, 264, 265
repressor binding sites, 264
segregation, definition, 253
sex determination, 259
sickle-cell anemia, 262
silent mutation, 261
structural genes, 264
testcross, 255–256
trisomy, 260–261
See also Bacterial genetics; DNA
Genotype, definition, 253
Geometric isomers, 584
Gestation, 388–389
Gibbs functions for equilibria, 508
Gigantism, 369
Global questions, 813, 817
Globular proteins, 790
Glucagon, 372
Glucocorticoids, 368, 369, 372
Gluconeogenesis, 368, 372
Glucose catabolism, 240–244
Glutamic acid, 262, 785, 786
Glyceraldehyde 3-phosphate (PGAL), 241
Glycerol from hydrolysis of fats, 245
Glycerophospholipids, 796
Glycine, 771, 779, 781–783, 783, 786
Glycolysis, 240–242
Glycoproteins, 790
Golden rule of equations, 884
Golgi apparatus, 223, 381
Gonadotropin-releasing hormone (GnRH), 382
Gonads, 379

Graham's law of diffusion and effusion, 525–526
Gram-equivalent weight (GEW), 448–449
Grammar and form
  clear modifiers, 51–52
  colloquialisms, 52–53
  faulty parallelism, 46–48
  matching verb and subject, 46–48
  principles of consistency, 43–52
  pronouns, agreement with antecedents, 48–51
  run-on sentences, 53, 54–55
  shifting narrative voice, 44–45
  See also Punctuation; Usage and style
Gram negative bacteria, 286
Gram positive bacteria, 286
Gram staining, 286
Granulocytes, 301
Graphing equations
  absolute value equations, 917
  domains of functions, 918
  linear functions and equations, 917
  piecewise functions, 917
  polynomial equations, 917
  quadratic equations, 917
  radical functions, 917
  ranges of functions, 917
  steps in graphing equations, 917–921
  x-intercept, 918
  y-intercept, 918
Grignard reagents, 695, 699, 723, 728
Ground state, 398
Growth, definition, 239
Growth hormone (GH, somatotropin), 369
Guanine, 768, 771
Guanine cap, 773

H

Hair, 299
Half-life ($T_{1/2}$) of radioactive decay, 560
Halogens (Group VIIA), 416
Haploid (1*N*) cells, 231, 233, 381, 382
Haversian canals, 325
Heart, 338–340
Heartbeat, 339
Heart rate, 339
Heart rate regulation, 339–340
Heisenberg uncertainty principle, 400
Helminths, 289
Heme group, 790
Hemiacetals, 682–683
Hemiketals, 682–683
Hemoglobin, 341, 343, 790
Hemophilia, 260
Henderson-Hasselbalch equation, 543, 782–783
Heterocyclic aromatic compounds, 649–650
Hetero-nuclear RNA (hnRNA) or pre-RNA, 773
Heterotrophs, definition, 290
Heterozygous, definition, 253
Hindbrain (rhombencephalon), 316
Histamine, 301
Histones, 223
HMG-CoA reductase inhibitors, 798
Hofmann elimination, 743
Hofmann rearrangement, 727
Homeostasis, definition, 239
Homogeneous mixtures, 461, 506
Homozygous, definition, 253
Hückel's rule, 647
Human chorionic gonadotropin (hCG), 383
Human immunodeficiency virus (HIV), 287, 295–296
Humoral immunity, 300, 304–305
Hund's rule, 403
Hybrid orbitals, 607–609
Hydration, 461

Hydration complexes, 418
Hydrazones, 680, 684
Hydroboration, 634–635, 640
Hydrogen, 416
Hydrogen bonding, 436, 437
Hydrogen ions, 449
Hydrolysis reactions, definition, 539–540
Hydrolytic enzymes in lysosomes, 224
Hydroxyl groups, 449, 659, 660–661
Hypercholesterolemia, 798–799
Hyperpolarization of neurons, 312
Hyperthyroidism, 371
Hypertonic solutions, 225
Hyphens, 58–59
Hypothalamus, 315, 369, 370–371
Hypothyroidism, 371
Hypotonic solutions, 225–226
H zone (muscle), 329

I

I band (muscle), 329
Ideal gases, 517–523
Ideal gas law, 520–523
Ideal solutions, 511
Idiomatic errors, 67
Ileum, 353
Illustration keywords, 808
Imaginary numbers, 921
Imines, 683–684, 737, 742
Immiscible liquids, 506
Immune system
  acquired or specific immunity, 305
  active immunity, 294, 304
  adaptive immunity, 305
  antibodies (immunoglobulins), 303, 304
  antigens, 300, 342
  basophils, 302
  B lymphocytes (B cells), 303
  cell-mediated immunity, 301, 301–303
  cytotoxic T (T_C) cells (CD8$^+$ T cells), 302
  dendritic cells, 302
  eosinophils, 302
  fever, 301
  granulocytes, 301
  histamine, 301
  humoral immunity, 300, 304–305
  immunization, 293–294
  immunocompromised patients, 306
  inflammatory response, 301
  innate immunity, 305
  leukocytes, 301–303, 341
  lymphatic system, 301, 341
  lymph nodes, 301, 341
  macrophages, 302
  mast cells, 302
  memory T cells, 302
  monocytes, 302
  natural killer T (NKT) cells, 302
  neutrophils, 301–302
  passive immunity, 294, 305
  regulatory or suppressor T (T_{reg}) cells, 302
  spleen, immune function, 301
  T helper (T_H) cells (CD4+ T cells), 302
  thymus, 303
  T lymphocytes (T cells), 302–303
  transplant rejection, 306
  types of immunity, 305–306
  vaccination, 304
Immunization, 293–294
Immunocompromised patients, 306
Incomplete dominance, 258
Inequalities, definition, 877
Inference questions, 815
Inflammatory response, 301

Infrared (IR) spectroscopy
  application, 751
  basic theory, 749–750
  characteristic absorptions of functional
    groups, 750
  fingerprint region, 750
  stretching, bending, and rotation vibrations,
    749–750
  summary, 751
  wavenumbers, 749
  See also Spectroscopy
Ingestion, definition, 239
Inhalation, 345
Innate immunity, 305
Insertion (muscles), 327
Inspiratory reserve volume, 347
Insulin, 372
Integers, 851
Integrals
  definite integrals, 939–942
  functions, 938
  graphical interpretation, 940
  integral of a number, 938
  limits of integration, 939
  meaning of the constant, 938
  of the sum of a number of functions, 939
  theory of integration, 941–942
  See also Calculus
Integumentary system, 299–300
Integument, definition, 299
Intermolecular forces, 425, 436–437
Interphase, 228, 231
Intracellular digestion, definition, 351
Intramembranous ossification, 326
Intrinsic factor, 353, 354
Introns, 773
Ionic bonds, 425–426, 605
Ionic equations, 472
Ionic radii, 412
Ionic solids, 506
Ionization energy (IE), 412–413
Ion product (Q_{sp}) of a compound in solution,
  499
Ions, 395, 415–416
Irreversible reactions, 480, 495
Irritability, definition, 239
Islets of Langerhans, 372
Isocyanates, 727
Isomers
  absolute configuration, 587–588
  achiral molecules, definition, 585
  anti conformation, 591
  asymmetric (chiral) carbon atoms, 585
  boat conformation, 592
  chair conformation, 592
  chirality, 585–590
  chiral molecules, definition, 585
  cis-trans isomers, 584, 629
  configuration, definition, 586
  conformational isomers, 590–593
  cyclic conformations, 592–593
  dextrorotatory compounds, 588
  diastereomers, 589–590
  eclipsed conformation, 591
  (*E*) isomers, 584
  enantiomers, definition, 585
  envelope conformation, 592
  Fischer projections, 586
  gauche conformation, 591, 592
  geometric isomers, 584
  levorotatory compounds, 588–589
  meso compounds, 590
  Newman projections, 590–591
  optical activity, 588–589

plane of symmetry, 590
  relative configuration, 586–587
  R/S naming convention, 587–588
  specific rotation, 589
  staggered conformation, 591
  stereoisomers, definition, 584
  structural isomers (constitutional isomers),
    583–584
  twist boat conformation, 592
  (*Z*) isomers, 584
Isometric contraction, 330
Isotonic contraction, 329
Isotonic solutions, 225–226
Isotopes, 395, 396, 397
Isotopic notation, 553

J

Jargon, avoiding, 41–42
Jejunum, 353
Joints, 326–327
Junk phrases, avoiding, 36

K

Karyokinesis (nuclear division), 228
Kelvin temperature (K), 517
Keratin, 788
Ketals, 682–683
Keto-enol tautomerism, 640
Ketones
  addition reactions, 681–684
  Clemmensen reduction, 680
  common names, 675–676
  condensation with ammonium derivatives,
    683–684
  cyanohydrin formation, 683
  enol form, 680–681
  enolization, 680–681
  hemiketal formation, 682–683
  hydration to form geminal diols, 682
  ketal formation, 682–683
  keto form, 680–681
  Michael addition, 681
  nomenclature, 675–676
  nucleophilic addition to carbonyl, 681
  overview, 677–678
  oxidation reactions, 679
  physical properties, 677
  reduction reactions, 679–680
  synthesis, 678–679
  Wittig reaction, 686
  Wolff-Kishner reduction, 680
Keywords
  Conclusion keywords, 808–809
  Continuation keywords, 110, 807
  Contrast keywords, 110, 808
  Emphasis keywords, 110, 808
  Evidence keywords, 808
  Illustration keywords, 808
  Sequence keywords, 807–808
  structural keywords, 110
  using keywords in reading, 807–809
Kidneys
  aldosterone, 363, 368, 373, 374
  and urethra, 360
  and urinary bladder, 360
  antidiuretic hormone (ADH; vasopressin),
    363, 370
  aquaporins (water channels), 363
  Bowman's capsule, 360, 361
  collecting duct, 360, 362–363, 370
  concentrated urine formation, 362–363
  cortex, 360, 363
  counter-current-multiplier system, 363
  distal convoluted tubule, 360, 362–363

effect of diuretics, 363
erythropoietin (EPO), 342, 373
filtrate, 361
filtration, 361
glomerulus, 360, 361
hyperosmolar spaces, 363
loop of Henle, 360, 362–363
medulla, 360, 363
nephron structure, 360–362
osmolarity gradient, 362, 363
osmosis, 363
passive and active transport, 361
peritubular capillaries, 361
pH maintenance, 363–364
proximal convoluted tubule, 360, 362
reabsorption of water and nutrients, 363, 368
renal pelvis, 360
renin, 373
secretion of waste, 362
selective permeability of nephrons, 362, 363
structure, 360–362
urine formation, 361–362
Kinetic energy, 398
Kinetic molecular theory of gases, 524–526
Kinetochore, 229, 233
Kingdoms of life, 222
Krebs cycle (citric acid cycle), 243

L

Labor and childbirth, 389
Lactase, 249, 354
Lacteals, 341
Lactic acid fermentation, 242
Lactose intolerance, 354
Lamarckian evolution, 271
Lamellae, 325
Lanthanides, 411
Large intestine, 352, 355
Lawn (plated bacteria culture), 287
Law of conservation of mass, 451
Law of constant composition, 449
Law of Independent Assortment (Mendel's second law), 256–258
Law of mass action, 495–496
Law of Segregation (Mendel's first law), 253–256
Le Châtelier's principle, 497–498
Leukocytes (white blood cells), 301–303, 341
Levorotatory compounds, 588–589
Lewis acids as electron acceptors, 432, 534, 633
Lewis bases as electron donors, 432, 534, 633
Lewis dot symbols, 427
Lewis structures, 427–431
Ligaments, 327
Limiting reactants, 453
Limits (calculus), 927–930
Line spectra, 399
Lipases, 245, 249, 354
Lipid (fat)-soluble vitamins, 798–799
Lipids
    amphipathic molecules, 795
    bilayers in cell membrane, 222–223, 795–796
    cholesterol, 797–798
    energy storage, 799–800
    glycerophospholipids, 796
    lipid (fat)-soluble vitamins, 798–799
    liposomes, 795–796
    phosphoglycerides, 796
    phospholipids, 222–223, 795–797
    prostaglandins, 798
    saponification, 722, 800
    signaling lipids, 797–800
    sphingolipids, 796
    structural lipids, 795–797

triacylglycerols (fats or triglycerides), 722, 799–800
    waxes, 797
    See also Fatty acids; Steroids
Lipoproteins, 790
Liposomes, 795–796
Liquid-solid equilibrium, 508
Liquids, properties, 505, 506
Lithium aluminum hydride, 663, 679–680, 700, 742
Litmus paper, 533
Liver
    detoxification, 355
    digestive function, 351, 354
    excretion of wastes, 360
    glycogen storage, 245, 355
Logarithms
    characteristic, 872
    exponents, 870–871
    log base 10, 866
    mantissa, 872
    pH and pOH, 535–537, 543, 782–783
    properties, 871
London dispersion forces (LDF), 436, 437
Lower esophageal (cardiac) sphincter, 353
Lungs
    capacities, 347
    excretion of wastes, 360
    gas exchange, 337, 344, 346
    pulmonary circulation, 338, 340
    ventilation, 345–346
Luteal phase, 383
Luteinizing hormone (LH), 369, 382
Lymph, 301, 341
Lymphatic system, 301, 341
Lymph nodes, 301, 341
Lymphocytes, 302–303, 341
Lymph vessels, 301, 341
Lysine, 786, 787
Lysosomes, 224

M

Macrophages, 302
Magnetic quantum number, 401
Male reproductive system, 380–381
Mantissa, 872
Markovnikov's rule, 633, 634, 639
Marsupials, 278
Mass defect, 553, 554–555
Mass number (A), 397, 553
Mass spectrometry, 758–759
Mass to charge ratio (*m/e* or *m/z*), 758–759
Mast cells, 302
Mastication, 352
Maxwell-Boltzmann distribution curve, 525
Mechanical digestion, 352
Median (statistics), 904
Medical microbiology
    active immunity, 294
    antibacterial agents, 294
    antifungal agents, 295
    antiparasitic agents, 295
    antiseptics, 293
    antiviral agents, 294–295
    attenuated pathogens, 294
    bactericidal agents, 294
    bacteriostatic agents, 294
    broad-spectrum antimicrobials, 296
    direct contact, 293
    disinfection, 293
    immunization, 293–294
    indirect contact, 293
    passive immunity, 294
    pasteurization, 293

pharmaceuticals, 294–296
    resistance (bacterial), 294, 295–296
    sterilization, 293
    transmission, 293
    transmission prevention, 293–294
    vaccines, 295
    vectors, 293
Medulla (medulla oblongata), 316
Meiosis, 231–233
Melanocyte-stimulating hormone (MSH), 369
Melatonin, 373
Melting, 508
Melting point, 508
Memory T cells, 302
Mendeleev, Dmitri, 411
Mendel's first law (Law of Segregation), 253–256
Mendel's Law of Dominance, 253–254
Mendel's second law (Law of Independent Assortment), 256–258
Menses, 383
Menstrual cycle, 382–384
Menstruation, 383
Meso compounds, 590
Mesoderm, 386, 387
Messenger RNA (mRNA), 772
Metabolism, definition, 239
Metallic solids, 506
Metalloids (semimetals), 414–415
Metals, 414
Metaphase, 229, 233
Metaphase plate, 229
Metathesis reactions, 472
Micelles, 703–704, 795–796, 800
Michael addition, 681
Microbial ecology, 289–290
Microevolution, 275–276
Microfilaments, 224
Microorganisms
    bacillus bacteria, 286
    bacteria, 285–286
    coccus bacteria, 285
    fungi, 288–289
    Gram staining, 286
    microbial ecology, 289–290
    parasites, 289
    spirillum bacteria, 286
    viruses, 287–288
Microtubules, 224, 229
Midbrain (mesencephalon), 316
Mineralocorticoids, 368
Miscibility of liquids, 506
Missense mutation, 261
Mitochondria, 224
Mitosis, 228–230
Mitral valve, 339
Mixed numbers, 858–860
Mixed-order reactions, 484
M line (muscle), 329
Mode (statistics), 905
Modifiers and modifying phrases, 51–52
Molality (*m*), 464, 510
Molarity (*M*), 463
Molar mass (molar weight), 522–523
Molecular biology
    alternate energy sources, 245–247
    cellular respiration, 242–244
    central dogma of molecular genetics, 767
    citric acid cycle (Krebs cycle), 243, 244
    electron transport chain, 240, 242, 243, 244
    fermentation, 242
    glucose catabolism, 240–244
    glycolysis, 240–242
    physiological regulation, 239
    respiration, overview, 239, 240

Molecular formulas, 449
Molecular geometry, 432–434
Molecular ion peak (parent ion peak, M$^+$), 758
Molecular mass (molecular weight), 397, 447–448
Molecular orbitals, 436, 606–607
Mole, definition, 397, 448
Mole fraction (X), 463
Monocytes, 302
Monohybrid crosses, 254
Monosomy, 260–261
Monozygotic (identical) twins, 385
Morula, 386
Motor neurons, 314
M phase (cell cycle), 228
Mucous secretions, 300
Mucus, 353
Multiple births, 385
Muscular system
    A band, 329
    absolute refractory period, 330
    and extrapyramidal system, 327
    and pyramidal system, 327
    ATP and muscle contraction, 329, 331, 332
    cardiac muscle, 331, 332
    concentric contraction, 330
    Cori cycle, 331
    creatine phosphate, 332
    dynamic contraction, 329–330
    eccentric contraction, 330
    energy reserves of muscles, 332
    H zone, 329
    isometric contraction, 330
    isotonic contraction, 329
    M line, 329
    muscle contraction, 329–330
    myofibrils, 328
    myoglobin, 332
    neuromuscular junction, 329
    rigor mortis, 329
    sarcolemma, 328
    sarcomeres, 328, 329
    sarcoplasmic reticulum, 328
    simple twitch, 330
    skeletal muscle, 328–331, 332
    smooth muscle, 331, 332
    stimulus and muscle response, 330–331
    striated muscle, 328
    temporal summation, 330
    tetanus, 330
    tonus, 331
    T system (transverse tubules in muscle fibers), 328
    Z lines, 329
Musculoskeletal system
    A band, 329
    absolute refractory period, 330
    appendicular skeleton, 326
    ATP and muscle contraction, 329, 331, 332
    axial skeleton, 326
    bone, 325–326
    bone formation, 326
    cardiac muscle, 331, 332
    cartilage, 325
    chrondrocytes, 325
    compact bone, 325
    concentric contraction, 330
    Cori cycle, 331
    creatine phosphate, 332
    dynamic contraction, 329–330
    eccentric contraction, 330
    endochondral ossification, 326
    energy reserves of muscles, 332
    extension (joints), 327

    extrapyramidal system, 327
    flexion (joints), 327
    Haversian canals, 325
    H zone, 329
    insertion (muscles), 327
    intramembranous ossification, 326
    isometric contraction, 330
    isotonic contraction, 329
    joints, 326–327
    lamellae, 325
    ligaments, 327
    M line, 329
    muscle contraction, 329–330
    muscular system, 327–332
    myofibrils, 328
    myoglobin, 332
    neuromuscular junction, 329
    origin (muscles), 327
    osteoblasts, 326
    osteoclasts, 326
    osteocytes, 326
    osteons (Haversian systems), 325
    pyramidal system (motor cortex), 327
    red marrow, 326
    rigor mortis, 329
    sarcolemma, 328
    sarcomeres, 328, 329
    sarcoplasmic reticulum, 328
    simple twitch, 330
    skeletal muscle, 328–331, 332
    skeletal system, 325–327
    smooth muscle, 331, 332
    spicules (trabeculae), 326
    spongy bone, 326
    stimulus and muscle response, 330–331
    striated muscle, 328
    sutures (immovable joints), 326
    temporal summation, 330
    tendons, 327
    tetanus, 330
    tonus, 331
    T system (transverse tubules in muscle fibers), 328
    yellow marrow, 326
    Z lines, 329
Mutation
    added, deleted, or substituted bases in, 261
    and evolution, 277, 767
    DNA, 767
    frameshift mutation, 261
    in phenylketonuria (PKU), 262
    in sickle-cell anemia, 262
    missense mutation, 261
    nonsense mutation, 261
    point mutation, 261
    silent mutation, 261
Myelin, 309, 312
Myofibrils, 328
Myoglobin, 332, 790

N

Nails (fingers and toes), 300
Narrative voice, 43–44
Natural killer T (NKT) cells, 302
Natural selection, 271–272, 276
Negative numbers, 852
Nervous system
    acetylcholine as neurotransmitter, 317
    autonomic nervous system (ANS), 317–318, 340
    brain, 315–316
    brainstem, 316
    central nervous system (CNS), 309, 315–317
    cerebellum, 316

    cerebral cortex, 315
    diencephalon, 315
    dorsal horn, 316
    dorsal root ganglia, 316
    electrochemical signals, 309
    epinephrine as neurotransmitter, 368
    extrapyramidal system, 327
    "flight or fight" responses, 317
    forebrain (prosencephalon), 315
    hindbrain (rhombencephalon), 316
    hypothalamus, 315
    medulla (medulla oblongata), 316
    medulla oblongata, 346
    midbrain (mesencephalon), 316
    neuroglia, 309
    norepinephrine as neurotransmitter, 317, 368
    olfactory bulb, 315
    organization of, 315–318
    parasympathetic nervous system, 317–318
    peripheral nervous system (PNS), 309, 317–318
    pons, 316
    pyramidal system (motor cortex), 327
    reflexes, 316
    "rest and digest" responses, 317
    somatic nervous system (SNS), 317
    spinal cord, 316–317
    stimuli and responses, 309
    sympathetic nervous system, 317, 318
    telencephalon, 315
    thalamus, 315
    types of cells, 310–311
    vagus nerve, 340
    ventral horn, 316
    See also Neurons
Net ionic equations, 472
Neural crest cells, 387
Neural tube, 387
Neuroglia, 309
Neuromuscular junction, 329
Neurons
    action potentials, 309, 310–311
    afferent neurons, 314
    axons, 309
    cell body (soma), 309
    dendrites, 309
    depolarized cells, 311
    effect of drugs, 314
    effector cells, 313
    efferent neurons, 314
    electrochemical signals and, 309
    function, 310–314
    ganglia, 315
    hyperpolarization, 312
    impulse propagation and speed, 312–313
    motor neurons, 314
    myelin, 309, 312
    neurotransmitters and, 227, 309–310, 311, 313–314, 329
    nodes of Ranvier, 309
    nuclei (central nervous system), 315
    oligodendrocytes, 309
    plexus, 315
    polarization, 311
    presynaptic neuron, 313
    refractory period, 312
    repolarization, 312
    resting potential, 310–311
    Schwann cells, 309, 387
    sensory neurons, 314
    structure, 309–310
    synapses (synaptic clefts), 309, 312–313
    synaptic terminals (boutons or knobs), 309
    synaptic vesicles, 311

threshold potential, 311
types of, 314–315
voltage-gated ion channels, 311
See also Nervous system
Neurosecretory cells (hypothalamus), 369, 370, 371
Neurotransmitters
acetylcholine, 317
and neurons, 227, 309–310, 312, 313–314, 329
endorphins, 369
epinephrine, 368
norepinephrine, 317, 368
Neurulation, 387
Neutralization reactions, 472, 539
Neutrons, 396
Neutrophils, 301–302
Newman projections, 590–591
Niches (biology), 274
Nitrenes, 727
Nitriles, 699, 742
Nitrogen-containing organic compounds, 738–739
Nitrogen cycle, 289
Nitrogen family (pnictogens, Group VA), 417
Noble gases (inert gases, Group VIIIA), 411, 414, 417
Nodes of Ranvier, 309
Nomenclature
acyl halides, 711–712
alcohols, 573, 659–660
aldehydes, 574–575, 675–676
alkanes, 615–616
alkenes, 570–571, 629–630
alkyl halides (haloalkanes), 572
alkynes, 572, 637
amides, 725
amines, 576, 737–738
anhydrides, 715
aromatic compounds, 648–650
Arrhenius acids, 534
carboxylic acids, 575–576, 696–697
cycloalkanes, 570
cycloalkenes, 571
esters, 719
ethers, 573–574, 666–667
ionic compounds, 415–416
ketones, 575, 676–677
prefixes for number of carbon atoms, 567, 615
prefixes for number of equivalent groups, 569
substituted alkanes, 572–576
Nondisjunction, 233, 260–261
Nonelectrolytes, 462
Non-Mendelian inheritance patterns, 258–260
Nonmetals, 414
Nonpolar covalent bonds, 432
Nonrepresentative elements, 411
Nonsense mutation, 261
Nonsteroidal anti-inflammatory drugs (NSAIDs), 798
Norepinephrine (noradrenaline), 317, 368
Normality (*N*), 464, 540–541
Noteboard strategies
asking for new noteboard or marker, 26
elimination table, 24, 25
passage maps, 809–810
practice and study tips, 17
Stop-Think-Predict-Match strategy, 20, 21
test strategies, 24–25, 26
Notochord, 387
Nuclear chemistry
alpha decay, 556–557
alpha particle (α-particle), 556–557
beta decay, 557–558
beta particle (β-particle), 556–557

binding energy, 553, 554–555
chain reactions, 555–556
daughter isotopes, 556
decay channels or decay modes, 556
decay constant, 560
electron capture, 559
exponential decay, 560–561
fission reactions, 553, 555–556
fusion reactions, 553, 555
gamma decay, 558–559
half-life ($T_{1/2}$) of radioactive decay, 560
isotopic notation, 553
mass defect, 553, 554–555
mass number (*A*), 397, 553
nuclear *vs.* chemical reactions, 553–554
nuclei, 553
nucleon or baryon number conservation, 555
nucleons, 553
parent isotopes, 556
positrons, 557
radioactive decay, 556–561
radioactivity, 553
radionucleotides, 553
rate of radioactive decay, 560
thermonuclear reactions, 555
Nuclear division (karyokinesis), 228
Nuclear magnetic resonance (NMR)
^{1}H NMR (proton NMR), 752–755
^{13}C NMR (carbon NMR), 755–757
basic theory, 752
chemical shift (δ), by type of proton, 754
chemical shift (δ), overview, 752
coupling (peak splitting, spin coupling), 754–755, 756
doublets, 754
peak location, 752–754
resonating, 752
singlets, 756
spin decoupling, 756
See also Spectroscopy
α-state, 752
β-state, 752
Nuclei (central nervous system), 315
Nucleon or baryon number conservation, 555
Nucleons, 553
Nucleophiles, properties, 616–617
Nucleophilic addition to carbonyl, reaction mechanism, 681
Nucleophilic substitution reactions
alcohol synthesis, 663
carbocation formation, S_N1 reactions, 617
carboxylic acids, 700–701
first-order kinetics, S_N1 reactions, 619
leaving groups, 617
mechanism, S_N1 reactions, 617–618
mechanism, S_N2 reactions, 619–620
rate-determining step, S_N1 reactions, 617, 618
reaction rates, S_N1 reactions, 618–619
reaction rates, S_N2 reactions, 620
second-order kinetics, S_N2 reactions, 620
size and polarizability of nucleophiles, 617
S_N1 (unimolecular nucleophilic substitution) reactions, 617–619, 621, 631
S_N2 (bimolecular nucleophilic substitution) reactions, 619–621, 632
stereochemistry, S_N1 reactions, 619
stereochemistry, S_N2 reactions, 620–621
transition state, S_N2 reactions, 619
See also Alkanes
Nucleoproteins, 790
Nucleotides, definition and structure, 768
Nucleus (atomic), 395, 553
Nucleus (cell), 223
Numbers and number operations

associative laws of addition and multiplication, 852–853
commutative laws of addition and multiplication, 852
difference, 851
distributive laws of multiplication and division, 853
integers, 851
negative numbers, 852
number line, 851–852
one (1) and negative one (–1), properties of, 855
operations, definition, 851
operations with signed numbers, 853–854
order of operations (PEMDAS), 856
positive numbers, 852
product, 851
real numbers, 851
reciprocals, 851, 853
sum, 851
zero (0), properties of, 852, 854–855
Numerator, 857

O

Octet rule, 425
Octet rule exceptions, 431
Okazaki fragments, 770
Olefins. *See* Alkenes
Olfactory bulb (brain), 315
Oligodendrocytes, 309
Omega-3 fatty acid, 798
Oogenesis, 379, 382
Operons, 265
Optical activity, 588–589
Oral cavity, 352
Orbitals
antibonding orbitals, 436
atomic orbitals, 400, 435–436, 605–606
bonding orbitals, 436
hybridization, 607–609
molecular orbitals, 436, 606–607
nodes, 605
orbital filling, 402–403
orbital radius, 398
sp^2 hybrid orbitals, 608–609
sp^3 hybrid orbitals, 607–608, 608
sp hybrid orbitals, 609
Order of operations (PEMDAS), 856
Organogenesis, 387
Organometallic reagents, 662, 699
Origin (muscles), 327
Origin of life, 278–279
Osmosis, 225–226, 363
Osmotic pressure (*Π*), 510
Osteoblasts, 326
Osteoclasts, 326
Osteocytes, 326
Osteons (Haversian systems), 325
Ovaries, 367, 379, 381–382, 383
Overpopulation, 272
Oviducts, 381
Ovulation, 383
Ovum, 381
Oxidation numbers, 417, 473–474
Oxidation-reduction (redox) reactions
balancing redox reactions, 474–476
electrolysis, 471
half-reaction method (ion-electron method), 474–476
net ionic equations, 472
oxidation, definition, 473
oxidation numbers, 473–474
oxidizing agents, 473
reducing agents, 474
reduction, definition, 473

Oxidation states, 417
Oxidative deamination, 246
Oxidative phosphorylation, 243, 244
Oxidizing agents, 473
Oximes, 684
Oxiranes, 574, 636, 667, 668
Oxygenated blood, 338
Oxyhemoglobin, 341
Oxytocin, 369, 371
Ozonolysis, 636

P
Pancreas
    digestive function, 351, 354, 372
    endocrine function, 372
    islets of Langerhans, 372
Parallel evolution, 273
Parallelogram rule, 922–923
Parasites, 289
Parasympathetic nervous system, 317–318
Parathyroid glands, 372
Parathyroid hormone (PTH), 372
Parental or P generation, 254
Parent isotopes, 556
Part-to-part and part-to-whole ratios, 860
Passage maps
    Global questions, 813
    purpose, 809, 813
    scope, 809, 813
    tone, 809, 814
    topic, 809, 813
Passive immunity, 294, 305
Passive voice, avoiding, 39–40
Pasteurization, 293
Pauli exclusion principle, 400
Pauling electronegativity scale, 414
Pepsin, 248, 353
Peptide bonds, 786–787
Peptide hormones, 373–374
Peptides
    amino acid residues, 786
    amino-terminal or N-terminal residue, 787
    dipeptides, 786
    hydrolysis, 787
    peptide bonds, 786–787
    polypeptides, 787
    properties, 787
    reactions, 786–787
    synthesis via RNA translation, 767, 773–774
    tripeptides, 786
    See also Amino acids; Proteins
Percent composition, 449–450
Percent composition by mass, 462
Percents (math)
    changing fractions to percents, 866–867
    changing percents to fractions, 866
    percent formula, 867
    translating word problems, 867–868
Percent yield, 453–454
Periodic table
    actinides, 411
    alkali metals (Group IA), 416
    alkaline earth metals (Group IIA), 413, 416
    anions, 415
    atomic number (Z), 411
    atomic radii, 412
    carbon group (Group IVA), 417
    cations, 415
    chalcogens (nitrogen family, Group VIA), 417
    effective nuclear charge (Z_{eff}), 412
    electron affinity, 413–414
    electronegativity, 414
    first ionization energy (IE), 412–413
    groups (columns), 411

halogens (Group VIIA), 416
hydrogen, 416
ionic radii, 412
ionization energy (IE), 412–413
ions, 415–416
lanthanides, 411
metalloids (semimetals), 414–415
metals, 414
noble gases (inert gases, Group VIIIA), 411, 414, 417
nonmetals, 414
nonrepresentative elements, 411
oxidation states, 417
Pauling electronegativity scale, 414
periodic law, 411
periodic properties, 411–414
periods (rows), 411
pnictogens (nitrogen family, Group VA), 417
polyatomic ions, 415–416
representative elements, 411
second ionization energy (IE), 413
transition elements, 411, 417–418
valence, 411
valence electrons, 411
Peripheral nervous system (PNS), 309, 317–318
Peristalsis, 353
Permutations (statistics), 906–907, 908–909, 909–911
Peroxycarboxylic acids, 636
Petrification, 276
pH, 535–536
Phagocytosis, 226
Pharmaceuticals, 294–296
Pharmacy College Admissions Test (PCAT)
    basic principles of good test mentality, 11–12
    Biology section, 5
    Chemistry section, 6
    composite score, 8
    computer-based test (CBT), 4
    content, 4–7
    introduction, 3
    mindset, 10–12, 26
    percentiles, 8
    Quantitative Ability section, 7
    raw score, 7–8
    Reading Comprehension section, 6
    scaled scores, 8
    scoring, overview, 7–8
    Verbal Ability section, 5
    Writing sections, 5, 7
Pharynx, 352
Phase changes
    boiling point, 508
    boiling-point elevation (ΔT_b), 510
    condensation, 507
    critical point, 509
    deposition, 508
    diffusion, 510
    evaporation, 507
    freezing point, 508
    freezing-point depression (ΔT_f), 509–510
    fusion or melting, 508
    gas-liquid equilibrium, 507–508
    gas-solid equilibrium, 508
    Gibbs functions for equilibria, 508
    liquid-solid equilibrium, 508
    melting point, 508
    phase diagrams, mixtures, 508
    phase diagrams, single component, 508–509
    phase equilibria, 507–508
    Raoult's law, 509, 511
    solidification, crystallization, or freezing, 508
    sublimation, 508
    triple point, 509

van 't Hoff factor (i), 510
vaporization, 507
vapor pressure, 507–508
vapor pressure lowering, 509, 511
Phase diagrams, 508–509
Phase equilibria, 507–508
Phases of matter
    amorphous solids, 506
    body-centered cubic unit cells (crystals), 507
    condensed phases, 505
    crystalline solids, 506
    emulsions, 506
    face-centered cubic unit cells (crystals), 507
    gases, properties, 505–506
    immiscible liquids, 506
    ionic solids, 506
    liquids, properties, 505, 506
    metallic solids, 506
    miscibility of liquids, 506
    simple cubic unit cells (crystals), 507
    solids, properties, 505, 506–507
    unit cells (crystals), 507
    vibrational energy, 506
Phenols, 660, 661, 663, 665, 666, 668
Phenotype, definition, 253
Phenylalanine, 262, 787
Phenyl group (Ph), 648
Phenylketonuria (PKU), 262
Phosphoglycerides, 796
Phospholipids
    amphipathic molecules, 795
    bilayers in cell membrane, 222–223, 795–796
    fatty acids in, 796
    glycerophospholipids, 796
    liposomes, 795–796
    micelles, 795–796
    phosphoglycerides, 796
    sphingolipids, 796
Phospholipids (phosphoglycerides), 724–725
Phosphoranes, 686
Photosynthesis, 290
Phylogeny, 273
Picking Numbers strategy
    answers that are fractions of an unknown value, 840–841
    manageable numbers, 838, 840, 842
    number property questions, 842
    percents in the answer choices, 840
    permissible numbers, 837, 838, 842
    rules, 837–838
    signals to use Picking Numbers approach, 838
    variables in the answer choices, 838–840
Pineal gland, 373
Pinocytosis, 226
Pituitary gland, 369–370
Pi (π) bonds, 436, 607
Placenta, 294, 305, 343, 374, 383, 385, 387–388
Placental development, 387–388
Planck's constant, 398, 399
Plane of symmetry, 590
Plane-polarized light, 588
Plasma, 341
Plasmids, 260, 262
Plasmolysis, 225–226
Platelet plug, 343
Platelets, 341
Plexus, 315
Pnictogens (nitrogen family, Group VA), 417
pOH, 535–536
Point mutation, 261
Polar body, 382
Polar covalent bonds, 431–432
Polarization, 311
Polar molecules, 432, 434–435

Polyatomic ions, 415–416
Polycyclic aromatic compounds, 649–650
Polymerization of alkenes, 637
Polynomial equations, graphing, 917
Polynomials, adding, subtracting, or
   multiplying, 879–880
Polynomials, dividing, 880–881
Polynomials, factoring, 881–883
Polyprotic bases, 544
Polyribosomes, 773
Pons, 316
Population genetics, 274–275
Positive numbers, 852
Positrons, 557
Posterior pituitary (neurohypophysis), 369–370
Potassium permanganate oxidation of alcohols,
   665, 678
Potassium permanganate oxidation of alkenes,
   635–636, 679
Potassium permanganate oxidation of alkynes,
   641
Potential energy diagrams, 485
Practice passages (Reading Comprehension)
   Foxglove, 823–825
   Relationships Between Food Resources and
      Population Size, 820–823
   Simultaneous Discovery, 826–828
Precalculus, 917–926
   See also Complex numbers; Graphing
      equations; Vectors (math)
Pregnancy and Rh factor, 342–343
Pressure units, 517
Presynaptic neuron, 313
Primary oocytes, 382
Primary sex cells, 231
Primary spermatocytes, 381
Primordial soup, 278
Principal quantum number, 400–401
Probability
   at least one of two events occurs, $P(A$ or $B)$,
      903
   describing probability, 898–900
   elementary events, 898
   empty set, 898
   events, 898
   experiments, 897
   independent events, 902–903
   multiple-event probability, 900–901
   mutually exclusive events, $P(A$ or $B)$, 900–901,
      904
   notation, 898
   outcomes, 897
   probability an event does not occur, 900
   probability two events occur (A and B),
      901–903
   sample space, 897
Product (numbers), 851
Products of chemical reactions, 472
Progesterone, 382, 383
Prokaryotes, definition, 222, 285
Prolactin, 369
Proline, 269, 790
Pronouns, agreement with antecedents, 48–51
Prophase, 229, 231
Prostaglandins, 798
Prosthetic groups, 249
Proteases, 249
Proteins
   as fuel molecules in cells, 246
   collagen, 343, 790
   conjugated proteins, 790
   cystine, 789
   denaturation, 790
   disulfide bonds, 789

fibrous proteins, 790
globular proteins, 790
glycoproteins, 790
hemoglobin, 790
keratin, 788
lipoproteins, 790
melting, 790
myoglobin, 332, 790
nucleoproteins, 790
peptide bonds, 786–787
primary structure, 788
prosthetic groups, 790
quaternary structure, 790
random-coil, 790
secondary structure, 788–789
sequencing, 788
synthesis via RNA translation, 767, 773–774
tertiary structure, 789–790
α-helix, 788
β-pleated sheets, 788–789
Prothrombin, 343, 799
Protons, 395–396
Protozoa, 225, 289
Proviruses, 287
Pulmonary arteries, 340
Pulmonary circulation, 338
Pulmonary veins, 340
Punctuation
   apostrophes, 60–62
   colons, 57–58
   commas, 55–57
   dashes, 59
   hyphens, 58–59
   semicolons, 57, 110, 119, 121
   See also Grammar and form; Usage and
      style
Punnett square diagrams, 254–255
Purines, 768
Purkinje fibers, 339
Pyloric sphincter, 353
Pyramidal system (motor cortex), 327
Pyridinium chlorochromate (PCC), 665
Pyrimidines, 768
Pyrolysis (cracking) of alkanes, 623
Pyruvate decarboxylation, 240–243, 244

Q

Quadratic equations, 886–888, 917
Quadratic formula, 887
Qualification, avoiding needless, 37–38
Quanta, 397–398
Quantitative Ability section of PCAT
   Backsolving strategy, 842–843
   estimation strategy, 843–844
   Picking Numbers strategy, 837–842
   strategic guessing, 843–844
   timing requirements and tips, 24
   See also Picking Numbers strategy
Quantized energy, 398
Quantum mechanical model of atoms, 400–404
Quantum numbers, 400–402, 605
Quantum theory, 397, 398–399
Quaternary ammonium compounds, 737
Question types
   comprehension questions, 813
   Detail questions, 813–814, 816
   Effectiveness questions, 815–816, 816
   Evaluation questions, 814–815, 815
   Function questions, 815
   Global questions, 813, 817
   Inference questions, 815
   Scattered detail questions, 814, 816
   Structure questions, 814–815
   Tone questions, 814, 816

triaging questions by type, 816
Vocab-in-Context questions, 814, 816

R

Radioactive decay, 556–561
Radioactivity, definition, 553
Radionucleotides, 553
Raoult's law, 509, 511
Rate constants, 480–482
Rate-determining step, 479, 480
Rate laws, 480–482
Ratios (numbers), 860–861
Raw score, PCAT, 7–8
Reactants, 471
Reaction coordinate, 485
Reaction mechanisms, 479
Reaction orders, 480–481, 482–484
Reaction quotient (Q), 496
Reaction rates. *See also* Reaction rates. *See*
   Chemical kinetics
Reading Comprehension section of PCAT
   comprehension questions, 813
   Conclusion keywords, 808–809
   Continuation keywords, 807
   Contrast keywords, 808
   Detail questions, 813–814, 816
   Effectiveness questions, 815–816, 816
   Emphasis keywords, 808
   Evaluation questions, 814–815, 815
   Evidence keywords, 808
   Extreme answer choices, 817
   Faulty Use of Detail, 817
   Function questions, 815
   Global questions, 813, 817
   Illustration keywords, 808
   Inference questions, 815
   Opposite choices, 817
   Out of Scope answer choices, 817
   passages, 805
   practice passages, 819–828
   reading critically, 806–807
   reading the PCAT, 805
   scattered detail questions, 814
   Scattered detail questions, 814, 816
   Sequence keywords, 807–808
   Structure questions, 814–815
   timing requirements and tips, 24
   Tone questions, 814, 816
   triaging questions by type, 816
   using keywords, 807–809
   Vocab-in-Context questions, 814, 816
   wrong answer pathologies, 816–817
   See also Dissecting an argument; Passage maps
Real gases, 523
Real numbers, 851
Recessive alleles, definition, 253
Reciprocals, 851, 853
Recombination (bacteria), 264
Rectum, 355
Red blood cells (RBCs or erythrocytes), 341–342
Red marrow, 326
Reducing agents, 474
Reduction, definition, 473
Redundancy, avoiding, 37
Reflexes, 316
Refractory period, 312
Regulatory or suppressor T (T_{reg}) cells, 302
Relative configuration, 586–587
Renal pelvis, 360
Renin, 373
Repolarization, 312
Representative elements, 411
Reproduction, definition, 239
Reproductive isolation, 273, 278

Reproductive system
  acrosomal process, 383
  acrosome, 381
  birth, 389
  cervix, 381
  corona radiata, 382
  corpus luteum, 369, 382, 383
  cortical reaction, 383
  dizygotic (fraternal) twins, 385
  ejaculatory duct, 380
  estrogens, 369, 374, 382
  female reproductive system, 381–385
  fertilization, 379–380, 383–384
  fertilization membrane, 383–384
  follicles, 381
  follicle stimulating hormone (FSH), 369, 382
  follicular phase, 382
  gametogenesis, 379, 387
  gestation, 388–389
  gonads, 379
  human chorionic gonadotropin (hCG), 383
  labor, 389
  luteal phase, 383
  luteinizing hormone (LH), 369, 382
  male reproductive system, 380–381
  menses, 383
  menstrual cycle, 382–384
  menstruation, 383
  monozygotic (identical) twins, 385
  multiple births, 385
  oogenesis, 379, 382
  ovaries, 367, 379, 381–382, 383
  oviducts, 381
  ovulation, 383
  ovum, 381
  polar body, 382
  primary oocytes, 382
  primary spermatocytes, 381
  progesterone, 382, 383
  secondary oocytes, 382
  secondary spermatocytes, 381
  sexual reproduction, overview, 379–380
  spermatids, 381
  spermatogenesis, 379, 381
  spermatogonia, 381
  sperm (spermatozoa), 381
  testes, 367, 368, 369, 374, 379, 380
  testosterone, 369, 380
  urethra, 380
  uterus, 381
  vagina, 381
  vas deferens, 380
  zona pellucida, 382
  See also Embryology
Residual lung capacity, 347
Resistance (bacterial), 294, 295–296
Resonance, 429–431
Resonance hybrids, 429
Resonance structures, 429–431
Respiration
  and carbohydrates, 240
  cellular respiration, 242–244
  development of aerobic respiration, 279
  excretion of respiration products, 239, 360
  external respiration, 240
  in mitochondria, 224
  internal respiration, 240
  primary goal, 346
Respiration, definition, 239
Respiratory system
  airways, 344
  and peripheral chemoreceptors, 345
  control of ventilation, 346
  exhalation, 345

expiratory reserve volume, 347
function of, 344–345
gas exchange, 337, 344, 346
inhalation, 345
inspiratory reserve volume, 347
lung capacities, 347
lungs, 337, 344
pulmonary capillaries, 346
residual volume, 347
respiratory centers in medulla oblongata, 346
surfactant, 345
tidal volume (TV), 347
total lung capacity, 347
ventilation, 345–346
vital capacity, 347
See also Cardiovascular system
"Rest and digest" responses, 317
Resting potential, 310–311
Reversible reactions
  and equilibrium, 495, 498, 507
  definition, 495
  enzyme-catalyzed reactions, 246
  redox reactions, 243
Rh factor, 342–343
Rhogam, 343
Ribosomal RNA (rRNA), 223, 772
Ribosomes, 223, 249, 772, 773, 775
Rigor mortis, 329
RNA polymerase, 264, 265, 772–773
RNA (ribonucleic acid)
  anticodons, 772
  A site (aminoacyl-tRNA complex binding site)
    of ribosome, 775
  elongation step of translation, 773
  exons, 773
  guanine cap, 773
  hetero-nuclear RNA (hnRNA) or pre-RNA,
    773
  initiation of translation, 773
  introns, 773
  messenger RNA (mRNA), 772
  poly-A tail, 773
  P site (peptidyl-tRNA binding site) of
    ribosome, 775
  ribosomal RNA (rRNA), 772
  start codon, 773
  stop codons, 773
  structure, 772
  termination step of translation, 773
  transcription from DNA, 772–773
  transfer RNA (tRNA), 772
  translation into proteins, 772, 773
  translocation step of translation, 773
  uracil, 772, 773
  See also DNA
Rotation vibration, 749, 750
Rough endoplasmic reticulum, 223
R/S naming convention, 587–588
Run-on sentences, 53, 54–55
Rydberg constant, 398

S
Saliva, 352
Salivary amylase (ptyalin), 352
Salivary glands, 352
Salt formation, 539–540
Sample student essays, 73–82
Saponification, 722, 800
Sarcolemma, 328
Sarcomeres, 328, 329
Sarcoplasmic reticulum, 328
Saturated fatty acids, 796
Saturated solutions, 461–462
Scaled scores, PCAT, 8

Scattered detail questions, 814, 816
Schwann cells, 309, 387
Scoring
  composite score, 8
  evaluation of practice essay samples, 73–82
  good scores, 8
  raw score, 7–8
  scaled scores, 8
  writing samples in PCAT, 7, 29, 32–33, 35
Sebaceous glands, 299
Secondary oocytes, 382
Secondary spermatocytes, 381
Second ionization energy (IE), 413
Second messenger, 373–374
Second-order reactions, 484
Second trimester of pregnancy, 388
Secretin, 354, 373
Segregation, definition, 253
Self-reference, avoiding excessive, 39, 43
Semicarbazones, 684
Semicolons, 57, 110, 119, 121
Semilunar valves, 339
Sensory ganglia, 387
Sensory neurons, 314
Sentence completion
  Continuation keywords, 110
  Contrast keywords, 110
  Emphasis keywords, 110
  meaning of the sentence, 115–116
  one-blank sentences, question strategy,
    109–112
  relationship between blanks, 116
  structural keywords, 110
  tips for sentence completions, 114–116
  two-blank sentences, question strategy,
    112–114
  word charge, 110–111, 112, 113, 115
  word clues, 114–115
Sentence fragments, 53–54
Sequence keywords, 807–808
Sex determination, 259
Sexual reproduction
  gametogenesis, 379, 387
  meiosis, 231–233
Sexual selection, 276
Shells, 401, 605
Sickle-cell anemia, 262
Sigma (σ) bonds, 436, 607
Silent mutation, 261
Simple cubic unit cells (crystals), 507
Simple sugars, transport by circulatory system,
  343
Simple twitch (muscles), 330
Simultaneous equations, 888
Single displacement reactions, 472, 477
Sinoatrial (SA) node (the pacemaker), 339
Sister chromatids, 228–229, 231, 233, 260
Skeletal muscle, 328–331, 332
Skeletal system, 325–327
Skin, 299–300
Skin microbiome, 299
Small intestine, 352, 353–354
Smooth endoplasmic reticulum, 223
Smooth muscle, 331, 332
S_N1 (unimolecular nucleophilic substitution)
  reactions, 617–619, 621, 631
S_N2 (bimolecular nucleophilic substitution)
  reactions, 619–621, 632
Soaps, 702, 722, 800
Sodium borohydride, 636, 663, 679
Sodium-potassium pump (Na^+/K^+ pump), 226
Solidification, crystallization, or freezing, 508
Solids, properties, 505, 506–507
Solubility, 461–462, 465, 499–502

Solubility product constant (K_{sp}), 499–500
Solutes, 461
Solution equilibria, 498–501
Solutions
    aqueous solutions, 462, 465
    common ion effect, 500–501
    concentrated solutions, 462
    concentration units (solutions), 462–464
    crystallization, 462
    dilute solutions, 462
    dilution, 464–465
    dissolution, 461
    electrolytes, 462
    homogeneous mixtures, 461, 506
    hydration, 461
    ideal solutions, 511
    ion product (Q_{sp}) of a compound in solution, 499
    miscibility of liquids, 506
    molality (m), 464, 510
    molarity (M), 463
    mole fraction (X), 463
    nonelectrolytes, 462
    normality (N), 464
    percent composition by mass, 462
    saturated solutions, 461–462
    solubility, 461–462, 465
    solubility product constant (K_{sp}), 499–500
    solutes, 461
    solution equilibria, 498–501
    solvation, 461
    strong electrolytes, 462
    supersaturated solutions, 462
    weak electrolytes, 462
Solution task in writing, 31
Solvation, 461
Somatic nervous system (SNS), 317
Speciation, 272–273
Specific rotation, 589
Spectator ions, 472
Spectroscopy
    atomic absorption spectra, 400, 758
    atomic emission spectra, 399, 758
    Balmer series, 399
    line spectra, 399
    Lyman series, 399
    mass spectrometry, 758–759
    ultraviolet-visible (UV-vis) spectroscopy, 757–758
    See also Infrared (IR) spectroscopy; Nuclear magnetic resonance
Spermatids, 381
Spermatogenesis, 379, 381
Spermatogonia, 381
Sperm (spermatozoa), 381
S phase (cell cycle), 228
Sphingolipids, 796
Spicules (trabeculae), 326
Spinal cord, 316–317
Spin quantum number, 401
Spirillum bacteria, 286
Spleen, immune function, 301
Spongy bone, 326
Spores (fungi), 289
Staggered conformation, 591
Standard atomic weight, 397
Standard conditions, 517
Standard deviation, 905–906
Start codon, 773
States of matter. *See also* Phases of matter
Statins (atorvastatin and simvastatin), 798
Statistics
    average (arithmetic mean, μ), 904
    combinations, 906–908

hybrids of combinations and permutations, 909–911
    median, 904
    mode, 905
    ordered selection, 906–907
    permutations, 906–907, 908–909
    range, 905
    standard deviation, 905–906
    unordered selection, 907
Stereoisomers, definition, 584
Sterilization (microbiology), 293
Steroids
    adrenocortical steroids, 368
    aldosterone, 363, 368, 373, 374
    androgens, 368
    cholesterol, 797–798
    corticosteroids, 368
    estrogens, 369, 374, 382
    mineralocorticoids, 368
    progesterone, 382, 383
    steroid hormones, mechanism of action, 374
    structure, 797
Stoichiometry
    actual yield, 453–454
    applications of, 452–454
    Avogadro's number, 397, 448
    equivalents, 448–449
    excess reactants, 453
    formula mass, 447
    gram-equivalent weight (GEW), 448–449
    limiting reactants, 453
    molecular mass (molecular weight), 397, 447–448
    mole, definition, 397, 448
    percent composition, 449–450
    percent yield, 453–454
    reversible reactions, 453
    stoichiometric coefficients, 451–452, 474, 480
    theoretical yield, 453–454
Stomach, 352, 353
Stop codons, 773
Stop-Think-Predict-Match strategy
    Analogies, 95–97
    Match, 21
    noteboard strategies, 21
    one-blank sentence completion, 109–112
    Predict, 20–21
    Stop, 20
    Think, 20
    two-blank sentence completion, 112–114
    Verbal Ability section of PCAT, 89, 95–97
Strategic guessing, 843–844
Stretching vibration, 749–750
Striated muscle, 328
Stroke volume (left ventricle), 339
Strong electrolytes, 462
Structural genes, 264
Structural isomers (constitutional isomers), 583–584
Structural keywords, 110
Structure questions, 814–815
Studying effectively
    how to study, 15–18
    study blocks, 14–15
    study breaks, 14–15
    study plans, 13–15, 16
    time off, 15
    where to study, 16–18
    Why I Missed It Sheet (WIMIS), 16
    See Usage and style
Subatomic particles, 395–396
Subject-verb agreement, 46–48
Sublimation, 508
Substrate-level phosphorylation, 243, 244

Substrates, 246
Subtraction frequencies, 418
Sum (numbers), 851
Superinfection, 287
Supersaturated solutions, 462
Suppressor or regulatory T (T_{reg}) cells, 302
Surfactant, 345
Surfactants, 345, 800
"Survival of the fittest," 264
    unstable gene pools, 275
    variations among offspring, 272
Sutures (immovable joints), 326
Sweat glands, 299, 359
Sympathetic nervous system, 317, 318
Symporters, 226
Synapses (synaptic clefts), 309, 312–313
Synapsis, 231
Synaptic terminals (boutons or knobs), 309
Synaptic vesicles, 311
Synthesis reactions, 239, 249
Systemic circulation, 338
Systole, 339

T

Tautomers, 680–681
Telencephalon, 315
Telophase, 229, 233
Temporal summation (muscles), 330
Tendons, 327
Testcross, 255–256
Testes, 367, 368, 369, 374, 379, 380
Testosterone, 369, 380
Test strategies
    Backsolving strategy, 842–843
    estimation strategy, 843–844
    identify easy or difficult questions, 22–23
    noteboard strategies, 4, 24–25, 26
    passage maps, 809–810, 813, 814
    Picking Numbers strategy, 837–842
    process of elimination, 19, 23, 23–24, 26, 814
    section-specific pacing, 24
    skip around, 10, 22
    Stop-Think-Predict-Match, 19–21, 26
    strategic guessing, 843–844
    test timing, 21–24, 26
    top ten PCAT strategies, 26
    triaging questions by type, 816
    using keywords, 807–809
    wrong answer pathologies, 816–817
Tetanus, 330
Thalamus, 315
T helper (TH) cells (CD4+ T cells), 302
Theoretical yield, 453–454
Thermonuclear reactions, 555
Third trimester of pregnancy, 389
Thoracic cavity, 345, 353
Threshold potential, 311
Thrombin, 343
Thromboplastin, 343
Thymine, 768, 771
Thymus, 303
Thyroglobulin, 371
Thyroid, 371–372
Thyroid-stimulating hormone (TSH), 369
Thyroxine (T4), 371
Tidal volume (TV) of lungs, 347
Timing strategies, 21–24
Titration
    end point, 541
    equivalence points, 541–542, 544
    indicators, 541
    See also Acids; Bases
T lymphocytes (T cells), 302–303
Tone questions, 814, 816

Tonus, 331
Topoisomerase, 769
Total lung capacity, 347
Transamination reactions, 246
Transcortins, 368
Transduction (bacteria), 263–264, 286
trans-fatty acids, 796
Transfer RNA (tRNA), 772
Transformation (bacteria), 262, 286
trans isomers, 584, 629
Transition elements, 411, 417–418
Transition states, 485
Transition state theory, 485–486
Transplant rejection, 306
Triacylglycerols (fats or triglycerides), 722, 799–800
Triaging questions by type, 816
Tricuspid valve, 339
Triiodothyronine (T3), 371
Triple point, 509
Trisomy, 260–261
Trypsin, 355, 787
Tryptophan, 787
T system (transverse tubules in muscle fibers), 328
Tubulin, 224
Twist boat conformation, 592
Type I and Type II diabetes, 372
Tyrosine, 262, 787

U

Ultraviolet-visible (UV-vis) spectroscopy, 757–758
Umbilical cord, 387, 389
Unified atomic mass unit (amu or u), 395
Unimolecular elimination (E1) reactions, 631
Unimolecular nucleophilic substitution (S_N1) reactions, 617–619, 631
Unit cells (crystals), 507
Unit conversions, 870
Unnecessary sentences, avoiding, 38
Unordered selection. *See also* Probability
Unsaturated fatty acids, 796–797
Uracil, 772, 773
Urethra, 360, 380
Urinary bladder, 360
Usage and style
  and scoring of essays, 35
  clear modification, 51–52
  clichés, 41
  colloquialisms, 52–53
  commonly misused words, 67–70
  concise writing, 35–38
  correctness in writing, 35–36, 43
  diction errors, 67
  faulty parallelism, 46–48
  forceful writing, 35–36, 39–43
  idiomatic errors, 67
  jargon, 41–42
  junk phrases, 36
  matching verb and subject, 46–48
  needless qualification, 37–38
  needless self-reference, 39, 43
  passive voice, 39–40
  principles of consistency, 43–52
  pronouns, agreement with antecedents, 48–51
  redundancy, 37
  run-on sentences, 53, 54–55

  sentence fragments, 53–54
  shifting narrative voice, 44–45
  unnecessary sentences, 38
  vague language, 40–41
  weak openings, 40
  See also Grammar and form; Punctuation
Uterus, 381

V

Vaccination, 304
Vaccines, 295
Vacuoles and vesicles, 224
Vagina, 381
Vague language, avoiding, 40–41
Vagus nerve, 317, 340
Valence, 411
Valence electrons, 396, 403–404, 411
Valence shell electron-pair repulsion (VSEPR) theory, 432–434
Valine, 262, 771, 772
Van der Waals forces, 436
van 't Hoff factor (*i*), 510
Vaporization, 507
Vapor pressure, 507–508
Vapor pressure lowering, 509, 511
Vas deferens, 380
Vasopressin (antidiuretic hormone; ADH), 363, 370
Vectors (math)
  adding and subtracting vectors, 925
  cross product, 926
  dot product, 926
  multiplying vectors, 925–926
  polar form, 924
  rectangular form, 924
Vectors (microbiology), 293
Veins, 337, 340
Ventricles, 338
Venules, 337
Verbal Ability section of PCAT
  best practices for studying, 90–91
  building your vocabulary, 89–93
  Stop-Think-Predict-Match strategy, 89, 95–97
  timing requirements and tips, 24
  See also Analogies; Sentence completion; Vocabulary
Vibrational energy, 506
Villi in small intestine, 353
Viruses
  human immunodeficiency virus (HIV), 287
  latent infection, 287
  lysogenic cycle, 287
  lytic cycle, 287
  plaque formation on bacterial lawn, 287
  protein capsid, 287
  proviruses, 287
  superinfection, 287
  virulent viruses, 287
Vital lung capacity, 347
Vitamin A, 799
Vitamin D (cholecalciferol, calcitriol), 799
Vitamin E, 799
Vitamin K, 343, 799
Vitamins, lipid (fat)-soluble, 798–799
Vocab-in-Context questions, 814, 816
Vocabulary
  best practices for studying, 90–91

  building your vocabulary, 89–93
  commonly misused words, 67–70
  vocabulary exercises, context, 181, 186, 191, 196
  vocabulary exercises, definitions, 179–180, 184–185, 189–190, 193–195, 199–200
  vocabulary exercises, word charge, 182–183, 186–187, 192–193, 197–198, 201–205
  vocabulary list, 91–92, 137–177
  word roots and their meanings, 124–135
  word roots, learning, 91, 123
  word roots, tips for using effectively, 90, 123–124
Voltage-gated ion channels, 311
Volume units, 517

W

Warfarin, 343, 799
Watson-Crick DNA model, 768, 768–769
Wavenumbers, 749
Waxes, 797
Weak electrolytes, 462
Weak openings, avoiding, 40
White blood cells (leukocytes), 301–303, 341
Williamson ether synthesis, 668
Wittig reaction, 686
Wolff-Kishner reduction, 680
Word charge
  and sentence completion, 110–111, 112, 113, 115
  vocabulary exercises, 182–183, 186–187, 192–193, 197–198, 201–205
Word clues, 114–115
Word problems (algebra), 867–868, 877–878
Word roots
  learning, 91, 123
  list of roots and meanings, 124–135
Words commonly misused, 67–70
Writing sections of PCAT
  evaluation of practice essay samples, 73–82
  practice prompts, 72
  practice tips, 33–34, 71
  sample student essays, 71–82, 73–82
  scoring, 7, 32–33
  writing tasks, 29, 31
  See also Usage and style
Writing steps
  clarify main idea and plan step, 31
  Kaplan's Five-Step Method, 30–32
  read and explain step, 30
  sample student essays, 73–82
  writing step, 31
Writing tasks, 29, 31
Wrong answer pathologies, 816–817

Y

Yellow marrow, 326
Ylides, 686
Yolk sac, 387

Z

(*Z*) isomers, 584
Zaitsev's rule, 632
Zero (0), properties of, 852, 854–855
Zero-order reactions, 482–483
Z lines (muscle), 329
Zona pellucida, 382

PCAT STUDY SHEET – TEST DAY STRATEGIES

PCAT
STUDY SHEETS

Use these sheets to help you remember the Kaplan Methods and the most important elements of each subject on the PCAT.

TEST DAY STRATEGIES

- Triage within every section.
- Get your easy points first.
- Answer every question.
- Mark questions that you want to return to if you have time later.
- Use your dry erase booklet for scratch work.

TEST DAY OUTLINE

Section Name	Time	Questions	Topics
Writing	30 min.	1 essay	Discuss a solution to a given world problem
Verbal Ability	25 min.	40	Analogies (62.5%), Sentence Completion (37.5%)
Biology	35 min.	48	General Biology (50%), Microbiology (20%), Human Anatomy and Physiology (30%)
Chemistry	35 min.	48	General Chemistry (50%), Organic Chemistry (32%), Biochemistry (18%)
BREAK	15 min.	-----	-----
Reading Comprehension	50 min.	48 (6 passages with 8 questions each)	6 Passages from medical and natural sciences, social sciences, and humanities
Quantitative Ability	40 min.	48	Basic Math (14%), Algebra (19%), Probability and Statistics (19%), Pre-calculus (24%), Calculus (24%)

STPM	Biology & Chemistry	Reading Comprehension	Quantitative Ability	Analogies	Sentence Completion
STOP Triage: Should you do this question now, later, or never?	Characterize the format of the answer choices (e.g., calculation, sentences, Roman Numerals, one word answers, graphs, etc.).	Characterize the question type: Global, Tone, Vocab-in-Context, Detail, Evaluation, Inference, Application.	Read the question stem and characterize the answer choices (e.g., numbers, equations, graphs, set-ups, words).	Scan the words used in the question for familiarity.	Determine if the question has one blank or two blanks.
THINK What is the question really asking?	Read the question. Paraphrase the question stem. If question asks for what is true/false, characterize the 1 right answer and 3 wrong answers.	Paraphrase the question stem. Where is the relevant information in the passage? How does the passage map help to answer the question?	Determine which strategy should be used to quickly and accurately solve the problem: Traditional Math, Picking Numbers, Backsolving, Estimation, Educated Guessing. Consider what is given and what is needed.	Read the question. What is the bridge between the stem words? Bridge Types: Synonym, Antonym, Association, Classification, Part/Whole, Characteristic	Read the sentence looking for clues. Two blanks: Which blank is easier? Both types: What is the blank referring to?
PREDICT Formulate a framework or prediction for your answer.	Predict the answer, ensuring your answer is in the format of the answer choices.	Research the relevant area in the map and/or passage and predict an answer.	Solve the problem using your chosen strategy.	Apply the bridge to the prompt word, predicting an answer.	Predict a word to fit in the blank, using word charge to help formulate your prediction.
MATCH Select the answer that truly meets the requirements of your prediction.	Select the answer that matches the prediction, avoiding answer choices that are half-right/half-wrong, distortions, or extreme.	Select the answer that matches the prediction based on the proof found in the passage. Avoid out of scope and faulty use of detail answers.	Select the answer that matches your prediction, taking into account any errors due to rounding.	Select the word that matches the prediction, narrowing or broadening the bridge if necessary.	Two blanks: Eliminate any answers that do not match. Repeat THINK and PREDICT steps for remaining blank if necessary. Both types: Read the sentence with the chosen answer plugged in ensuring that it makes sense.

THE KAPLAN METHOD FOR WRITING SAMPLE

Step	Timing
Read and Explain	1 min
Prewrite	6 min
Clarify Main Idea and Plan	1 min
Write	20 min
Proofread	2 min
Total	30 min/essay

PACING BY SECTION

	Section			
Timing	Verbal Ability	Sciences	Reading Comp.	Quant. Ability
	Analogies–30 sec/Q Sent. Comp.–45 sec/Q 90 sec for Review	43 sec/Q	8 min/passage Read and map: 4 min Qs: 4 min = 30 sec/Q 2 min for Review	50 sec/Q

THE KAPLAN METHOD FOR READING COMPREHENSION

Read Strategically

- Preview the passage for Topic.
- Anticipate while reading using Keywords.
- Map each paragraph's Scope.
- Determine the author's Tone.
- Identify the author's overall Purpose.

Keyword Types: Continuation, Sequence, Illustration, Evidence, Contrast, Emphasis, Conclusion

Purpose Verbs: Explain, Evaluate, Argue, Compare

Tone: Positive (+), Negative (−), Neutral (/)

THE READING COMPREHENSION QUESTION TYPES

Type	Task
Global	Identify the general purpose or main idea of the passage.
Tone	Determine the author's tone in the passage.
Vocab-in-Context	Identify the meaning of a word or phrase as used in the passage.
Detail	Research the passage for the detail and stick closely to it in the answers.
Evaluation	Determine why or how the author constructed the argument.
Inference	Deduce what must be true based on the passage.
Application	Apply the passage to new information and determine the effect.

WRONG ANSWER PATHOLOGIES

Pathology	Why It's Wrong
Faulty Use of Detail	May be a true detail, but it does not answer question at hand
Opposite	Opposite of credited answer, oftentimes due to one word (e.g., not or except)
Distortion	Slightly twists the correct answer or is too extreme
Out of Scope	Brings in new information, even though the new information could be true
Miscalculation	Incorrect value or relationship oftentimes from using the wrong equation or missing a step or sign

DEALING WITH UNFAMILIAR VOCABULARY IN VERBAL ABILITY

Word Roots: Determine the meaning of the word by identifying its word root.

Cognates: Think of words in other languages that you know that seem similar to this word.

Tone: Trust your ear to determine if a word is positive or negative in tone.

Eliminate: Eliminate answers that definitely do not make sense.

Work Backwards: Try to plug in the answer choices to see what answers may make sense.

ANALOGY BRIDGE TYPES

Type	Relationship
Synonym	words having same or similar meaning
Antonym	words having opposite or contrasting meaning
Association	function of, cause/effect, by-product, tool used by, transformation
Classification	type, hierarchy, two members of the same class
Part/Whole	one word is a component of another (or vice versa)
Characteristic	attribute or quality that is present or lacking

WORD ROOTS

Root	Meaning
a, an	not, without
ab, a	from, away, apart
ad, a	to, toward
ali, altr	another
ambi, amphi	both
ante, ant	before
auto	self
bene, ben	good
bi	two
bio	life
chron	time
circum	around
co, com, con	with, together
cogn, gno	know
contra	against
cresc, cret	grow
culp	blame
dis, dif, di	not, apart, away
en, em	in, into
ex, e	out, out of
fac, fic, fect, fy, fea	make, do
gen	birth, class, kin
hetero	other
homo	same
hyper	too much, excess
hypo	too little, under
in, ig, il, im, ir	not
in, il, im, ir	in, on, into
inter	between, among
intra, intr	within
it, iter	between, among
loqu, loc, log	speech, thought

Root	Meaning
mal	bad
medi	middle
mono	one
neo	new
ob	against
omni	all
pan	all
pen	almost
phil	love
phob	fear
pre	before
prim, pri	first
pro	ahead, forth
prox, prop	near
retro	backward
sacr, sanct	holy
sec, sect, seg	cut
sent, sens	feel, think
sim, sem	similar, same
soph	wisdom
sub	under
summ	highest
super, sur	above
syn, sym	together
term	end
trans	across, over, through, beyond
uni, un	one
ven, vent	come
ver	true
vict, vinc	conquer
viv, vit	life

PCAT STUDY SHEET – BIOCHEMISTRY AND BIOLOGY

BIOCHEMISTRY

Triplet Codon Code for Amino Acids

		Second Nucleotide Position		
	U	**C**	**A**	**G**
U	UUU Phenylalanine UUC Phenylalanine UUA Leucine UUG Leucine	UCU Serine UCC Serine UCA Serine UCG Serine	UAU Tyrosine UAC Tyrosine UAA STOP UAG STOP	UGU Cysteine UGC Cysteine UGA STOP UGG Tryptophan
C	CUU Leucine CUC Leucine CUA Leucine CUG Leucine	CCU Proline CCC Proline CCA Proline CCG Proline	CAU Histidine CAC Histidine CAA Glutamine CAG Glutamine	CGU Arginine CGC Arginine CGA Arginine CGG Arginine
A	AUU Isoleucine AUC Isoleucine AUA Isoleucine AUG Methionine	ACU Threonine ACC Threonine ACA Threonine ACG Threonine	AAU Asparagine AAC Asparagine AAA Lysine AAG Lysine	AGU Serine AGC Serine AGA Arginine AGG Arginine
G	GUU Valine GUC Valine GUA Valine GUG Valine	GCU Alanine GCC Alanine GCA Alanine GCG Alanine	GAU Aspartate GAC Aspartate GAA Glutamate GAG Glutamate	GGU Glycine GGC Glycine GGA Glycine GGG Glycine

First Nucleotide Position

Amino Acid Structures and Names

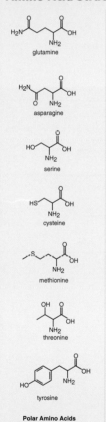
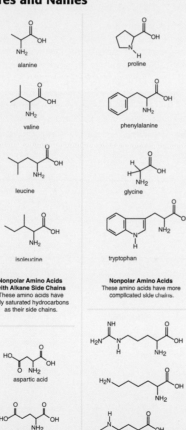

glutamine

alanine

proline

asparagine

valine

phenylalanine

serine

leucine

glycine

cysteine

isoleucine

tryptophan

methionine

Nonpolar Amino Acids with Alkane Side Chains
These amino acids have fully saturated hydrocarbons as their side chains.

Nonpolar Amino Acids
These amino acids have more complicated side chains.

threonine

arginine

aspartic acid

lysine

tyrosine

Polar Amino Acids

glutamic acid

histidine

Acidic Amino Acids

Basic Amino Acids

PROTEINS

Peptide Bonds (Amide Links)

The 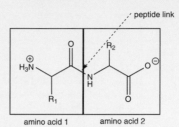 (amide) linkage that forms between the amino acids is known as a **peptide bond** or **peptide linkage**.

amino acid 1   amino acid 2

peptide link

Three-Dimensional Shape of Protein

Primary Structure Unique sequence of amino acids

Secondary Structure α-helix and β-pleated sheet

Tertiary Structure Interactions between the various side chains of amino acids

Quaternary Structure Interaction of two or more polypeptides

LIPIDS

Fatty Acids

Fatty acids contain a straight alkyl chain (hydrophobic) portion, and a terminal carboxylic acid (hydrophilic) group.

carboxylic acid   hydrophobic alkyl chain
saturated fatty acid

double bond   **unsaturated fatty acid**

Triacylglycerols

Triacylglycerols are esters of glycerol.

glycerol   carboxylic acid   triacylglycerol

MICROBIOLOGY

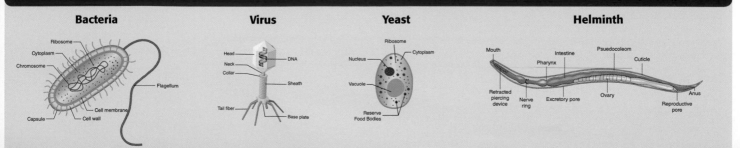

Bacteria

Ribosome, Cytoplasm, Chromosome, Flagellum, Cell membrane, Cell wall, Capsule

Virus

Head, Neck, Collar, Sheath, Tail fiber, Base plate, DNA

Yeast

Ribosome, Cytoplasm, Nucleus, Vacuole, Reserve Food Bodies

Helminth

Mouth, Pharynx, Intestine, Psuedocoeloem, Cuticle, Retracted piercing device, Nerve ring, Excretory pore, Ovary, Anus, Reproductive pore

PCAT STUDY SHEET – QUANTITATIVE ABILITY

Quantitative Ability Strategies Summary

Test Day Strategy	When to Use
Traditional Math	Use when you can quickly see how to set up and execute an equation.
Picking Numbers	Use when the question asks about number properties or when the answer choices are variables or percents with unknown values.
Backsolving	Use when the question asks for the specific value of one term and there are numbers in the answer choices.
Estimation	Use when there are large numbers involved in the calculations and the answer choices are spread apart.
Educated Guessing	Use when you do not see an efficient way to solve the problem or if you're running out of time.

Picking Numbers

HOW TO PICK NUMBERS
Pick easy, manageable numbers such as 2 and 3.
Avoid numbers with unusual properties such as 1 and 0.
On number properties questions, you may need to try both positive and negative or both odd and even numbers.
Pick numbers that are permissible according to the question stem.
For percent questions, use 100.

Backsolving
Plug the answer choice into the question stem to determine the answer.
Start with answer (B).
If (B) is correct, you are done.
If (B) is too big, (A) is the correct answer.
If (B) is too small, try (C) or (D), based on which answer is more manageable.
If you try (C) and it is too small, the correct answer is (D).
If you try (D) and it is too big, the correct answer is (C).
Only try a maximum of two answer choices.

Estimation
Round decimals or large numbers.
Account for rounding when selecting your answer.

Educated Guessing
Don't spend too much time on a single question.
Avoid answers that come from numbers in the question stem.
Think critically to eliminate illogical answers.

QUANTITATIVE ABILITY FORMULAS

Order of Operations: PEMDAS

$$\text{Average} = \frac{\text{Sum of the terms}}{\text{Number of terms}}$$

$$\text{Probability} = \frac{\text{Number of desired outcomes}}{\text{Number of possible outcomes}}$$

$y = mx + b$

$m = \text{slope} = \frac{\Delta y}{\Delta x}$

$b = y\text{-intercept}$

Percent Increase:
Original value • (1 + Percent increase/100)
Percent Decrease:
Original value • (1 – Percent increase/100)

Position, $s(t)$
Velocity, $v(t)$, $v(t) = s'(t)$
Acceleration, $a(t)$, $a(t) = v'(t) = s''(t)$

Quadratic Identities

$a^2 + 2ab + b^2 = (a + b)^2$

$a^2 - 2ab + b^2 = (a - b)^2$

$a^2 - b^2 = (a - b)(a + b)$

Area Between Two Curves

$$\text{Area} = \int_{x=a}^{x=b} [f(x) - g(x)]dx$$

Mean Value Theorem

If $f(x)$ is continuous on $[a,b]$ and differentiable on (a,b), then there exists a point c in (a,b) such that:

$$f'(c) = \frac{f(b) - f(a)}{b - a}$$

The "i" Pattern

Raise i to	1	2	3	4	5	6	7	8
Result	i	-1	$-i$	1	i	-1	$-i$	1

Power Rules

$x^0 = 1$

$x^{-n} = \frac{1}{x^n}$

$x^a \bullet x^b = x^{a+b}$

$(x^a)^b = x^{ab}$

$\frac{x^a}{x^b} = x^{a-b}$

$(xy)^a = x^a y^a$

Logarithms

$\log(ab) = \log(a) + \log(b)$

$\log\frac{a}{b} = \log(a) - \log(b)$

$\log\frac{1}{a} = -\log(a)$

$\log(a^b) = b\log(a)$

Variance:

$$\sigma^2 = \frac{1}{n}\sum_{i=1}^{n}(X_i - \bar{X})^2$$

Standard Deviation:

$$\sigma = \sqrt{\frac{1}{n}\sum_{i=1}^{n}(X_i - \bar{X})^2}$$

Radicals

$\sqrt{a} \times \sqrt{b} = \sqrt{a \times b}$

$a\sqrt{c} + b\sqrt{c} = (a + b)\sqrt{c}$

$\frac{\sqrt{a}}{\sqrt{b}} = \sqrt{\frac{a}{b}}$

But:

$\sqrt{a} + \sqrt{b} \neq \sqrt{a + b}$

Integrals

Trigonometric Functions

$\int\cos(x)dx = \sin(x) + C$

$\int\sin(x)dx = -\cos(x) + C$

$\int\sec^2(x)dx = \tan(x) + C$

$\int\csc(x)\cot(x)dx = -\csc(x) + C$

$\int\sec(x)\tan(x)dx = \sec(x) + C$

$\int\csc^2(x)dx = -\cot(x) + C$

$\int(f'(x)\ dx) = f(x)$

Inverse Trigonometric Functions

$\arcsin(x) = \sin^{-1}(x)$

$\arccos(x) = \cos^{-1}(x)$

$\arctan(x) = \tan^{-1}(x)$

Reciprocal Trigonometric Functions

$\csc(x) = \frac{1}{\sin(x)}$

$\sec(x) = \frac{1}{\cos(x)}$

$\cot(x) = \frac{1}{\tan(x)}$

Derivatives

Derivative of a constant is zero

$\frac{d}{dx}(k) = 0$

Sum Rule

$\frac{d}{dx}(u + v) = \frac{du}{dx} + \frac{dv}{dx}$

Power Rule/Chain Rule

$\frac{d}{dx}(u^n) = nu^{n-1}\frac{du}{dx}$

Product Rule

$\frac{d}{dx}(uv) = u\frac{dv}{dx} + v\frac{du}{dx}$

Quotient Rule

$$\frac{d}{dx}\left(\frac{u}{v}\right) = \frac{v\frac{du}{dx} - u\frac{dv}{dx}}{v^2}$$

Logarithmic Functions

$\frac{d}{dx}(\ln u) = \frac{1}{u}\frac{du}{dx}$

Exponential Functions

$\frac{d}{dx}(e^u) = e^u\frac{du}{dx}$

Trigonometric Functions

$\frac{d}{dx}\sin(x) = \cos(x)$

$\frac{d}{dx}\cos(x) = -\sin(x)$

$\frac{d}{dx}\tan(x) = \sec^2(x)$

$\frac{d}{dx}\csc(x) = -\csc(x)\cot(x)$

$\frac{d}{dx}\sec(x) = \sec(x)\tan(x)$

$\frac{d}{dx}\cot(x) = -\csc^2(x)$

PCAT STUDY SHEET – BIOLOGY

THE CELL

FLUID MOSAIC MODEL AND MEMBRANE TRAFFIC

- Phospholipid bilayer with cholesterol and embedded proteins
- Exterior: hydrophilic, phosphoric-acid region
- Interior: hydrophobic, fatty-acid region

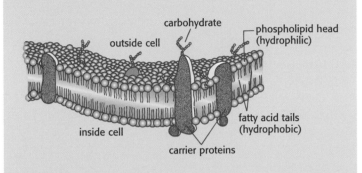

carbohydrate

phospholipid head (hydrophilic)

outside cell

inside cell

fatty acid tails (hydrophobic)

carrier proteins

HOMEOSTASIS

HORMONAL REGULATION

Aldosterone

- Stimulates Na^+ reabsorption and K^+ secretion, increasing water reabsorption, blood volume, and blood pressure
- Secreted from adrenal cortex
- Regulated by renin-angiotensin system

ADH

- Increases collecting duct's permeability to water to increase water reabsorption
- Secreted from posterior pituitary with high [solute] in the blood

THE LIVER'S ROLES IN HOMEOSTASIS

1. Gluconeogenesis
2. Processing of nitrogenous wastes (urea)
3. Detoxification of wastes/chemicals/drugs
4. Storage of iron and vitamin B_{12}
5. Synthesis of bile and blood proteins
6. Beta-oxidation of fatty acids to ketones
7. Interconversion of carbs, fat, and amino acids

ENZYMES

REGULATION

- **Allosteric**: Binding of an effector molecule at allosteric site.
- **Feedback inhibition**: End product inhibits initial enzyme pathway.
- **Reversible inhibition**: Competitive inhibitors bind to active site; noncompetitive inhibitors bind to allosteric site.

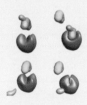

GLUCOSE CATABOLISM

Glycolysis occurs in the cytoplasm: $C_6H_{12}O_6 + 2\ ADP + 2\ P_i + 2\ NAD^+ \rightarrow$ 2 Pyruvate + 2 ATP + 2 NADH + 2 H^+ + 2 H_2O.

Fermentation occurs in anaerobic conditions. Pyruvate is converted into lactic acid (in muscle) or ethanol (in yeast).

Respiration occurs in aerobic conditions.

- **Pyruvate decarboxylation**: Pyruvate converted to acetyl CoA in the mitochondrial matrix.
- **Citric acid cycle**: Acetyl CoA enters; coenzymes exit.
- **Electron transport chain**: Coenzymes are oxidized; energy is released as electrons are transferred from carrier to carrier.
- **Oxidative phosphorylation**: Electrochemical gradient caused by NADH and $FADH_2$ oxidation provides energy for ATP synthase to phosphorylate ADP into ATP.

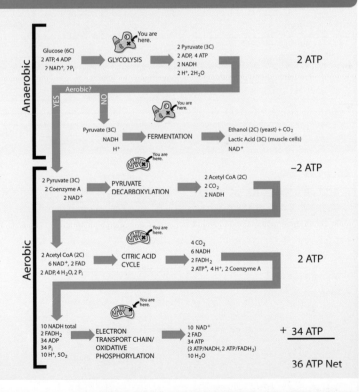

MUSCULOSKELETAL SYSTEM

Sarcomere

- Contractile unit of the fibers in skeletal muscle.
- Contains thin actin and thick myosin filaments.

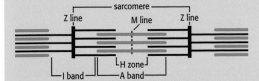

sarcomere

Z line   M line   Z line

H zone

I band   A band

CONTRACTION

Initiation

- Depolarization of a neuron leads to action potential.

BONE FORMATION AND REMODELING

- **Osteoblast**: Builds bone.
- **Osteoclast**: Breaks down bone.
- **Reformation**: Inorganic ions are absorbed from the blood for use in bone.
- **Resorption**: Inorganic ions are released into the blood.

ENDOCRINE SYSTEM

Direct hormones directly stimulate organs. **Tropic** hormones stimulate other glands.
Mechanisms of hormone action: **Peptides** act via secondary messengers. **Steroids** act via a hormone/receptor binding to DNA. **Monoamines** may do either.

Hormone	Source	Action
Follicle-stimulating (FSH)	Anterior pituitary	Stimulates follicle maturation, spermatogenesis
Luteinizing (LH)		Stimulates ovulation, testosterone synthesis
Adrenocorticotropic (ACTH)		Stimulates adrenal cortex to make and secrete corticosteroids
Thyroid-stimulating (TSH)		Stimulates thyroid to produce thyroid hormones
Prolactin		Stimulates milk production and secretion
Endorphins		Inhibit the perception of pain in the brain
Growth hormone		Stimulates bone and muscle growth, lipolysis
Oxytocin	Hypothalamus; stored in posterior pituitary	Stimulates uterine conteractions during labor, milk secretion during lactation
Vasopressin (ADH)		Stimulates water reabsorption in kidneys
Thyroid hormones (T_4, T_3)	Thyroid	Stimulate metabolic activity
Calcitonin		Decreases (tones down) blood calcium level
Parathyroid hormone	Parathyroid	Increases blood calcium level
Glucocorticoids	Adrenal cortex	Increase blood glucose level, decrease protein synthesis
Mineralocorticoids		Increase water reabsorption in kidneys
Epinephrine, Norepinephrine	Adrenal medulla	Increases blood glucose level, heart rate
Glucagon	Pancreas	Stimulates conversion of glycogen to glucose in the liver, increases blood glucose
Insulin		Lowers blood glucose, increases glycogen stores
Somatostatin		Suppresses secretion of glucagon and insulin
Testosterone	Testes	Maintains male secondary sexual characteristics
Estrogen	Ovary/Placenta	Maintains female secondary sexual characteristics
Progesterone		Promotes growth/maintenance of endometrium
Melatonin	Pineal	Maintains circadian rhythms
Atrial natriuretic peptide	Heart	Involved in osmoregulation and vasodilation
Thymosin	Thymus	Stimulates T lymphocyte development

REPRODUCTION

CELL DIVISION

- **G_1:** Cell doubles its organelles and cytoplasm
- **S:** DNA replication
- **G_2:** Same as G_1
- **M:** Cell divides in two
- Mitosis = PMAT
- Meiosis = PMAT × 2

Mitosis

centrosome — centriole
nuclear membrane — chromatin
interphase — 2N
spindle, aster — mitosis
2 chromosomes — prophase
metaphase plate
2 chromosomes — metaphase
4 chromosomes — anaphase
4 chromosomes — telophase
daughter cell
2N 2N
2 chromosomes 2 chromosomes

Meiosis

centrosome — centriole
nuclear membrane — chromatin
interphase — 2N
meiosis
prophase I — 2 chromosomes
metaphase I — 2 chromosomes
disjunction
anaphase I — 2 chromosomes
telophase I — 2 chromosomes
1 chromosome metaphase II — 1 chromosome daughter cells
2 chromosomes anaphase II — 2 chromosomes
telophase II
1 chromosome in each daughter cell
N N N N
gametes

SEXUAL REPRODUCTION

Meiosis I

- Two pairs of sister chromatids form tetrads during prophase I.
- Crossing over leads to genetic recombination in prophase I.

Meiosis II

- Identical to mitosis but without replication.
- Meiosis occurs in **spermatogenesis** (sperm formation) and **oogenesis** (egg formation).

FOUR STAGES OF EARLY DEVELOPMENT

Cleavage: Mitotic divisions
Implantation: Embryo implants during blastulation
Gastrulation: Ectoderm, endoderm, and mesoderm form
Neurulation: Germ layers develop a nervous system

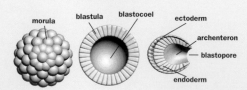

morula
blastula — blastocoel
ectoderm
archenteron
blastopore
endoderm

Ectoderm "Attract-o-derm"	Nervous system, epidermis, lens of eye, inner ear	**Endoderm** "Endernal" organs	Lining of digestive tract, lungs, liver, pancreas	**Mesoderm** "Means-o-derm"	Muscles, skeleton, circulatory system, gonads, kidney

DIGESTION

CARBOHYDRATE DIGESTION

Enzyme	Site of Production	Site of Function	Hydrolysis Reaction
Salivary amylase (ptyalin)	Salivary glands	Mouth	Starch → maltose
Pancreatic amylase	Pancreas	Small Intestine	Starch → maltose
Maltase	Intestinal glands	Small Intestine	Maltose → 2 glucoses
Sucrase	Intestinal glands	Small Intestine	Sucrose → glucose, fructose
Lactase	Intestinal glands	Small Intestine	Lactose → glucose, galactose

PROTEIN DIGESTION

Enzyme	Production Site	Function Site	Function
Pepsin	Gastric glands (chief cells)	Stomach	Hydrolyzes specific peptide bonds
Trypsin	Pancreas	Small Intestine	Hydrolyzes specific peptide bonds Converts chymotrypsinogen to chymotrypsin
Chymotrypsin	Pancreas	Small Intestine	Hydrolyzes specific peptide bonds
Carboxypeptidase	Pancreas	Small Intestine	Hydrolyzes terminal peptide bond at carboxyl
Aminopeptidase	Intestinal glands	Small Intestine	Hydrolyzes terminal peptide bond at amino
Dipeptidases	Intestinal glands	Small Intestine	Hydrolyzes pairs of amino acids
Enterokinase	Intestinal glands	Small Intestine	Converts trypsinogen to trypsin

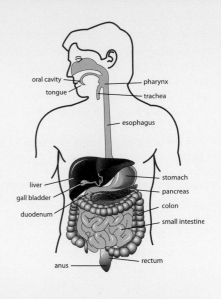

IMMUNE SYSTEM

- The body distinguishes between "self" and "nonself" (antigens).

HUMORAL IMMUNITY (specific defense)

B lymphocytes

Memory cells
remember antigen,
speed up secondary
response

Plasma cells
make and release antibodies
(**IgG, IgA, IgM, IgD, IgE**), which
induce antigen phagocytosis

- **Active immunity**: Antibodies are produced during an immune response.
- **Passive immunity**: Antibodies produced by one organism are transferred to another organism.

CELL-MEDIATED IMMUNITY

T lymphocytes

Cytotoxic T cells
destroy cells directly

Suppressor cells
regulate B and T cells to
decrease anti-antigen activity

Helper T cells
activate B and T cells
and macrophages by
secreting lymphokines

Memory cells

NONSPECIFIC IMMUNE RESPONSE

Includes skin, passages lined with cilia, macrophages, inflammatory response, and interferons (proteins that help prevent the spread of a virus).

LYMPHATIC SYSTEM

- Lymph vessels meet at the thoracic duct in the upper chest and neck, draining into the veins of the cardiovascular system.
- Vessels carry **lymph** (excess interstitial fluid), and capillaries (**lacteals**) collect fats by absorbing chylomicrons in the small intestine.
- **Lymph nodes** are swellings along the vessels with phagocytic cells (leukocytes) that remove foreign particles from lymph.

CIRCULATION

BLOOD TYPING

Antigens are located on the surface of red blood cells.

Blood type	RBC antigen	Antibodies	Donates to:	Receives From:
A	A	Anti-B	A, AB	A, O
B	B	Anti-A	B, AB	B, O
AB	A, B	None	AB only	All
O	None	Anti-A, B	All	O

Blood cells with Rh factor are Rh⁺ and produce no antibody. Rh⁻ lack antigen and produce an antibody.

MOLECULAR GENETICS

NUCLEIC ACID

- Basic unit: nucleotide (sugar, nitrogenous base, phosphate)
- DNA's sugar: deoxyribose. RNA's sugar: ribose.
- 2 types of bases: double-ringed **purines** (adenine, guanine) and single-ringed **pyrimidines** (cytosine, thymine, uracil).
- **DNA double helix:** antiparallel strands joined by base pairs (AT, GC).
- RNA is usually single-stranded: A pairs with U, not T.

TRANSCRIPTION REGULATION, PROKARYOTES
Regulated by the **operon**
- **Structural genes:** have DNA that codes for protein
- **Operator gene:** repressor binding site
- **Promoter gene:** RNA polyermase's 1st binding site
- **Inducible systems:** need an inducer for transcription to occur
- **Repressible systems:** need a corepressor to inhibit transcription

MUTATIONS

- **Point:** One nucleotide is substituted by another; they are silent if the sequence doesn't change.
- **Frameshift:** Insertions or deletions shift reading frame. Protein doesn't form or is nonfunctional.

VIRUSES

- Acellular structures of double- or single-stranded DNA or RNA in a protein coat.
- **Lytic cycle:** Virus kills the host.
- **Lysogenic cycle:** Virus enters host genome.

DNA REPLICATION

- **Semiconservative:** each new helix has an intact strand from the parent helix and a newly synthesized strand.

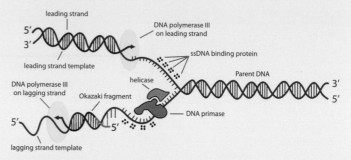

EUKARYOTIC PROTEIN SYNTHESIS

- **Transcription:** RNA polymerase synthesizes hnRNA using a DNA, "antisense strand" as a template.
- **Post-transcriptional processing:** Introns cut out of hnRNA, exons spliced to form mRNA.
- **Translation:** Occurs on ribosomes in the cytoplasm.

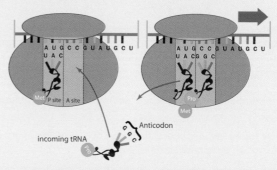

- **Post-translational modifications:** (e.g., disulfide bonds) made before the polypeptide becomes a functional protein.

EVOLUTION

- When frequencies are stable, the population is in Hardy-Weinberg equilibrium: no mutations, large population, random mating, no net migration, and equal reproductive success.

$$p + q = 1; p^2 + 2pq + q^2 = 1$$

p = freq. of dom. allele q = freq. of rec. allele

p^2 = freq. of dom homozygotes

$2pq$ = freq. of heterozygotes

q^2 = freq. of recessive homozygotes

CLASSICAL GENETICS

- If both parents are Rr, the alleles separate to give a genotypic ratio of 1:2:1 and a phenotypic ratio of 3:1.

Law of independent assortment: Alleles of unlinked genes assort independently in meiosis.
- For two traits: AaBb parents will produce AB, Ab, aB, and ab gametes.
- The phenotypic ratio for this cross is 9:3:3:1.

STATISTICAL CALCULATIONS

- The probability of producing a genotype that requires multiple events to occur equals the *product* of the probability of each event.
- The probability of producing a genotype that can be the result of multiple events equals the *sum* of each probability.

GENETIC MAPPING

- Crossing over during meiosis I can unlink genes during prophase I.
- Genes are most likely unlinked when far apart.
- One map unit is 1% recombinant frequency.

Given recombination frequencies

X and Y: 8%

X and Z: 12%

Y and Z: 4%

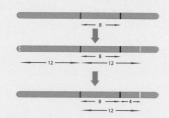

INHERITED DISORDERS in PEDIGREES

- **Autosomal recessive:** Skips generations
- **Autosomal dominant:** Appears in every generation
- **X-linked (sex-linked):** No male-to-male transmission, more males are affected.

PCAT STUDY SHEET – GENERAL CHEMISTRY

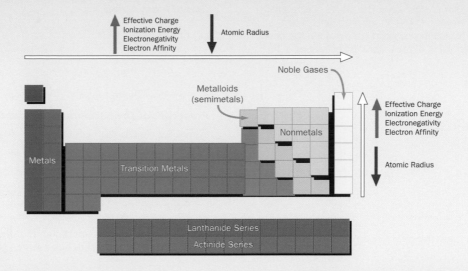

ATOMIC STRUCTURE

Atomic weight: The weight in grams of one mole (mol) of a given element and is expressed in terms of g/mol.

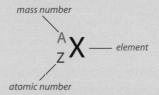

$$_{Z}^{A}X$$

mass number — A

element — X

atomic number — Z

A **mole** is a unit used to count particles and is represented by **Avogadro's number**, 6×10^{23} particles.

$$\text{Moles} = \frac{\text{grams}}{\text{atomic or molecular weight}}$$

Isotopes: For a given element, multiple species of atoms with the same number of protons (same atomic number) but different numbers of neutrons (different mass numbers).

Planck's quantum theory: Energy emitted as electromagnetic radiation from matter exists in discrete bundles called quanta.

Bohr's Model of the Hydrogen Atom

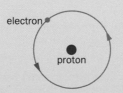

electron

proton

Angular momentum: $\frac{nh}{2\pi}$

Energy of electron: $E = \frac{-RH}{n^2}$

Electromagnetic energy of photons: $E = \frac{hc}{\lambda}$

The group of hydrogen emission lines corresponding to transitions from upper levels $n > 2$ to $n = 2$ is known as the **Balmer series**. The group corresponding to transitions between upper levels $n > 1$ to $n = 1$ is known as the **Lyman series.**

Absorption spectrum: Characteristic energy bands where electrons absorb energy.

Quantum Mechanical Model of Atoms

Heisenberg uncertainty principle: It is impossible to determine with perfect accuracy the momentum and the position of an electron simultaneously.

Quantum Numbers:

#	Character	Symbol	Value
1st	Shell	n	n
2nd	Subshell	l	From zero to $n - 1$
3rd	Orbital	m_ℓ	Between l and $-l$
4th	Spin	m_s	½ or $-$½

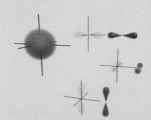

Principal Quantum Number (n): The larger the integer value of n, the higher the energy level and radius of the electron's orbit. The maximum number of electrons in energy level n is $2n^2$.

Azimuthal Quantum Number (l): Refers to subshells, or sublevels. The four subshells corresponding to $l = 0, 1, 2,$ and 3 are known as s, p, d and f, respectively. The maximum number of electrons that can exist within a subshell is given by the formula $4l + 2$.

Magnetic Quantum Number (m_ℓ): This specifies the particular orbital within a subshell where an electron is highly likely to be found at a given point in time.

Spin Quantum Number (m_s): The spin of a particle is its intrinsic angular momentum and is a characteristic of a particle.

Electron Configuration

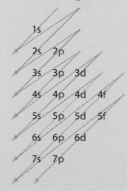

1s
2s 2p
3s 3p 3d
4s 4p 4d 4f
5s 5p 5d 5f
6s 6p 6d
7s 7p

Hund's rule: Within a given subshell, orbitals are filled such that there are a maximum number of half-filled orbitals with parallel spins.

Valence electrons: Electrons of an atom that are in its outer energy shell or that are available for bonding.

KINETICS AND EQUILIBRIUM

Experimental Determination of Rate Law: The values of k, x, and y in the rate law equation (rate $= k[A]^x[B]^y$) must be determined experimentally for a given reaction at a given temperature. The rate is usually measured as a function of the initial concentrations of the reactants, A and B.

Efficiency of Reactions

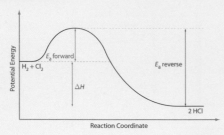

Factors affecting reaction rates: Reactant Concentrations, Temperature, Medium, Catalysts

Catalysts are unique substances that increase reaction rate without being consumed; they do this by lowering the activation energy.

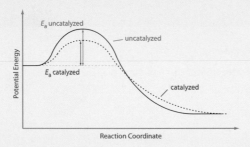

Law of Mass Action

$$aA + bB \rightleftharpoons cC + dD$$

$$K_c = \frac{[C]^c[D]^d}{[A]^a[B]^b}$$

K_c is the equilibrium constant. (c stands for concentration.)

Properties of The Equilibrium Constant

Pure solids/liquids don't appear in expression.

- K_{eq} is characteristic of a given system at a given temperature.
- If $K_{eq} > 1$, an equilibrium mixture of reactants and products will contain very little of the reactants compared to the products.
- If $K_{eq} < 1$, an equilibrium mixture of reactants and products will contain very little of the products compared to the reactants.
- If K_{eq} is close to 1, an equilibrium mixture of products and reactants will contain approximately equal amounts of the two.

$A + B \rightleftharpoons C +$ **heat**	
Will shift to **RIGHT:**	Will shift to **LEFT:**
1. if more A or B added	1. if more C added
2. if C taken away	2. if A or B taken away
3. if pressure applied or volume reduced (assuming A, B, and C are gases)	3 if pressure reduced or volume increased (assuming A, B, and C are gases)
4. if temperature reduced	4. if temperature increased

BONDING AND CHEMICAL INTERACTIONS

Formal Charges

Formal charge = Valence electrons $- \frac{1}{2} N_{bonding} - N_{nonbonding}$

Intermolecular Forces

1. **Hydrogen Bonding:** The partial positive charge of the hydrogen atom interacts with the partial negative charge located on the electronegative atoms (F, O, N) of nearby molecules.

2. **Dipole-Dipole Interactions:** Polar molecules orient themselves such that the positive region of one molecule is close to the negative region of another molecule.

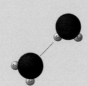

3. **Dispersion Forces:** The bonding electrons in covalent bonds may appear to be equally shared between two atoms, but at any particular point in time they will be located randomly throughout the orbital. This permits unequal sharing of electrons, causing rapid polarization and counter-polarization of the electron clouds of neighboring molecules, inducing the formation of more dipoles.

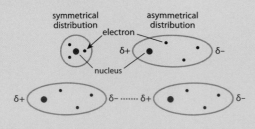

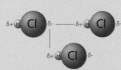

COMPOUNDS AND STOICHIOMETRY

A **compound** is a pure substance composed of two or more elements in a fixed proportion.

A **mole** is the amount of a substance that contains the same number of particles found in a 12.0 g sample of carbon-12.

Combination Reactions: two or more reactants form one product.

$$S\ (s) + O_2\ (g) \rightarrow SO_2\ (g)$$

Decomposition Reactions: A compound breaks down into two or more substances, usually as a result of heating or electrolysis.

$$2\ HgO\ (s) \rightarrow 2\ Hg\ (l) + O_2\ (g)$$

Single-Displacement Reactions: An atom (or ion) of one compound is replaced by an atom of another element.

$$Zn\ (s) + CuSO_4\ (aq) \rightarrow Cu\ (s) + ZnSO_4\ (aq)$$

Double-Displacement Reactions: Also called metathesis reactions, elements from two different compounds displace each other to form two new compounds.

$$CaCl_2\ (aq) + 2\ AgNO_3\ (aq) \rightarrow Ca(NO_3)_2\ (aq) + 2\ AgCl\ (s)$$

Net Ionic Equations: These types of equations are written showing only the species that actually participate in the reaction. So in the following equation,

$$Zn\ (s) + Cu^{2+}\ (aq) + SO_4^{2-}\ (aq) \rightarrow Cu\ (s) + Zn^{2+}\ (aq) + SO_4^{2-}\ (aq)$$

the spectator ion (SO_4^{2-}) does not take part in the overall reaction, but simply remains in solution throughout. The net ionic equation would be:

$$Zn\ (s) + Cu^{2+}\ (aq) \rightarrow Cu\ (s) + Zn^{2+}\ (aq)$$

Neutralization Reactions: These are a specific type of double displacements that occur when an acid reacts with a base to produce a solution of a salt and water:

$$HCl\ (aq) + NaOH\ (aq) \rightarrow NaCl\ (aq) + H_2O\ (l)$$

ACIDS AND BASES

Arrhenius: An acid is a species that produces H^+ (a proton) in an aqueous solution, and a base is a species that produces OH^- (a hydroxide ion).

Brønsted-Lowry: An acid is a species that donates protons, while a base is a species that accepts protons.

Lewis: An acid is an electron-pair acceptor, and a base is an electron-pair donor.

Properties of Acids and Bases

$$pH = -\log[H^+] = \log\left(\frac{1}{[H^+]}\right)$$

$$pOH = -\log[OH^-] = \log\left(\frac{1}{[OH^-]}\right)$$

$$H_2O\ (l) \rightleftharpoons H^+\ (aq) + OH^-\ (aq)$$

$$K_w = [H^+][OH^-] = 10^{-14}$$

$$pH + pOH = 14$$

Weak Acids and Bases

$$HA\ (aq) + H_2O\ (l) \rightleftharpoons H_3O^+\ (aq) + A^-\ (aq)$$

$$K_a = \frac{[H_3O^+][A^-]}{[HA]}$$

$$K_b = \frac{[B^+][OH^-]}{[BOH]}$$

Salt Formation: Acids and bases may react with each other, forming a salt and (often, but not always) water in a neutralization reaction.

$$HA + BOH \rightarrow BA + H_2O$$

Titration and Buffers

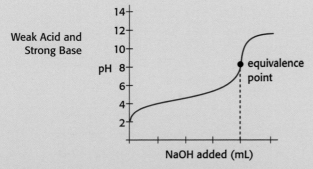

Strong Acid and Strong Base

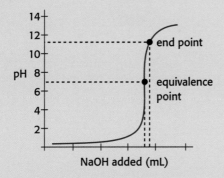

Weak Acid and Strong Base

Titration is a procedure used to determine the molarity of an acid or base by reacting a known volume of a solution of unknown concentration with a known volume of a solution of known concentration.

ACIDS AND BASES *(cont.)*

Henderson-Hasselbalch equation is used to estimate the pH of a solution in the buffer region where the concentrations of the species and its conjugate are present in approximately equal concentrations.

$$pH = pK_a + \log\frac{[\text{conjugate base}]}{[\text{weak acid}]}$$

$$pOH = pK_b + \log\frac{[\text{conjugate acid}]}{[\text{weak base}]}$$

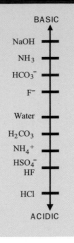

THE GAS PHASE

1 atm = 760 mm Hg = 760 torr

Do not confuse STP with standard conditions—the two standards involve different temperatures and are used for different purposes. STP (0°C or 273 K) is generally used for gas law calculations; standard conditions (25°C or 298 K) is used when measuring standard enthalpy, entropy, Gibbs free energy, and voltage.

Boyle's Law

$$PV = k \text{ or } P_1V_1 = P_2V_2$$

Charles's Law

$$\frac{V}{T} = k \text{ or } \frac{V_1}{T_1} = \frac{V_2}{T_2}$$

Avagadro's Principle

$$\frac{n}{T} = k \text{ or } \frac{n_1}{T_1} = \frac{n_2}{T_2}$$

Ideal Gas Law

$$PV = nRT$$

Deviations due to Pressure: As the pressure of a gas increases, the particles are pushed closer and closer together. At moderately high pressure a gas's volume is less than would be predicted by the ideal gas law, due to intermolecular attraction.

Deviations due to Temperature: As the temperature of a gas decreases, the average velocity of the gas molecules decreases, and the attractive intermolecular forces become increasingly significant. As the temperature of a gas is reduced, intermolecular attraction causes the gas to have a smaller volume than would be predicted.

SOLUTIONS

Units of Concentration

Percent Composition by Mass: $= \dfrac{\text{Mass of solute}}{\text{Mass of solution}} \times 100\ (\%)$

Mole Fraction: $\dfrac{\text{\# of mol of compound}}{\text{total \# of moles in system}}$

Molarity: $\dfrac{\text{\# of mol of solute}}{\text{liter of solution}}$

Molality: $\dfrac{\text{\# of mol of solute}}{\text{kg of solvent}}$

Normality: $\dfrac{\text{\# of gram equivalent weights of solute}}{\text{liter of solution}}$

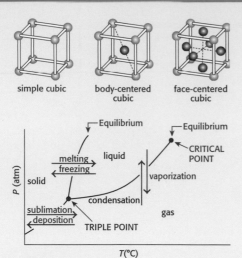

simple cubic   body-centered cubic   face-centered cubic

Colligative Properties: Physical properties derived solely from the number of particles present, not the nature of those particles, usually associated with dilute solutions.

Freezing Point Depression

$$\Delta T_f = K_f m$$

Boiling Point Elevation

$$\Delta T_b = K_b m$$

Osmotic Pressure

$$\Pi = MRT$$

Vapor-pressure Lowering (Raoult's Law)

$$P_A = X_A P^\circ_A;\ P_B = X_B P^\circ_B$$

Solutions that obey Raoult's Law are called ideal solutions.

Graham's Law of Diffusion and Effusion

Diffusion: occurs when gas molecules diffuse through a mixture.

Effusion: is the flow of gas particles under pressure from one compartment to another through a small opening.

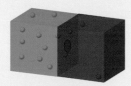

Effusion

Both diffusion and effusion have the same formula:

$$\frac{r_1}{r_2} = \left(\frac{MM_2}{MM_1}\right)^{\frac{1}{2}}$$

Oxidation: Loss of electrons

Reduction: Gain of electrons

Oxidizing agent: Causes another atom to undergo oxidation, and is itself reduced

Reducing agent: Causes another atom to be reduced, and is itself oxidized

Constant-volume and constant-pressure calorimetry: used to indicate conditions under which the heat changes are measured.

$Q = mc\Delta T$, where Q is the heat absorbed or released in a given process, m is the mass, c is the specific heat, and ΔT is the change in temperature.

States and State Functions: are described by the macroscopic properties of the system. These are properties whose magnitude depends only on the initial and final states of the system, and not on the path of the change.

Enthalpy (H): is used to express heat changes at constant pressure.

Standard Heat of Formation (ΔH°_f): the enthalpy change that would occur if one mole of a compound were formed directly from its elements in their standard states.

Standard Heat of Reaction (ΔH°_{rxn}): the hypothetical enthalpy change that would occur if the reaction were carried out under standard conditions.

$$\Delta H^\circ_{rxn} = \text{(sum of } \Delta H^\circ_{rxn} \text{ of products)} - \text{(sum of } \Delta H^\circ_{rxn} \text{ of reactants)}$$

Hess's Law: Enthalpies of reactions are additive.

The reverse of any reaction has an enthalpy of the same magnitude as that of the forward reaction, but its sign is opposite.

Bond Dissociation Energy: Average of the energy required to break a particular type of bond in one mole of gaseous molecules:

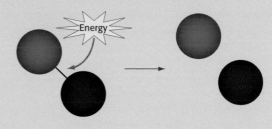

Entropy (S): Measure of the disorder, or randomness, of a system.

$$\Delta S_{universe} = \Delta S_{system} + \Delta S_{surroundings}$$

Gibbs Free Energy (G): combines the two factors that affect the spontaneity of a reaction—changes in enthalpy, ΔH, and changes in entropy, ΔS.

$$\Delta G = \Delta H - T\Delta S$$

if ΔG is negative, the rxn is spontaneous

if ΔG is positive, the rxn is not spontaneous

if ΔG is zero, the system is in a state of equilibrium; thus, $\Delta G = 0$ and $\Delta H = T\Delta S$

ΔH	ΔS	Outcome
−	+	Spontaneous at all temps.
+	−	Nonspontaneous at all temps.
+	+	Spontaneous only at high temps.
−	−	Spontaneous only at low temps.

Reaction Quotient (Q): Once a reaction commences, the standard state conditions no longer hold. For the reaction,

$$aA + bB \rightleftharpoons cC + dD$$

$$Q = \frac{[C]^c[D]^d}{[A]^a[B]^b}$$

PCAT STUDY SHEET – ORGANIC CHEMISTRY

NOMENCLATURE

1. Find the longest carbon chain containing the principle functional group (highest priority groups are generally more oxidized).
2. Number the carbon chain so the principle functional group gets lowest number (1).
3. Proceed to number the chain so the lowest set of numbers is obtained for the substituents.
4. Name the substituents and assign each a number.
5. Complete the name by listing substituents in alphabetical order; place commas between numbers and dashes between numbers and words.

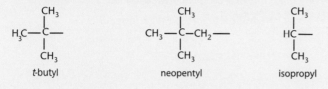

t-butyl   neopentyl   isopropyl

sec-butyl   isobutyl

Functional Group	Suffix
Carboxylic Acid	-oic acid
Ester	-oate
Acyl halide	-oyl halide
Amide	-amide
Nitrile/Cyanide	-nitrile
Aldehyde	-al

Functional Group	Suffix
Ketone	-one
Thiol	-thiol
Alcohol	-ol
Amine	-amine
Imine	-imine
Ether	-ether

ISOMERS

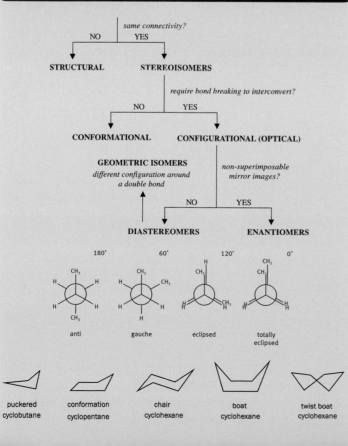

same connectivity?

NO / YES

STRUCTURAL   STEREOISOMERS

require bond breaking to interconvert?

NO / YES

CONFORMATIONAL   CONFIGURATIONAL (OPTICAL)

GEOMETRIC ISOMERS
different configuration around a double bond

non-superimposable mirror images?

NO / YES

DIASTEREOMERS   ENANTIOMERS

180°   60°   120°   0°

anti   gauche   eclipsed   totally eclipsed

puckered cyclobutane   conformation cyclopentane   chair cyclohexane   boat cyclohexane   twist boat cyclohexane

BONDING

Bond order	single	double	triple
Bond type	sigma	sigma pi	sigma 2 pi
Hybridization	sp^3	sp^2	sp
Angles	109.5°	120°	180°
Example	C–C	C=C	C≡C

ALKANES

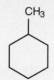

Free radical halogenation
- Initiation
- Propagation
- Termination

Combustion
$$C_3H_8 + 5\,O_2 \rightarrow 3\,CO_2 + 4\,H_2O + heat$$

Nucleophilicity and basicity
$$RO^- > HO^- > RCO_2^- > ROH > H_2O$$

Nucleophilicity, size, and polarity
$$CN^- > I^- > RO^- > HO^- > Br^- > Cl^- > F^- > H_2O$$

Leaving groups (weak bases best)
$$I^- > Br^- > Cl^- > F^-$$

S_N1	S_N2
2 steps	1 step
Favored in polar protic solvents	Favored in polar aprotic solvents
3° > 2° > 1° > Methyl	Methyl > 1° > 2° > 3°
Rate = k[RX]	Rate = k[Nu][RX]
Racemic products	Optically active and inverted products
Strong nucleophile not required	Favored with strong nucleophile

AMINO ACIDS, PEPTIDES, AND PROTEINS

Amino acids have four substituents: amine group, carboxyl group, hydrogen, and R group. Amino acids are **amphoteric**—they can act as either acids or bases and often take the form of **zwitterions** (dipolar ions).

amino acid   →(neutral solution)→   zwitterion

Structure
Primary: Sequence of amino acids
Secondary: α-helix, β-pleated sheet
Tertiary: Disulfide bridges, hydrophobic/hydrophilic interactions
Quaternary: Arrangement of polypeptides

Henderson–Hasselbalch Equation
$$pH = pK_a + \log \frac{[\text{conj. base}]}{[\text{conj. acid}]}$$

ALKYNES

Alkynes have a terminal hydrogen that is appreciably more acidic than hydrogens on alkanes and alkenes.

Synthesis via double elimination of geminal or vicinal dihalide

$$\text{Heat, Base} \rightarrow CH_3C\equiv CCH_3 + 2\ HBr$$

Oxidation with KMnO$_4$, O$_3$

1) KMnO$_4$, OH$^-$
2) H$^+$

1) O$_3$, CCl$_4$
2) H$_2$O

Reduction with Lindlar's catalyst or liquid ammonia

$$CH_3C\equiv CCH_3 \xrightarrow[\text{Quinoline (Lindlar's catalyst)}]{H_2, Pd/BaSO_4} \text{cis-2-butene}$$

2-butyne → cis-2-butene

$$CH_3C\equiv CCH_3 \xrightarrow{Na,\ NH_3\ (liq)} \text{trans-2-butene}$$

2-butyne → trans-2-butene

Free radical addition

$$CH_3CH_2C\equiv CH + X\cdot \rightarrow$$

Electrophilic addition (anti orientation)

$$CH_3C\equiv CH \xrightarrow{Br_2}$$

$$CH_3C\equiv CH \xrightarrow{2\ Br_2} CH_3CBr_2CBr_2H$$

Hydroboration (cis alkene formed)

$$3\ H_3CC\equiv CCH_3 + \tfrac{1}{2}\ B_2H_6 \rightarrow$$

$$\xrightarrow{CH_3COOH} 3$$

ALKENES

Catalytic Reduction

$$\xrightarrow[Pd]{H_2}$$

Electrophilic Addition of HX

$$\xrightarrow{+H^+} \xrightarrow{Br^-}$$

Electrophilic Addition of X$_2$

anti-addition

Electrophilic Addition of H$_2$O

$$\xrightarrow[H_2O]{H^+} \xrightarrow{H_2O} \xrightarrow[-H^+]{H_3O^+}$$

Free Radical Addition (anti-Markovnikov)

$$\xrightarrow{Br\cdot} \xrightarrow{HBr} + Br\cdot$$

most stable radical

Hydroboration (anti-Markovnikov, syn orientation)

$$3 \xrightarrow{BH_3} \xrightarrow[OH^-]{H_2O_2} 3$$

Oxidation with KMnO$_4$

$$\xrightarrow[KMnO_4]{\text{cold, dilute}} + MnO_2(s)$$

Oxidation with O$_3$

1) O$_3$, CH$_2$Cl$_2$
2) Zn/H$_2$O → 2

ALDEHYDES

The dipole moment of aldehydes causes an elevation of boiling point, but not as high as alcohols since there is no hydrogen bonding.

Synthesis

- Oxidation of primary alcohols
- Ozonolysis of alkenes
- Friedel-Crafts acylation

Reactions

Reactions of Enols (Michael additions)

$$\xrightarrow{Base} + H{:}Base$$

$$+ \rightarrow + Base$$

Nucleophilic Addition to a Carbonyl

$$\xrightarrow{H^+}$$

Aldol condensation

An aldehyde acts both as nucleophile (enol form) and target (keto form).

CARBOXYLIC ACIDS

Carboxylic acids have pK_as of around 4.5 due to resonance stabilization of the conjugate base. Electronegative atoms increase acidity with inductive effects. Boiling point is higher than alcohols because of the ability to form two hydrogen bonds.

Synthesis

Oxidation of Primary Alcohols with $KMnO_4$

Organometallic Reagents with CO_2 (Grignard)

Hydrolysis of Nitriles

$$CH_3Cl \longrightarrow CH_3CN \longrightarrow CH_3\overset{O}{\overset{\|}{C}}OH + NH_4^+$$

Reactions

Formation of soap by reacting carboxylic acids with NaOH; arrange in micelles.

nonpolar tail   polar head

Nucleophilic Acyl Substitution

Ester formation

Acyl halide formation

Reduction to alcohols

carboxylic acid   aldehyde

alcohol

ALCOHOLS

- Higher boiling points than alkanes
- Weakly acidic hydroxyl hydrogen

Synthesis

- Addition of water to double bonds
- S_N1 and S_N2 reactions
- Reduction of carboxylic acids, aldehydes, ketones, and esters
  - Aldehydes and ketones with $NaBH_4$
  - Esters and carboxylic acids with $LiAlH_4$

Reactions

E1 dehydration reactions in strongly acidic solutions

Hoffman product — minor

Zaitsev product — major

Substitution reactions after protonation or leaving group conversion

tosyl chloride

Oxidation

- PCC takes a primary alcohol to an aldehyde.

- Jones's reagent, $KMnO_4$, and alkali dichromate salts will convert secondary alcohols to ketones and primary alcohols to carboxylic acids.

- Tertiary alcohols cannot be oxidized without breaking a carbon-to-carbon bond.

Oxidation and Reduction

Wittig Reaction

$$(C_6H_5)_3P + CH_3Br \longrightarrow (C_6H_5)_3\overset{+}{P}CH_3 + Br^-$$

$(C_6H_5)_3\overset{+}{P}$—CH_3 $\xrightarrow{\text{Base}}$ $(C_6H_5)_3P$=CH_2 $\longleftrightarrow$ $(C_6H_5)_3\overset{+}{P}$—$\overset{-}{C}H_2$

phosphonium salt   ylide

CARBOXLIC ACID DERIVATIVES

Acyl halides

Nucleophilic acyl substitution

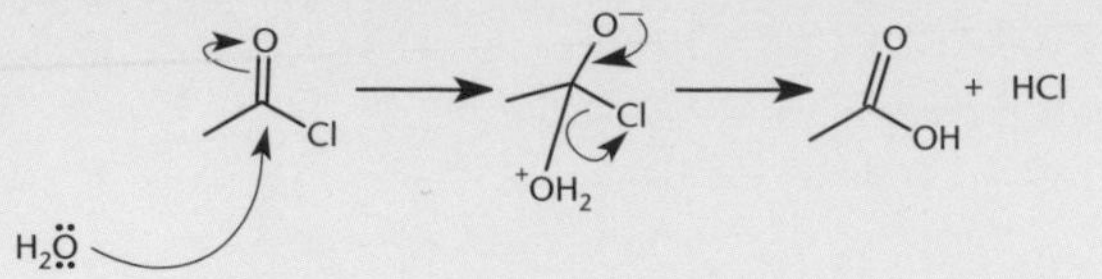

Friedel–Crafts acylation

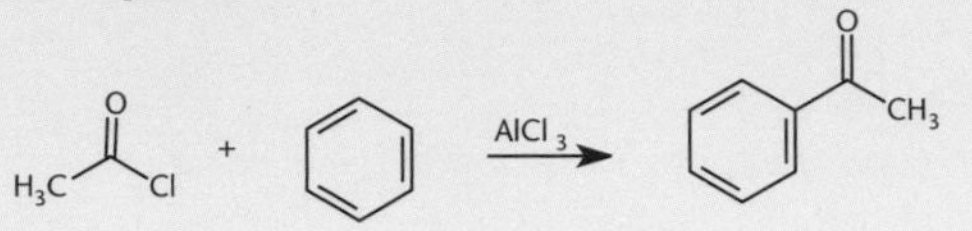

Reduction

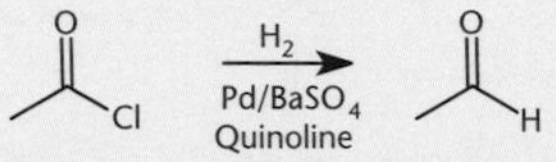

Anhydrides

Synthesis via reaction of carboxylic acid with an acid chloride

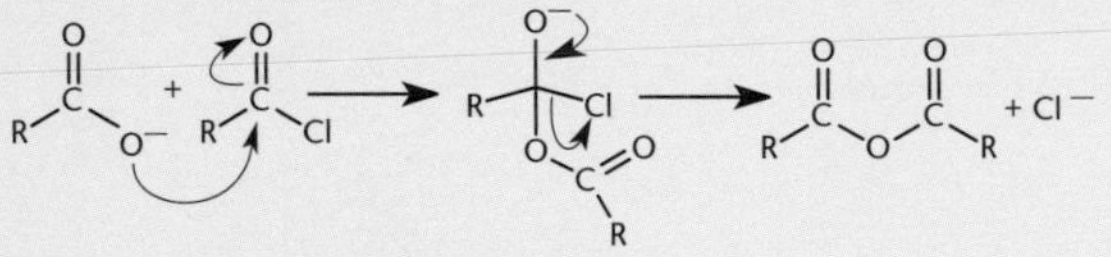

Addition of ammonia to form amides

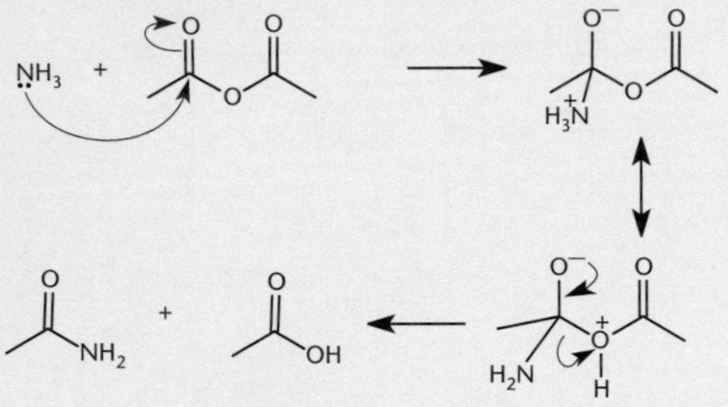

Friedel–Crafts acylation

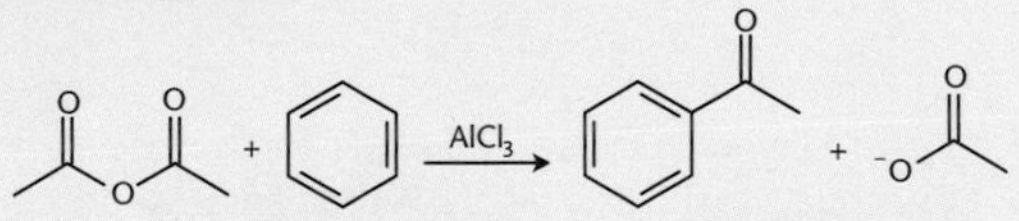

Amines and Nitrogen-Containing Compounds

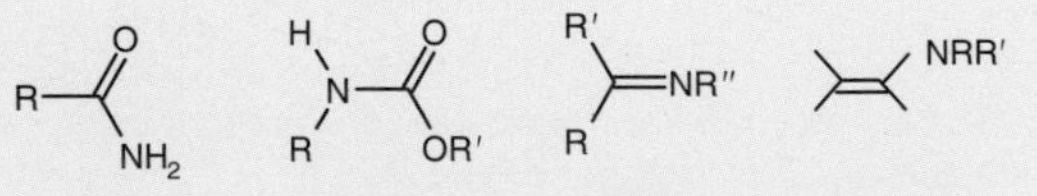

Amide   Carbamate   Imine   Enamine

Azide   Nitrile   Isocyanate

Direct alkylation of ammonia

$$CH_3Br + NH_3 \longrightarrow CH_3\overset{+}{N}H_3Br^- \xrightarrow{NaOH} CH_3NH_2 + NaBr + H_2O$$

Reduction from nitro compounds, nitriles, imines, and amides

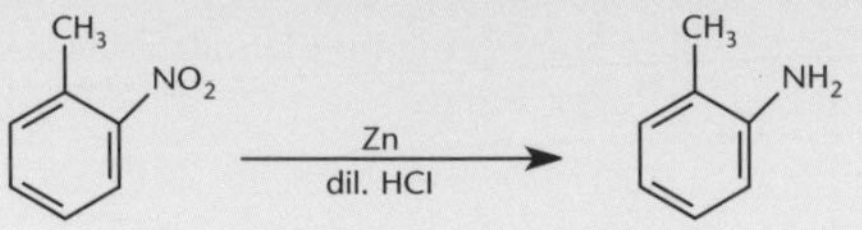

$$CH_3CH_2C\equiv N \xrightarrow{LAH} CH_3CH_2CH_2NH_2$$

Exhaustive methylation (Hoffman elimination)

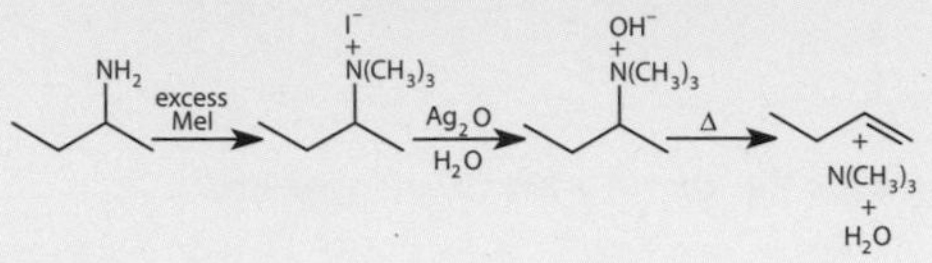

Gabriel Synthesis

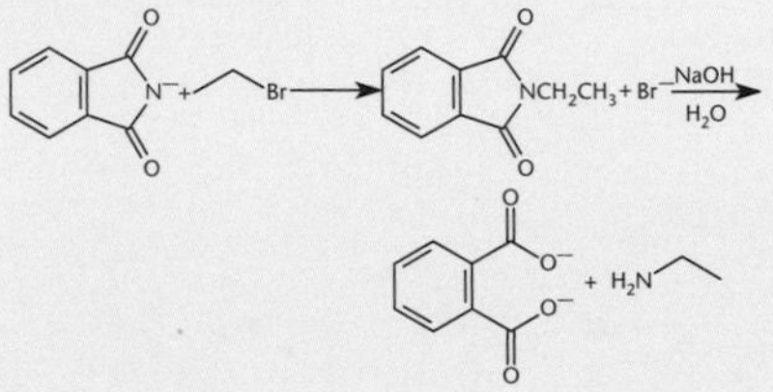

Amides

Hoffman rearrangement converts amides to primary amines

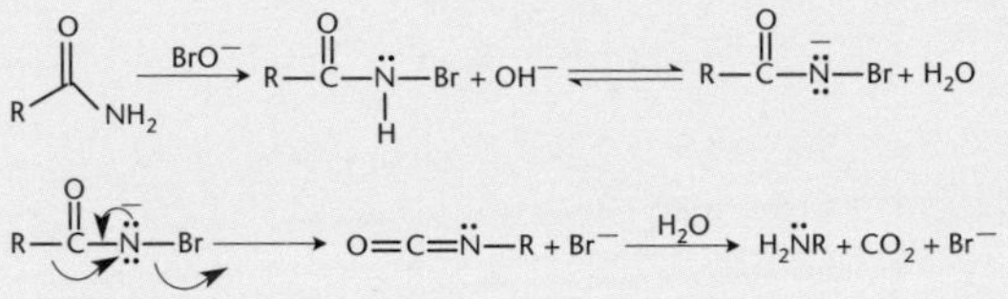

nitrene   isocyanate

Reduction with LAH

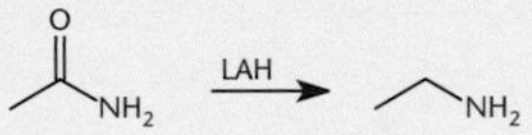

Esters

Synthesis via condensation of carboxylic acids and alcohols

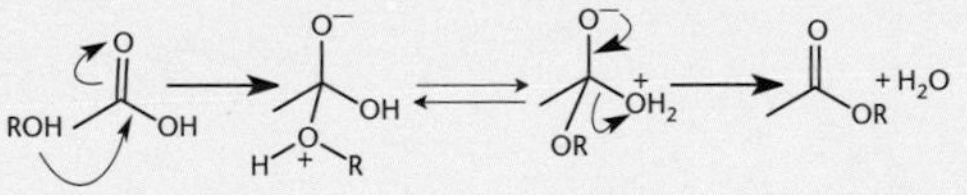

Conversion to amides

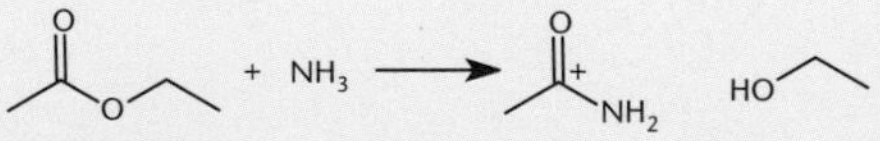

Claisen condensation

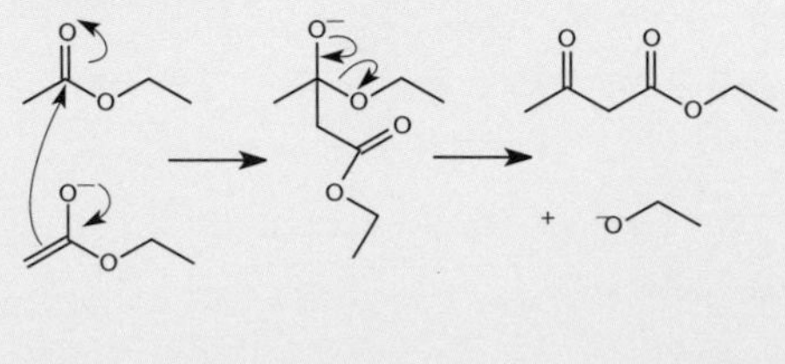